3-D Radiation Treatment Planning and Conformal Therapy

Proceedings of an International Symposium

April 21-23, 1993

Edited by

James A. Purdy, Ph.D &
Bahman Emami, M.D.

Mallinckrodt Institute of Radiology
Washington University School of Medicine
St, Louis, Missouri

Published by
Medical Physics Publishing
Madison, Wisconsin

International Standard Book Number: 0-944838-51-0

Library of Congress Card Number: 95-80190

For information, address the publisher:

Medical Physics Publishing
4513 Vernon Blvd.
Madison, Wisconsin, 53705

Printed in the United States of America

Preface

An international conference on 3-D Radiation Treatment Planning and Conformal Therapy was held on April 21-23, 1993 in St. Louis, Missouri, USA. The conference was sponsored by the Radiation Oncology Center, Mallinckrodt Institute of Radiology, Washington University School of Medicine in St. Louis.

The comprehensive two and a half day program encompassed a broad range of topics in 3-D radiation treatment planning (RTP) and conformal radiation therapy (CRT). The primary objective was to present up to date information on the use of 3-D RTP and to create an intellectual environment for discussion of new and innovative approaches to conformal therapy. Topics discussed included 3-D computerized RTP for external beam and brachytherapy, 3-D dose calculation algorithms, 3-D RTP quality assurance, CT-simulation, CRT delivery equipment and techniques, on-line portal imaging, computer networking, and preliminary clinical information. The faculty included many nationally and internationally known experts in the field of radiation oncology actively engaged in advancing 3-D CRT.

These proceedings are being published to disseminate what we believe to be much needed information to the radiation oncology community. In some cases, the articles included are lengthy review type articles; while others are short and more anecdotal. The editors chose to include both types to insure the reader the most up to date information on 3-D RTP and CRT and to capture the enthusiasm and stimulating intellectual discourse the symposium generated. The editors wish to thank all of the authors who took time out of their busy schedule to contribute to this book. We thank Cheryl Zmaila, Dr. Purdy's secretary, who worked hard in helping reformat the submitted articles to a common word processing program. We also wish to thank Eileen Healy and Elizabeth Seaman, managing editors of Medical Physics Publishing Co., who provided editorial support for this book. We hope that this book will be helpful to all within the radiation oncology community in understanding and utilizing 3-D RTP as we begin this new and exciting era of conformal radiation therapy.

James A. Purdy, Ph.D.
Bahman Emami, M.D.

Table of Contents

Chapter 1

3-D Radiation Treatment Planning: NCI Perspective

Sandra Zink, Ph.D.

Radiation Research Program, National Cancer Institute, Bethesda, Maryland

The National Cancer Institute and the American Cancer Society estimate that there will be approximately 1.2 million new cancer patients in 1993. About 48% of those patients will undergo radiation therapy during the course of their treatment and half of those will be treated with curative intent [1]. Treatment-related morbidity and complications to normal tissues, however, are frequently the limiting factor in delivering a high radiation dose to tumor targets, reducing the probability of tumor control [2,3]. A review of the literature on survival and local control for patients undergoing radiotherapy at a number of disease sites discussed the potential gain in survival in patients with reduced local regional failure [4]. In addition, the correlation of local failure to the incidence of distant metastases is well documented [5,6,7].

The technical advances that have been achieved over the last decade in the area of 3-D treatment planning capabilities and new and more flexible hardware capabilities, such as computer-controlled treatments, multi-leaf collimators and real-time portal imaging devices, have brought about the promise of a new technology, 3-D Conformal Radiation Therapy, or 3-D CRT. With these new technologically advanced capabilities, conventional high energy external photon beams can achieve highly focused radiation dose distributions that spare the normal tissues to a greater degree than has ever before been possible. The potential of delivering a higher radiation dose, with no increase in normal tissue morbidity, is an attractive prospect for improved local tumor control, increased patient survival and an enhanced quality of life.

Sophisticated 3-D CRT techniques make use of the entire three dimensional aspect of the anatomy in the treatment planning process, and the employment of more complex beam geometries and beam-shaping techniques that reduce the dose to normal tissues. The improved technology has the potential to deliver a 10 to 20% higher dose to the tumor target with no increase in radiation-induced complications [5,8,9]. This improvement in technological capability is not unlike the advances that were achieved in physical dose distributions as a result of megavoltage equipment replacing Cobalt units. A Patterns of Care study showed a remarkable gain in survival and therapeutic results that correlated with the use of megavoltage equipment [10].

In recognition of the importance of 3-D treatment planning in radiation therapy and the promise of improved technological capabilities, the National Cancer Institute (NCI) launched a series of research initiatives in the early 1980s to evaluate the potential of 3-D treatment planning and to make recommendations to the NCI for future research. Five Collaborative Working Groups (CWGs) were funded between 1982 and 1994 to focus on 3-D treatment planning and interstitial brachytherapy (see Table 1). Several reports as well as a special issue of the *International Journal of Radiation Oncology and Physics* and a textbook resulted from these efforts (see following section). In addition to documenting the results of their treatment planning evaluations, the reports contained recommendations for future research and consensus guidelines for the radiation therapy research community.

The NCI has also funded over the last decade several other investigators through the NIH grant mechanism. Examples include 3-D dynamic conformal or segmented therapy, photon dose calculation algorithms, computer controlled treatments, real-time portal imaging and others. Many of these efforts have resulted in spin-off technology that has been further developed by the industrial/vendor community.

Table 1-1.   *NCI-Supported Collaborative Working Groups (1982-94)*

Particle CWG: Evaluation of Treatment Planning for Particle Beam Radiotherapy (1982-86)
Massachusetts General Hospital, Harvard University, Boston
Lawrence Berkeley Laboratory, Department of Energy, Berkeley, CA
University of Pennsylvania, Philadelphia
University of Texas, M.D. Anderson Hospital, Houston

Photon CWG: Evaluation of High Energy Photon External Beam Treatment Planning (1984-87)
Massachusetts General Hospital, Harvard University, Boston
Memorial Sloan-Kettering Institute, New York City
University of Pennsylvania, Philadelphia
Washington University at St. Louis

Interstitial CWG: Evaluation of Dosimetry, Calculations and Afterloading Techniques for
Interstitial Radiotherapy (1985-88)
Memorial Sloan-Kettering Institute, New York City
University of California, San Francisco
Yale University School of Medicine

Electron CWG: Evaluation of High Energy Electron External Beam Treatment Planning (1986-89)
University of Michigan, Ann Arbor
University of Texas, M.D. Anderson Hospital, Houston
Washington University at St. Louis

Tools CWG: Radiotherapy Treatment Planning Tools (1989-94)
University of North Carolina, Chapel Hill
University of Washington, Seattle
Washington University at St. Louis

CWG Accomplishments

The Collaborative Working Groups (CWGs) have been enormously productive due to (1) interactions that occurred as a result of regular working group meetings; (2) the need to reach consensus in a timely manner to meet contract deadlines; (3) the multi-disciplinary involvement of everyone involved in the treatment planning process, including radiation oncologists, medical physicists, dosimetrists, software engineers and computer specialists; and (4) sharing of resources, ideas and expertise between members of the CWGs. Except for the first group, each CWG has been able to build on the accomplishments of the previous groups, which has been instrumental in making major advances in 3-D treatment planning. By funding the several Collaborative Working Groups (Table 1-1), the NCI not only provided resources to various institutions to explore 3-D developments and applications, each CWG provided a focus for the radiotherapy community at large that was not present prior to the NCI commitment. Many of the treatment planning capabilities that are now incorporated as standard features in modern 3-D treatment planning systems were first proposed, modeled and prototyped in the NCI working groups. A summary of some of the accomplishments of each of the CWGs follows.

Particle CWG

The Particle CWG had the most difficult job as they first had to develop the framework of the collaborative group that was to be used by subsequent CWGs. In addition, the investigators needed to develop a vocabulary for communicating the concepts of treatment planning, such as "mobile" target volume and "immobile" target volume, to distinguish between known tumor with adjacent tissues at risk, from that target volume that was needed to take account of patient motion and setup error. These concepts, initially spawned and developed in the CWGs, are now part of standard radiotherapy clinical practice, although the names have been modified by the International Commission on Radiation Units (ICRU) to be gross tumor volume (GTV), clinical tumor volume (CTV) and planning target volume (PTV). In addition, the Particle CWG developed (1) the first treatment planning protocols for simultaneous treatment planning experiments between institutions using actual patient data, (2) the first formats for exchanging data by magnetic tape, (3) the first models for evaluating competing plans, such as dose-volume-histograms (DVH), tumor control probability and complication probability, and (4) many of the first 3-D tools that are now part of every modern 3-D treatment planning system, such as color-wash displays, beam's-eye-view and others. Five hundred copies of a large report quickly disappeared into the hands and onto the shelves of the radiotherapy 3-D treatment planning community [11].

Photon CWG

The Photon CWG built on the accomplishments of the Particle CWG and two of the participating institutions in this CWG overlapped both groups, increasing the sharing of expertise and resources. This CWG brought the needs of routine clinical practice and conventional photon radiotherapy to the 3-D treatment planning process. The institutional participants added and enlarged upon existing 3-D capabilities and tools in anatomical reconstruction, dose distribution display and plan evaluation. The group expanded the models for tumor control probability and normal tissue control probability. A number of pilot studies were carried out in which 3-D CRT techniques were applied to a variety of patient configurations and tumor sites to more fully explore the full potential of 3-D conformal therapy. The accomplishments of this group were so great that an entire volume of a scientific journal was devoted solely to the collective accomplishments of this CWG [12].

Interstitial CWG

The Interstitial CWG was funded to establish standards and guidelines for interstitial radiotherapy through a consensus process and to develop a report that would address (1) accepted standard brachytherapy procedures; (2) uncertainty in dose calculations; and (3) lack of agreement on dose specification conventions. The group was immensely productive, carrying out many difficult and exacting measurements that were then correlated with dose calculations. But the real contribution to the radiotherapy community was a published textbook [13] which includes chapters on radioactive sources, radiobiology of brachytherapy, dose computation and evaluation, clinical procedures to be followed in brachytherapy, and two sections on quality assurance and radiation protection. This consolidation of a large amount of material, combining the physics of brachytherapy with the clinical considerations, was a significant and unique contribution to the radiotherapy literature.

Electron CWG

The Electron CWG addressed the formidable task of evaluating electron beam dose models and algorithms by carrying out hundreds of calculations, comparing them with measurements in realistic phantoms and evaluating them for their appropriate usage and implementation in an external beam 3-D electron treatment planning system. The algorithms were evaluated not only for dose verification and accuracy, but were also applied in treatment plans to actual patient cases and evaluated as to their utility. The advantages and drawbacks of 3-D treatment planning for electron beams were thoroughly explored. The group also developed new 3-D tools that were specific to electron treatment planning, as well as expanded tools that had been developed earlier. The accomplishments of this group are published as individual articles in various journals in the scientific literature [14,15,16].

Tools CWG

The last group, the Tools CWG, was given the dual tasks of (1) developing software tools that would make 3-D CRT less labor intensive so that it could be adapted into routine clinical practice; and (2) providing a means for sharing software between institutions in a seamless and user-friendly manner. A typical treatment planning system requires somewhere between 30 and 50 man-years of effort to develop. It is rare, however, that the software is portable to another institution and/or hardware configuration without modification, unless virtually every component of the entire system is duplicated at the new site, from the model of computer and system software being used down to the style and model of the digitizing tablet. The Tools effort has focused on software engineering techniques that separate out the site-specific components of a treatment planning system (operating system, hardware configuration, graphics software, data formats) so that the universal components (dose algorithms, kinds of display, plan evaluation models, etc.) can be shared between institutions and between treatment planning systems. The accomplishments of this group will make it possible to very quickly take advantage of new treatment planning capabilities, such as a very fast dose calculating algorithm or a computer generated (digitized reconstructed) radiograph, in a broad spectrum of commercial products, treatment planning systems and hardware configurations. This capability of sharing and transporting software, eliminating the necessity of "reinventing the wheel," may be the most profound and lasting contribution of the NCI-supported CWG efforts. The progress of this CWG is documented in several Technical Reports.[1]

Decade of 3-D Accomplishments

The advances that have been achieved over the last decade in 3-D treatment planning are too extensive to be described in detail here. The reader is referred to two journals in particular for a summary and review of the state-of-the-art in 3-D treatment planning. The first is the special issue dedicated to the results of the Photon Treatment Planning CWG [12] and the second is a special issue of Seminars in Radiation Oncology [17]. Some highlights of the decade's accomplishments are given here.

New Software Tools

Software is now available that (a) delineates anatomy using a variety of techniques [18]; (b) produces a planning treatment volume from a gross tumor volume [19]; (c) offers high quality digitially reconstructed or computer generated radiographs that reproduce the portal film (or on-line image) of the patient in the treatment position [20]; (d) displays 3-D images of anatomy, tumor and dose using a wide variety of techniques that enable better visualization of the relationship of the tumor and normal structures to the high-dose regions [21-24]; (e) registers MRI and CT images for improved visualization and delineation of the tumor [25-28]; (f) comprehensive collection of tools for evaluating and scoring competing treatment plans [29]; and (g) comparison of on-line digital portal images with digitized simulation films for rapid and accurate placement of the patient in the

---

[1] Technical Report (TR) 90-1: Radiotherapy Treatment Planning Tools (RTPT) First Year Progress Report (August 1990); TR90-2: Standards and Practices of the Collaborative Working Group on RTPT (March 1990); TR91-1: Foundation Library Specification and Virtual Machine Platform (VMP) Specification (June 1991); TR91-2: RTPT Second Year Progress Report (December 1991); TR92-1: ANSI C Language Bindings to the Foundation and VMP; TR92-2: Common Lisp Language Bindings to the Foundation and VMP; and TR92-3: RTPT Third Year Progress Report (December 1992).

treatment position [30]. While this list is by no means comprehensive or all-inclusive, it is astonishing that less than five years ago, none of these tools existed, or they existed as primitive, prototype examples. These software tools are now at a level of proficiency to be used routinely and in many cases, are being used, for clinical applications.

New Software Engineering

The currently funded NCI-CWG, Radiotherapy Treatment Planning Tools, has developed and implemented a new software engineering technology that allows for seamless portability across different computer hardware, various operating systems and diverse computer languages.[1] The accomplishments of this CWG have the potential for one group or institution to very quickly take advantage of new treatment planning capabilities developed by another group, without having to rewrite the original software. Examples might include an automatic segmentation tool for delineating anatomical structures, a very fast dose calculating algorithm or an image registration tool that registers a CT image accurately on its corresponding MRI image. This capability of not having to reinvent the wheel has the potential to revolutionize software development standards in radiation therapy treatment planning.

New Conceptualizations, Models

Many of the advances have come about through an improved understanding of the treatment planning process and the development of new models, that both conceptually and computationally, enhance the capabilities of the user, whether that individual is a physician, physicist or dosimetrist. The dose-volume histogram [31]; beam's eye view [32]; and the computer generated or digitally reconstructed radiograph [33] are examples of new tools that have come about to improve the treatment planner's conceptualization and realization of a complex 3-D plan. Improved dose calculation algorithms have not only improved the speed with which the radiation dose is calculated in large treatment volumes, they have also improved the accuracy by taking into account inhomogeneties, not only of the tumor region, but of adjacent tissue that affect the distribution of radiation dose in the irradiated volume [34-39]. New models have emerged to grapple with the overwhelming volume of data that a full 3-D planning exercise generates. Dose-volume-histograms were an early development to distill a vast collection of 3-D data to a two-dimensional format. Models were developed to assess tumor control probability [40-42] and normal tissue complications [43-46] and these have provided the treatment planner with additional tools for assessing the relative merits of competing plans. Evaluation and scoring of competing treatment plans [47-49] are examples of other techniques to reduce a complex treatment plan to a single number or characteristic that reflects it overall desirability. Goitein has written a comprehensive review of the techniques in use today [29].

Computer Hardware

Dramatic advancements in computer hardware capabilities over the last 10 years have increased the speed of computations by orders of magnitude and increased computer memory at an ever decreasing and more affordable cost. Such advancements now make rapid computations of complex 3-D treatment plans not only feasible, but highly desirable to enable the exploration of new beam and treatment configurations and to explore the potential for computer-controlled complex treatments.

Clinical Implementations

The progress of the last decade has been so profound that the first tentative, labor-intensive efforts to apply 3-D treatment planning techniques to real patients have now advanced into full-scale routine clinical activities [50-52]. With the development of new hardware capabilities, such as multi-leaf collimators [53-56] and on-line portal imaging [57-58], the technology has reached a new level of capability that allows for the treatment of a large number of patients with new and advanced technology at several of the major cancer centers. As with any new technology, it must be demonstrated that there is a clinical advantage and that it can be used safely and effectively.

3-D Clinical Trials

Studies on patterns of failure after curative local-regional therapy for carcinoma of the prostate (i.e., surgery and/or radiotherapy) show that the incidence of metastatic disease significantly increases as a result of failure to control the primary tumor [59]. The high doses that were achieved through radioactive implants were correlated with local control. In an analysis of Patterns of Care data presented at an NCI consensus conference in 1988 on the treatment of prostate cancer, Hanks found that the incidence of in-field recurrence decreased as dose was increased [60]. A reduction in treatment-related morbidity can be tested with relatively modest numbers of patients [61]. Several pilot studies have already showed the feasibility of increasing dose for prostate cancer treatments beyond those normally used for this disease [8,62,63].

In recognition of the profound advances in 3-D treatment planning technology, the improved computer hardware and software capabilities, and the existence of newly developed hardware to assist in the clinical treatments, the National Cancer Institute approved a set-aside of funds in 1991 to fund a Cooperative Group to explore dose escalation studies for prostate cancer, using 3-D conformal radiation therapy (3-D CRT). The new Cooperative Group, which consists of a headquarters, providing operations and statistical support, a quality control center, and several therapy centers, has recently been formed to conduct Phase I and II dose escalation studies in prostate cancer and to then proceed to a Phase III trial. The headquarters will be located at the offices of the Radiation Therapy Oncology Group (RTOG) with 3-D treatment planning support and quality assurance oversight provided through a subcontract with Washington University at St. Louis. The task of the Cooperative Group will be to determine a new maximum tolerated dose to the prostate using 3-D conformal radiotherapy techniques. It is planned that the Phase I/Phase II dose-searching studies will then proceed to Phase III studies, in which patients will be randomized to receive conventional radiotherapy or 3-D conformal therapy at the higher dose. The completion of a Phase III study can potentially influence the future of radiotherapy by showing whether 3-D conformal therapy techniques have a measurable clinical impact on survival and quality of life. An important additional research objective for the Cooperative Group will be the development of a 3-D database documenting dose as a function of volume in partially irradiated organs and sensitive structures.

Future Efforts

The National Cancer Institute will continue to be interested in clinical applications that assess how 3-D technology impacts the cancer patient, both in terms of survival and outcome, but also quality of life. The evaluation of 3-D technology in the oncology clinic with respect to the process of diagnosis and therapy planning for all modalities (surgery, chemotherapy and radiotherapy) is also of interest. As with all new medical technologies, it must be demonstrated that 3-D technology provides a clinical advantage, that it can be carried out safely in routine clinical practice, that its appropriate use is well understood and safely applied and that it is cost effective in an environment of rising health care costs. Evaluation of all these aspects of how 3-D technology impacts the cancer patient's therapy process, from diagnosis to treatment to follow-up and measures of quality of life, will all constitute important research activities for the future.

References

1.   Owen J, Hanks G., *Patterns of Care in Radiation Oncology*. 1993, National Cancer Institute Contract N01-CM87275, Internal NCI Report.

2. Moore JV, H.J., Hunter RD, *Dose-incidence curves for tumour control and normal tissue injury, in relation to the response of clonogenic cells.* Radiother Oncolo, 1983. **1**(2): p. 143-57.

3. Emami B, L.J., Brown A, Coia L, Goitein M, Munzenrider JE, Shank B, Solin LJ, Wesson M, *Tolerance of normal tissue to therapeutic irradiation.* Int. J Radiat Oncol Biol Phys, 1991. **21**: p. 109-123.

4. Suit HD, W.S., *Impact of improved local control on survival.* Int J Radiation Oncol Biol Phys, 1986. **12**: p. 453-58.

5. Fuks Z, L.S., Kutcher GJ, Mohan R, Ling CC, ed. *Three dimensional conformal treatment: a new frontier in radiation therapy.* Important Advances in Oncology, ed. H.S. DeVita VT Jr Rosenberg SA. 1991, Lippincott: Philadelphia, PA. 151-172.

6. Zagars GK, v.E.A., Ayala AG, et al, *The influence of local control on metastatic dissemination of prostate cancer treated by external beam megavoltage radiation therapy.* Cancer, 1991. **68**: p. 2370-77.

7. Ramsay J, S.H., Sedlacek R, *Experimental studies on the incidence of metastases after failure of radiation treatment and the effect of salvage surgery.* Int J Radiat Oncol Biol Phys, 1983. **14**: p. 1165-68.

8. Sandler HM, P.-T.C., Ten Haken RK, et al, *Dose escalation for stage C(T3) prostate cancer: minimal rectal toxicity observed using conformal therapy.* Radiat Oncol, 1992. **23**: p. 1-64.

9. Leibel SA, K.G., Harrison LB, Fass DE, Burman CM, Hunt MA, Mohan R, Brewster MS, Ling CC, *Improved dose distributions for 3-D conformal boost treatments in carcinoma of the nasopharynx.* Int J Radiat Oncol Biol Phys, 1993. **in press**.

10. Hanks GE, D.J., Kramer S, *The need for complex technology in radiation oncology. Correlations of facility characteristics and structure with outcome.* Cancer, 1985. **55**: p. 2198-2201.

11. Particle Treatment Planning Collaborative Working Group, *Evaluation of Treatment Planning for Particle Beam Radiotherapy.* 1987, National Cancer Institute: Bethesda, MD.

12. Photon Treatment Planning Collaborative Working Group, *International Journal of Radiation Oncology Biology and Physics.*, Three-Dimensional Photon Treatment Planning: Report of the Collaborative Working Group on the Evaluation of Treatment Planning for External Photon Beam Radiotherapy, Phil Rubin, Editor; Alfred R. Smith and James A. Purdy, Guest Editors, May 15, 1991, Vol. 21 (1), pp. 1-266.

13. Interstitial Collaborative Working Group, *Interstitial Brachytherapy: physical, biological and clinical considerations.* Editors: Lowell L. Anderson, Ravinder Nath, Keith A. Weaver, Dattatreyudu Nori, Theodore L. Phillips and Yung H. Son, 1990, New York: Raven Press.

14. Shiu AS, T.S., Hogstrom KR, Wong JW, Gerber RL, Harms WB, Purdy JA, Ten Haken RK, McShan DL, Fraass BA, *Verification data for electron beam dose algorithms.* Med Phys, 1992. **19**(3): p. 623-36.

15. Shiu AS, H.K., *Pencil-beam redefinition algorithm for electron dose distributions.* Med Phys, 1991. **18**(1): p. 7-18.

16. Hogstrom KR, *Treatment planning in electron beam therapy.* Front Radiat Ther Oncol, 1991. **25**: p. 30-52.

17. *Seminars in Radiation Oncology,* Three-Dimensional Treatment Planning, Edward L. Chaney, Guest Editor, October 1992, Vol 2, pp 213-312.

18. Chaney EL, P.S., *Defining anatomical structures from medical images.* Seminars in Radiat Oncol, 1992. **2**(4): p. 215-225.

19. Radiotherapy Treatment Planning Tools Collaborative Working Group, *RTPT Third Year Progress Report (December 1992).* 1992, University of North Carolina, University of Washington and Washington University at St. Louis:

20. Rosenman JG, C.E., Cullip TJ, Symon JR, Chi VL, Fuchs H, Stevenson DS, *VISTAnet: interactive real-time calculation and display of 3-dimensional radiation dose: an application of gigabit networking.* Int J Radiat Oncol Biol Phys, 1993. **25**(1): p. 123-9.

21. Kessler ML, M.D., Fraass BA, *Displays for three-dimensional treatment planning.* Seminars Radiat Oncol, 1992. **2**(4): p. 226-234.

22. Photon Treatment Planning Collaborative Working Group, *Three-dimensional displays in planning radiation therapy: A clinical perspective.* Int J Radiat Oncol Biol Phys, 1991. **21**: p. 79-89.

23. Purdy JA, W.J., Harms WB, Emami B, Matthews JW, *State of the art of high energy photon treatment planning.* Front. Radiat Ther Oncol, 1987. **21**: p. 4-24.

24. Rosenman J, S.G., Fuchs H, et al, *Three-dimensional display techniques in radiation therapy treatment planning.* Int J Rad Oncol Biol Phys, 1989. **16**: p. 263-269.

25. Kessler ML, P.S., Pettit P, et al., *Integration of multimodality imaging data for radiotherapy treatment planning.* Int J Rad Oncol Biol Phys, 1991. **21**: p. 1653-1667.

26. Fraas BA, M.D., Diaz RF, et. al, *Integration of MRI into radiation therapy treatment planning.* Int J Rad Oncol Biol Phys, 1987. **13**: p. 1897-1908.

27. Judnick JW, K.M., Fleming T, Petti P, Castro JR, *Radiotherapy technique integrates MRI into CT.* Radiol Technol, 1992. **64**(2): p. 89-9?.

28. Ten Haken RK, T.A.J., Sandler HM, LaVigne ML, Quint DJ, Fraass BA, Kessler ML, McShan DL, *A quantitative assessment of the addition of MRI to CT-based, 3-D treatment planning of brain tumors.* Radiother Oncol, 1992. **25**(2): p. 121-33.

29. Goitein M, *The comparison of treatment plans.* Seminars Radiat Oncol, 1992. **2**(4): p. 246-256.

30. Bosch WR, Low DA, Gerber RL, Graham MV, Michalski JM, Perez CA and Purdy JA, An electronic viewbox tool for radiation therapy treatment verification. Med. Phys. (Abst.) 1993, **20**: p. 897.

31. Chen GTY, *Dose volume histograms in treatment planning.* Int J Radiat Oncol Biol Phys, 1988. **14**: p. 1319-1320.

32. Goitein M, Abrams M, Rowell D, et al, *Multi-dimensional treatment planning II: beam's eye-view, back projection and projection through CT sections.* Int J Radiat Oncol Biol Phys, 1983. **9**: p. 789-97.

33. Sherouse GW, N.K., Chaney EL, *Computation of digitally reconstructed radiographs for use in radiotherapy treatment design.* Int J Radiat Oncol Biol Phys, 1990. **18**: p. 671-658.

34. Bourland JD, C.E., *A finite-size pencil beam model for photon dose calculations in three dimensions.* Med Phys, 1992. **19**(6): p. 1401-12.

35. Boyer AL, M.E., *Calculation of photon dose distributions in an inhomogeneous medium using convolutions.* Med Phys, 1986. **13**: p. 503.

36. Chui CS, M.R., *Extraction of pencil beam kernels by the deconvolution method.* Med Phys, 1988. **15**: p. 138-144.

37. Mohan R, C.C., Lidofsky L, *Differential pencil beam dose computation model for photons.* Med Phys, 1986. **13**: p. 64-73.

38. Mohan R, C.C., *Use of fast fourier transforms in calculating dose distributions for irregularly shaped fields for three-dimensional treatment planning.* Med Phys, 1987. **14**: p. 70-77.

39. Purdy JA, *Photon dose calculations for three-dimensional radiation treatment planning.* Seminars Radiat Oncol, 1992. **2**(4): p. 235-245.

40. Goitein M, *The probability of controlling an inhomogeneously irradiated tumor.* Particle Treatment Planning Collaborative Working Group, *Evaluation of Treatment Planning for Particle Beam Radiotherapy.* 1987, National Cancer Institute: Bethesda, MD.

41. Niemierko A, G.M., *Modeling of normal tissue response to radiation: the critical volume model.* Int J Radiat Oncol Biol Phys, 1993. **25**(1): p. 135-45.

42. Yaes RJ, *Some implications of the Linear Quadratic model for tumor control probability.* Int J Radiat Oncol Biol Phys, 1988. **14**(1): p. 147-57.

43. Burman C, K.G., Emami B, Goitein M, *Fitting of normal tissue tolerance data to an analytic function.* Int J Radiat Oncol Biol Phys, 1991. **21**(1): p. 123-35.

44. Lyman JT, W.A., *Optimization of radiotherapy III: A method of assessing complication probabilities from dose volume histograms.* Int J Radiat Oncol Biol Phys, 1987. **13**, p. 103-109.

45. Kutcher GJ, B.C., *Calculation of complication probability factors for non-uniform normal tissue irradiation: the effective volume method.* Int J Radiat Oncol Biol Phys, 1989. **16**: p. 1623-30.

46. Niemierko G, G.M., *Calculation of normal tissue complication probability and dose-volume histogram reduction schemes for tissues with a critical element architecture.* Radiother Oncol, 1991. **20**: p. 166-176.

47. Shalev S, V.D., Carey M, et al, *The objective evaluation of alternative treatment plans II: Score functions.* Int J Radiat Oncol Biol Phys, 1991. **20**: p. 1067-1073.

48. Viggars DA, S.S., Stewart M, et al, *The objective evaluation of alternative treatment plans. III: The quantitative analysis of dose volume histograms.* Int J Radiat Oncol Biol Phys, 1992. : p. in press.

49. Munzenrider JE, B.A., Chu JC, et al, *Numerical scoring of treatment plans.* Int J Radiat Oncol Bios Phys, 1991. **21**: p. 147-163.

50. Leibel SA, K.G., Mohan R, Harrison LB, Armstrong JG, Zelefsky MJ, LoSasso TJ, Burman CM, Mageras GS, Chiu CS, Brewster LJ, Masterson ME, Lo YC, Ling CC, Fuks Z, *Three-dimensional conformal radiation therapy at the Memorial Sloan-Kettering Cancer Center.* Seminars Radiat Oncol, 1992. **2**(4): p. 274-289.

51. Lichter AS, S.H., Robertson JM, et al, *Clinical experience with three-dimensional treatment planning.* Seminars Radiat Oncol, 1992. **2**: p. 267-273.

52. Hanks GE, *Conformal radiation in prostate cancer: reduced morbidity with hope of increased local control.* Int J Radiat Oncol Biol Phys, 1993. **15**(25): p. 3.

53. Boesecke R, B.G., Alandt K, Pastyr O, Doll J, Schlegel W, Lorenz WJ, *Modification of a three-dimensional treatment planning system for the use of multi-leaf collimators in conformation radiotherapy.* Radiother Oncol, 1991. **21**(4): p. 261-8.

54. Galvin JM, S.A., Lally B, *Characterization of a multi-leaf collimator system.* Int J Radiat Oncol Biol Phys, 1993. **25**(2): p. 181-92.

55. LoSasso T, C.C., Kutcher GJ, Leibel SA, Fuks Z, Ling CC, *The use of a multi-leaf collimator for conformal radiotherapy of carcinomas of the prostate and nasopharynx.* Int J Radiat Oncol Biol Phys, 1993. **25**(2): p. 161-70.

56. Powlis WD, S.A., Cheng E, Galvin JM, Villari F, Bloch P, Kligerman MM, *Initiation of multi-leaf collimator conformal radiation therapy.* Int J Radiat Oncol Biol Phys, 1993. **25**(2): p. 171-9.

57. DeNeve, W., F. Van den Heuvel, M. DeBeukeleer, M. Coghe, L. Thon, P. DeRoover, M. VanLancker and G. Storme, *Routine clinical on-line portal imaging followed by immediate field adjustment using a tele-controlled patient couch.* Radiotherapy and Oncology, 1992. **24**: p. 45-54.

58. Wong JW, B.W., Cheng AY, Geer LY, Epstein JW, Klarmann J, Purdy JA, *On-line radiotherapy imaging with an array of fiber-optic image reducers.* Int J Radiat Oncol Biol Phys, 1990. **18**(6): p. 1477-84.

59. Fuks Z, L.S., Wallner KE, Begg CB, Fair WR, Anderson LL, Hilaris BS, Whitmore WF, *The effect of local control on metastatic dissemination in carcinoma of the prostate: long-term results in patients treated with ^{125}I implantation.* Int. J Radiat. Oncol. Biol. Phys, 1991. **21**: p. 549-566.

60. Hanks, G., *External-beam radiation therapy for clinically localized prostate cancer: Patterns of care studies in the United States.* NCI Monographs, 1988. **7**: p. 75-84.

61. Thames HD, S.T., Hendy JH, et.al., *Can modest escalations of dose be detected as increased tumor control?* Int J Rad Oncol Biol Phys, 1992. (22): p. 241-246.

62. Hanks GE, *Conformal radiation in prostate cancer: reduced morbidity with hope of increased local control.* Int J Radiat Oncol Biol Phys, 1993. **15**(25): p. 3.

63. Schimizu T, T.Y., Takeshita N, Matsuda T, *Conformation radiotherapy of carcinoma of the prostate.* Nippon Igaku Hoshasen Gakkai Zasshi, 1992. **52**(7): p. 993-1000.

Chapter 2

Volume and Dose Specification for Three-Dimensional Conformal Radiation Therapy

James A. Purdy, Ph.D.

Mallinckrodt Institute of Radiology, Washington University School of Medicine, St. Louis, Missouri

Prescription, specification, and reporting of radiation treatments are not uniform throughout most centers worldwide. While the policies and procedures of treatment delivery may be well understood by the staff in any individual center, the ability to communicate treatment reports in an unambiguous and comprehensible manner is poor. In the published literature, it is rare to find a description of treatment detailed sufficiently to facilitate correct interpretation by others.

The International Commission on Radiation Units and Measurements (ICRU) Report 29 [1] and its successor, ICRU Report 50 [2], have addressed the issue of consistent volume and dose specification in radiation therapy. However, the proposed methodology has not been universally accepted and there continues to be a lack of rigor and compliance worldwide, particularly with regard to three-dimensional conformal radiation therapy (3-D CRT).

The dose/volume specification dilemma has been pointed out by several authors [3, 4, 5]; for example, is the prescription dose the minimum dose to the target volume? Is it the maximum dose to the target volume? Or is the prescription dose that at or near the center of the tumor? The question is clearly not trivial, as there can be significant differences in the above numbers. Frequently, the difference is 10% or greater. There are risks of serious errors, both in under and overdosage, if published schema are adopted without first standardizing reporting definitions. Clear definitions of the method for specifying the dose and dose homogeneity throughout the target volume are essential to facilitate communication and to improve the knowledge of dose-effect relationships.

ICRU 50 Definitions

Several centers have now implemented 3-D radiation treatment planning systems and commercial systems are rapidly becoming available. Treatment techniques are thus becoming more complex. Therefore the rather simple set of recommendations proposed in ICRU Report 29 had to be modified. In 1987, the ICRU formed a new working group (which led to ICRU Report 50), under the chairmanship of Dr. T. Landsberg, to address the topic of dose and volume specification for reporting in external beam therapy with photons and electrons. The purpose of ICRU Report 50 is to define important volumes and absorbed dose patterns and to recommend methods for specifying the dose for reporting external beam therapy with photons and electrons. If the recommendations are followed uniformly by all facilities, then it will be possible to have meaningful interpretations and evaluations of the outcome of treatments.

The ICRU Report 29 definition of target volume included the oncological safety margin and the planning safety margin. A clear separation between these two concepts was made in ICRU Report 50 to ensure that all tissues included in the target volume receive the appropriate dose. It was clear that the inaccuracy of patient and/or beam positioning must be taken into account. It was also recognized that the target volume(s) can move internally and that the size and shape of the target volume can change (e.g., rectum, bladder).

Three new volumes have been introduced in ICRU 50 to account for these factors. (See Figure 2-1). The *gross tumor volume (GTV)* is the gross palpable or visible/demonstrable extent and location of the malignant growth. The *clinical target volume (CTV)* is the tissue volume that contains a GTV and/or subclinical microscopic malignant disease that must be treated to achieve the aim of therapy, cure or palliation. The CTV is thus an anatomical-clinical concept that must be defined before a choice of treatment modality and technique is made. The *planning target volume (PTV)* is defined by the margins that must be added around the CTV to compensate for the effects of organ and patient movements and inaccuracies in beam and patient setup. PTV is defined to select appropriate beam sizes and beam arrangements, taking into consideration the net effect of all possible geometrical variations and inaccuracies to ensure that the prescribed dose is actually delivered to the CTV. The PTV is thus a static, geometrical concept used for treatment planning and for specification of dose. Its size and shape depend primarily on the CTV and the effect caused by internal motions of organs as well as the treatment technique (including immobilization) used.

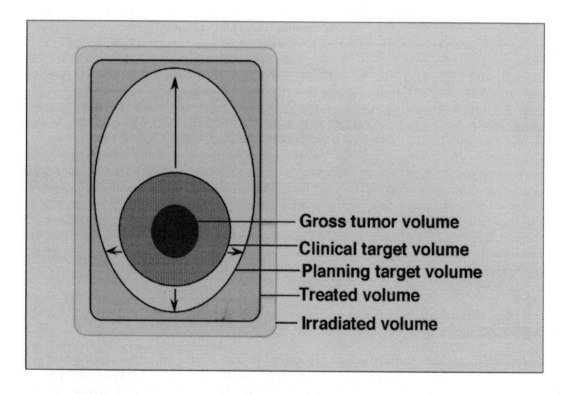

Gross tumor volume

Clinical target volume

Planning target volume

Treated volume

Irradiated volume

Figure 2-1. Schematic illustration of the different volumes as defined by ICRU Report 50

Two other volumes have been retained from ICRU Report 29. They are the *treated volume*, which is the volume enclosed by an isodose surface, selected and specified by the radiation oncologist as being appropriate to achieve the purpose of treatment (e.g., tumor eradication, palliation), and the *irradiated volume*, which is the volume that receives a dose considered significant in relation to normal tissue tolerance.

Organs at risk (OAR) are defined as normal tissues whose radiation sensitivity may significantly influence treatment planning and/or prescribed dose.

The physical treatment planning process is dependent on the delineation of the three volumes (GTV, CTV, and PTV) and the prescription of the target dose. These factors constitute the medical decision that must precede the determination of the dose distribution in the patient. The target volumes must always be described, independent of the dose distributions, in terms of the patient's anatomy and topography and the margins to account for geometrical uncertainty, and the physical dimensions must be stated. The extent of the treated volume, as well as the irradiated volume, depends on the treatment technique used. In general, because of limitations in treatment techniques, the treated volume cannot be made to conform exactly with the target volume and will often be larger and of a similar shape. However, with 3-D CRT techniques, this goal is much more likely to be attained.

ICRU 50 recommends that dose be reported for a reference point (called *ICRU Reference Point*) which is selected based on the following criteria. First, the point must be clinically relevant and be defined in an unambiguous way. Second, it must be located where the dose can be accurately determined, and third, it cannot be located in a region where there are steep dose gradients. In general, the reference point is in the central part of the target volume. In cases where the beams intersect at a given point, the intersection point is recommended to be the ICRU Reference Point.

The minimum and the maximum dose to the PTV must also be reported. For 3-D CRT, the mean dose to the PTV should also be given. However, information should be added about how it was computed to ensure consistency among reported mean dose values. Finally, dose-volume histograms (DVHs) for PTV(s) and for organs at risk should be reported to facilitate the interpretation of the treatment outcome and the comparison of the relative merits of different techniques.

Using ICRU 50 Methodology

A volumetric computed tomography (CT) scan series of the patient is typically used for 3-D CRT planning. However, magnetic resonance imaging (MRI), single photon emission computed tomography (SPECT), or even photon emission computed tomography (PET) are often needed to supplement the CT data set to accurately define the GTV and CTV. The CT study must be performed with the patient in the treatment position, using any immobilization devices required for treatment. Skin marks used as an aid in repositioning the patient for treatment can be made visible on the CT images by the use of radioopaque markers. CT scan protocols for 3-D planning are tumor site dependent and typically require slice thicknesses ranging from 2 to 8 mm and consist of 40 to 100 images. More recently, the total number of slices has increased to improve digital reconstructed radiograph (DRR) quality and in some cases has approached 200.

Determining GTV, CTV, PTV, and organs at risk by drawing contours on the CT image on a slice-by-slice basis as opposed to drawing portals on a radiograph is a major paradigm shift for the radiation oncologist and treatment planner. Experience has shown that several factors influence the delineation of these volumes. For example, when the GTV is delineated, it is important to use the appropriate CT window and level settings to determine the maximum dimension of what is considered to be potential gross disease. A diagnostic radiologist working with the radiation oncologist at the 3-D RTP system display monitor can be of significant value in delineating the target volumes and some critical structures that are difficult to distinguish on the CT image. Also, a fiducial grid superimposed on the CT display aids in adding the appropriate margins for the PTV. Software that creates the PTV based on a defined CTV and specific margin inputs for all dimensions would be useful.

Automatic contouring of the CT data can be done only for those structures with distinct boundaries (skin, lung, etc.). For medium and low contrast structures, this task must be accomplished manually using a digitizer. This process can take 1 to 2 hours, depending on the site of the disease, for a complete 3-D CT series. Much of this task is performed by treatment planning staff. However, there are critical structures that require the efforts of the radiation oncologist (brachial plexus, esophagus, etc.).

The radiation oncologist is responsible for defining the GTV, CTV, and PTV, whereas a treatment planner may enter most of the organs at risk contours. CTV delineation is more complicated than either organ structure or GTV delineation because the CTV is not based solely on imaged data and has no well-defined shape. For example, the CTV may change from case to case according to grade, stage, and histology of the tumor, and the natural avenues of spread for the particular disease and site. The boundary of the CTV must be defined by the radiation oncologist based on clinical experience.

Presently one of the most time consuming steps in 3-D planning is the manual contouring of the CT data. Although some software tools are available for this task, improved tools in this area are still needed. In the future, an improved user interface similar to popular painting and drawing programs available for personal computers would help in the critical structure, tumor volume and target volume delineation process. Also, expert systems technology could play an important role. For example, the system could suggest the volume needed to include a particular nodal chain and the target volume automatically drawn onto the CT or MRI data set in 3-D, which could be either accepted or modified by the radiation oncologist using an interactive edit program.

Specifying the boundary of the PTV must also be done by the radiation oncologist, in consultation with the radiation oncology physicist, based on clinical experience. Unfortunately solid data for setup error and internal organ motion for most sites are sorely lacking although several uncertainty studies addressing these issues are underway.

The DRR calculated from the CT data is an extremely useful tool in appreciating the drawn contours. The various target volumes and corgans at risk, as well as the beam defining apertures, can be superimposed on the DRR, thus providing the radiation oncologist and/or therapist with a plane film representation with the same perspective as a simulator or portal film.

Problems with ICRU 50

There are some problems with the PTV concept. However, none outweigh the usefulness of the ICRU 50 methodology. First, there is not a similar methodology for accounting for normal tissue geometrical uncertainty. Second, the PTV treats all points within the PTV as equally likely for the CTV to occupy all of the time, and that obviously does not occur in practice. Third, when the PTV overlaps with a critical normal structure, which volume should the overlapping voxels be assigned for DVH calculations. We have chosen to double count the overlapping voxel elements, assigning them to both volumes. This is a conservative approach and results in a higher dose being assigned to the normal structure than is likely to occur.

While these problems should encourage researchers to continue to seek improved methods of specifying dose and volume, the author hopes that the radiation oncology community will adopt the ICRU 50 methodology and build on its foundation during the remaining years of this decade. This will allow institutions throughout the world to share more easily their results and clearly help 3-D CRT progress in a most efficient manner.

References

1. ICRU Report 29: Dose Specifications for Reporting External Beam Therapy with Photons and Electrons, International Commission on Radiation Units and Measurements, Bethesda, MD, 1978.

2. ICRU Report 50: Prescribing, Recording, and Reporting Photon Beam Therapy. International Commission on Radiation Units and Measurements, Bethesda, MD, 1993.

3. Dutriex A: Prescription, Precision and Decision in Treatment Planning ASTRO (Keynote Address). Int. J. Rad. Oncol. Biol. Phys. 1987;13:1291.

4. Hendrickson F: Dose Prescription Dilemma, Editorial Int. J. Rad. Oncol. Biol. Phys. 1988;14:595.

5. Suntharalingam N and Purdy JA: Dose Specification: External and Brachytherapy, in Purdy JA (ed): Advances in Radiation Oncology Physics - Dosimetry, Treatment Planning, and Brachytherapy. New York, American Institute of Physics, Inc., 1992, pp 573-595.

Chapter 3

The Impact of Local Tumor Control on the Outcome in Human Cancer

Steven A. Leibel, M.D. and Zvi Fuks, M.D.

Department of Radiation Oncology, Memorial Sloan-Kettering Cancer Center, New York, New York

The impact of local tumor control on the outcome in human cancer has been an issue of debate in the recent literature. Obviously, this question is primarily relevant in patients receiving treatment for tumors still confined to their original local or local-regional sites. While it is obvious that eradication of the primary tumor is essential for the achievement of cure, several investigators have argued that the presence of incurable micrometastases from spread before initial diagnosis is the most important determinant of the ultimate fate in early stage patients (DEVITA et al. 1986; SUIT 1982). Concerns have, therefore, been raised that efforts to improve local control will be offset by the eventual development of metastatic disease and will thus represent a futile endeavor in many types of tumors. However, while relapse due to early micrometastatic dissemination is a relevant pattern of failure in a fraction of locally controlled patients, recent retrospective studies have demonstrated that local recurrence at the primary tumor site is associated with a significant increase of metastatic disease in nearly every type of tumor tested (FUKS et al. 1991a; LEIBEL et al. 1991b). Some investigators have interpreted these data as indicating that local failure represents a "marker" for tumors with a high propensity for metastatic dissemination, and therefore, improvements in local control are unlikely to affect the outcome in a major way (FISHER et al. 1991; WALSH 1987). On the other hand, recent studies on the temporal relationship between local recurrence and the first detection of metastatic disease in the same patients are most consistent with the hypothesis that distant metastases in such patients are derived from residual tumor clonogens which acquire a metastatic potential after the failure to eradicate the primary tumor (FUKS et al. 1991a; LEIBEL et al. 1991b). These observations indicate a possible causative relationship between local relapse and metastatic spread and highlight the relative importance of local control as a biological determinant that impacts on the metastatic outcome and the likelihood of survival. This review discusses some of these issues in the context of the need to develop new therapeutic methods for improving local control in human tumors.

The Curative Potential of Localized Modes of Cancer Therapy

While chemotherapy has occasionally been used to eradicate localized tumors, especially in the malignant lymphomas, surgery and/or radiation therapy have been the mainstays of localized treatment aimed at attaining a local cure in the great majority of human tumors. Data from the National Cancer Institute Surveillance, Epidemiology, and End Results (SEER) program (U.S. DEPARTMENT of HEALTH and HUMAN SERVICES 1988) and the National Cancer Data Base (NCDB) (MENICK, et al. 1991) indicate that approximately 65% of invasive cancer patients initially present with tumors still confined to their original local or local-regional sites and without clinical evidence of distant spread. Only two-thirds of such patients attain a permanent local control with the current modes of radiation and/or surgery (MYERS and RIES 1989). An accurate assessment of the patterns of failure in those who relapse are not available, but published estimates suggest that approximately one-third of the patients fail at the primary tumor sites alone, one-third recur at primary sites with concurrent or subsequent failures at distant sites, and one-third relapse at distant metastatic sites only (DEVITA 1983; SUIT 1982; PEREZ and BRADY 1992). Obviously, patients who recur at local sites alone are those who would be the primary candidates for gains from improved local tumor control. However, some of the patients who relapse at both local and distant sites may also benefit from treatments that improve local control since, as discussed later in this review, clinical and experimental studies suggest that metastatic disease in patients who fail local-regional therapy frequently occurs significantly later than the local recurrence and probably secondary to the re-growth process of the residual primary tumor (FUKS et al. 1991a; LEIBEL et al. 1991b). Based on these considerations, it is estimated that if local relapses were to be completely eliminated, an increment of up to one-third of the cancer patients who currently succumb to metastatic disease could perhaps be rescued by the prevention of metastatic dissemination due to the spread of clonogenic tumor cells with freshly acquired metastatic potential, arising from locally relapsing tumors.

Causes of Local Failure in Clinical Radiation Therapy

Analysis of the causes for local failure in radiation therapy requires consideration of multiple biological and treatment related factors. There is good evidence that the radiosensitivity of human tumors varies from one tumor type to another (FERTIL and MALAISE 1981; FERTIL and MALAISE 1985; DEACON et al. 1984, WEICHSELBAUM et al. 1989). This heterogeneity is a function of inherent factors, such as the tumor cell radiosensitivity, the size of the clonogenic stem cell pool, tumor cell kinetics during the course of radiation therapy, and the prevalence of various microenvironmental factors. These factors determine the potential and proficiency of radiation damage repair, which have been shown to correlate with the relative response of tumors to ionizing irradiation (MCMILLAN 1992). Unfortunately, at the present time it is not possible to effectively modulate these parameters and, hence, affect the local outcome in clinical radiation therapy. However, because of the random nature in which lethal radiation lesions are produced, the inactivation of tumor clonogens by ionizing irradiation is dose dependent, mathematically described as an exponential function (ALPER 1980). Hence, dose related factors, including the size of the dose per fraction, the overall treatment duration, and the total dose, as well as the homogeneity of the dose distribution within the tumor (in particular the presence of geographical volumes of tumor underdosage), strongly affect the therapeutic outcome. If optimized, these treatment related factors may serve to partially or completely overcome the relative radiation resistance in some types of human tumors.

In animal experiments, where all variables can be carefully controlled, there is a distinctive relationship between dose and tumor control that is best described by Poisson distributions (MUNRO and GILBERT 1961; HENDRY and MOORE 1984). Accordingly, at low radiation dose levels, tumor control probabilities are small, but at higher doses there is a sigmoid shape to the curve relating tumor control to dose, with a steep increase in control from 10% to 90% over a relatively narrow dose range until a plateau is reached (PORTER 1980). A similar dose-response pattern has been observed for radiation induced damage in normal tissues. Dose-response studies in human tumors have been rare, but available clinical data confirm the sigmoidal nature of dose-tumor control curves (FISCHER and MOULDER 1975; THAMES et al. 1980; METZ et al. 1982; PETERS and FLETCHER 1983; ZAGARS et al. 1987). The steepness of published curves varies significantly between reported series, suggesting the existence of significant variations in the sensitivity of the clonogenic cell populations within human tumors, but treatment related inaccuracies have also contributed to the flattening of dose-response curves in human tumors (DUTREIX et al. 1988; PETERS et al. 1981). In early stage tumors where the accuracy of target coverage is more certain, dose-response curves have been relatively steep. For example, FOWLER (1986) reported on dose-response relationships in T1-2 head and neck tumors and found that in the steep segments of the curves a 10% increase in dose lead to an 8-20% increase (full range 5-50%) in local control. On the other hand, THAMES et al. (1980) showed that in T3 and T4 pharyngeal wall tumors, in which the technical aspects of treatment are more challenging, a 30% dose increment was required to increase local control from 37% to 50% (i.e., 13% increase). Because the curves flattened at the 50% control level, a further increase in local control could not be achieved without exceeding unacceptably toxic dose levels. Similarly, METZ et al. (1982) found a steep dose-response curve for T1-T2 nasopharyngeal lesions, but a flatter dose-response relationship in T3 and T4 lesions.

While the number of patient series which have analyzed dose-response relationships are too small to provide detailed definitions of tumor control probabilities and curve steepness, existing data suggest that the range of doses necessary to increase tumor control by about 1% varies from 10 cGy to 60 cGy (Taylor and Withers to be published; Thames et al. 1992). The slope of the dose-response curve is defined by the gfactor, which describes the percentage increase in tumor control for a 1% increase in dose (Brahme 1984). Representative clinical series suggest that the median value for gis approximately 1.8 (Taylor and Withers to be published; Thames et al. 1992) while the gfactor for normal tissue complications has been estimated at 4 (Thames et al. 1992), demonstrating the overall relative flatness of tumor response curves. If treatment related factors (e.g., increasing the accuracy of dose distribution and eliminating geographical underdosage) were optimized, the change in tumor control probability with dose would be steeper than suggested by the retrospective studies. Under such circumstances the effect of dose escalation on the probability of local control will be maximized.

The application of new methods for accurate radiation treatment planning and delivery, together with improved staging and better assessment of tumor characteristics (e.g., DNA ploidy, proliferative profiles, and radiosensitivity), are expected to improve tumor control probabilities even without the use of dose escalation. Recent comparative studies of CT-assisted two-dimensional with the new techniques of three-dimensional (3-D) treatment planning, capable of providing complete anatomical and dose information for the entire tumor volume and its surrounding normal tissues (PHOTON TREATMENT PLANNING COLLABORATIVE WORKING GROUP 1991), have in fact documented significant improvements in target coverage and dose homogeneity with 3-D techniques (TEN HAKEN et al. 1989; LEIBEL et al. 1991a). An open question remains as to the need for dose escalation to overcome the inherent radiation resistance of tumor stem cells. Clinical studies currently underway have been designed to test the effect of dose on the probability of local tumor control using the high precision techniques of 3-D conformal photon beam radiation therapy (LEIBEL et al. 1992). These techniques are capable of not only avoiding underdosed regions within the tumor and outright marginal misses, but also enable tumor dose escalation due to meticulous removal of normal tissues from the volume receiving high radiation doses. The feasibility of dose escalation has been demonstrated in several types of human tumors, but its effect on the outcome still needs to be established (LEIBEL et al. 1992). Indeed, there have been concerns that in many human tumors a significant escalation of dose will be necessary before an effect on local control can be detected (THAMES et al. 1992).

Local Control and Metastatic Dissemination in Experimental Tumors

Several experimental studies in animal models have demonstrated that failure to control the primary tumor leads to increased rates of distant metastases. Early experiments by KAPLAN and MURPHY (1949) and by VON ESSEN and KAPLAN (1952) demonstrated that sub-curative irradiation of a transplanted mammary carcinoma in C57BL mice resulted not only in local recurrences but also in an increased incidence of pulmonary metastases when compared to unirradiated controls. Subsequently, SHELDON et al. (1974) showed that the incidence of distant metastases after locally curative irradiation was reduced compared to animals in whom a local cure was not achieved. Using first generation transplants of a spontaneous mammary carcinoma in C3H/He mice, they found that the incidence of lung metastases increased from 8% when mice were locally cured by high dose radiation therapy to 35% in animals with local failure after irradiation. While the rate of metastasis was found to be identical after local cure with either surgery or irradiation, the ultimate incidence of distant metastases was dependent on the size of the tumor at the time of definitive therapy (SHELDON et al. 1974; TODOROKI and SUIT 1985; RAMSAY et al. 1988).

RAMSAY et al. (1988) reported data which demonstrated an association between local relapse and an increase in distant metastases. C3Hf/Sed mice were transplanted with early generation transplantable tumors into their limbs. When the transplanted tumor reached a diameter of 6 mm, the tumor bearing limb was either amputated or treated with a TCD$_{50}$ dose of radiation. Animals that recurred locally after irradiation underwent a salvage amputation when the recurrent tumor regained the size of 6 mm. Mice transplanted with SCVII squamous cell carcinoma exhibited a 6-fold increase in the incidence of metastases (43%) when local relapse occurred, as compared to animals with successful initial local treatment (6.9%). A 4-fold increase in distant metastases was also observed in a transplanted FSaII spontaneous fibrosarcoma in the same experimental system. A similar phenomenon was observed in experiments published by PETERS (1975), who irradiated transplanted squamous cell carcinoma in WHT/Ht mice with doses of approximately the TCD50. Both the incidence and the probability of death from lung metastases were found to significantly correlate with the probability of local control at the primary site. Furthermore, the slope of the survival curves published in this study for mice who had a local relapse was significantly steeper than that observed when a permanent local control was achieved, suggesting that local failure was associated in this system not only with an increased incidence, but also with accelerated dissemination of metastatic clonogens.

Local Control and Metastatic Dissemination in Human Tumors

Until recently there have been few reports which specifically focused on the impact of local control on the incidence of distant metastases in human tumors. However, retrospective studies of patterns of failure in patients undergoing curative local-regional therapy indicate that human tumors conform in general with the patterns of relapse observed in animal models, exhibiting increased metastatic dissemination after failure to control the primary tumor.

To analyze the effect of local control on metastatic dissemination, human cancers can be divided into three categories. The first, exemplified by carcinomas of the prostate and breast, includes tumors in which survival is determined by the development of metastatic disease, whereas local tumor progression only rarely impacts on the outcome. The second group includes tumors arising in sites such as the head and neck, in which local failure is frequently the direct cause of the patient's death, while metastatic disease becomes a factor that impacts on the outcome mostly in locally controlled patients. Finally, there are those tumors, including non-small cell lung carcinoma, in which both local failure and distant metastases affect the survival outcome.

The first category is the most relevant model for examining the impact of local control on the metastatic outcome, as locally failing patients survive long enough to evaluate a possible association with metastatic disease. An analysis of 679 patients with surgically staged B-CN0 prostatic carcinoma treated at the Memorial Sloan-Kettering Cancer Center with interstitial ^{125}I source implants showed that the actuarial 15-year distant metastasis-free survival rate in 351 locally controlled patients was 77%, compared to 24% in 328 patients who relapsed locally (p < 0.00001) (FUKS et al. 1991b). Thus, in addition to metastases arising from micrometastatic spread before initial treatment (observed in locally controlled patients), there was a 2-fold increment in metastatic disease which was associated with the failure to control the primary tumor within the prostate. To test the biological significance of this association, a Cox proportional regression analysis of factors affecting the probability of distant metastases-free survival was performed. Local control was found to be the most significant factor affecting the metastatic outcome. The relative risk of metastatic disease subsequent to local relapse was four times greater than the risk without evidence of local failure. Since local control is a potentially transient state, it was necessary to use a period analysis to determine accurately the annual and cumulative risks of distant metastases. The difference in metastatic disease was highly significant with an $11 \pm 0.8\%$ annual mean incidence during the three to ten year interval for locally relapsing patients as compared to $1.7 \pm 0.3\%$ per year for those in local control. The relationship between local failure and the development of metastatic disease was uniformly observed across the spectrum of biological variants, from the less aggressive B1N0-grade 1 lesions to the highly malignant stage B3-C and grade 3 tumors. The median local relapse-free survival for patients with local recurrences who did not receive hormonal therapy before distant metastases were detected was 51 months, compared to a median of 71 months for distant metastases-free survival in the same patients (p < 0.001), supporting the hypothesis that in patients with local residual tumors metastases are formed and disseminated secondary to re-growth of the occult local residuum (FUKS et al. 1991b).

In contrast to patients without pelvic lymph node metastases, a Cox proportional hazard analysis of 345 patients with pelvic lymph node involvement showed that control of the primary tumor had no impact on the development of distant metastases. The most important covariate affecting distant metastasis-free survival in this group of patients was the number of tumor containing pelvic lymph nodes, followed by tumor grade and stage, indicating that nodal involvement is an important marker of disseminated disease in prostate carcinoma (LEIBEL and FUKS in preparation).

Increased metastases in patients with locally recurring prostatic carcinoma has also been reported by others, although no other study has separated patients according to pelvic lymph node status. KUBAN et al. (1989) showed that 68% of patients treated with either ^{125}I implantation or external beam irradiation who developed local recurrence ultimately developed distant metastases, whereas only 19% of those who had no evidence of local relapse developed distant metastatic dissemination (p < 0.001). When the primary tumor was controlled, the metastatic rate increased with lesser degrees of tumor differentiation and higher stage, suggesting that disease dissemination had preceded therapy in high grade and advanced stage tumors. However, when local failure occurred, the incidence of metastases was consistently high across grade and stage categories, suggesting a significant contribution of dissemination from the recurring local tumor. Similarly, ZAGARS et al. (1991) reported a 70% 13-year actuarial incidence of distant metastases in 93 patients with locally recurring stage A2-C prostate carcinoma, compared to 40% in 508 locally controlled patients (p < 0.001). Factors that are predictive of metastatic disease were equally distributed between the locally controlled and relapsed patients. The differences in metastatic outcome was most striking in patients with early stage disease who were less likely to have micrometastatic dissemination at the time of initial diagnosis. In a series of patients who underwent biopsies after external beam radiotherapy, FREIHA and BAGSHAW (1984) observed that 28 of 39 patients (72%) with positive biopsies subsequently developed metastases compared with 6 of 25 (24%) with negative biopsies.

A similar relationship between metastatic disease and the local outcome was reported in carcinoma of the breast. Fisher et al. (1991) examined the impact of ipsilateral breast tumor recurrences on the development of distant metastatic disease in patients accrued to the National Surgical Adjuvant Breast and Bowel Project (NSABP) trial B-06 (Fisher et al. 1989). This study comprised 1857 women with N0-1M0 breast tumors measuring 4 cm or less in size, randomly assigned to treatment by total mastectomy, lumpectomy and radiation therapy, or lumpectomy alone. Follow-up at 5, 8, and 9 years demonstrated no significant difference in distant disease-free survival or overall survival rates between the three treatment arms. However, by 9 years 43% of women treated by lumpectomy alone and 12% of those treated by lumpectomy and radiation therapy recurred in the ipsilateral breast. A Cox proportional hazards regression analysis revealed that local recurrence, age, nodal status, nuclear grade and tumor type were independent covariates that affected the time to distant metastases. However, ipsilateral breast tumor recurrence had the highest regression coefficient, with locally failing patients having a 3.41 fold greater risk of metastatic disease than those who were locally controlled. Ipsilateral breast tumor recurrences impacted on the time to distant disease in both node negative and node positive patients (Fisher et al. 1991). The authors did not present a period analysis of the incidence of distant metastases according to local disease and axillary lymph node status, or other stratifications by covariates that also affect the metastatic outcome. Hence, the conclusion offered by the authors that ipsilateral breast tumor recurrence represents a high risk marker for metastatic disease rather than a cause of distant spread is not completely substantiated. It is possible that in the ipsilaterally controlled patients, other risk factors such as nodal status and grade outweighed the beneficial impact of local control on the metastatic outcome, leading to an equal rate of metastatic dissemination as observed in the ipsilateral failing patients.

Another recent study on the association of a breast relapse and metastatic disease in axillary lymph node negative patients was reported by CHAUVET et al. (1990). This study comprised a relatively homogeneous group of 202 patients with pT1pN0 breast carcinoma treated by lumpectomy, axillary dissection and radiation therapy, without adjuvant chemotherapy. Both the overall survival and distant metastasis-free survival rates were significantly increased in locally controlled patients. The 5-year overall survival rates were 87.5% for relapsed and 98.3% for controlled patients (p < 0.001), whereas the 5-year distant metastases-free survival rates were 80.2% for relapsed and 91.3% for controlled patients (p < 0.001).

The effect of local relapse on the metastatic outcome was also demonstrated in the categories of patients who frequently succumb to locally recurrent disease. The analysis of this group of patients is, however, complicated due to an attrition by early death from local relapse before metastatic disease has had a chance to become clinically apparent. LEIBEL et al. (1991c) reported the treatment results in 2648 head and neck cancer patients retrieved from the database of the Radiation Therapy Oncology Group (RTOG). A Cox proportional hazards regression analysis showed that local-regional failure had a 3.9- to 15-fold greater effect on increasing the incidence of metastatic disease than tumor site, N-stage, and T-stage, all of which were independent variables affecting the metastatic outcome. Patients who were in local-regional control at 6 months after the beginning of treatment (1874 patients) were compared with surviving patients who relapsed locally by that time point (774 patients). The 5-year time-adjusted distant metastasis-free survival rate was 79% for patients who were in local-regional control at 6 months and 62% for relapsed patients (p < 0.001). A period analysis for patients at risk between 6 months and 2.5 years after treatment showed that the incidence of distant metastases was significantly reduced in locally controlled patients (p < 0.001). The difference in metastatic risk was highly significant for patients with tumors of the oral cavity, oropharynx, supraglottic larynx, and glottis (19% distant metastases after local-regional failure vs. 7% in patients with local-regional control; p < 0.001), but was not significant for those with carcinoma of the nasopharynx or hypopharynx (20% distant metastases after local-regional failure vs. 23% in patients with local-regional control; p = 0.455). As the likelihood of distant metastases in locally controlled nasopharynx and hypopharynx primaries (23%) was significantly higher than for locally controlled patients at other head and neck sites (7%), it seems that nasopharyngeal and hypopharyngeal carcinomas have a greater propensity for micrometastatic spread at the time of initial diagnosis. Whether local control affects the metastatic outcome in patients with nasopharynx and hypopharynx tumors who do not develop micrometastatic dissemination before diagnosis remains to be studied. However, LEE et al. (1989), reported that in 196 patients with stage I nasopharyngeal carcinoma, the risk of distant metastasis was 20% in patients with local-regional failure compared to 3% in controlled patients.

Similar difficulties in the analysis of the effects of local failure on the metastatic outcome have been encountered in patients with non-small cell lung carcinoma (NSCLC). PEREZ et al. (1987) found little difference in the overall incidence of distant metastases between locally controlled or locally failing patients (46% vs. 58%, respectively). However, at 6 months the incidence of distant metastases in patients with thoracic tumor control was 16.7%, compared to 37.8% in those who relapsed in the thorax. At longer follow-up periods (2 and 3 years), a significant attrition had occurred due to death from either local failure, distant metastases, or both, and a difference could no longer be demonstrated due to small patient numbers (PEREZ et al. 1986a). CHUNG et al. (1982) reported that in surgically staged T1-2 NSCLC, patients who did not have regional lymph node involvement and who relapsed locally had a significantly greater risk of metastatic disease than those who were locally controlled (90% vs. 24%, respectively, p = 0.001). Local control did not, however, appear to affect the incidence of distant metastases in patients with N1-2 disease. A similar trend was reported by MALISSARD et al. (1991) in a retrospective study of 186 patients with primary adenocarcinoma of the lung. Local control was not found to have an effect on the risk of distant metastases in node positive patients, but in node negative patients, those who were locally controlled had a 17% incidence of distant metastases at 1 year, whereas in those who relapsed locally, the risk was 67%.

Similar associations between local failure and metastatic disease have been reported in carcinoma of the rectum (SCHILD et al. 1989; VIGLIOTTI et al. 1987), uterine cervix (PAUNIER et al. 1967; ANDERSON and DISCHE 1981; Perez et al. 1988b; FAGUNDES et al. 1992), endometrium and vagina (STOKES et al. 1986; PEREZ et al. 1988a), and in soft tissue sarcoma (MARKHEDE et al. 1982; SUIT et al. 1988; GUSTAFSON et al. 1991. Some of these databases reported only crude overall incidence rates, with no distinction made between node negative and node positive patients, and in some cases there was no stratification for biological covariates, such as grade and stage. Nonetheless, these studies provide strong evidence that the association of metastatic disease and local relapse represents a general phenomenon across the spectrum of human tumors, even in tumors with an inherent propensity for early and frequent metastatic dissemination (i.e., carcinomas of the breast, lung, and nasopharynx), or tumors that lead to an early death from local recurrences (i.e., carcinomas of the head and neck and lung). Furthermore, this generalized association suggests, although it does not prove, a causative rather than an incidental association between the two phenomena.

Generation and Nature of Metastatic Clonogens in Primary and in Locally Relapsing Tumors

The association between local relapse and metastatic disease can be interpreted as evidence that neoplastic clonogens within locally relapsing tumors are subjected to biological pressures that lead to an accelerated acquisition of a metastatic competence and to an increased potential for metastatic dissemination. The experimental data of RAMSAY et al. (1988) described above are consistent with this hypothesis, as they show that equi-size primary and locally relapsing tumors are associated with different rates of lung metastases in two types of transplantable murine tumors. However, this postulate applies only if it is assumed that the ability to metastasize is not a random property equally shared by all tumor cells, but that metastatogenic clonogens are phenotypically and functionally distinct from non-metastatic tumor cells. The paradigm of existence of specific tumor phenotypes with metastatic competence was, in fact, introduced by FIDLER in 1973 and has since been confirmed by many investigators (FIDLER 1990). Furthermore, recent investigations on the generation of metastatic phenotypes have indicated that metastatic competence is a product of a mutational process that occurs in tumor clonogens which are primarily non-metastatic. There is compelling evidence that malignant transformation and tumor progression result from a multi-stage process of pleiotropic mutagenic events (FEARON and VOGELSTEIN 1990). Alterations in positive and negative regulatory genes seem equally prevalent among human cancers (BISHOP 1991). Genetic instability apparently leads to a series of mutational events, altered transcriptional activations and phenotypic alterations, granting selective advantage to specific neoplastic cells. Metastasis is the ultimate outcome of tumor progression in this selective process (FEARON and VOGELSTEIN 1990; BISHOP 1991; VOGELSTEIN et al. 1989; HOLLSTEIN et al. 1991; KERBEL 1989; SOBEL 1990).

The full details of the mutational processes that leads to maturation of the metastatic phenotype are still unknown. However, existing data indicate that it apparently involves several recessive suppressor genes, dominant regulatory genes and oncogenes (VOGELSTEIN et al. 1989; HOLLSTEIN et al. 1991; KERBEL 1989; SOBEL 1990; STEEG et al. 1988; LIOTTA et al. 1991a), and is also associated with over-expression or suppression of several normal genes (LIOTTA et al. 1991a; VLODAVSKY et al. 1988; SLOANE et al. 1981). It appears that it is the accumulation rather than the order of these pleiotropic events that confers in tumor cells the ability to invade and metastasize, thus creating an uncontrollable widespread disease.

The simplest approach to characterizing metastatic phenotypes is by identifying differential gene expressions in primary versus metastatic lesions. In animal models there is evidence that metastasis is associated with alterations in the function of the major histocompatibility complex (MHC) (FELDMAN and EISENBACH 1991). The metastatic competence of mouse 3LL Lewis lung carcinoma cells was found to correlate with suppression of the $H\text{-}2K^b$ gene expression (EISENBACH et al. 1984), and this association appeared to be a causal relationship, since transfection of metastatic clones with the H-2K^b genes abrogated their metastatic competence (PLASKIN et al. 1988). Alterations in MHC gene expression were also demonstrated in human tumors. CORDON-CARDO et al. (1991) recorded the expression of determinants of the HLA Class I (HLA A, B, and C) antigens in fresh-frozen tissue specimens obtained from 70 breast, colon, bladder and renal primary tumor lesions, and from either synchronous or metachronous lymph node, lung or liver metastases available in 44 of the patients. The majority (>70%) of tumor cells in the primary lesions were HLA-positive (observed in 38/70 patients; 54%), especially in patients who did not have clinical evidence of metastatic disease (8/11 patients; 73%). Various degrees of loss of expression were observed in 32 (46%) of the primary lesions, although the neoplastic cells were nearly exclusively HLA nonexpressors in only 8 (12%) (7 of these were obtained from patients with clinically proven metastatic disease). In contrast, the majority of the metastatic lesions consisted either of predominantly HLA negative cells (33/44 specimens; 75%) or of mixed populations (10/44 specimens; 23%), and only one metastatic lesion manifested HLA class I antigen expression in more than 70% of its tumor cells (p = 0.0005). Of particular interest was the finding that intravascular clusters of tumor cells, representing metastatic tumor phenotypes enroute to metastatic colonization at remote target organs, consisted predominantly of HLA class I nonexpressors. The pattern of HLA class I suppression in human tumors suggests that it is a characteristic feature of the metastatic phenotype, although occasionally, under undefined paracrine tissue conditions, expression of this gene may be re-induced in metastatic cells.

Other normal genes which exhibit altered functions in metastatic variants are the enzymes involved in the metastatic cascade. These genes are either over-expressed or ectopically expressed in cells with metastatic competence leading to production and release of the enzymes that participate in the biochemical degradation of extracellular matrix and basement membranes during invasion and metastasis (LIOTTA et al. 1991b; VLODAVSKY et al. 1990). This category includes tissue plasminogen activator (VLODAVSKY et al. 1988), collagenase type IV (LIOTTA et al. 1991b; LIOTTA et al. 1989), heparanase (VLODAVSKY et al. 1988; VLODAVSKY et al. 1990; NAKAJIMA et al. 1988), and the cathepsin proteases (SLOANE et al. 1981; TANDON et al. 1990), and their demonstration in tumor cells has been considered as evidence for the presence of metastatic phenotypes.

Another approach to characterize metastasis genes has been by transfection of tested gene constructs into the genome of tumor cells, and testing their effect on the acquisition of metastatic competence. Transfection with one of several oncogenes, including myc, ras, fos, fms and src, was shown to confer metastatogenicity in various cell systems (Muschel and Liotta 1988; Greenberg et al. 1989). The most relevant of these oncogenes to human tumors has been the myc oncogene. Transfection of myc into a neuroblstoma cell line induced metastatic competence (Bernards et al. 1989). These data complement clinical studies which have reported amplification of N-myc in advanced metastatic neuroblastoma, as compared to the normal levels observed in early and non-metastatic stage I and II tumors (Seeger et al. 1985). Similarly, amplification and over-expression of N-myc and L-myc have been associated with metastases an small cell lung cancer (Gemma et al. 1989).

Some genes have been shown to suppress, rather than induce, the metastatic competence upon transfection. For example, transfection with the Adenovirus 2 E1a suppressor gene abrogated the metastatic competence of ras transfected rat embryo fibroblasts (Pozzati et al. 1986). Based on these and similar observations, it was postulated that mutagenic deactivation or deletion of recessive suppressor genes may be involved in the metastatogenic transformation. Steeg et al. (1988) reported that mRNA levels of the nm23-H1 suppressor gene were approximately 10-fold higher in two K-1735 murine melanoma lines with low metastatic potential as compared with five highly metastatic K-1735 melanoma cell lines. The human nm23-H1 gene maps to the 17q21 chromosome, and it encodes for a 17 kD nucleoside diphosphate (NDP) kinase (Biggs et al. 1990; Stahl et al. 1991). A study by Bevilacqua et al. (1989) of 27 primary breast tumors showed reductions in cytoplasmic nm23-mRNA levels and in immunoperoxidase detectable 17 kD nm23 protein in specimens from patients with histological and clinical evidence of highly metastatic tumors. These observations were confirmed by Hennessy et al. (1991) who reported that patients with high levels of nm23 mRNA in their primary breast tumors exhibited significantly longer disease-free ($p < 0.002$) and overall ($p < 0.003$) survivals than patients with low levels of nm23 mRNA.

In contrast to breast cancer, high rather than low levels of p19/nm23-H1 protein were found in advanced stage neuroblastoma associated N-myc gene amplification and metastasis (Hailat et al. 1991). Similarly, Haut et al. (1991) reported that nm23 mRNA was increased in 13 colonic tumor specimens relative to morphologically normal colon mucosa in the same patients. The latter data are surprising in view of the fact that the same group reported somatic allelic deletions of nm23 in DNA extracts from a variety of human tumors, including carcinoma of the colon (Leone et al. 1991). Indeed, Cohn et al. (1991) found allelic deletions of the nm23-H1 gene in 11 of 21 human colonic tumors and a significant correlation between nm23/H1 allelic deletion in the primary tumors and the eventual development of metastatic spread. The enigma of nm23 and the metastatic competence in carcinoma of the colon is as yet unresolved. It is possible that the increased levels of nm23 gene products detected in some tumors are produced by a mutated gene which lacks suppressor activity. A similar phenomenon has been described for the p53 suppressor gene in colonic tumors (Baker et al. 1989).

The p53 gene is another suppressor gene associated with the metastatic potential in several types of tumors (LEVINE et al. 1991). It is located on the chromosome 17p13.1 and encodes a phosphoprotein which localizes to the nucleus and appears to play an essential role in the negative regulation of the G0-G1 transition of the cell cycle (LEVINE et al. 1991). The p53 protein does not normally accumulate in the cell, but missense mutations significantly increase its half-life, thereby leading to its accumulation and detectability by immunohistochemical analysis.

Somatic mutations of the p53 gene have been described in patients with tumors of the breast (THOR et al. 1992; ELLEDGE et al. 1992), colon (BAKER et al. 1989; CAMPO et al. 1991), prostate (EFFERT et al. 1992; VISAKORPI et al. 1992), and the urinary bladder (PRESTI et al. 1991; DALBAGNI et al. to be published). In a recent study, THOR et al. (1992) reported that patients with mutated p53 in primary breast tumors had a shorter metastases-free survival ($p = 0.003$) and poorer overall survival ($p = 0.0008$) than patients negative for this protein. VISAKORPI et al. (1992) reported that only 6% of 137 primary prostatic tumors exhibited intense immunostaining for mutated p53, but high levels of mutated p53 accumulation predicted for both a significantly shortened progression-free interval ($p < 0.01$) and poor survival ($p < 0.001$) as compared to patients without evidence of mutated p53 in their tumors. DALBAGNI et al. reported that p53 mutations and 17p allelic deletions significantly correlated with vascular invasion ($p = 0.021$) and the presence of lymph node metastases ($p = 0.007$) in 60 patients with carcinoma of the bladder.

A third suppressor gene associated with the metastatic potential is the retinoblastoma susceptibility (Rb) gene, located on chromosome 13q14 (Friend et al. 1986; Lee et al. 1987). It encodes a 110 kD nuclear phosphoprotein, believed to function as a cell cycle regulator. Historically, Rb gene deletions were initially described in heritable retinoblastoma (Friend et al. 1986). Subsequently, either deletions, rearrangements, or altered expressions of the Rb gene have been described in several types of tumors, including soft tissue and bone sarcomas (Friend et al. 1986; Reissman et al. 1989; Cance et al. 1990; Wunder et al. 1991), bladder (Presti et al. 1991; Cairns et al. 1991; Cordon-Cardo et al. 1992; Ishikawa et al. 1991), renal (Ishikawa et al. 1991; Anglard et al. 1991), testicular (Strohmeyer et al. 1991), breast (Lee et al. 1988; Varley et al. 1989) and small cell lung tumors (Harbour et al. 1988; Minna et al. 1989). Cance et al. (1990) demonstrated an inverse correlation between the expression of Rb gene and both the metastatic spread and prognosis in patients with soft tissue sarcomas. When the nuclear Rb protein was partially or completely deleted, there was an increased incidence of patients succumbing to metastatic disease, compared to patients in whom the tumor cells exhibited homogeneous and intensive staining of the Rb protein. Examination of 12 metastatic lesions showed a complete or significant deletion of the Rb gene product in all tumor specimens. Cordon-Cardo et al. (1992) evaluated the Rb gene expression in 48 primary bladder tumors from radical cystectomy specimens and reported that survival was significantly decreased in Rb negative patients compared to those with normal Rb expression (p < 0.001). Since mortality in this group of patients resulted from distant metastases, these data suggest an association between altered Rb protein expression and metastatic disease in bladder tumors.

Taken together, these data strongly suggest that suppressor genes are associated with progression of tumors to the metastatic phase. However, the data also demonstrate that none of these genes is uniformly altered in metastatic phenotypes, disclosing occasionally normal gene expressions in metastatic lesions. This phenomenon indicates that perturbation in the function of any of these genes alone is not sufficient to induce the metastatic phenotype, and it appears that either concurrent or stepwise processes in several suppressor and other metastasis genes are required for the progression of the metastatic conversion.

The realization that a multi-step mutational process is associated with the acquisition of the metastatic competence may elucidate the mechanism by which local failure enhances the rate of metastatic disease. It is likely that tumor cell clonogens remaining in residual tumors after failure to eradicate the primary lesion are primed with at least some of the initial genetic events required for completion of the metastatic conversion. The increased mitotic activity and enhanced growth fraction that are typical for the early phases of the regrowth of locally failing primary residual lesions (TUBIANA 1988; WITHERS et al. 1988) provide an opportunity for an accelerated accumulation of the mutations required for completion of the metastatic transformation. Hence, the incomplete eradication of the primary tumor in patients in whom the multi-stage metastatic conversion has not been completed before the initial diagnosis leaves behind a small volume residual tumor that initiates an intensive mitotic activity, and thus, creates a highly favorable condition for the maturation of premetastatic clonogens and the subsequent development of metastatic disease. This model is consistent with the observations on the temporal development of local relapse and metastatic disease when occurring in the same patients described by FUKS et al. (1991b) in carcinoma of the prostate. It is also consistent with the pattern of the temporal appearance of metastatic disease in patients with local control versus those with local relapse described in the same series (FUKS et al. 1991b). This hypothesis also emphasizes the need for complete eradication of the primary tumor during the initial attempt at curative therapy, and serves as a biological basis for the development of studies on the effect of improved local control on the metastatic outcome (FUKS et al. 1991a; LEIBEL et al. 1991b).

Conclusions

The need to improve local control while minimizing treatment related toxicities continues to represent a major challenge in the management of localized human cancer. The limited success in controlling localized disease with the current available modalities and the association of local failure with incurable metastatic disease have stimulated a search for improved methods to accomplish a permanent control of the primary tumor at the initial therapeutic attempt. Whereas the maximal potential benefits from modern surgical approaches have probably been realized, recent technological advances in computerized radiation treatment planning and delivery systems have produced opportunities for the application of new high precision techniques to improve the likelihood of local control (FUKS et al. 1991a; Suit and Urie 1992; LEIBEL et al. 1992). In addition to brachytherapy, intraoperative radiotherapy, chemical modifiers of the radiation response and altered fractionation schemes, techniques that improve external beam targeting and the differential dose distribution between tumor and normal tissues exemplify several of the more advanced strategies that are being actively explored. However, such efforts can only be justified if an improvement in local control has a significant impact on the outcome in patients with several different cancers.

Based on the biological considerations discussed in this review, we have proposed the hypothesis that improved local control is likely to decrease the ultimate rates of metastatic disease in several types of tumors (Fuks et al. 1991a; Leibel et al. 1991b). The recently introduced modality of three-dimensional conformal radiation therapy using either protons (Suit and Urie 1992) or photons (Fuks et al. 1991a; Leibel et al. 1992) provide a tool for testing this hypothesis. The studies required to test the hypothesis would be greatly assisted by the availability of predictive indicators to distinguish prospectively between patients who are candidates for cure by local treatment modalities from those who already have micrometastatic dissemination at the time of initial diagnosis, who would also require adjuvant systemic treatments. Based on the demonstration that tumor cells which metastasize are phenotypically distinct from the non-metastatic variants, the development of such assays may be feasible. Accordingly, at the Memorial Sloan-Kettering Cancer Center we are currently examining primary tumor specimens using a panel of biological and immunological markers to enumerate the frequency of neoplastic cells bearing metastatic phenotype markers and correlate the frequency of such phenotypes with the eventual metastatic outcome. The successful establishment of criteria for predictive indicators of the probability of micrometastatic spread before initial treatment would improve the ability to select the most appropriate therapy for the individual patient and facilitate studies designed to test the impact of local control on the outcome.

References

1. Alper T (1980) Survival curve models. In: Meyn RE, Withers HR (eds) Radiobiology in Cancer Research, Raven Press, New York, pp 3-18.

2. Anderson P, Dische S (1981) Local tumor control and subsequent incidence of distant metastatic disease. Int J Radiat Oncol Biol Phys 7: 1645-1648.

3. Anglard P, Tory K, Brauch H, et al. (1991) Molecular analysis of genetic changes in the origin and development of renal cell carcinoma. Cancer Res 51: 1071.

4. Baker S, Fearon E, Nigro J, et al. (1989) Chromosome 17 deletions and p53 gene mutations in colorectal carcinoma. Science 244: 217-221.

5. Bentzen SM, Thames HD (1991) Clinical evidence for tumor clonogen regeneration: implications of the data. Radiother and Oncol 22: 161-166.

6. Bernards R, Dessain SK, Weinberg RA (1989) N-myc amplification causes down-modulation MHC class I antigen expression in neuroblastoma. Cell 47: 667-674.

7. Bevilacqua G, Sobel ME, Liotta LA, Steeg PS (1989) Association of low nm 23 RNA levels in human primary infiltrating breast carcinoma with lymph node involvement and other histopathological indicators of high metastatic potential. Cancer Res 49: 5185-5199.

8. Biggs J, Hersperger E, Steeg PS, et al. (1990) A drosophila gene that is homologous to a mammalian gene associated with tumor metastasis codes a nucleoside diphosphate kinase. Cell 63: 933.

9. Bishop JM (1991) Molecular themes in oncogenesis. Cell 64: 235-249.

10. Brahme A (1984) A. Dosimetric precision requirements in radiation therapy. Acta Radiol Oncol 23: 379-391.

11. Cairns P, Proctor AJ, Knowles MA (1991) Loss of heterozygosity at the RB locus is frequent and correlates with muscle invasion in bladder carcinoma. Oncogene 6: 2305.

12. Campo E, Calle-Martin O, Miquel R, Palacin A, Romero M, Fabregat V, Vives J, Cardesa A, Yague J (1991) Loss of heterozygosity of p53 gene and p53 protein in human colorectal carcinoma. Canc Res 51: 4436-4442.

13. Cance WG, Brennan MF, Dudas ME, Huang C-M, Cordon-Cardo C (1990) Altered expression of the retinblastoma gene product in human sarcomas. N Eng J Med 323: 1457-1462.

14. Chauvet B, Reynaud-Bougnoux A, Calais G, Panel N, Lansac J, Bougnoux P, Le Floch O (1990) Prognostic significance of breast relapse after conservative treatment in node-negative early breast cancer. Int J Radiat Oncol Biol Phys 19: 1125-1130.

15. Chung CK, Stryker JA, O'Neill M, DeMuth WE (1982) Evaluation of adjuvant postoperative radiotherapy for lung cancer. Int J Radiat Oncol Biol Phys 8: 1877-1880.

16. Cohn KH, Wang F, DeSoto-LaPaix F, Solomon WB, Patterson LG, Arnold MR, Weimer J, Feldman JG, Levy AT, Leona A, Steeg PT (1991) Association of nm23-H1 allelic deletions with distant metastatses in colorectal carcinoma. Lancet 338: 722-724.

17. Cordon-Cardo C, Wartinger D, Petrylak D, Dalbagni G, Fair WR, Fuks Z, Reuter VE (1992) Altered expression of the retinoblastoma gene product: prognostic indicator in bladder cancer. J Natl Cancer Inst 84: 1251-1256.

18. Cordon-Cordo C, Fuks Z, Eisenbach L, Feldman M (1991) Expression of HLA-A,B,C antigens on primary and metastatic tumor cell populations of human carcinomas. Cancer Res 51: 6372-6380.

19. Dalbagni G, Presti JC, Reuter VE, et al. (1993) Molecular genetic alterations of chromosome 17 and p53 expression in human bladder cancer. Diag Mol Pathol 2: 4-13.

20. Deacon JM, Peckham MJ, Steel GG (1984) The radioresponsiveness of human tumours and the initial slope of the cell survival curve. Radiother and Oncol 2: 317-323.

21. DeVita VT (1983) Progress in cancer management. Cancer 51: 2401-2409.

22. DeVita VT, Lippman M, Hubbard S.A, Idhe DC, Rosenberg SA (1986) The effect of combined modality therapy on local control and survival. Int J Radiat Oncol Biol Phys 12: 487-501.

23. Dutreix J, Tubiana M, Dutreix A (1988) An approach to the interpretation of clinical data on tumour control probability-dose relationship. Radiother and Oncol 11: 239-258.

24. Effert PJ, Neubauer A, Walter PJ, Liu E (1992) Alterations of the p53 gene are associated with the progression of human prostate carcinoma. J Urol 147: 789-793.

25. Eisenbach L, Hollander N, Greenfeld L, Yakor H., Segal S, and Feldman M (1984) The differential expression of H-2K versus H-2-D antigens distinguishing low metastatic from high metastatic clones is correlated with the immunogenic properties of the tumor cells. Int J Cancer 34: 567-573.

26. Elledge RM, Fukua SAW, Clarck GM, Allerd DC, McGuire WL (1992) Prognostic significance of mutations in the p53 gene in node-negative breast cancer. Proc Am Assoc Cancer Res 33: 253.

27. Fagundes H, Perez CA, Grigsby PW, Lockett MA (1992) Distant metastases after irradiation alone in carcinoma of the uterine cervix. Int J Radiat Oncol Biol Phys 24: 197-204.

28. Fearon ER, Vogelstein B (1990) A genetic model for colorectal tumorigenesis. Cell 61: 759-767.

29. Feldman M, and Eisenbach L (1991) MHC class I genes controlling the metastatic phenotype of tumor cells. Semin Cancer Biol 2: 337-346.

30. Fertil B, Malaise EP (1981) Inherent cellular radiosensitivity as a basic concept for human tumor radiotherapy. Int J Radiat Oncol Biol Phys 7: 621-629.

31. Fertil B, Malaise EP (1985) Intrinsic radiosensitivity of human cell lines is correlated with radioresponsiveness of human tumors analysis of 101 published survival curves. Int J Radiat Oncol Biol Phys 11: 1699-1707.

32. Fidler IJ (1990) Critical features in the biology of human metastasis: G.H.A. Clowes Memorial Award Lecture. Cancer Res 50: 6130-6138.

33. Fidler IJ (1973) Selection of succesive tumor lines for metastasis. Nat New Biol 242: 148-149.

34. Fischer JJ, Moulder JE (1975) The steepness of the dose-response curve in radiation therapy. Rad Biol 117: 179-184.

35. Fisher B, Anderson S, Fisher ER, Redmond C, Wickerham DL, Wolmark N, Mamounas EP, Deutsch M, Margolese R (1991) Significance of ipsilateral breast tumor recurrence after lumpectomy. Lancet 338: 327-331.

36. Fisher B, Redmond C, Poisson R, Margolese R, Wolmark N, Wickerham L, Fisher E, Deutsch M, Caplan R, Pilch Y, Glass A, Shibata H, Lerner H, Terz J, Sidorovich L (1989) Eight-year results of a randomized clinical trial comparing total mastectomy and lumpectomy with or without irradiation in the treatment of breast cancer. N Eng J Med 320: 822-828.

37. Fowler JF (1986) Potential for increasing the differential response between tumors and normal tissues: can proliferation rate be used? Int J Radiat Oncol Biol Phys 12: 641-645.

38. Freiha FS, Bagshaw MA (1984) Carcinoma of the prostate: results of post-irradiation biopsy. The Prostate 5: 19-25.

39. Friend SH, Bernards R, Rogelj S, Weinberg RA, Rapaport JM, Albert DM, Dryja TP (1986) A human DNA segment with properties of the gene that predisposes to retinoblastoma and osteosarcoma. Nature 323: 643-646.

40. Fuks Z, Leibel SA, Kutcher GE, Mohan R, Ling CC (1991a) Three dimensional conformal treatment: a new frontier in radiation therapy. In: DeVita VT Jr, Hellman S, Rosenberg SA (eds) Important Advances in Oncology, Lippincot, Philadelphia, pp 151-172.

41. Fuks Z, Leibel SA, Wallner KE, Begg CB, Fair WR, Anderson LL, Hilaris BS, Whitmore WF (1991b) The effect of local control on metastatic dissemination in carcinoma of the prostate: long term results in patients treated with ^{125}I implantation. Int J Radiat Oncol Biol Phys 21: 537-547.

42. Gemma A, Nakajima T, Shiraishi M, et al. (1989) Myc family gene abnormality in lung cancer and its relation to xenotransplantability. Cancer Res 48: 6025-6028.

43. Greenberg AH, Egan SE, Wright LA (1989) Oncogenes and metastatic progression. Inv Metas 9: 350-378.

44. Gustafson P, Rooser B, Rydholm A (1991) Is local recurrence of minor importance for metastases in soft tissue sarcoma? Cancer 67: 2083-2086.

45. Hailat N, Keim DR, Melhem RF, Zhu XX, Eckerskorn C, Brodeur GM, Reynolds CP, Seeger RC, Lottspeich F, Stahler JR and Hanash SM (1991) High levels of p19/nm23 in neuroblastoma are associted with advanced stage disease and with N-myc gene amplification. J Clin Inv 88: 341-345.

46. Harbour JW, Lai S-L, Whang-Peng J, et al. (1988) Abnormalities in structure and expression of the human retinoblastoma gene in small cell lung cancer. Science 241: 353.

47. Haut M, Steeg PT, Wilson KJV, Markowitz SD (1991) Induction of nm23 expression in human colonic neoplasms and equal expression in colon tumors of high and low metastatic potential. J Natl Cancer Inst 83: 712-716.

48. Hendry JH, Moore JV (1984) Is the steepness of dose-incidence curves for tumour control or complications due to variation before or as a result of irradiation? Brit J Rad 57: 1045-1046.

49. Hennessy C, Henry JA, May FEB, et al. (1991) Expression of the anti-metastatic gene nm23 in human breast cancer: association with good prognosis. J Natl Cancer Inst 83: 281-285.

50. Hollstein M, Sidransky D, Vogelstein B, et al. (1991) p53 mutations in human cancers. Science 253: 49-53.

51. Ishikawa J, Xu H-J, Hu S-X, Yandell DW, Maeda S, Kamidono S, Benedict WF, Takahashi R (1991) Inactivation of the retinoblastoma gene in human bladder and renal cell carcinomas. Cancer Res 51: 5736-5743.

52. Kaplan HS, Murphy ED (1949) The effect of local roentgen irradiation on the biological behavior of a transplantable mouse carcinoma. I. Increased frequency of pulmonary metastasis. J Natl Cancer Inst 9: 407-414.

53. Kerbel RS (1989) Towards an understanding of the molecular basis of the metastatic phenotype. Inv Metast 9: 329-337.

54. Kuban DA, El-Mahdi AM, Schellhammer PF (1989) Prognosis in patients with local recurrence after definitive irradiation for prostatic cancer Cancer 63: 2421-2425.

55. Lee EYH, To H, Shew J-Y, et al. (1988) Inactivation of the retinoblastoma susceptibility gene in human breast cancers. Science 241: 218.

56. Lee WH, Bookstein R, Hong F, Young LJ, Shew J-Y, Lee EYH (1987) Human retinoblastoma susceptibility gene: cloning, identification and sequence. Science 235: 1394-1399.

57. Lee AW, Sham JS., Poon YF, Ho JH (1989) Treatment of stage I nasopharyngeal carcinoma: analysis of the patterns of relapse and the results of withholding elective neck irradiation. Int J Radiat Oncol Biol Phys 17: 1183-1190.

58. Leibel SA., Kutcher GJ., Harrison LB, Fass DE, Burman CM, Hunt MA, Mohan R, Brewster MS, Ling CC Fuks Z (1991a) Improved dose distributions for 3-D conformal boost treatments in carcinoma of the nasopharynx. Int J Radiat Oncol Biol Phys 20: 823-833.

59. Leibel SA, Kutcher GJ, Mohan R, Harrison LB, Armstrong JG, Zelefsky MJ, LoSasso TJ, Burman CM, Mageras GS, Masterson ME, Lo Y-C, Ling CC, Fuks (1992) Three-dimensional conformal radiation therapy at the Memorial Sloan-Kettering Cancer Center. Seminars in Radiat Oncol 2: 274-289.

60. Leibel SA, Ling CC, Kutcher GJ, Mohan R, Cordon-Cardo C, Fuks Z (1991b) The biological basis of conformal three-dimensional radiation therapy. Int J Radiat Oncol Biol Phys 21: 805-811.

61. Leibel SA, Scott CB, Mohiuddin M, Marcial V, Coia LR, Davis LW, Fuks Z (1991c) The effect of local-regional control on distant metastatic dissemination in carcinoma of the head and neck: results of an analysis from the RTOG head and neck database. Int J Radiat Oncol Biol Phys 21: 549-556.

62. Leibel SA, Fuks Z, Zelelfsky MJ, Whitmore WF Jr., (1994). The effects of local and regional treatments on the metastatic outcome in prostatic carcinoma with pelvic lymph node involvement. Int J Radiat Oncol Biol Phys 28:7-16.

63. Leone A, McBride OW, Weston A, Wang MG, Anglard P, Cropp CS, Goepel JR, Lidereau R, Callahan R, Linehan WM, et al. (1991) Somatic allelic deletion of nm23 in human cancer. Cancer Res 51: 2490-2493.

64. Levine AJ, Momand J, Finalay CA (1991) The p53 tumor suppressor gene. Nature 250: 435-456.

65. Liotta LA, Steeg PS, Stettler-Stevenson WG (1991a) Cancer metastasis and angiogenesis: an imbalance of positive and negative regulation. Cell 64: 327-336.

66. Liotta LA and Stetler-Stevenson WG (1991b) Tumor invasion and metastatsis: an imbalance of positive and negative regulation. Cancer Res 51: 5054s-5059s.

67. Liotta LA, Wewer U, Rao NC, Schiffman E, Starcke M, Guirguis R, Thorgirsson U, Muschel R, Sobel M (1989) Biochemical mechanisms of tumor invasion and metastases. Adv Exp Med Biol 233: 161-169.

68. Malissard L, Nguyen TD, Jung GM, Forçard JJ, Castelain B, Tuchais C, Allain YM, Denepoux R, Lagrange JL, Panis X, Rathelot P, Chaplain G, Koechlin M, Rozan R (1991) Localized adenocarcinoma of the lung: a retrospective study of 186 non-metastatic patients from the French Federation of Cancer Institutes-The Radiotherapy Cooperative Group. Int J Radiat Oncol Biol Phys 21: 369-373.

69. Markhede G, Angervall L, Stener B (1982) A multivariate analysis of the prognosis after surgical treatment of soft tissue tumors. Cancer 49: 1721-1733.

70. McMillan TJ (1992) Residual DNA damage: what is left over and how does this determine cell fate? Europ J Cancer 28: 267-269.

71. Menick HR, Garfinkel L, Dodd GD (1991) Preliminary report of the National Cancer Data Base. CA 41: 7-18.

72. Metz CE, Tokars RP, Kronman HB, Griem ML (1982) Maximum likelihood estimation of dose-response parameters for therapeutic operating characteristic (TOC) analysis of carcinoma of the nasopharynx. Int J Radiat Oncol Biol Phys 8: 1185-1192.

73. Merino OR, Lindberg RD, Fletcher GH (1977) An analysis of distant metastases from squamous cell carcinoma of the upper respiratory and digestive tracts. Cancer 40: 145-151.

74. Minna JD, Schütte, Viallet J, et al. (1989) Transcription factors and recessive oncogenes in the pathogenesis of human lung cancer Int J Cancer 4: 32.

75. Munro TR, Gilbert CW (1961) The relation between tumour lethal doses and the radiosensitivity of tumour cells. Brit J Rad 34: 246-250.

76. Muschel R, Liotta RA (1988) Role of oncogenes in metastasis. Carcinogenesis 9: 705-710

77. Myers MH, Ries LA (1989) Cancer patient survival rates: SEER program results for 10 years of follow-up. CA 39: 21-32.

78. Nakajima M, Irimura T, Nicolson GL (1988) Heparanase and tumor metastasis. J Cell Bioch 36: 157-167.

79. Paunier JP, Delclos L, Fletcher GH (1967) Cause, time of death, and sites of failure in squamous cell carcinoma of the uterine cervix on intact uterus. Radiology 88: 552-562.

80. Perez CA, Bauer M, Edelstein S, Gillespie BW, Birch R (1986a) Impact of tumor control on survival in carcinoma of the lung treated with irradiation. Int J Radiat Oncol Biol Phys 12: 539-547.

81. Perez CA, Brady LW (1992) Overview. In: Perez CA, Brady LW (eds) Principles and Practice of Radiation Oncology, 2nd edn. JB Lippincott, Philadelphia, pp 25-26.

82. Perez CA, Camel HM, Galakatos AE, Grigsby PW, Kuske R, Buchsbaum G, Hederman MA (1988a) Definitive irradiation in carcinoma of the vagina: long-term evaluation of results. Int J Radiat Oncol Biol Phys 15: 1283-1290.

83. Perez CA, Kuske RR, Camel HM, Galakatos AE, Hederman MA, Kao MS, Walz BJ (1988b) Analysis of pelvic tumor control and impact on survival in carcinoma of the uterine cervix treated with radiation therapy alone. Int J Radiat Oncol Biol Phys 14: 613-621.

84. Perez CA, Pajak TF, Rubin P, Simpson JR, Mohiuddin M, Brady LW, Perez-Tamayo R, Rotman M (1987) Long term observations of the pattern of failure in patients with unresectable non-oat cell carcinoma of the lung treated with definitive radiotherapy. Report by the Radiation Therapy Oncology Group. Cancer 59: 1874-1881.

85. Perez CA, Pilepich MV, Zivnuska F (1986b) Tumor control in definitive irradiation of localized carcinoma of the prostate. Int J Radiat Oncol Biol Phys 12: 523-531.

86. Peters LJ (1975) A study of the influence of various diagnostic and therapeutic procedures applied to a murine squamous carcinoma and its metastatic behaviour. Brit J Cancer 32: 355-365.

87. Peters LJ, Fletcher GH (1983) Causes of failure of radiotherapy in head and neck cancer. Radiother and Oncol 1: 53-63.

88. Peters LJ, Withers HR, Thames HD, Fletcher GH (1981) Keynote address - The problem: tumor radioresistance in clinical radiotherapy. Int J Radiat Oncol Biol Phys 8: 101-108.

89. Photon Treatment Planning Collaborative Working Group (1991) State of the art of external photon beam radiation treatment planning. Int J Radiat Oncol Biol Phys 21: 9-23.

90. Plaksin D, Gelber C, Feldman M, Eisenbach L (1988) Reversal of the metastatic phenotype in Lewis lung carcinoma cells after transfection with syngeneic H-2K^b gene. Proc Natl Acad Sci USA 85: 4463-4467.

91. Porter EH (1980) The statistical dose-cure relationships for irradiated tumors. Brit J Radiol 53: 336-345.

92. Pozzati R, Muschel RJ, Williams JE, Padmanhabhan R, Howard B, Liotta LA, Khoury G (1986) Primary rat embryo cells transformed by one or two oncogenes show different metastatic potentials. Science 232: 223-227.

93. Presti JC, Reuter VE, Galan T, Fair WR, Cordon-Cardo C (1991) Molecular genetic alterations in superficial and locally advanced human bladder cancer. Cancer Res 51: 5405-5409.

94. Ramsay J, Suit HD, Sedlacek R (1983) Experimental studies on the incidence of metastases.after failure of radiation treatment and the effect of salvage surgery. Int J Radiat Oncol Biol Phys 14: 1165-1168.

95. Reissman PT, Simon MA, Lee W-H, Slamon DJ. (1989) Studies of the retinoblastoma gene in human sarcomas. Oncogene 4: 839-842.

96. Schild SE, Martenson JA Jr, Gunderson LL, Ilstrup DM, Berg KK, O'Connell MJ, Weiland LH (1989) Postoperative adjuvant therapy of rectal cancer: An analysis of disease control, survival and prognostic factors. Int J Radiat Oncol Biol Phys 17: 55-62.

97. Seeger R, Brodeur G, Sather H, et al. (1985) Association of multiple copies of N-*myc* oncogene with rapid progression of neuroblastoma. N Engl J Med 313: 1111-1116.

98. Sheldon PW, Begg AC, Fowler JF, Lansley IF (1974) The incidence of lung metastases in C3H mice after treatment of implanted tumors with X-rays or surgery. Brit J Cancer 30: 342-348.

99. Sloane BF, Dunn TR, Honn KV (1981) Lysosomal cathepsin B: Correlation with metastatic potential. Science 212: 1151-1153.

100. Sobel ME (1990) Metastasis suppressor genes. J Natl Cancer Inst 82: 267-276.

101. Stahl JA, Leone A, Rosengard AM, et al. (1991) Identification of a second human nm23 gene, nm23-H2. Cancer Res 51: 445-449.

102. Steeg PS, Bevilacqua G, Kopper L, et al. (1988) Evidence for a novel gene associated with low tumor metastatic potential. J Natl Cancer Inst 89: 200-203.

103. Stokes S, Bedwinek J, Kao MS, Camel HM, Perez CA (1986) Treatment of Stage I adenocarcinoma of the endometrium by hysterectomy and adjuvant irradiation: a retrospective analysis of 304 patients. Int J Radiat Oncol Biol Phys 12: 339-344.

104. Strohmeyer T, Reissmann P, Cordon-Cardo C, et al. (1991) Correlation between retinoblastoma gene expression and differentiation in human testicular tumors. Proc Natl Acad Sci 88: 6662.

105. Suit HD (1982) Potential for improving survival rates for the cancer patient by increasing the efficacy of treatment of the primary lesion. Cancer 50: 1227-1234.

106. Suit HD, Mankin HJ, Wood WC, Gebhardt MC, Harmon DC, Rosenberg A, Tepper JE, Rosenthal D (1988) Treatment of the patient with stage M0 soft tissue sarcoma. J Clin Oncol 6: 854-862.

107. Suit H, Urie M (1992) Proton beams in radiation therapy. J Natl Cancer Inst 84: 155-164.

108. Tandon, AK, Clark G.M, Chamnes GC, Chirgwin JM, McGuire WI (1990) Cathepsin D and prognosis in breast cancer. N Engl J Med 322: 297-302.

109. Taylor JMC, Withers HR (1992) Dose-time factors in head and neck data. Radiother and Oncol 25: 313-315.

110. Ten Haken RK, Perez-Tamayo C, Tesser RJ, McShan DL, Fraass BA, Lichter AS (1989) Boost treatment of the prostate using shaped fixed beams. Int J Radiat Oncol Biol Phys 16: 193-200.

111. Thames HD Jr, Peters LJ, Spanos WS Jr, Fletcher GF (1980) Dose response of squamous cell carcinomas of the upper respiratory and digestive tracts. Br J Cancer 41Suppl IV: 35-38.

112. Thames HD, Schulthheiss TE, Hendy JH, Tucker SL, Dubray BM, Brock WA (1992) Can modest escalations of dose be detected as increased tumor control? Int J Radiat Oncol Biol Phys 22: 241-246.

113. Thomlinson RH, Gray LH (1955) The histological structure of some human lung cancers and the possible implications for radiotherapy. Brit J Cancer 9: 539-549.

114. Thor AD, Moore DH, Edgerton SM (1992) Accumulation of p53 tumor suppresor protein: an independent marker of prognosis in breast cancer. J Natl Cancer Inst 84: 845-855.

115. Todoroki T, Suit HD (1985) Therapeutic advantage in preoperative single dose radiation combined with conservative and radical surgery in different size murine fibrosarcoma. J Surg Oncol 29: 207-215.

116. Tubiana M (1988) Repopulation in human tumors. Acta Oncol 27: 83-88.

117. Department of Health and Human Services (1988) Cancer Trends: 1950-1985 In: 1987 Annual Cancer Statistics Review, NIH Publication No. 88-2789, Bethesda, Maryland, pp II.1-II.203.

118. Varley JM, Armour J, Swallow JE, Jeffreys AJ, Ponder BAJ, T'Ang A, Fung Y-K, Brammar WJ, Walker RA (1989) The retinoblastoma gene is freuqently altered leading to loss of expression in primary breast tumors. Oncogene 4: 725-729.

119. Vigliotti A, Rich TA, Romsdahl MM, Withers HR, Oswald MJ (1987) Postoperative adjuvant radiotherapy for adenocarcinoma of the rectum and rectosigmoid. Int J Radiat Oncol Biol Phys 13: 999-1006.

120. Visakorpi T, Kallioniemi OP, Heikkinen A, Koivula T, Isola J (1992) Small group of aggressive, highly proliferative prostatic carcinoma defined by p53 accumulation. J Natl Cancer Inst 84: 883-887.

121. Vlodavsky I, Michaeli RI, Bar-Ner M, Friedman R, Howowitz AT, Fuks Z, Biran S (1988) Involvement of heparanase in tumor metastasis and angiogenesis. Isr J Med Sci 24: 464-470.

122. Vlodavsky I, Korner G, Ishai-Michaeli R, Bashkin P, Bar-Shavit R, Fuks Z (1990) Extracellular matrix-resident growth factors and enzymes: possible involvement in tumor metastasis and angiogenesis. Cancer Metastasis Rev 9: 203-226.

123. Vogelstein B, Fearon ER, Kern SE, et al. (1989) Allelotype of colorectal carcinomas. Science 244: 207-211.

124. Von Essen CF, Kaplan HS (1952) Further studies of metastasis of a transplantable mouse mammary carcinoma after roentgen irradiation. J Natl Cancer Inst 12: 883-890.

125. Walsh PC (1987) Adjuvant radiotherapy after radical prostatectomy: is it indicated? J Urol 138: 1427-1428.

126. Weichselbaum RR, Rotmensch J, Swan SA, Beckett MA (1989) Radiobiological characterization of 53 human tumor cell lines. Int J Radiat Biol 56: 553-560.

127. Withers HR, Taylor JMG, Maciejewski B (1988) The hazards of accelerated tumor clonogens repopulation during radiotherapy. Acta Oncol 27: 131-146, 1988.

128. Wunder JS, Czitrom AA, Kandel R, Andrulis IL (1991) Analysis of alterations in the retinoblastoma gene and tumor grade in bone and soft-tissue sarcomas. J Natl Cancer Inst 83: 194.

129. Zagars GK, Schultheiss TE, Peters LJ (1987) Inter-tumor heterogeneity and radiation dose-control curves. Radiother and Oncol 8: 353-362.

130. Zagars GK, von Eschenbach AC, Ayala AG, Schultheiss TE, Sherman NE (1991) The influence of local control on metastatic dissemination of prostate cancer treated by external beam megavoltage radiation therapy. Cancer 68: 2370-2377.

Chapter 4

Conformal Therapy Using Proton Beams

Lynn J. Verhey, Ph.D.

Department of Radiation Oncology, University of California, San Francisco, California

Three-dimensional conformal radiotherapy (3-D CRT), defined as the treatment of a target volume using multiple beams from carefully selected directions, each one shaped to the projection of the target volume, had its beginnings in proton and heavy ion radiotherapy [1, 2]. Unlike photons, proton therapy was always required to be three dimensional [3, 4] to account for the need to predict the stopping point along each particle's trajectory [5]. Many of the techniques which make 3-D CRT possible with photons today, were developed by physicists working in proton radiotherapy during the past two decades [5-8].

As first described by R. R. Wilson in a seminal paper in 1946 [9], the physical properties of protons which make it possible to conform the dose distribution to a target in three dimensions include: (1) a well-defined range that can be adjusted so that little or no dose is deposited distal to the target volume [10], (2) an initial region of lower dose at beam entrance (the plateau) followed by a higher dose (the Bragg peak) at or near the end of beam range, producing depth dose distributions for each incident energy which can be combined to produce a uniform dose in depth (spread-out Bragg peak) with a width which can be tailored to the thickness of the target [11], and (3) very sharp lateral beam falloff which permits collimated beam cross-sections which conform tightly to the projected target contour. In contrast, photon depth doses are characterized by a low entrance dose followed by a rapid rise to a dose maximum and then a slow, exponential falloff in dose at deeper depths. Figure 4-1 shows the comparison between the depth dose of a 6 MV x-ray beam and a spread out Bragg peak from a proton beam. The lateral beam falloff in a well-collimated high energy linear accelerator beam can be nearly as good as that observed with protons. Figure 4-2 shows the field edges of an 18 MV x-ray beam compared to the edge of a collimated proton beam, both at a depth of 10 cm in water and both defined by a cerrobend block.

Given these properties, for a fixed number of beam entrance angles, the dose localization to the target volume for protons will clearly be superior to that achievable with photons, simply on the basis of exit dose comparisons. Figure 4-3 compares the doses achievable with protons and 6 MV x-rays, using 4 opposed fields on a 20 cm thick patient section. If a large number of entrance angles with multiple fixed photon beams are used, very low doses to normal tissue can be achieved in spite of the high exit dose of each individual beam, assuming each beam is designed to conform to the projected target contour.

The primary advantage of protons for conformal therapy is the ability to reduce the dose in each beam from 100% to essentially zero in a distance of a few mm distal to the target volume (see Figure 4-1). By using a spread-out Bragg peak of width adequate to cover the thickest portion of the target, the dose inside the target can be made uniform to within 5% or better. The lateral edges of the beam at depth are at least as sharp as that of a well-collimated linear accelerator photon beam, and so the dose to normal tissues lateral to the target can be made small beyond a safety margin of a few mm. In the entrance region of each proton beam, the dose is equal to, or less than the target dose. So if **n** proton beam angles are used to treat a target, the maximum dose outside the intersection region of the beams will be approximately **100%/n**, a number which might be clinically acceptable if 4 or more widely separated beams are used. In fact, the dose to normal tissue for **n** opposed proton fields would be approximately the same as for **2n** opposed x-ray fields.

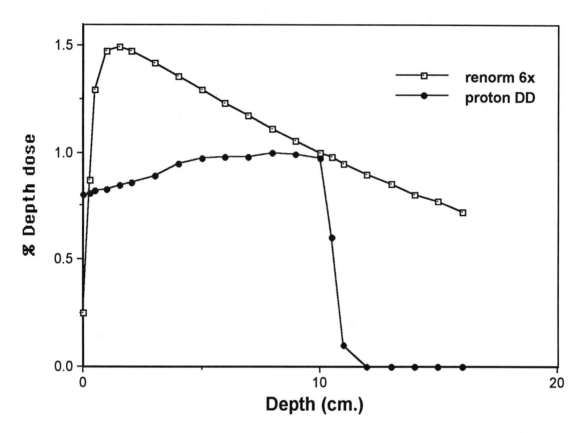

6x vs. proton depth dose

Figure 4-1. *Comparison of single field depth doses for 6 MV x-ray beam and a 5 cm spread out Bragg peak proton beam, normalized to the distal edge of a target assumed at 10 cm depth.*

It is important to recognize that this is a geometric argument which assumes the target is approximately in the center of a cross section of uniformly sensitive normal tissue. Protons have proven their worth in situations where many potential beam directions are unacceptable due to the configuration of target and normal tissues and where the well-defined range of the proton beam is critically important. [12, 13] For these types of situations, conformal therapy with x-rays might not be practical.

The primary disadvantage of protons relative to photons is also a result of the finite range of the protons. In order to accurately predict the stopping point of a particular proton in tissue, it is necessary to know the initial proton energy and the integrated stopping power of the tissues traversed [5, 14]. Although the proton stopping powers of tissues are quite well predicted from the x-ray attenuation coefficients which are measured by computed tomography (CT) [4], the use of these stopping powers in a clinical treatment requires that the position and angle of each beam be well known relative to the patient's tissues. That is, the patient position in the treatment room must be accurately controlled in both translation and rotation, to be nearly identical to that of the treatment planning CT scan [8]. If an error is made in the stopping power prediction, the dose to the target volume could be zero in some portions of the target volume, or the dose to a sensitive distal structure could be unexpectedly high [14]. With photon treatments, errors induced by unsuspected rotations of the patient in the treatment room would produce only small changes in the dose delivered to the target.

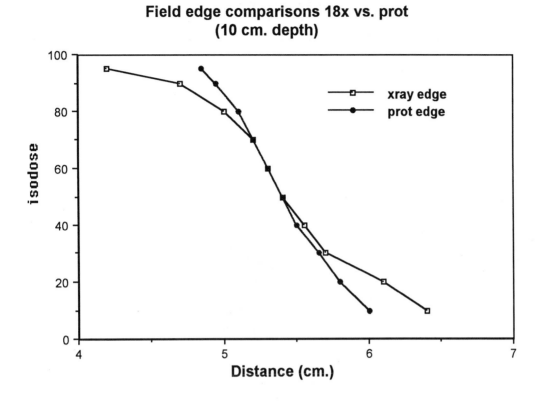

Figure 4-2. *A comparison of the field edges of an 18 MV x-ray beam and a proton beam at a depth of 10 cm, both defined by secondary cerrobend block.*

Historically, the requirement to verify the patient's position and angle very precisely before each treatment has been primarily responsible for keeping the cost of treatment very high and the throughput of patients rather small in existing proton facilities. The recent development of proton gantry delivery systems at Loma Linda University Medical Center [15] has made the rapid delivery of multiple proton fields much simpler, although the pretreatment radiographic verification of position and angle has remained labor intensive. However, recent work on semi-automatic position verification of patients using implanted markers [16] plus the development of digital imaging promise to make the delivery of proton beams much more efficient.

The clinical implementation of multi-leaf collimators (MLC) on linear accelerators [17] is making it possible to rapidly deliver x-ray beams from many different angles. Work is underway to allow the individual leaf positions in the MLC to vary their position either at a fixed gantry position (static) or during gantry motion (dynamic) to allow even more flexibility in treatment delivery [18].

Recent developments in 3-D treatment planning algorithms and in the computers used for radiotherapy planning promise to significantly reduce the effort required to develop a treatment plan for either protons or photons. The problem of devising an optimal conformal plan for either modality requires the understanding of the interplay of the dose constraints to normal tissues and the prescribed dose to the target. The desire to minimize the volume of normal tissue in the high dose region, makes conformal photons and protons similarly labor intensive.

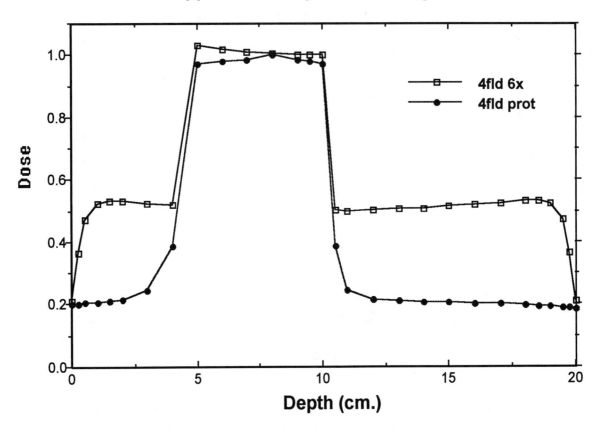

Figure 4-3. *A comparison of doses from a 4-field x-ray and proton plan for a 20 cm thick patient section. Note that the entrance doses become smaller for increased numbers of fields, though for the same number of fields, protons will always deliver less dose to normal tissue than x-rays.*

In summary, the technologies associated with planning, delivering and verifying conformal fields for protons and photons have advanced to a similar point. The costs of these two types of treatments will soon be fairly similar for equal degrees of target- normal tissue complexity. The clinical comparison of the efficacy of conformal protons and photons can now proceed, unencumbered by perceived differences in cost or ease of implementation. Although theoretical dose-volume histogram comparisons of practical proton and photon conformal plans will help to determine the optimal situations for each modality, only clinical studies can adequately define their relative roles.

References

1. Suit, H., et al., Evaluation of the clinical appicability of proton beams in definitive fractionated radiation therapy. Int. J. Radiat. Oncol. Biol. Phys., 1982. 8: p. 2199-2205.

2. Austin-Seymour, M., et al., Progress in low-LET heavy particle therapy: Intracranial and paracranial tumors and uveal melanoms. Radiat. Res., 1985. 104: p. S219-226.

3. Goitein, M., et al., Planning treatment with heavy charged particles. Int. J. Radiat. Oncol. Biol. Phys., 1982. 8: p. 2065-2070.

4. Chen, G.T.Y., et al., Treatment planning for heavy ion radiotherapy. Int. J. Radiat. Oncol. Biol. Phys., 1979. 5: p. 1809-1819.

5. Goitein, M., Compensation for inhomogeneities in charged particle radiotherapy using computed tomography. Int. J. Radiat. Oncol. Biol. Phys., 1978. 4: p. 499-508.

6. Goitein, M. and M. Abrams, Multi-dimensional treatment planning. I. Delineation of anatomy. Int. J. Radiat. Oncol. Biol. Phys., 1983. 9: p. 777-787.

7. Goitein, M., et al., Multi-dimensional treatment planning. II Beam's eye-view, back projection and projection through CT sections. Int. J. Radiat. Oncol. Biol. Phys., 1983. 9: p. 789-797.

8. Verhey, L., et al., Precise positioning of patients for radiation therapy. Int. J. Radiat. Oncol. Biol. Phys., 1982. 8: p. 289-294.

9. Wilson, R.R., Radiological use of fast protons. Radiology, 1946. 47: p. 487-491.

10. Koehler, A.M., R.J. Schneider, and J.M. Sisterson, Range modulators for protons and heavy ions. Nucl. Instrum. Methods, 1975. 131: p. 437-440.

11. Koehler, A.M., R.J. Schneider, and J.M. Sisterson, Flattening of proton dose distributions for large-field radiotherapy. Med. Phys., 1977. 4: p. 297-301.

12. Gragoudas, E.S., et al., Proton irradiation of small choroidal malignant melanomas. Am. J. Ophthalmol, 1977. 83: p. 665-673.

13. Austin-Seymour, M., et al., Fractionated proton radiation therapy of chordoma and low-grade chondrosarcoma of the base of the skull. J. Neurosurg., 1989. 70: p. 13-17.

14. Goitein, M., Calculation of the uncertainty in the dose delivered during radiation therapy. Med. Phys., 1985. 12: p. 608-612.

15. Slater, J.M., D.W. Miller, and J.O. Archambeau, Development of a hospital-based proton beam treatment center. Int. J. Radiat. Oncol. Biol. Phys., 1988. 14: p. 761-775.

16. Gall, K., L. Verhey, and M. Wagner, Computer-assisted positioning of radiotherapy patients using implanted radiopaque fiducials. Int. J. Radiat. Oncol. Biol. Phys., 1993. 20(4): p. 000-000.

17. LoSasso, T., et al., The use of a multi-leaf collimator for conformal radiotherapy of carcinomas of the prostate and nasopharynx. Int. J. Radiat. Oncol. Biol. Phys., 1993. 25: p. 161-170.

18. Carol, M.P., et al., An automatic 3-D treatment planning and implementation system for optimized conformal therapy. Int. J. Radiat. Oncol. Biol. Phys., (Submitted).

Chapter 5

Quantitative Analysis of Treatment Plans

Robert E. Drzymala, Ph.D.

Washington University School of Medicine, Mallinckrodt Institute of Radiology, St. Louis, Missouri.

When planning a radiotherapy treatment, one attempts to find the best therapeutic ratio by maximizing the dose to the target tissue, while minimizing irradiation of the surrounding normal tissue for a specific patient. It is usually the avoidance of unacceptable injury to the radiosensitive normal tissue that imposes a limitation on the dose that is prescribed to the target, which in turn may be insufficient for eradication of the that tissue. In cases like these, it is desireable to have an objective, comprehensive approach to optimizing the therapeutic ratio for the patient. Ideally, all dose information within the full three-dimensional (3-D) volume of the patient must be examined, which increases the complexity of the process many-fold. The task is compounded by the fact that one wishes to arrive at a "best plan" from an suitably large set of candidates that will fulfill the treatment goals for the patient. The sheer amount of data to be analyzed in 3-D treatment planning, as well as assuring that no important aspect of the treatment plan is overlooked or improperly emphasized, makes for difficult evaluation and comparison of rival plans.

The use of computerized tools that predict the effects of radiation on biological tissue can aid in the objective evaluation of plans by providing a quantitative basis for the analysis. Computerized 3-D treatment planning systems, being able to accurately calculate volumetric dose distributions, make possible obtaining, storing and processing radiotherapy data from many patients. Conceptually, one would like to learn from the accumulated biological data in order to develop and test predictive mathematic models and to find the appropriate parameters for these models that fit patient data. These results ultimately feed back to the treatment planning system and allow one to predict, with sufficient accuracy, the tumor control probabilities (TCPs) and normal tissue complication probabilities (NTCPs) for specific tissues, patients and plans.

A good mathematic model needs to make reasonable biological sense and standardize the various data derived from multiple patients. This requires quantitative adjustment for the differences in individual patient treatments and correlating these with patient outcome. For example, the model may need to account for the effect of non-uniform irradiation, different time-dose-fractionation schemes, partial volume effects, health status of the patient, histology of the tumor, etc. The ultimate goal would be to arrive at a numerical score that ranks one treatment plan relative to others based on sound biological and mathematical principles. In practice, this is difficult and the heueristic models that we currently employ are quite controversial and there is usually a lack of complete biological data to provide a rigorous confirmation of the model. The task may not be so honorous if we take the accept the following, however. A model is acceptable, although it may not be based on obvious biological principles, if it will fit the accumulated observable biological data to an acceptable degree of accuracy. One could then adjust the parameters affecting the model's goodness-of-fit with the data in order to obtain acceptable agreement with the data for a particular organ, tumor pathology, or group of patients. This would imply that, not only must the model be flexible and have enough parameters to "tweek," but also we must understand the limits of acceptance in the model's error and identify those instances where the error may be more or less tolerable.

Biological Effect

A huge body of literature exists, which attempts to standardize the biological effects of radiation on biological tissue in mathematical terms. Among the variables that appear to be important in defining an equivalent biological doses are the total dose given, the volume irradiated, the overall time of irradiation and the number of fractions. Accounting for these variables is important when reviewing treatment plans, because practically all have non-uniformly irradiated regions, resulting from overlapping beams, beam penumbra, etc. These localized effects need to be incorporated in order to attain a true appreciation of the treatment plan. One way to incorporate this information is to use the dose matrix computed for individual organs or tissues and obtain the radiobiological effect for each volume element (voxel) or each functional subgrouping of voxels of the patient according to its response to the dose, timing and volume of irradiation. The individual partial volume effects can then be recombined to obtain the overall effect for the organ.

The capability of generating a dose volume histogram (DVH) is found in many state-of-the-art 3-D treatment planning systems (3, 5). The DVH is a data reduction and display method that subdivides any delineated anatomical structure into its constituent voxels, computes the dose to each voxel, and sums the volume of each voxel into bins corresponding to this dose. The resultant data is then plotted as volume versus dose. There are two plot types for DVH data: cumulative and differential. The cumulative plot depicts the volume accumulated going from the high dose bins to those of lower value until eventually the total volume is accumulated at zero dose. The differential DVH is simply a plot of the amount of volume summed within each bin. The DVH can be viewed directly to screen treatment plans for excessively high doses in critical organs or unacceptably low doses in target volumes. In some TCP and NTCP models, DVHs are used to provide the basic input data for their computations.

Although the DVH loses the spatial relationship of the voxels, it provides a convenient construct with which one can assign a radiobiological effect to each voxel of an anatomical structure to estimate their combined effects on the entire structure. This would require a way to estimate the radiobiological effect for each voxel.

From a consideration of biological isoeffect relationships in clinical radiotherapy, Ellis (6, 7) proposed that the tolerance dose of normal tissue (D) could be related to the overall treatment time (T) and and the number of radiation dose fractions (N) according,

$$D = (NSD)T^{0.11}N^{0.24} .$$

This power law formulation has come to be known as the Ellis nominal standard dose (NSD) equation. It is based on the isoeffect curve for skin tolerance. By knowing the biologically effective dose, the NSD, for a certain fractionation scheme, equivalent doses can be computed for other times and fractions. The proposed unit for NSD is the ret, which stands for rad equivalent therapy and its dimensions include dose and time. This equation has been generalized by Wara et al. (29) in order to fit tissues other than skin by replacing the the exponents with arbitrary fitting parameters a and b according

$$D = EDn^aT^b \quad or, \quad d = EDn^{a-1}T^b ,$$

when ED is the estmated single dose. By fitting this equation to biological data, Wara found the exponent values for irradiated mouse lung tolerance to be a = 0.377 and b = 0.058. Likewise, a similar equation has been found to apply to CNS tissue. Called the Neuret Equation, the relationship is expressed as

$$neuret = DT^aN^b ,$$

when D is in megavoltage rad equivalents (MRE). The exponent values found in the literature for CNS tissue range from -0.377 for a to -0.46 and -0.03 to -0.09 for b, as reviewed by Leibel and Sheline (17).

Another model that has recently received great interest is the linear-quadratic (LQ) equation (1, 8-11, 19, 21-28, 30-32). It incorporates two components of cell killing by radiation, one of which is proportional to dose , the other of which is proportional to the square of the dose. It has been formulated (26) to include a time component to account for proliferation or slow repair during therapy and can be written as the following:

$$E = \left(\alpha d + \beta d^2\right)n - \gamma T$$

where E is the response of a tissue or organ, d is the dose per fraction, n is the number of fractions, T is overall treatment duration, and α, β, γ are fitting parameters. The application of this equation and its variants to biological data has been recently reviewed (9, 19).

One can employ the LQ equation to modify the dose bins of the DVH during the histogram reduction process in order to obtain the bioeffectve dose for each voxel in the entire volume of an anatomical structure. Since all of the voxels in a structure experience the same overall treatment time, this term can be dropped. Then solving for the total dose (D_1) at fraction size (d_1) that is equivalent to a total dose (D_0) at fraction size (d_0) one can obtain the relationship:

$$\frac{D_1}{D_0} = \frac{d_0 + \alpha/\beta}{d_1 + \alpha/\beta} .$$

When dealing with an organized cellular unit within the body, such as an organ or tumor, it is convenient to treat it as a population of cells having an "average" sensitivity to radiation. Each cell in the population would have an individual sensitivity that is normally distributed about the average. This concept allows us to apply certain phenomenologically-based and statistically-based models to predict cellular damage. These would demonstrate a sigmoidal relationship, when a manifestation of such damage (e.g., tumor control) is plotted versus dose. To account for partial volume effects and the effect of non-uniformly irradiated tissue, a family of sigmoidal curves, one at each partial volume would exist in theory to describe the overall radiosensitivity of an organ, for example. (See Figure 5-1.) Combining the damage to the partial volumes in an appropriate way would give the damage to organ as a whole. This reasoning may be applied to either computation of TCP or NTCP.

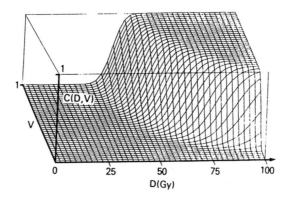

Figure 5-1. *The theoretical response of biological tissue to radiation as a function of dose and partial volume irradiated (Reprinted with permission from the International Journal of Radiation Oncology Biology and Physics.)*

Tumor Control Probability

Goitein (12, 13) has proposed that, in the instance of uniform dose within a tumor volume, TCP may be computed using the equation,

$$TCP = \frac{1}{\left(1 + \left(\dfrac{Dose}{D_{50}}\right)^{-K}\right)}$$

where

$$K = 4 / \Gamma$$

and

$$\Gamma = \text{slope of the dose response curve at 50\% cell death.}$$

For a non-uniform dose distribution, the total volume is reduced to smaller volumes having "uniform" doses within. The TCP is computed for these volume elements as stated above. They are then weighted according to their volume-fractions and summed according to the equation:

$$\ln TCP = \sum \left(\frac{\Delta V}{V_0}\right) \ln TCP \left(V_0, D(x,y,z)\right),$$

where

$$V_0 = \text{total tumor volume;}$$

and

$$\Delta V = \text{volume element of dose } D.$$

A plot of the model as TCP versus dose would appear as a sigmoidal shape.

Normal Tissue Complication Probability

Ongoing studies attempt to predict normal tissue complications using the following equation developed by Lyman (18).

$$NTCP = \frac{1}{\sqrt{2p}} \int_{-\infty}^{t} exp(-t^2 / 2) \, dt$$

where

$$t = \left(D - TD_{50}(V)\right) / m * TD_{50}(V),$$

and

$$TD_{50}(1) = TD_{50}(V) * V^{-n}$$

$TD_{50}(1)$ is the tolerance dose for 50% complications for uniform whole organ irradiation, whereas $TD_{50}(V)$ is the 50% tolerance dose for uniform partial organ irradiation to the partial volume V. The arbitrary variables m and n are found by fitting tolerance doses for uniform whole and partial organ irradiation, where m is the slope of the dose response function at TD_{50} and n is the volume effect parameter. This equation also demonstrates a sigmoidal shape when NTCP is plotted against dose.

Kutcher and Burman have modified this algorithm to account for non-uniform doses in the volumes of interest using what they call the Effective Volume Method (16). In this data reduction procedure, a uniformly-irradiated dose equivalent is calculated for each tissue that contains dose heterogeneities. For example, each step in the histogram of height ΔV_i and extension D_i is assumed to satisfy a power law relationship so that it adjusts to one of smaller volume V_{eff} and extension D_{max} using

$$V_{eff} = \Delta V_{max} + \Delta V_1 \left(D_1 / D_{max}\right)^{\frac{1}{n}} + \Delta V_2 \left(D_2 / D_{max}\right)^{\frac{1}{n}} + ...$$

where n is a size parameter.

Other models for predicting normal tissue complications have been proposed that build upon the foregoing. Niemierko and Goitein have proposed what they call the Critical Volume Model (20) which they have applied to the appearance of nephritis. Its form is similar to that by Lyman (18), but includes additional terms to account for the radiosensitivity of functional or structural subunits in the kidney. The group at the University of Michigan has proposed a simple phenomenological model for normal tissue complication, based on the sigmoidal realtionship derived by Goitein (12). In their model, however, they have nested the sigmoidal cell-killing function into another sigmoidal relationship describing complication or functional damage of an organ. (For a more detailed description of their approach, see another paper in this publication by T.S. Lwarence.)

There are other factors to be considered, when designing models that predict the manifestation of complications resulting for irradiation. Some tissues may appear to have a critical volume below which they may be irradiated to any dose, and show no detrimental effect. One may also need to consider the capacity of one organ in a pair to compensate for damage to the other. Furthermore there may be a demonstrable effect resulting internal structure of an organ or comparmentalization and redundancy in function. The appropriate mathematical model should be flexible enough to account for these if necessary.

Obtaining the Fitting Parameters

When a model is chosen, one needs to accrue sufficient clinical data to test its applicability and arrive at suitable fitting parameters. This could proceed as schematically outlined in Figure 5-2. In the process, 3-D treatment plans would be generated for many individual patients that represent the configuration of beams, modifiers, etc. as the patients were treated. Doses would be computed and processed by the appropriate data reduction methods and mathematic models to arrive at esimates for tumor control and/or tissue complications. Relevant conditions pertaining to the patient (e.g. possible effect of chemotherapy or on complications, health status) would be recorded. Each patient would then be followed for an appropriate period of time after treatment and the occurrence of acute and chronic clinical endpoints (e.g. pneumonitis, necrosis, etc.) would be noted. Finally, a comparison of the computed values with those observed would permit successive refinement of the fitting parameters for the model under study until computed and clinical results agreed to the best of the model's ability. Burman et al. (2) have taken a similar approach to arrive at fitting parameters for their NTCP model.

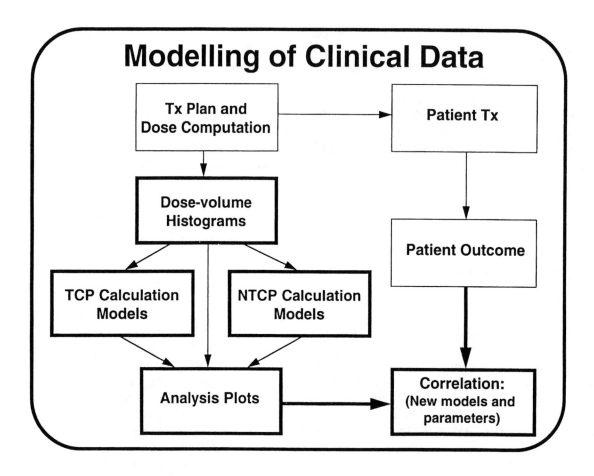

Figure 5-2. The process of mathematically modelling clinical results for radiotherapy patients

Agreement between calculated and observed results can be analyzed graphically. The type of plot that would be useful to evaluate the curve-fitting will depend on the model being tested. One approach may be to probe the internal workings and assumptions of the model by looking at how well it accounts for partial volume effects. This would require gathering sufficient data over a broad range of partial volumes that were irradiated and correlating the results with demonstrable complications. Another approach would be to review the final outcome of the calculation. A simple example is to plot complications computed versus those observed. Observed data for a simple linear relationship such as this could be grouped into 4 equal subdivisions of patients, according a rank-ascending order of complications, as shown in Figure 5-3. Perfect agreement would result in all points lying on a line, having a slope equal to 1 and going through the origin. The fitting parameters could then be adjusted so that the clinical data points lie close to the line.

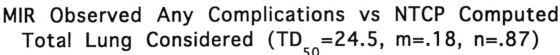

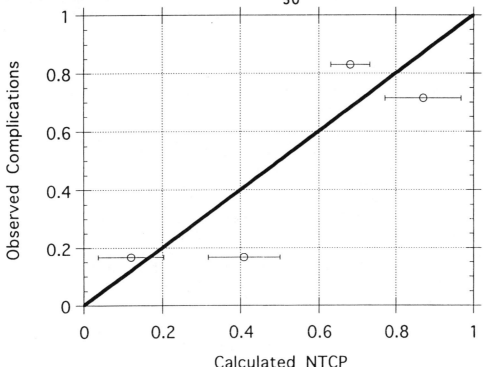

Figure 5-3. *An analysis plot that could be used to verify a mathematic model, which predicts complications, and its fitting parameters.*

Analysis of Treatment Plans

Ultimately, one would like to employ useful mathematical models to evaluate specific 3-D treatment plans. In order to appropriately consider all of the computed results, a software tool that manages and presents the data in a unified format would be useful. To satisfy this need, the Graphical Plan Evaluation Tool (GPET) (4) was developed for the National Cancer Institute (NCI) Radiotherapy Tools Contract.[1] Briefly, GPET controls the computation of DVHs, NTCPs, TCPs, and other statistics in order to display the results graphically and in tables. Up to three treatment plans and 30 anatomical structures can be considered at one time. Associated with GPET is the Figure of Merit Tool (FOM), which ranks each plan according to a numerical score. FOM uses a decision-analytic model (14, 15) that combines not only all of the computed statistics for each plan, but also includes treatment preferences of the radiation oncologist.

Summary

With the increased use of 3-D radiotherapy treatment planning systems, new opportunities have arisen for extracting the dose-volume relationships for observable clinical endpoints. Access to this

---

[1] NCI Contract N01-CM-97564.

data has the potential to help refine mathematic models that predict the radiosensitivities of biological tissue in humans based on time-dose-volume considerations. Models that show merit would eventually be incorporated into 3-D radiotherapy treatment planning systems for the clinical evaluation of competing plans in the management of patients. These models would then have the potential to provide an objective and quantitative means of comprehensively evaluating 3-D treatment plans.

References

1. Bentzen, S.M.; Thames, H.D. Is there an influence of overall treatment time in the response of lung to fractionated radiotherapy? Radiother. Oncol. 14:171-173; 1989.

2. Burman, C.; Kutcher, G.J.; Emami, B.; Goitein, M. Fitting of normal tissue tolerance data to an analytic function. Int. J. Radiat. Oncol. Biol. Phys 21:123-135; 1991.

3. Chen, G.T.Y.; Austin-Seymour, M.; Castro, J.R.; Collier, J.M.; Lyman, J.T.; Pitluck, S.; Saunders, W.M.; Zink, S.R. Dose volume histograms in treatment planning evaluation of carcinoma of the pancreas. In: Eighth International Conference on the Use of Computer in Radiation Therapy. IEEE Computer Society Press; 1984:264-268.

4. Drzymala, R.E.; Holman, M.D.; Yan, D.; Harms, W.B.; Jain, N.L.; Kahn, M.G.; Emami, B.; Purdy, J.A. Integrated software tools for the evaluation of radiotherapy treatment plans. Int. J. Radiat. Oncol. Biol. Phys. in press:1994.

5. Drzymala, R.E.; Mohan, R.; Brewster, L.; Chu, J.; Goitein, M.; Harms, W.; Urie, M. Dose volume histograms. Int. J. Radiat. Oncol. Biol. Phys. 21:71-78; 1991.

6. Ellis, F.The relationship of biological effect to dose-time fractionation factors in radiotherapy. In: Howard, E.M. Current Topics in Radiation Research. Amsterdam: North Holland Publishing Company; 1968:

7. Ellis, F. Dose, time and fractionation. A clinical hypothesis. Clin. Radiol. 20:1-7; 1969.

8. Fowler, J.; Stern, B.E. Dose-rate effects: some theoretical and practical considerations. Br. J. Radiol. 33:389-395; 1960.

9. Fowler, J.F. The first James Kirk memorial lecture. What next in fractionated radiotherapy? Br. J. Cancer 49:285-300; 1984.

10. Fowler, J.F. Fractionated radiation therapy after Strandqvist. Acta Raiol. (Oncol.) 23:209-216; 1984.

11. Fowler, J.F. The linear-quadratic formula and progress in fractionated radiotherapy [Review]. Br. J. Radiol. 62:679-694; 1989.

12. Goitein, M. The utility of computed tomography in radiation therapy: an estimate of outcome. Int. J. Radiat. Oncol. Biol. Phys. 5:1799-1807; 1979.

13. Goitein, M. The comparison of treatment plans. Semin. Radiat. Oncol. 2:246-256; 1992.

14. Jain, N.L.; Kahn, M.G. Ranking radiotherapy treatment plans using decision-analytic and heuristic techniques. Comp. Biomed. Res. 25:374-383; 1992.

15. Jain, N.L.; Kahn, M.G.; Drzymala, R.E.; Emami, B.; Purdy, J.A. Objective evaluation of 3-D radiation treatment plans: A decision-analytic tool incorporating treatment preferences of radiation oncologists. Int. J. Radiat. Oncol. Biol. Phys. 26:321-333; 1993.

16. Kutcher, G.J.; Burman, C. Calculation of complication probability factors for non-uniform normal tissue irradiation: The effective volume method. Int. J. Radiat. Oncol. Biol. Phys. 16:1623-1630; 1989.

17. Leibel, S.A.; Sheline, G.E.Tolerance of the brain and spinal cord to conventional irradiation. In: Gutin, P.H., Leibel, S.A.; Sheline, G.E. Radiation Injury to the Nervous System. New York, NY: Raven Press, Ltd.; 1991:239-256.

18. Lyman, J.T.; Wolbarst, A.B. Optimization of radiation therapy, III: a method of assessing complication probabilities from dose-volume histograms. Int. J. Radiat. Oncol. Biol. Phys. 12:103-109; 1987.

19. Newcomb, C.H.; Van Dyk, J.; Hill, R.P. Evaluation of isoeffect formulae for predicting radiation-induced lung damage. Radiother. and Oncol. 26:51-63; 1993.

20. Niemierko, A.; Goitein, M. Modeling of normal tissue response to radition: the critical volume model. Int. J. Radiat. Oncol. Biol. Phys. 25:135-145; 1993.

21. Scalliet, P.; Cosset, J.-M.; Wambersie, A. Application of the LQ model to the interpretation of absorbed dose distribution in the daily practice of radiotherapy. Radiother. Oncol. 22:180-189; 1991.

22. Schultheiss, T.E.; Zagars, G.K.; Peters, L.J. An explanatory hypothesis for early- and late-effect parameter values in the LQ model. Radiother. Oncol. 9:241-248; 1987.

23. Shukovsky, L.J. Dose, time, volume relationship s in squamous cell carcinoma of the supraglottic larynx. Roentgen. 108:27-29; 1970.

24. Strandqvist, M. Studien uber die kumulative wirkung der Rontgenstrahlen bei fraktionierung. Ergahungen aus dem Radiumhemmet an 280 Haut- und Lippenkarzionomen. Acta Radiol. (Stock.) 55(Suppl.):1-318; 1944.

25. Thames, H.D.; Withers, H.R.; Peters, L.J.; Fletcher, G.H. Changes in early and late radiation responses with altered dose fractionation: implications for dose survival relationships. Int. J. Radiat. Oncol. Biol. Phys. 8:219-226; 1982.

26. Travis, E.L.; Tucker, S.L. Isoefect models and fractionated radiotherapy. Int. J. Radiat.

27. Tucker, S.L.; Travis, E.L. Comments on a time-dependent version of the linear-quadratic model. Radiother. Oncol. 18:155-163; 1990.

28. Van Dyk, J.; Mah, K.; Keane, T.J. Radiation-induce lung damage: dose-time-fractionation considerations. Radiothep. Oncol. 14:55-69; 1989.

29. Wara, W.M.; Phillips, T.L.; Margolis, L.W.; Smith, V. Radiation pneumonitis: a new approach to the derivation of time-dose factors. Cancer 32:547-552; 1973.

30. Williams, M.V.; Denekamp, J.; Fowler, J.F. A review of alpha/beta ratios for experimental tumors: implications for clinical studies of altered fractionation. [Review]. Int. J. Radiat. Oncol. Biol. Phys. 11:87-96; 1985.

31. Withers, H.R.; Thames, H.D.; Peters, L.J.Differences in the fractionation response of acutely and late-responding tissues. In: Karcher, K.H., Kogelnik, H.D.; Reinartz, G. Progress in radio-oncolgy. New York, NY: Raven Press; 1982:287-296.

32. Wollin, M.; Kagan, A.R. Modification of the biological dose to normal tissue by daily fractionation. Model for calculating normal tissue tolerance. Acta Radiol. Thera. Phys. Biol. 15:481-492; 1976.

Chapter 6

Treatment Plan Optimization[1]

Andrzej Niemierko, Ph.D.

Dept. of Rad. Oncology, Massachusetts General Hospital, Harvard Med. School, Boston, Massachusetts

What is treatment plan optimization? Treatment plan optimization is a process where an enormous space of possible treatment plans is explored to find a plan which, according to selected criteria, is judged to be the best of all analyzed plans. The term "plan" underscores that not only can the dose distribution be optimized, but also the manner in which a dose distribution is delivered. For example, the fractionation scheme can be optimized too.

Do we need computer optimization? Recent advances in computer technology such as parallel processing, gigabit networking, transputers and other high-tech gadgets may make us wonder: why bother with computer plan optimization, if we can calculate and display a complete 3-D dose distribution in a few seconds, and play with various plan parameters almost in real time?

Compared with 2-D planning, in the 3-D case the planner has to deal with a much larger amount of data (such as CT and/or MRI scans, 3-D dose distributions, dose-volume histograms). Displaying 3-D data is much more complex and displayed 3-D objects are more difficult to comprehend and to analyze quantitatively. On the other hand technical advances, such as these provided by multi-leaf collimators and computer controlled treatment units, allow the delivery of more complex and more sophisticated treatments with conformal, non-coplanar, and dynamic beams with individualized apertures and beam intensity profiles. Simply, there are too many options to be explored fully by the conventional trial and error approach to planning. Therefore, answering the question, it is not a matter of how fast is the dose calculation, but how limited is the human mind in exploring a huge multidimensional space of possible treatment plans.

It seems almost inescapable that computer plan optimization is going to play an increasingly important role in 3-D treatment planning because of its potential to explore and to take full advantage of new treatment techniques and new technical developments.

The next question that must be addressed is what to optimize. Optimization can be applied (at least theoretically) to all plan parameters including beam parameters (such as size, position, intensity profile, wedge angle and wedge orientation, filters, blocks and boluses, relative weight, energy or even radiation modality) and fractionation parameters (such as total dose, dose per fraction, number of fractions and their distribution in time). The exploration of all of these is computationally a very demanding and time consuming process. Impressive results have been achieved with much fewer parameters being considered; for example when the beam weights have been the only optimized parameters.

[1] Supported in part by Grant CA 50628 and Grant CA 21239 from the National Cancer Institute, DHHS.

Components of the Optimization System

There are two major components of any optimization system: (1) the description of the plan goals (optimization model) and (2) the method of achieving the desired goal(s) (optimization algorithm).

Plan Goals (optimization model)

An optimization model is usually expressed in a form of the *objective (score) function* which describes a figure of merit of a particular plan and is to be maximized or minimized, and/or a set of *constraints* (requirements) which have to be satisfied by the optimal plan and which define the domain of all feasible (that is, satisfying all constraints) solutions.

Objective function: An objective function provides a single number (a score) for the plan and is used for judging which one of all rival plans is the best. It is quite awkward and uncomfortable to many practitioners of radiotherapy to reduce a plan to a single number. However, this must be both possible, and doable, if one is to pick the better of two plans. That is, radiotherapists or planners rank plans (which mathematically is equivalent to assigning scores) routinely.

Although the main goal of radical therapy is usually straightforward - sterilization of tumor tissue while sparing normal tissues - this does not translate easily into a quantitative description of an optimal plan which has to be physically and technically feasible. Several types of objective function have been investigated and shown to be useful in some clinical situations but unsuitable in others.

In the past scoring has been based entirely on dose criteria. However, because the optimization model should describe as realistically as possible the patient's response to radiation it is desirable that the model allows an objective function (and constraints) to be expressed in terms of tumor control probability and normal tissue complication probability. Only recently this has been made possible by developments in modelling radiobiological response of tumor and normal tissues.

The following is a list of the objective functions we have investigated at MGH and have judged to be clinically useful [8]:

- Tumor Control Probability (TCP)

- Normal Tissue Complication Probability (NTCP)

- Weighted Uncomplicated Local Control

- The maximum or minimum dose to a volume or given proportion of the volume (e.g., maximization of the dose to 90% of the target volume)

- The volume receiving dose smaller or larger than a certain limit (e.g., minimization of the volume of the critical organ receiving more than 50 Gy)

- The range of doses to the target volume (e.g., minimization of variance of the mean target dose)

- The maximum/minimum/mean/integral dose to a region of interest (e.g., minimization of the integral dose outside the target volume)

The objective function can be also a combination of such functions. Combining functions has advantages and disadvantages. A planner faces a very difficult problem of assigning the relative weights to each component of the objective function. On the other hand, it allows a planner to make his/her own subjective judgements about importance of various characteristics of the plan to be optimized.

Although, by definition, only one objective function (made up of one or more components) can be used at a time, the user can switch objective functions or change the relative weights of its components for another optimization trial. If the optimization program is fast enough (say, minutes for one trial) trying out several objective functions and constraints is a reasonable and recommended procedure. Because there is not a single universally adequate objective function, the optimization component of the 3-D treatment planning system should be an interactive tool for the planner - not a "black box" gadget.

Constraints: Constraints define a minimum requirements for a plan to be accepted. In mathematical terms, they define the domain in which the optimal solution is to be sought. The most common type of constraint is a <u>dose constraint</u> such as, for example, the requirement for the maximum dose to a normal tissue to be less than 50 Gy or, the requirement that the minimum target dose is 60 Gy. Dose constraints can be specified for a selected point or points or for the entire organ/volume of interest in which case they are automatically applied to a set of calculational points uniformly distributed within the specified structure.

Another type of constraint is a <u>dose-volume constraint</u>. For example, the requirement that no more than 40% of a kidney can receive a dose larger than 30 Gy. This type of constraint is very useful since it is thought that essentially all organs and tumors exhibit volume effects. Dose-volume constraints allow the optimized dose distribution to have small hot or cold spots which might be inevitable or clinically insignificant. They also avoid specifying the maximum (or minimum) dose of the hot/cold spot. Of course, if some parts of the organ at risk are more important than, or are known to respond differently from, the others, the organ can be divided into smaller sub-volumes each with its own constraints.

Models of tissue response to radiation can be implemented as <u>biophysical constraints</u>. They allow a planner to define the plan requirements in a more clinically relevant manner. For example, the planner may specify that the maximum tolerable complication probability for the kidney is 5%. Biophysical constraints permit considerable flexibility in the plans they give rise to. For example, they may permit the target dose distribution to be inhomogeneous (although this is not a property of biophysical constraints alone). Inhomogeneity of the target dose distribution may be either desirable, or unavoidable.

Optimization Algorithm

The optimization algorithm searches the domain of plan variables to find the optimal plan, that is, the set of plan variables (parameters) which maximize/minimize the chosen objective function subject to specified constraints. A variety of optimization algorithms have been investigated in planning radiotherapy; they can be grouped into the following categories:

• Exhaustive search techniques [3].

These brute force techniques evaluate each possible combination of (quantized) treatment parameters. A score is calculated for each analyzed set of treatment plan parameters, possibly derived from sub-scores combined with subjectively chosen weight factors. Constraints can be taken into account by setting the score to zero if the constraints are not satisfied. The plan which is found to have the lowest/largest score is the optimal plan. Because of the truly vast number of possible combinations of parameters (for example, for 4 beams with 4 possible wedges, 20 quantized weights and only 36 orientations of each beam, the number of possible plans exceeds 10^{15}), this procedure is feasible only for very small problems. The approach has been used with simplistic dose calculation models for 2-dimensional cases.

- Linear and quadratic mathematical programming [5, 10].

If the scoring function and constraints can be written as a linear (or quadratic) function of the plan parameters, then very elegant mathematical techniques can be applied which are guaranteed to find the optimum score. The most popular techniques are the Simplex algorithm (for linear problems) and the Wolfe, or Beale, or matrix transformation algorithms (for quadratic objective functions - with, nevertheless, linear constraints). These techniques can solve, with reasonable speed, relatively small problems (say, up to 200 constraints with up to 20 variables). A <u>combinatorial linear programming</u> algorithm has also been investigated and successfully applied for problems with a few hundred constraints. The combinatorial algorithm allows some of the variables to have only integer (or, in general, discrete) values but otherwise suffers from the same limitations as linear or quadratic programming algorithms.

- Non-linear mathematical programming [2].

If the scoring function or constraints are not linear or quadratic in the parameters of interest, then non-linear search techniques have to be used. Their limitations are that, with the exception of some unimodal functions, they are susceptible to getting trapped in a local extremum of the score function, they are sensitive to the starting conditions, and their performance dramatically decreases as problems become larger. The non-linear algorithms with the best performance require calculations of the first or even higher derivatives of the objective function and constraints and, in general, belong to one of two families of algorithms: conjugate gradient algorithms and variable metric algorithms. Because of the large size and mathematical difficulties of practical clinical problems, none of the standard non-linear programming algorithms have so far been found clinically useful.

- Finding a feasible solution [9].

One class of solutions that has been proposed involves stating the problem as a set of a dose constraints without an objective function. An iterative approach then solves the possibly many thousands of linear inequalities (constraints) and the solution is the first case encountered that satisfies all the constraints. In this approach (which is not, as such, an optimization algorithm because nothing is maximized or minimized) it is assumed that every feasible solution is clinically satisfactory and that all feasible solutions are of more or less equal quality. This approach requires constraints to be defined in a such way that the space of feasible solutions is relatively small or flat. This is possible when the planner or the clinician designing treatment plan has a knowledge about the physically obtainable optimal dose distribution, and set ups constraints (i.e., dose limits) which quite closely define this optimal distribution. If the constraints are too tight (which is not known a priori) there is no solution. If the constraints are too loose, there is a near-infinite space of solutions and the probability that the first solution found is the best one is equal to probability that the solution is the worst one (of all feasible solutions).

- Inverse solution approach [1].

The inverse approach posits an ideal dose distribution and attempts to determine beam weights and compensator shapes that lead to a physical solution that is "as close as possible" to the ideal. The idea is similar to the problem of reconstructing a tomographic image from projections at many angles. In principle, there are some one-pass solutions to this problem but, in practice, the algorithms used to solve inverse problems tend to be iterative in nature and, therefore, not self-evidently faster then other iterative search techniques. Besides the well known problems with the mathematics of deconvolution (for example, the convolution kernel is assumed to be spatially invariant - which is not the case in radiation therapy for inhomogeneous media and with scatter effects taken into account), there are other, more fundamental problems. It has not been proved, nor do there seem to be mathematical grounds for the assertion, that the truncation of negative weights (which are the result of an unconstrained deconvolution) gives the "closest" physically obtainable solution to the ideal solution. Indeed, the concept of the "closest" solution is not rigorously defined. The physical solution obtained by truncation of negative beam intensities does not satisfy the ideal prescription and does not appear to maximize or minimize any score of clinical interest (for example, it does not minimize the integral dose outside the target volume).

Apart from theoretical issues, the real concern with the inverse approach is in the way the problem is defined. It is not, a priori, possible, to prescribe (i.e., to define using equalities) a "best" physically obtainable dose distribution. Practical dose distributions are always non-uniform (often for good reasons) and, contrary to the problem of reconstructing tomographic images, have regions that are clinically more important than others. It is easy to show that the idea of matching the dose distribution to a specified one rejects, as worse, solutions (i.e., dose distributions) that by any clinically sound measure are superior to the prescribed one. For example, of two solutions with the same dose to the target but with different doses to an organ at risk, the solution with higher dose to the organ at risk will be judged by the algorithm as the better if its dose is closer to the prescribed dose. All this having been said, the dose distributions developed in the "inverse problem" papers are undoubtedly interesting. Perhaps their main interest is in showing the advantages that may accrue from designing non-uniform beam profiles.

- Artificial intelligence [4, 12].

Another interesting optimization approach that seems to be potentially useful in radiotherapy treatment planning is based on artificial intelligence (AI) or, more precisely, the use of knowledge-based systems that represent in the computer the knowledge of "experts" in radiotherapy. Some techniques of AI, especially these concerning the problem of exploring alternatives (e.g., alpha-beta pruning or branch and bound methods), can be also used in some mathematical programming techniques, particularly those that use a heuristic methodology.

- Heuristic algorithms [6, 7, 11].

Most of the heuristic algorithms are based on Monte Carlo techniques. One good example is the simulated annealing algorithm which has been successfully applied to optimization of large and difficult non-linear problems. Simulated annealing is based on an analogy with the way that liquids crystallize - that is, the way liquids reach a state of minimum energy. In the case of planning radiotherapy, energy is equated with some objective function. The major problem with simulated annealing is that the system must be cooling (i.e., converging to the optimum) slowly. To overcome this problem various techniques have been investigated. For example, the RONSC algorithm [7] renormalizes the beam weights each time a new solution is generated so that all constraints are satisfied. The simulated annealing algorithm is a promising and a powerful tool for optimization of large and difficult problems which cannot be solved with other algorithms. The algorithm has been a subject of intensive research and its performance has recently been significantly improved.

Which group of algorithms is best suited for optimization of radiation therapy plans? There is no agreement among experts on this subject. However, because clinically meaningful optimization models are non-linear, the search algorithm should be able to handle non-linear score functions and constraints. The most flexible are the heuristic algorithms which can be specifically designed for optimization of radiation treatment plans. These algorithms can be applied to any form of the objective function and constraints (even for non-continuous or discrete variable domains). They have a potential to find the global extremum (although this might not be necessary in many clinical cases), and they are easy to implement. On the other hand, the promising feature of the inverse approach is that it can handle thousands or even hundreds of thousands variables. Handling of that many variables may be necessary for optimization of beam intensity profiles.

Conclusion

We are observing new and very encouraging developments in the treatment plan optimization. The new generation of 3-D planning systems based on faster computers, the general availability of computed tomography (CT and MRI), and better understanding of biological effects of radiation have given a new impetus to investigating the enticing idea of having computers search for the "best" plan.

References

1. Brahme, A.; Kallman, P.; Lind, B.K. Optimization of proton and heavy ion therapy using an adaptive inversion algorithm. Radiotherapy and Oncology, 15:189-197, 1989.

2. Cooper, R.E.M. A gradient method of optimizing external-beam radiotherapy treatment plans. Radiology, 128:235-243, 1978.

3. Hope, C.S.; Orr, J.S. Computer optimization of 4 MeV treatment planning. Phys. Med. Biol. 10:365-370, 1965.

4. Jain, N. L.; Kahn, M. G.; Drzymala, R. E.; Emami, B. E.; Purdy, J. A. Objective evaluation of 3-D radiation treatment plans: a decision-analytic tool incorporating treatment preferences of radiation oncologists. Int. J. Radiat. Oncol. Biol. Phys. 26(2):321-333, 1993.

5. Langer, M.; Brown, R.; Urie, M.; Leong, J.; Stracher, M.; Shapiro, J. Large scale optimization of beam weights under dose-volume restrictions. Int. J. Radiat. Oncol. Biol. Phys. 18:887-893, 1990.

6. Mageras, G.S.; Mohan, R. Application of fast simulated annealing to optimization of conformal radiation treatment. Med. Phys. 20(3):639-647, 1993.

7. Niemierko, A. Random search algorithm (RONSC) for optimization of radiation therapy with both physical and biological end points and constraints. Int. J. Radiat. Oncol. Biol. Phys. 23(1):89-98, 1992.

8. Niemierko, A.; Urie, M.; Goitein, M. Optimization of 3-D radiation therapy with both physical and biological end points and constraints. Int. J. Radiat. Oncol. Biol. Phys. 23(1):99-108, 1992.

9. Powlis, W.D.; Altschuler, M.D.; Censor, Y.; Buhle, E.L. Semi-automated radiotherapy treatment planning with a mathematical model to satisfy treatment goals. Int. J. Radiat. Oncol. Biol. Phys. 16:271-276, 1989.

10. Rosen, I.I.; Lane, R.G.; Morill, S.M.; Belli, J.A. Treatment plan optimization using linear programming. Medical Physics, 18:141-152, 1991.

11. Webb, S. Optimization by simulated annealing of three-dimensional treatment planning for radiation fields defined by a multileaf collimator. Phys. Med. Biol. 36:1201-1226, 1991.

12. Zink, S. The promise of a new technology: knowledge-based systems in radiation oncology and diagnostic radiology. Computerized Medical Imaging and Graphics. 13:281-293, 1989.

Chapter 7

Few Field Radiation Therapy Optimization in the Phase Space of Complication Free Tumor Control

Svante Söderström, Anders Eklöf, M.Sc. and Anders Brahme, Ph.D.

Department of Medical Radiation Physics, Karolinska Institutet and University of Stockholm, Stockholm, Sweden

Since the beginning of radiation therapy selection of the most suitable beam entrance portals have been performed based on the knowledge and experience of the dose planning personnel. Preferably the collective knowledge of physicians, physicists, and dosimetrists should be used in the optimization of a radiation treatment. Despite the accumulated knowledge of the whole radiotherapeutic team, the selection of the best beam entry directions and the number of beam portals are almost always dependent on a trial and error like search in the entire phase space of possible beam combinations. The fact that no simple and universal method have yet been presented for selection of optimal beam portals is in itself an indication on how difficult this task really is. The difficulties are further increased if the selection is limited to a small number of beam portals. This is due to the increasing relative importance of each beam as the number of beams decrease. A further increase in complexity arises if the primary fluence profiles are also allowed to vary across the beam. Variations of the primary fluence over the beam have until recently only been considered when using wedged or partly blocked beams. With the introduction of dynamic multileaf collimation, automatic compensator design or scanned electron and photon beams, it has become possible to shape the primary fluence profile across the beam in an accurate and advantageous manner.

In general treatment optimization the degrees of freedom are immense. First each beam may consist of some 100 by 100, that is 10^4 "bixels" or beam elements. A complete plan using dynamic dose delivery may in its turn consist of hundreds of beam portals, so the number of free variables are then already up in the 10^6 region without having considered different radiation modalities such as electrons, protons, photons, and neutrons. In addition, the different beam modalities can have different energy spectra and time dose fractionation patterns. A fullblown optimization may therefore contain as many as 10^{10} free variables (Lind and Brahme 1992). To get a feeling for the shape of this huge phase space it has to be projected down to some subspace that can be visualized. First of all it is then important to use some scalar quantity such as P+ which describes the probability to achieve tumor control without causing severe complications in healthy tissues to allow a strict comparison of different treatment techniques. In this presentation, we have chosen to only look at the highest P+ value for the best possible beam profiles $\hat{\Psi}_\Omega$ from given directions of incidence W and to disregard all other sub-optimal beam profiles. To simplify the presentation even further we do not even look at the beam shape itself, but only its associate P+ value.

In the present paper the probability of achieving tumor control without causing severe complications is investigated for different one, two, and three-field techniques. In the different field combinations investigated the incident fluence profiles, $\Psi(\xi)$, are optimized with the treatment objective to maximize P_+. Optimizations using homogeneous and wedged beams are also investigated. The phase space of maximal P_+ values for each combination of beam entry directions $\Omega_1, \Omega_2, \Omega_3$:

$$P_+\left(\hat{\Psi}_{\Omega_1}, \hat{\Psi}_{\Omega_2}, \hat{\Psi}_{\Omega_3} \right) \text{ or } P_+^3$$

for short has been investigated for three different target geometries.

General properties of the P_+ phase space are described as well as details due to the three target geometries chosen for illustration. The influence of different number of beam portals on the treatment result is considered as well as the effect of different degrees of freedom in the beam profiles during the optimization procedure.

Materials and Methods

Target Geometries

Three target geometries have been used in the examination of the properties of the P_+ phase space. The tumors are assumed to have varying properties of clonogenic tumor cells and normal tissue stroma inside their target volumes.

The first case is a head and neck target consisting of the locally involved lymph nodes of a larynx cancer. In this patient geometry the normal tissue stroma and the spinal cord are the principal organs at risk. The target volume is assumed to consist of 90% normal tissue stroma infiltrated by 10% clonogenic cells.

In the second case an esophageal cancer in the thorax region is used. This target volume is assumed to consist of 50% normal tissue stroma infiltrated to 50% by a the tumor cell population. In this target geometry there are four major organs at risk; the lungs, the heart, the spinal cord, and the normal tissue stroma. The right and left lung are here treated as one single organ at risk. This organization of the lungs is used since the right and left lung treated as two separate organs will result in a fatal treatment if either of the lungs are damaged. This is not a realistic treatment complication unless the other lung of the patient was already damaged.

Finally, the last target geometry is an advanced cervix cancer with involved local lymph nodes. In this case the organs at risk are the bladder, the rectum, the small bowel, and the normal tissue stroma. In this last case the gross cervix tumor and the involved lymph nodes are regarded as separate biological structures and therefore they are associated with different biological responses. The gross cervix tumor is assumed to have a 50% clonogenic cell population and the involved local lymph nodes are assumed to contain 10% of clonogenic cells. The remaining tissue in the two target volumes are regarded as normal tissue stroma infiltrated by tumor. The radiobiological parameters for the different tissue types used in this study are presented in Table 7-1.

Energy Deposition Kernels

All the energy deposition kernels used here to calculate the dose distributions are pencil beam kernels defined on a square matrix with 25 cm side length and discretized in 128 x 128 voxels. Calculations are performed assuming semi-3-D geometry with a 10 mm cylindrical extension of the patient geometry in the third dimension. The pencil beam kernels are calculated through convolution of Monte-Carlo calculated point spread function (Ahnesjö *et al.* 1987) with the energy fluence of the primary photons (Eklöf *et al.* 1990).

Table 7-1. *The radiobiological data set used in the calculations. The normalized gradient of the dose response relation, γ, the 50% response dose, D_{50}, and the relative seriality, s.*

Organ type	γ	D_{50} [Gy]	s
Head and Neck geometry			
Normal tissue stroma	2.76	65.0	1.00
Spinal cord	1.78	60.0	1.00
Tumor	3.00	52.0	-
Thorax geometry			
Normal tissue stroma	2.76	65.0	1.00
Spinal cord	1.78	60.0	1.00
Lung	2.10	24.5	0.006
Heart	3.00	49.2	0.20
Tumor	3.00	52.0	-
Cervix geometry			
Small bowel	1.50	80.0	2.60
Bladder	3.00	80.0	1.30
Rectum	3.00	55.0	0.69
Lymph nodes	3.00	39.0	-
Tumor	4.00	52.0	-

The kernels are of two main categories; monoenergetic photon kernels and bremsstrahlung kernels. The bremsstrahlung kernels are obtained by adding monoenergetic kernels weighted by the energy bins of the bremsstrahlung spectrum.

A 50 MV bremsstrahlung pencil beam kernel has been used for optimizations performed on the cervix and the thorax geometry. For the head and neck geometry a ^{60}Co pencil beam kernel is used. A 10 MeV monoenergetic pencil beam kernel, corresponding to a 30MV bremsstrahlung beam, is used for the comparison of uniform, wedged, and general non-uniform beam profiles on the cervix geometry.

Biological Objective Function

With a reliable biological objective function the optimization will automatically be directed at the optimal combination of radiobiological responses in the tumor (eradication of all tumor clonogens) and the normal tissues (a minimum of severe complications). One such biological objective function is the probability of achieving tumor control without severe complications, P_+, defined as:

$$P_+ = P_B - P_B \cap P_I \tag{1}$$

where P_B is the probability of tumor control and P_I is the probability of severe injury to normal tissues. Ågren *et al.* (1990) studied P_+ values observed in clinical practice and they found that P_+ is well described by

$$P_+ = P_B - P_I + \delta(1 - P_B)P_I \qquad (2)$$

where P_B is the probability of benefit, P_I is the probability of injury, and the parameter d specifies the fractions of patients where the probability of benefit and the probability of injury are statistically independent endpoints. For small tumors and low doses $\delta \approx 0$ and for larger tumors and high dose levels $\delta \approx 0.2$. For simplicity $\delta = 0$ has been used in the present calculations. The Poisson statistical model has been used to describe the dose response of the different tissues and tumor types present in the calculations. The radiobiological model for the response of tumor and normal tissue reactions used here takes structural organization of the tissue into account.

In this model the probability of causing tissue injury or achieving tumor control may be approximated by

$$P(D) = 2^{-\exp[e\gamma(1 - D/D_{50})]} \qquad (3)$$

where D_{50} is the 50% response dose and g is the normalized gradient of the dose response relation. The structural organization of the tissue is considered by assuming the tissue consists of a continuous matrix of sub-units. Their functional organization is considered to be built up of parallel and serial structures as described by a single parameter namely their relative seriality, s (for further details see Källman *et al.* 1992).

The radiobiological parameters should preferably be taken from the patient himself using some type of predictive assay performed for example on biopsy specimens. This will allow the use of patient specific dose response relations for those tissues that have been analyzed. With accurate patient specific biological parameters the final optimized treatment plan will be truly individualized and more reliable. It may not be possible or even desirable to acquire biopsies from all important tissues of a patient. In many cases a library of radiobiological parameters for different organs and tumors can be used and adjusted depending on if the patient is found to have an efficient or deficient repair system for radiation damage.

Optimization Algorithm

The principal problem of radiation therapy planning can be formulated in the form of an integral equation that expresses the resultant dose distribution in the patient for a given incoming radiation field.

The most elementary incident radiation beam is a point monodirectional or pencil beam $p(E, \Omega, r, \rho)$, that describes the energy deposition at r for a given energy E, surface point ρ, and direction Ω of incidence of an uncharged radiation beam of for example photons or neutrons. The incident energy fluence differential in energy and angle of such incident beams on points ρ on the patient surface is denoted $\Psi_{E,\Omega}(\rho)$.

The absorbed dose at a point r in the patient due to an incident radiation field of neutral particles is then given by:

$$D(r) = \iint_S \iiint p(E, \Omega, r, \rho)\, \Psi_{E,\Omega}(\rho)\, \mathrm{d}E \mathrm{d}\Omega \mathrm{d}^2\rho \qquad (4)$$

where the spatial integrals have to be performed over the relevant entrance surface, S, of the patient. A similar equation for charged particles was formulated by Brahme (1992).

The principal unknown quantity to be determined in the optimization of a treatment plan is the incident energy fluence $\Psi_{E,\Omega}(\rho)$. As recently discussed by Lind (1990), it is generally not possible to find an exact solution to the above Fredholm equation of the first kind, Eq. (4). Thus, the aim is to find a solution that fulfills our treatment objective as well as possible.

Gustafsson *et al.* (1994) have developed an iterative algorithm suitable for optimization of the incident fluences in Eq. (4). To do so by numerical methods it is fundamental to discretize the functions concerned. During the calculations it is therefore assumed that a function of the spatial coordinates in the patient such as the dose $D(r)$ is sampled at n volume elements or voxels. The components of the vector representation d of the absorbed dose in the patient are thus given by

$$d_i = D\big(X(i), Y(i), Z(i)\big), \qquad\qquad\qquad i = 1,\, 2,\, ...,\, n \qquad\qquad (5)$$

where $X(i)$, $Y(i)$ and $Z(i)$ are the coordinates specified by the sampling functions along the x, y and z coordinates respectively for the i:th sampling point inside the patient.

Similarly, the photon pencil beams p can be sampled in a pencil beam matrix P, while the corresponding energy fluences $\Psi_{E,\Omega}$ can be sampled in a generalized fluence vector denoted Ξ (Gustafsson *et al.* 1994). The total number of bixels or beam elements on the patient surface used in the generalized fluence vector Ξ, is denoted v. In the case of external radiation the bixels may be distributed in v_Ω beams, the total number of bixels is however always v. The pencil beam belonging to each generalized fluence component is best discretized on the same grid as the resultant dose distribution vector d. The pencil beam matrix P will then obviously consist of $n \times v$ components, where n is the number of voxels in the vector representation of $D(r)$ as described above. In its discretized form Eq. (4) reduces to the simple matrix equation:

$$d = P\Xi \ . \qquad\qquad\qquad\qquad (6)$$

The mapping of Ξ by P on d and the geometrical structure of Eq. (6) is illustrated in color Plate 1.

Gustafsson *et al.* (1994) used a constrained iterative gradient method previously developed by Lind and Brahme (1987), where $\mathbf{C}$ is a constraint operator. In the work of Gustafsson *et al.* (1994) $\mathbf{C}$ only works as a positivity operator, whereas in this article $\mathbf{C}$ is used somewhat differently (cf Gustafsson *et al.* 1995). The optimization algorithm is written such that it minimizes a scalar objective function and therefore the complement of P_+, i.e. the probability $1 - P_+$ of getting severe complications and/or a recurrence, may be used in the algorithm.

An iterative scheme optimizing the biological objective function P_+ with steepest decent is then given by:

$$\Xi^{k+1} = \mathbf{C}\Big[\Xi^k - A\nabla_\Xi\big(1 - P_+(d^k)\big)\Big] = \mathbf{C}\Big[\Xi^k + A(\nabla_\Xi d)^{\mathrm{T}}\big(\nabla_d P_+(d^k)\big)\Big] \qquad (7)$$

where the $v \times v$-dimensional diagonal parameter matrix A controls the speed of convergence for the different energy deposition kernels. Notice that the chain rule has been used to get an expression of the gradient of P_+ with respect to d. Notice also that for an arbitrary generalized fluence vector Ξ the gradient of d with respect to Ξ reduces to P according to Eq. (6).

Using the iterative scheme Eq. (7), the optimized fields generally becomes highly non-uniform. Such fields are possible to reproduce using compensators, dynamic multileaf collimation (Källman *et al.* 1988, Svensson *et al.* 1994), scanned beams or a combination of the three. Since such technique for non-uniform dose delivery are not very widespread, it is of clinical interest that the algorithm Eq. (7) also can optimize more restricted beams, such as uniform or wedged beams. As shown by Gustafsson *et al.* (1995) it is also possible to optimize given functions of the generalized fluence Ξ. The generalized fluence vector Ξ can quite generally be expressed as a function $\Xi = \Xi(T, F, \dot{\Psi}, t)$, or more exactly,

$$\Xi = TF\dot{\Psi}t , \tag{8}$$

where T is a diagonal $v \times v$-dimensional transmission matrix of the adjustable collimators in the treatment head, F is similarly a diagonal $v \times v$-dimensional filter matrix describing the influence of the flattening filter in the accelerator, a wedge filter or compensating filter and $\dot{\Psi}$ is the $v \times v_\Omega$-dimensional accelerator energy fluence rate mapping the v_Ω-dimensional treatment time vector t onto the v bixels. T, F and $\dot{\Psi}$ are here considered time-independent. Time dependence is however easily incorporated, as discussed by Gustafsson *et al.* (1995).

Below one-dimensional uniform and wedged photon fields are considered for delivering two-dimensional dose distributions. Bixel ι, defined for beam Ω, is located at position x defined in the isocenter plane of the treatment unit. For all cases in this review it is assumed that the energy fluence rate $\dot{\Psi}$ of the accelerator is constant for all bixels and from all radiation fields and no flattening filter is needed.

The treatment time for each beam is given by the time components of t from direction Ω, denoted t_Ω. For uniform field radiation the filter matrix F is equal to unity, whereas for wedged fields the ι:th diagonal component $F(\iota)$ in the filter matrix F depends on the wedge isodose angle (ICRU 1976), i.e. the relative energy fluence slope $\left(\dfrac{\Psi'_0}{\Psi_0}\right)$ on the central axis of beam which from direction Ω is denoted ω_Ω, such that

$$F(\iota) = 1 - \omega_\Omega x . \tag{9}$$

A wedged field of an arbitrary isodose angle can be delivered using dynamic collimator blocks, multileaf collimation, the wedge selection technique (Svensson *et al.* 1977, Petti and Siddon 1985) or elementary bremsstrahlung beam scanning.

The projected positions of the right and left collimator edges for beam Ω are denoted x_Ω^- and x_Ω^+, respectively both defined in the isocenter "plane". The ι:th diagonal component $T(\iota)$ in the transmission matrix T is then given by:

$$T(\iota) = H(x - x_\Omega^-)H(x_\Omega^+ - x) , \tag{10}$$

where $H(x)$ is the so-called Heaviside step function, equal to unity when $x > 0$ and zero when $x < 0$. $H(x)$ accurately describes the transmission at the collimator edge when penumbra effects are negligible.

For simplicity x_Ω^- and x_Ω^+ are fixed throughout the calculations in this article, such that the photon beam from direction Ω completely irradiates the tumor region regardless of the location of the organs at risk. Gustafsson *et al.* (1995) recently used a more general approach to optimize also collimator edge positions and treatment time simultaneously using the same objective function.

The parameters of the generalized fluence vector Ξ to be optimized are in both the case of uniform and wedged fields the treatment time components t_Ω. Furthermore, in the case of wedged fields the relative slope components ω_Ω are to be optimized.

The components of the gradient $\nabla_\Xi d$ at voxel i corresponding to the generalized fluence parameters and the constraint operator for the parameters of the generalized fluence vector in the iterative scheme Eq. (7) can now be formulated. For uniform fields

$$\frac{\partial d_i}{\partial t_\Omega} = P_{il} H(x - x_\Omega^-) H(x_\Omega^+ - x) , \tag{11}$$

where P_{il} is the i:th energy deposition component of the l:th beam element, corresponding to x in the isocenter "plane", and

$$C t_\Omega = \begin{cases} t_\Omega, & t_\Omega > 0 \\ 0, & t_\Omega < 0 \end{cases} . \tag{12}$$

For wedged fields the constraint operator Eq. (12) still holds as the treatment time constraint. The treatment time gradient however should be written out for clarity:

$$\frac{\partial d_i}{\partial t_\Omega} = P_{il} H(x - x_\Omega^-) H(x_\Omega^+ - x)(1 - \omega_\Omega x) . \tag{13}$$

The relative slope gradient is given by

$$\frac{\partial d_i}{\partial \omega_\Omega} = -P_{il} H(x - x_\Omega^-) H(x_\Omega^+ - x) x t_\Omega \tag{14}$$

and the corresponding constraint operator is

$$C \omega_\Omega = \begin{cases} (x_\Omega^-)^{-1}, & 1 - \omega_\Omega x_\Omega^- < 0 \\ (x_\Omega^+)^{-1}, & 1 - \omega_\Omega x_\Omega^+ < 0 . \\ \omega_\Omega, & \text{otherwise} \end{cases} \tag{15}$$

For a general derivation of the gradient $\nabla_\Xi d$ the reader is referred to Gustafsson *et al.* (1995).

Calculations

Calculation of the complete three-dimensional P_+ phase space at an angular spacing of 15° were performed with the algorithm Eq. (7) presented above. In the simplest calculation only one free variable for each beam profile namely the treatment time for the uniform beam was used. In the second calculation of the three-dimensional P_+ phase space the number of free variables were increased to two by considering both beam weight and wedge angle during the optimization of each dose plan. To simulate completely non-uniform beam profiles in the third calculation 64 free variables have been used in each beam profile. Each of the 25 cm wide beam profiles are divided into 64 equal segments width of about 4 mm.

For k incident beams the general projected k-dimensional phase space, P_+^k, for a given patient geometry the number of dose plans N_k^n to be evaluated when searching for optimum beam entry directions is according to combinatorial theory given by the sum:

$$N_k^n = n + \binom{n}{2} + \binom{n}{3} + \ldots + \binom{n}{k} \tag{16}$$

where n is the number of possible beam portal orientations to be investigated and k is the maximum number of allowed beam portals in each case. The three-dimensional phase space P_+^3 for each target geometry have been investigated here using combinations of beam entry directions in increments of 15° requiring

$$N_3^{24} = 24 + \binom{24}{2} + \binom{24}{3} = 2324 \tag{17}$$

dose plans to be evaluated and individually optimized.

The influence of the number of beam portals used is investigated using all three patient geometries. Thus, 2324 different dose plans have been calculated and individually optimized with respect to beam profiles for each patient geometry. The maximum P_+ level is calculated for the optimum selection of beam entry directions for one, two, and three beam portals. When using more than three beam portals the beam entry directions are distributed at equidistant angles.

Results

General Properties of the Phase Space of P_+^k

As can be seen in color Plate 2, the calculated volume of the P_+^3 phase space is only one sixth of the complete cube of presented data. The presented cube of the P_+ phase space has therefore a six fold redundancy in its information content. The phase space is displayed in this way for clarity and to improve interpretation at the borders of the calculated volume.

When looking at the P_+^2 phase space one may observe several lines of symmetry (Söderström and Brahme 1993). The principal shape of these symmetry lines present in the P_+^2 phase space are to a certain extent independent of the location of the target volume and the organs at risk. Important symmetry lines are those that are related to a reduction of the number of beam portals where $\Omega_1 = \Omega_2$, but also those lines representing parallel opposed beams, i.e. where $\Omega_1 = \Omega_2 \pm \pi$. The corresponding lines and planes can also be observed in the three-dimensional P_+^3 phase space as seen in Figure 7-1 and color Plates 3 and 4.

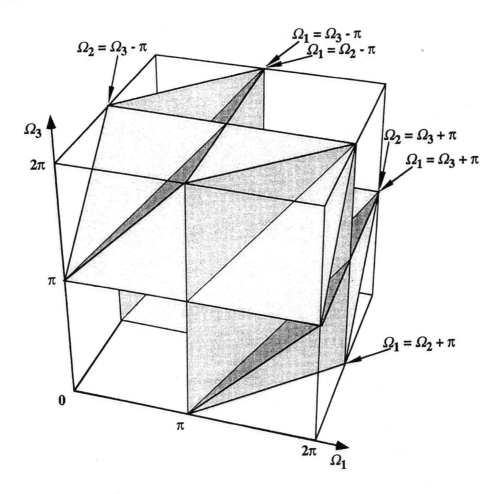

Figure 7-1. *The six planes in the three-dimensional P+ phase space representing parallel opposed beams.*

When the 2-D phase space P_+^2 is expanded to 3-D or P_+^3 by increasing the number of beam portals to three, symmetry lines representing a reduction of the number of used beam portals from two to one are expanded to symmetry planes representing a reduction of the number of used beam portals from three to two, see color Plate 3. Each one of these three planes are actually built up of the complete two-dimensional P_+ phase space. Symmetry lines in the P_+^2 phase space representing parallel opposed beams become six symmetry planes in the cube of the P_+^3 phase space, as shown in Figure 7-1. This is due to the fact that the number of possible combinations using three beam portals when any two of them are parallel opposed, is six since the order of application irrelevant. In the intersection between the planes representing a reduction of the number of used beam portals from three to two and the planes representing parallel opposed beams a more severe reduction of the P_+ level than otherwise will be observed. These intersection lines will be clearly visible in the P_+ phase space as intrinsic low P_+ regions (cf Figure 7-1 and color Plates 3 and 4). A symmetry line also appears at the intersection line of the three planes representing a reduction of the number of used beam portals corresponding to one single incident beam ($\Omega_1=\Omega_2=\Omega_3$). Along this line the lowest possible P_+ level will always appear corresponding to the degenerate case of one single field.

Comparison of the Merits of Uniform, Wedged and Non-uniform Beams

When only classical uniform beams are allowed during the optimization most of the above described structures of the three-dimensional P_+^3 phase space, due to the use of non-uniform beams, are lost as seen by comparing color Plates 6 to 8. High P_+ levels can only be found when the beam angle combination include some beam angle close to $\Omega=0°$. In the one-dimensional phase space for uniform beams as shown by the dashed line in color Plate 5 the maximum P_+ level ($P_+=37.3\%$) is located at $\Omega=0°$. Significant non-zero P_+ values can only be observed for beam entry directions in the vicinity of $\Omega=0°$. Very small, but still non-zero, P_+ values can also be observed for beam entry directions around $\Omega=180°$. Adding a second beam increases the P_+ level by no more than 2.0% ($P_+=39.3\%$) for the optimum combination of beam entry directions, $\Omega_1=75°$ and $\Omega_2=345°$ (see Figure 7-2). With the optimum three beam combination, $\Omega_1=15°$, $\Omega_2=270°$ and $\Omega_3=345°$, using classical uniform beams an increase of the P_+ level by as little as 0.3% ($P_+=39.6\%$) is obtained and no new internal structures in the P_+^3 phase space can be observed as seen in color Plate 6. The cervix target geometry is not very suitable for treatment using a few uniform beams partly because the tumor is surrounded by organs at risk but there are also two target volumes, the gross tumor and the microscopic invasion, requiring different dose levels for optimal treatment. It would thus be more suitable to use a coarse division of each beam into a small number of homogeneous beams from each beam entry direction as shown by Gustafsson *et al.* (1995).

In color Plate 5 the one-dimensional P_+^1 phase space due to treatment optimization using wedge shaped beams is also shown by dotted lines. Compared to the optimization using only uniform beams an increase of the P_+ level by 3.2% to 40.5% can be observed for the optimum wedged beam direction at, $\Omega=30°$. It can also be seen that it is possible to use a wider range of beam entry directions without reducing the P_+ level significantly with wedged beams. It is interesting to note in Figure 7-2 that the treatment outcome is better with one wedged beam than with three uniform beams even if the beam weights and beam entry directions are optimally selected. Optimization of the two wedged beams reveals a large amount of structure with two advantageous beam entry directions, around $\Omega=90°$ and $\Omega=270°$ as seen in Figure 7-2. The merits of these beam entry directions are related to the patient geometry. Using these beam entry directions when irradiating the cervix results in the longest possible radiation path through the gross tumor volume. Optimum settings of the beam entry directions are found at $\Omega_1=15°$ and $\Omega_2=90°$ resulting in an increase in the P_+ level by 9.7% to 50.2% when compared to the use of only one beam portal and an increase of 10.9% compared to the use of two uniform beams (cf Figure 7-2). The merit of these beam entry directions remains when the number of beams are increased to three. The internal structure of the three-dimensional P_+^3 phase space can be summarized as high levels in beam directions $\Omega=90°$ and $\Omega=270°$. The basic structure of the P_+ phase space described above for non uniform beams, with low P_+ levels in the planes and along lines representing a reduction of the number of used beam portals are also present when using wedged beams. However, opposing beams are not that critical with respect to reduction of the P_+ level. This may be seen in color Plate. 7. The optimum selection of beam entry directions in the P_+^3 phase space is found to be the three field combination $\Omega_1=90°$, $\Omega_2=135°$ and $\Omega_3=255°$ for which a P_+ level of 54.0% is reached.

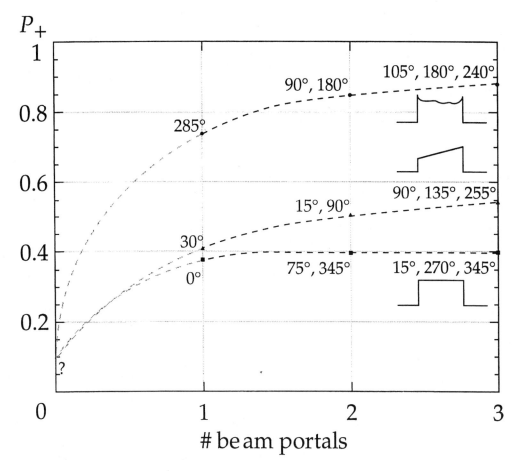

Figure 7-2. *The outcome of optimal treatments for the cervix target using increasing number of beam portals when using uniform, wedged and generally non uniform beam profiles. In each case the optimal beam angles of incidence are also given. The results obtained when using homogeneous, wedged and non-homogenous beams are indicated by squares, triangles and circles respectively. The question mark near the vertical axis may be interpreted as a clinically unobservable spontaneous healing probability without irradiation.*

When allowing non-uniform beam profiles in the optimization all the above described structures of the P_+^3 phase space are most clearly seen. For the one-dimensional P_+ phase space the optimum beam entry direction is around $\Omega=285°$ as can be seen in color Plate 5. It is seen that the amount of structure in the one-dimensional P_+ phase space is largest for non-uniform beams. The optimized dose plan using this beam portal reaches a P_+ level of 73.4% which is 19.4% more than using three optimized wedged beams and 38.8% more than obtained with three optimized uniform beams. When adding a second beam portal during the optimization, the P_+ level increases by 11.4% to $P_+=84.8\%$. The low P_+ levels pertaining to $\Omega_1=\Omega_2$, $\Omega_1=\Omega_2+\pi$ and $\Omega_1=\Omega_2-\pi$ are also clearly visible in color Plate 8. The best beam entry directions when using two non-homogeneous beams with optimized beam profiles are close to $\Omega_1=90°$, $\Omega_2=180°$. A further increase of the P_+ level by 3.0% to $P_+=87.8\%$ is achieved when the optimum three beam dose plan with $\Omega_1=105°$, $\Omega_2=180°$ and $\Omega_3=240°$ is used.

If each beam profile, instead of being divided into 64 3.9 mm wide bixels, is more coarsely divided so that only a few uniform beam segments are used for each beam entry direction the probability of achieving tumor control without severe complications is very close to the value found when using non-uniform beams (Gustafsson *et al.* 1994). For example, when the three optimal beam entry directions with non-uniform beam profiles are used, and if each beam is divided into three uniform beam segments, the P_+ value will drop by only 1.6% to P_+=86.2%. This shows that it is sometimes possible to perform highly conformal treatments with good treatment outcome without the need of fully non-uniform dose delivery (Gustafsson *et al.* 1994).

The Phase Space Gradient

The gradient in the P_+ phase space determines how densely the angles of incidence of the beams have to be sampled to find the true optimal beam portals. When studying the gradient of the P_+ phase space it is quite interesting to observe that an increasing number of allowed beam portals results in a more uniform high plateau region of P_+ in the phase space. In the one-dimensional phase space the gradient in the plateau region is approximately 0.3%/° requiring a 3.3° spacing between the beams to find the optimal angle of incidence. This corresponds to that 110 different beam entry directions have to be investigated, if the optimum P_+ level is to be found within about 0.5%. For the two-dimensional phase space the gradient in the plateau region is decreased slightly to 0.2%/°. This requires a 5° spacing between the beams if the accuracy in the determination of the optimum P_+ level should be found within 0.5%. When using three beams the gradient in the plateau region is decreased even further to approximately 0.1%/° or lower. This indicates that it is sufficient to try incident beams every 10 degrees to find the optimum P_+ level within 0.5%. This also means that the maximum gradient of the P_+ phase space surrounding low P_+ areas is increased as the number of beams are increased, from 2.0%/° for one beam to 5.6%/° for two beams and 6.9%/° for the three-dimensional P_+^3 phase space. If the complete three-dimensional P_+^3 phase space is to be searched within 1% accuracy at least 2400 different beam entry directions or $2.3 \cdot 10^9$ different combinations of beam entry directions have to be investigated. However as shown above, locally in a high level plateau region the gradient becomes smaller as the number of beam portals increase. This means that, as the number of beams gradually becomes larger the optimal beam entry directions becomes gradually less critical, provided coincident or parallel opposed beams are avoided and the fluence profiles are allowed to vary across the beam to find the optimal beam profiles using the biological objective function P_+ (Söderström *et al.* 1993). The above mentioned values for the gradient of the P_+ phase space are typical for all the presently investigated target geometries and beam energies.

The Role of Large Number of Beam Portals

It is quite clear from color Plate 9 that there is very little to be gained in the probability of achieving tumor control without severe complications when more than approximately three to five beam portals are used. The increase in P_+ when going from 3 to 72 non uniform beam portals is only between 0.5-2.2% for the different patient geometries. For the cervix target the gain is 1.8% when going from P_+=87.9%, for three fields with optimized beam entry directions, to P_+=89.7% for full 72-beam optimization with the beams being equidistant in angle. About the same amount of gain in P_+ (2.2%) results for the head and neck target when going from P_+=71.2% for three fields with optimized beam entry directions to P_+=73,4% for 72 equidistant beams. The smallest gain was obtained for the thorax target geometry where only a 0.5% increase in P_+ could be achieved when increasing the number of used beam portals from 3 (P_+=86.8%) to 72 (P_+=87.3%).

A low number (≈ 3) of non-uniform beams may thus be used without losing P_+ and unnecessarily increasing the total treatment time. It has been shown by Svensson *et al.* (1994) that the use of non-uniform fluence profiles generally increases the total treatment time by a factor of 1.5 - 2. The reduction of the number of beam portals that results by using non-uniform fluence profiles may thus decrease the total treatment time to approximately the same value as with uniform beams and at the same time a substantial gain in P_+ is achieved (cf Söderström *et al.* 1993).

Clinical Factors Determining the Optimum Treatment

As can be seen in Table 7-2, the increase in the probability to achieve tumor control without causing severe complications in normal tissues when increasing the number of beam portals for the cervix case, is due to a reduction of the probability of injury to the small bowel. Most of the improvement is obtained going from one ($P_I=21.0\%$) to two ($P_I=8.6\%$) beam portals. When going from two to three beam portals the improvement is mainly due to an improved probability of controlling in the local lymph nodes. The homogeneity of the dose distributions inside the target volumes are improved as the number of beam portals are increased and the maximum dose may thus be lowered. It is interesting to note that, when using three beams, the optimum beam entry directions are posterior-anterior oriented despite the fact that the most radiation sensitive organ at risk, the rectum, is located in the posterior region. Using these beam entry directions the different beams are directed to coincide behind the rectum in the gross tumor volume and thus in an efficient way shape the resultant dose distribution to spare the rectum.

A quite different situation occurs for the thorax target geometry. This can be seen in Table 7-3. In this case the heart is the most critical organ obtaining a 11.3% probability of injury when one beam is used. When going to two portals the optimal beams are displaced from the optimal single beam entry direction at 150°, to $\Omega_1=105°$ and $\Omega_2=180°$ thereby avoiding injury to the heart but increasing the probability of injury to the normal tissue stroma by 1.7%. Only minor further improvements can be observed when increasing the number of beam portals to three. It is interesting to observe that all the beams are irradiating the target through the left lung of the patient. The left lung is thus partly sacrificed in the treatment to achieve a high probability of tumor control. This is the result when considering the left and the right lung as one single organ. If the left and the right lung would have been considered as two separate organs a different dose plan and a lower probability of tumor control without severe complications would result. This is so since a large probability of injury to any one of the left or right lung would have resulted from any beam entry direction. A separate calculation verifies this conclusion and shows a 10% reduction of the probability of tumor control without severe complications for the optimum selection of beam entry directions.

The most interesting feature of the head and neck irradiation is the movement of the beam entry directions when increasing the number of beam portals (cf Table 7-4). The situation is quite similar to that of the cervix target. In this case much of the probability of injury to the spinal cord and some of that to the normal tissue stroma may be avoided and at the same time the probability of tumor control can be increased. This is achieved by irradiating the lymph nodes using a cross-fire technique with two ($\Omega_1=135°$, $\Omega_2=285°$) or three ($\Omega_1=135°$, $\Omega_1=225°$, $\Omega_3=285°$) anterior-posterior beams instead of one posterior-anterior beam ($\Omega=0°$).

Table 7-2. *The mean, minimum, and maximum dose and the standard deviation of the distribution for the different organs at risk and the target volumes for the cervix case.*

	$\langle D \rangle$ [Gy]	D_{min} [Gy]	D_{max} [Gy]	σ_D [Gy]	P_B, P_I
1 optimized beam, P_+ = 67.7%					
Small bowel	37.5	0.0	89.6	26.0	0.210
Rectum	42.9	40.1	47.9	2.1	0.017
Bladder	53.1	10.7	62.1	10.5	0.002
Lymph nodes	57.3	38.0	84.0	10.6	0.942
Gross tumor	66.3	59.0	73.8	3.8	0.957
2 optimized beams, P_+ = 85.6%					
Small bowel	35.0	0.0	72.5	20.5	0.086
Rectum	40.9	38.0	45.7	2.5	0.006
Bladder	46.7	18.6	58.0	7.4	0.000
Lymph nodes	56.7	39.8	69.3	5.4	0.970
Gross tumor	68.6	60.0	72.5	2.5	0.977
3 optimized beams, P_+ = 87.9%					
Small bowel	33.4	0.1	72.3	18.2	0.082
Rectum	39.1	36.3	43.1	2.1	0.001
Bladder	48.2	43.0	55.5	3.5	0.000
Lymph nodes	57.9	46.2	68.7	4.1	0.983
Gross tumor	68.7	63.5	72.3	2.1	0.979

Table 7-3. *The mean, minimum, and maximum dose and the standard deviation of the dose distribution for the different organs at risk and the target volumes for the thorax case.*

	$\langle D \rangle$ [Gy]	D_{min} [Gy]	D_{max} [Gy]	σ_D [Gy]	P_B, P_I
1 optimized beam, P_+ = 55.4%					
Normal tissue stroma	18.1	0.0	69.2	25.1	0.061
Spinal cord	0.2	0.1	0.2	0.0	0.000
Lung	15.6	0.0	74.6	25.0	0.021
Heart	32.8	0.2	53.6	19.7	0.113
Target volume	58.6	43.8	67.6	4.3	0.738
2 optimized beams, P_+ = 86.3%					
Normal tissue stroma	19.4	0.0	70.9	25.0	0.078
Spinal cord	8.3	3.0	13.8	6.1	0.000
Lung	14.3	0.0	67.4	15.0	0.002
Heart	28.6	0.6	67.8	13.3	0.002
Target volume	67.7	61.3	70.9	2.0	0.944
3 optimized beams, P_+ = 86.8%					
Normal tissue stroma	19.6	0.0	71.7	24.4	0.079
Spinal cord	8.4	3.0	14.0	6.2	0.000
Lung	14.3	0.1	70.2	14.2	0.009
Heart	27.9	1.2	62.6	12.0	0.005
Target volume	68.2	60.0	71.7	1.9	0.949

Table 7-4. *The mean, minimum, and maximum dose and the standard deviation of the dose distribution for the different organs at risk and the target volumes for the head and neck case.*

	$\langle D \rangle$ [Gy]	D_{min} [Gy]	D_{max} [Gy]	σ_D [Gy]	P_B, P_I
1 optimized beam, $P_+ = 60.3\%$					
Normal tissue stroma	48.2	0.0	71.0	15.1	0.158
Spinal cord	42.5	41.4	43.6	0.8	0.047
Target volume	61.4	47.8	71.0	5.4	0.800
2 optimized beams, $P_+ = 69.2\%$					
Normal tissue stroma	45.9	3.8	77.3	15.5	0.152
Spinal cord	35.2	32.3	39.1	2.5	0.005
Target volume	61.8	49.6	77.3	3.4	0.848
3 optimized beams, $P_+ = 71.2\%$					
Normal tissue stroma	44.9	2.5	70.5	16.1	0.146
Spinal cord	33.6	30.5	36.6	2.0	0.002
Target volume	61.9	54.4	70.5	2.6	0.860

Conclusions

The use of optimal non-uniform dose delivery can reduce the number of required beam portals to a low number (2-5) at the same time as the probability of achieving tumor control without causing severe complications is practically as high as it can be with an infinite number of beams. This requires that the beam profiles are optimized using a biological objective function such as P_+. An important consequence is that a few static fields can be used to deliver an optimal treatment plan without the need of complex rotation techniques. Since such objective functions are steadily being developed and the associated radiobiological data are being collected at many clinics all the essential requirements are fulfilled to perform an accurate radiobiological optimization on a routine clinical basis. Examples showing that the use of sophisticated equipment such as scanned photon or electron beams, dynamic multileaf collimators, and computer controlled compensator production, may not be necessary to obtain a good treatment outcome. It may thus be possible to achieve close to optimal treatment results by careful selection of the beam portals. We have also shown that the selection of optimal beam portals can significantly improve the treatment result. It is therefore an important task to develop algorithms for optimal selection of beam entry directions for treatments using a limited number of beam portals. With help of the new rules for selection of beam portals presented here and by Söderström *et al.* (1993) it should be possible for the therapeutic team to select clinically advantageous beam portals for most typical tumor and normal tissue combinations. Once the most important tumor groups have been investigated it is sufficient to optimize one single few field doseplan, at least if not an extremely strict optimization on the fractional percent level is called for.

Acknowledgments

The calculation of point energy deposition kernels and program development by Anders Ahnesjö and Anders Gustafsson are gratefully acknowledged.

References

1. Ahnesjö, A., Andreo, P. and Brahme, A. Calculation and application of point spread functions for treatment planning with high energy photon beams. Acta Oncol. **26**, 49-56 (1987).

2. Brahme, A. Treatment optimization using physical and radiobiological objective functions. In Radiation Therapy Physics, Chap. 11, A. Smith, ed. (Berlin-Springer 1992).

3. Eklöf, A., Ahnesjö, A. and Brahme, A. Photon beam energy deposition kernels for inverse radiotherpy planning. Acta Oncol. **29**, 447-454 (1990).

4. Gustafsson, A., Lind, B. K. and Brahme, A. A generalized pencil beam algorithm for optimization of radiation therapy. Med. Phys. **21**, 343-356 (1994).

5. Gustafsson, A., Lind, B. K. and Brahme, A. Simultaneous optimization of dynamic multileaf collimation and scanning patterns on compensation fitters using a generalized pencil beam algorithm. Med. Phys. **22**, 1141-1156 (1995).

6. ICRU 24 Determination of Absorbed Dose in a Patient Irradiated by Beams of X or Gamma rays in Radiotherapy Procedures (Bethesda, 1976).

7. Källman, P., Lind, B. K., Eklöf, A. and Brahme, A. Shaping of arbitrary dose distributions by dynamic multileaf collimation. Phys. Med. Biol. **33**, 1291-1300 (1988).

8. Källman, P., Lind, B. K. and Brahme, A. An algorithm for maximizing the probability of complication free tumor control in radiation therapy. Phys. Med. Biol. **37**, 871-890 (1992).

9. Källman, P. Optimization of radiation therapy planning using physical and biological objective functions. Thesis Stockholm University Sweden. (1992).

10. Lind, B. K. Properties of an algorithm for solving the inverse problem in radiation therapy. Inverse Problems **6**, 415-426 (1990).

11. Lind, B. K. and Brahme, A. Optimization of radiation therapy dose distributions with scanned photon beams. The Use of Computers in Radiation Therapy, pp 235-239, I A D Bruinvis *et al.*, ed. (Proc 9th ICCR, 1987).

12. Lind, B. K. and Brahme, A. Photon field quantities and units for kernel based radiation therapy planning and treatment optimization. Phys. Med. Biol. **37**, 891-909 (1992)

13. Petti, P. L. and Siddon, R. L. Effective wedge angles with a universal wedge. Phys. Med. Biol. **30**, 985-991 (1985).

14. Svensson, H., Jonsson, L., Larsson, L. G., Brahme, A., Lindberg, B. and Reistad, D. A 22MeV microtron for radiation therapy. Acta Radiol. Ther. Phys. Biol. **16**, 145-156 (1977).

15. Svensson, R., Källman, P. and Brahme, A. An Analytical solution for the dynamic control of multileaf collimators. Phys. Med. Biol. 39, 37-61 (1994).

16. Söderström, S. and Brahme, A. Optimization of the dose delivery in few field techniques using radiobiological objective functions. Med. Phys. **20**, 1201-1210 (1993).

17. Söderström, S., Gustafsson, A. and Brahme, A. The clinical value of different treatment objectives and degrees of freedom in radiation therapy optimization. Radiother. Oncol. **29**, 148-163 (1993).

18. Ågren, A-K., Brahme, A. and Turesson, I. Optimization of uncomplicated control for head and neck tumors. Int. J. Radiat. Oncol. Biol. Phys. **19**, 1077-1085 (1990).

Chapter 8

Quality Assurance for 3-D Treatment Planning

Benedick A. Fraass, Ph.D., Daniel L. McShan, Ph.D., Mary K. Martel, Ph.D.

Department of Radiation Oncology, University of Michigan Medical Center, Ann Arbor, Michigan

The creation and maintenance of comprehensive and effective quality assurance (QA) programs is one of the most important tasks of the clinical medical physicist in a Radiation Oncology clinic. The QA program should consider all of the technical and procedural aspects of activities related to patient treatment (see for example the report of AAPM Task Group 40 [1]). Treatment planning is one of the very important parts of the therapy process, and requires a significant amount of effort directed toward quality assurance. The development and clinical use of 3-dimensional treatment planning systems has significantly affected the scope and approach to treatment planning quality assurance.

In most 2-D treatment planning, many important decisions involved in patient treatments are made externally to the computerized treatment planning system. For example, if block shapes are not input into the planning system, QA of this important part of the therapy process is a mechanical and operational issue, unrelated to "treatment planning." If beam directions, field sizes, blocking, and other issues are determined during simulation, the main decisions made as part of so-called treatment planning involve possible use of wedges, and changing beam weights to make the dose to the target uniform. The accuracy of the dose calculations is of course an important issue, and most publications and work on QA for treatment planning has concentrated on this issue [2-5]. Recently, there has been some discussion of the broader issues associated with treatment planning [6,7].

A quality assurance program which can address this new situation should include a number of different components, including: (1) QA of the computerized treatment planning system, including its software, procedures, training, and other facets of its use; (2) Measurement, testing, and verification of the dosimetric aspects of the planning system; (3) Testing, documentation and characterization of the non-dosimetric aspects of planning; (4) QA of the clinical use of treatment planning throughout the entire planning and treatment processes.

Here we discuss one approach to organizing the large amount of work associated with QA of clinical 3-D treatment planning. Our experience in attempting to develop a QA program for 3-D treatment planning in our clinic is used to illustrate some of the advantages and pitfalls associated with this kind of work.

Materials and Methods

The information contained in this work is the result of our efforts to organize the QA efforts associated with the clinical use of the 3-D planning system developed in the department ("U-MPlan"). This system was clinically implemented in early 1986, and has been used for all clinical treatment planning in the department since that time. It has been described in a number of publications[8-20], and has been used for numerous clinical treatment planning studies (see references contained in references [10,21]). The QA approach described here has evolved over the last 9 years of use of the 3-D planning system.

Dosimetric measurements used for calculation model parameter determination, algorithm validation, and clinical dose calculation verification tests have been based on film, ion chamber and diode data. For the last several years, we have used 3-D dose distributions which are generated from 2-D planar dose distributions obtained with film, as described by Stern et al. [22]. Measurement techniques which are used for Ion chamber and diode measurements in water phantom systems have also been described for [23,24]. The generation of self-consistent dose distributions from measured data is a very important part of the measurement and analysis process, especially for 3-D planning system QA, and has been briefly described [22].

Results

Quality Assurance of the Treatment Planning Software

QA for software and hardware components of the treatment planning system are an important part of any QA program. The clinical user's approach to software QA will depend somewhat on whether the software is commercial software provided by a vendor, or software developed in-house. Even though in most cases the software QA for the planning software is not under the control of the user, the general approach the user should take with the provider of the planning software may be quite similar in either situation.

Although software engineering and QA are beyond the scope of this work, several comments about those subjects are relevant here. The user of commercial software-based products does have the ability to affect the software quality assurance programs of vendors. As suggested in a recent AAPM Task Group report on Accelerator Safety for Computer-Controlled Medical Accelerators [25], the user should require enough documentation from the vendor that the user can be convinced that the system design, implementation, and quality assurance program are robust enough for the clinical use that the user intends. This kind of documentation should be available to the user, as it can be of significant assistance to users as they design their own QA programs. There are numerous published descriptions of the standard software engineering tools and procedures which are used to meet the quality standards [26,27], and the user can exert pressure for as much information as can reasonably be provided by the vendor or assimilated by the user. The user should always expect that there are unreported errors in large software systems such as treatment planning systems [28].

Dosimetric Quality Assurance

Dose calculation verification and QA has been the primary kind of planning system QA which has been performed or discussed in the literature. Most workers have concentrated on the basic verification of 2-D dose calculations [2-5,28-30]. Most users of treatment planning systems have performed at least some tests of their systems themselves in order to show that the dose calculations presented by the system agree with the data measured at that institution. Considering the importance of dose calculations, this is not an unreasonable first step. However, to approach the planning system QA with an organized methodology, one must pursue the dosimetric checks of the planning system with a number of different operations.

a. The 3-D Measured Dataset:

The measurement of a complete and self-consistent dataset characterizing the dose distributions obtained on a particular machine is one of the most important activities needed in order to perform dosimetric testing on the planning system. With many 2-D systems, the only beam data needed was a few profile and depth dose curves for several square field sizes. As long as these few profiles could be renormalized to the values given by the depth doses, then the consistency of the data was not too important, since there were few checks of the internal consistency of the data.

The requirements for the measured data are much more rigorous for a 3-D planning system. The dose calculations are used to predict the dose throughout an entire volume of the patient. Therefore, the measured data should be obtained throughout the volume, and the comparison should also occur throughout the volume of interest. Since it is typically difficult to make measurements directly on a volumetric basis (although there have been some efforts [31]), measurements are still often made with 1-D curves (depth dose and profile measurements). When this kind of data is obtained, one curve at a time, it becomes very difficult to obtain a 3-D set of data curves that is all self-consistent. For example, even when 1-D measurements are made only on the principal sagittal and axial planes through the central axis of the beam, these data may themselves be inconsistent along the line (the central axis) where they should both agree [23].

One method which can be used to generate a complete 3-D dose distribution from measured data has been recently reported by Stern et al. [22]. This method uses film dosimetry to measure the dose distribution in a number of 2-D planes perpendicular to the beam central axis ("BEV planes"), and a depth dose curve (measured with ion chamber or other appropriate dosimeter). The depth dose curve is used to generate a non-linear interpolation between the BEV plane data, along divergent ray lines. This method, which uses the symmetry and physics of the divergent geometry generally followed by the photon beam, generates 3-D dose distributions (Figure 8-1) which can be directly compared to the calculated 3-D dose distributions obtained from the 3-D planning system. These kind of data are essential if the full 3-D dose distribution calculated by a 3-D system is to be fully characterized and verified.

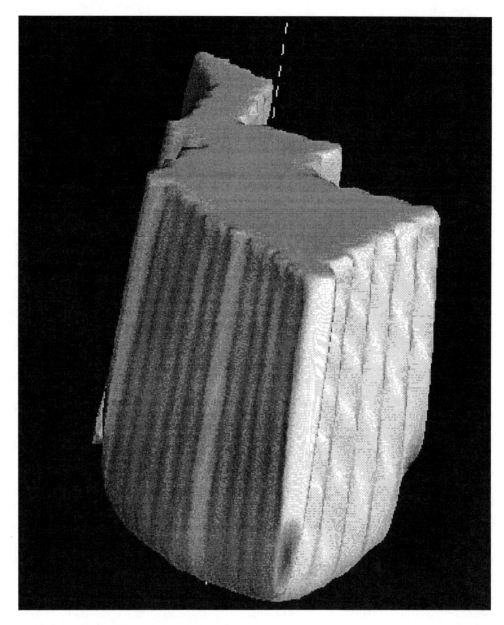

Figure 8-1. *50 % isodose surface from 3-D measured dose distribution for MLC shaped field. Field normalized at depth of 10 cm.*

b. Dose Distribution Comparison and Verification Checks:

Verification checks of 2-D dose distributions are often performed by overlaying two plots of profiles, depth doses, or an isodose chart measured on the central axial contour, but other techniques are often quite useful. One can summarize the depth dose behavior as a function of field size by creating tables of FDD (or TPR) for various field sizes and depths[32], and then subtracting the data and calculation results from each other. This difference table can show the overall quality of the agreement with statistics like the maximum deviation and/or the standard deviation over the table. Trends of discrepancies are also easily inspected.

For checks of the entire 3-D dose distribution, more sophisticated techniques are necessary. Use of isodose curve overlays on sagittal, coronal, and other axonometric displays illustrates the agreement between the distributions in 3-D. Coronal cuts are particularly useful, since they show the dosimetry relevant to the BEV displays which are used to design beam apertures. For a more detailed view, subtracting calculated results from the data generates a dose difference distribution (in 2-D or 3-D if available). Isodifference lines or colorwash dose displays effectively highlight the differences.

In order to summarize the results of the dose comparison throughout the 3-D volume of interest, the dose difference distribution can be histogrammed (creating a dose (difference) volume histogram (DVH)). This DVH can be used as a quantitative measure of the overall agreement between calculations and data. The DVH analysis can generate much more detailed information by separately histogramming the volumes inside the beam, outside the beam, and in the penumbra regions. Use of a distance map (the distance between particular isodose lines in the measured and calculated distributions can also be useful in high gradient regions (penumbra, electron depth dose)[33].

c. Verification of Input Test Data:

There are several kinds of calculation verification checks which are required. The first is to verify that the calculation model adequately reproduces the input data. In many 2-D calculation models, which are directly based on data or beam libraries, this is mostly a check on the software and the accuracy of the data entry. However, the situation is often different for the generally more complex calculation algorithms which are used in 3-D planning systems. Much more data is typically required for 3-D algorithms, and field shaping devices, wedges, oblique angulations and non-axial beams, compensators, and other devices and situations are more important. 3-D algorithms often contain more modeling of the real physics, so they can be used in situations where direct measurements are difficult to obtain. Since a number of these models are based on first principles theories and parameters (for example the Monte Carlo -based kernels used for the convolution techniques developed by Mackie [34], and Ahnesjo [35], often the reproduction of the usual input data (field flatness and details of the depth dose behavior) must be carefully checked. Differences between the basic field data and the calculations must be well-characterized and understood, because they will form the basis for some amount of the differences between calculations and data in other comparison situations also.

d. Applicability and Limits of the Dose Calculation Algorithm:

A very important point has been made by Jacky et al. [28] on QA testing for dose calculations. All current dose calculation algorithms contain approximations and limitations. Algorithm tests must be performed to confirm that it behaves as it was designed to work. If the algorithm is simple, the agreement between calculations and data may be very poor, even if the algorithm is working perfectly. Therefore, any analysis of calculation results must be analyzed with full knowledge of the results which should be expected, considering the effects which are modeled by the algorithm. Tests used to characterize these effects may be very different in scope, operation, or results than the tests (next section) used to verify that the algorithm predicts the dose well enough to be used for clinical planning. Design and operation of algorithm tests are individualized to each calculation algorithm.

e. Dose Verification over the Range of Clinical Usage:

One of the most traditional kinds of verification checks is comparison of calculation results with measured data over the range of clinical use expected. This is probably the most clinically relevant type of comparison. Errors in input data, fitting, algorithm coding and/or design, and various other kinds of errors are all incorporated in the results. This is a critical test since it shows the overall precision with which particular kinds of calculations may be performed. If there is a discrepancy, however, this test will likely not help explain the reasons for the problem.

f. Verification of Absolute Dose Output and Plan Normalization:

All of the tests above have concentrated on the relative dose distribution. However, absolute dose delivered to the prescription point in the patient is critical. Important parts of this process include plan prescription methods, dose and prescription point, relative beam normalizations, and monitor unit (MU) calculations. Although specific checks of each part of the process should be performed, a complete check can be performed by normalizing the same plan in several ways and comparing the MU obtained with each. One must also be assured the normalization process will perform as expected for any combination of situations, or even in the face of deliberate errors or mis-use. A careful analysis of the possible hazards associated with this aspect of the system is particularly appropriate. This is an important activity for the clinical physicist at each institution, since the plan prescription - normalization - monitor unit calculation methods vary quite a bit from institution to institution. To perform this kind of analysis requires detailed knowledge of the design, methodologies, algorithms, and safety checks which are part of the system design.

Tests of Non-Dosimetric Functions

Modern planning systems, especially 3-D systems, are involved in much more than dose calculations. These non-dosimetric parts of the planning process also need to be verified and quality assured. Although there have been preliminary reports in this area[36], a comprehensive set of tests has not been described. The scope of the required QA is extensive, since the scope of non-dosimetric features in a modern 3-D planning system is several orders of magnitude larger than those used in 2-D systems.

In this section, a series of areas which may require testing are listed and briefly discussed. The intent of the discussion which follows is not to provide a comprehensive list of things which should be verified, but rather to provide examples of kinds of functions which should be considered for clinical testing. At the least, the approach described here should help people pursue a similar strategy when designing QA tests relevant to the local situation.

a. Image Conversion:

Imaging information, particularly from CT, but also including MR, SPECT, PET, and others, is the basis of most anatomical information on which treatment planning is based. Other images, such as digitized radiographs from a video camera system or laser digitizer, may also be incorporated in the planning process. Typically, each image is transferred from a vendor-specific computer system, usually with vendor-specific image file format and/or transfer media or network, to the planning system. Tests of geometric, text, and imaging information from each study should verify that the data, as used inside the planning system, corresponds to the original data. If the planning system software is used to un-distort or otherwise modify the imaging data, this procedure must also be tested..

b. Anatomical Structures:

One of the few non-dosimetric tests which is often included in routine 2-D RTTP QA testing is the anatomical description of the patient. In 2-D planning, the entire anatomical description of the patient is provided by one or more axial contours of the external surface of the patient, perhaps with the addition of one or more internal contours which represent other parts of the anatomy. Typically, the contour accuracy is checked by performing a simple checks on the accuracy of the digitizer tablet which is used to enter the contours into the planning system [6]. Further checks of the contours may also include SSD and depth checks for points which are entered on the contour.

In a general 3-D planning system, however, the anatomical model used for the patient is a much more complex set of objects, which require a much more complete set of test procedures. The basic building block of the anatomical model in a 2-D system, the contour, has been superseded by a number of objects in the hierarchy, including 3-D structures, and perhaps the use of multiple datasets of self-consistent volumetric imaging information. Although the anatomical model may be particular to each planning system, the list of anatomically-related checks which follows can be generalized as needed for other systems.

(1) 3-D Structure Definition.

A 3-D structure is the main anatomical object, and consists is typically generated from a series of contours. Each structure may also include attributes such as the structure's bulk density (if CT-based density corrections are not used), the way the top and bottom of the structure should be capped or closed off above the last contour, and other attributes.

(2) Mechanical Contours.

Contours drawn with mechanical contouring devices, including the digitizer, the keyboard, or mouse/joystick type entry, must be verified for the input devices used. Devices like the digitizer must be checked for geometrical accuracy and stability routinely.

(3) Contours on Axial Images.

Contours are typically drawn based on images like CT slices. One should verify 1) the accuracy of the contour display with respect to the image display, 2) the 3-D location of the contour, 3) the coordinates of contour points with respect to the coordinate system used for dose calculation, and 4) the response of the contouring algorithm to too many points, or loops, or other uncommon situations.

(4) Autotracking Contours.

The use of autotracking (the computer tracks a density gradient like the external surface) to define contours is widespread. Careful checks of the response of the tracking algorithm must be made for situations in which there are different gradients in the image, different image formats, and the use of various gray scale gradient ranges (tracking MR images rather than CT). The robustness of the tracking algorithm in situations in which masks, markers, contrast, or artifacts exist on the images can be verified by routine use in any situation used clinically, followed by careful inspection of the results of the autotracking in the clinical cases.

(5) Generation of 3-D Surfaces.

Contours of a 3-D structure are typically used to generate a 3-D surface description which is used for display and calculations. This is usually a complex algorithm which may attempt to take into account the sharpness of corners which are allowed in 3-D, and even the bifurcation of one structure into two branches which have distinct contours on the same CT slices. Complete testing of such an algorithm may be quite difficult and will require detailed knowledge of the algorithmic approach. As described later, checks during routine treatment planning can help assure that problems due to patient-specific glitches in this algorithm can slip through the routine planning process.

(6) Structure Capping.

Most 3-D structures are defined by drawing contours on axial CT slices. When a structure is contoured on one CT slice, and not found on the next slice, what is the shape of the 3-D surface in that region? The shape may be critical for dose calculations and beam aperture shaping, and the way this works [37] must be carefully understood and verified.

(7) Use of Non-Axial Contours for Surface Generation.

Use of non-axial contours for surface generation must also be checked.

(8) Extraction of Contours from Surfaces.

In order to show how 3-D structures appear on a particular image plane, one can extract or "cut" a contour from a 3-D surface description onto a particular plane or image of interest. cuts the surface, and then to display that extracted contour onto the image. As this is important for displaying contour information on sagittal, coronal and oblique CT image reconstructions, it should be carefully verified.

(9) Surface Expansion.

In our clinical practice, a 3-D expansion of the target volume is used in virtually every case in order to allow for setup and treatment uncertainty (at least). As this expansion creates a 3-D surface which is used as the planning target volume, this algorithm must also be carefully verified. Since a 3-D expansion is performed, the verification must also be 3-D. Happily, this expansion is straightforward to check on each clinical case as part of the planning process, so the need for exhaustive testing of this feature is lessened.

(10) Bolus.

Different types of bolus, including 1) external bolus on the patient surface, 2) changing the CT densities in an internal region (to edit out the effects of contrast material, for example), and 3) use of bolus material in sinuses or cavities, are often used clinically and must be checked. In addition, automated bolus design features (for example, automatic use of the skin surface as the back of the skin bolus) must also be considered.

(11) Contours Drawn on Projection Images.

Contours drawn on projection images (computed or digitized radiographs), or CT scout images, cannot be used unless the contour information is correctly projected into other image displays. One must therefore verify the accuracy of projection of BEV-designed contours onto the relevant 2-D slices, and onto other 3-D displays.

(12) 3-D points.

The display and geometrical definition of any points defined inside the system must accurately reflect the geometrical location of the image on which the point is defined.

c. Dataset Registration:

One of the powerful advances associated with 3-D planning has been the use of imaging information from different imaging modalities, such as CT, MR, PET, SPECT, ultrasound, and radiographic imaging. To use this information, the planning system must contain tools which allow geometric registration of one set of data with another [11,38-40]. The general behavior of the coordinate system transforms which are used to implement this registration, as well as each of the various registration techniques used, must be characterized and verified.

d. Density Representation:

In addition to 3-D structures and surface descriptions, a full 3-D representation of the CT densities of the patient is important. Among features to consider for QA testing are 1) creation and maintenance of the CT density file(s), 2) verification of the density lookup mechanism, 3) ability to create a density matrix based on assigned bulk densities, 4) the various conversions from image gray level to CT number to relative electron density, and 5) bolus and density-editing routines.

e. Image Use:

The use of image information inside the planning system is distinct from simply converting the image format into the standard format used by the planning system. There are two different used of imaging data to consider. Most image display manipulation affects the visual presentation of the data, but is not critical so the planning effort. However, if target definition protocols depend on contours drawn under specific CT window and level parameters, and they are handled incorrectly, then a much more significant error occurs. The geometric identification of the image location is also of course critical.

(1) Grayscale Window and Level Settings.

Window and level transformations used for image display may occasionally be a high priority function for some particular treatment protocol situations, so it must be quantitatively checked.

(2) Creation of Reconstructions.

The use of sagittal, coronal, and oblique CT reconstructions obtained by reformatting CT data is quite important. Checks should include verifying the geometry of the resulting image (and its related plane through the patient) and the way in which the image was constructed. Details of the reconstructions algorithm may be important, for example, the way the algorithm interpolates between different axial slices.

(3) Geometrical Accuracy of Image Planes.

Often, a geometric cut, slice or plane is associated with each particular CT image. The geometrical location of image cuts is critical and must be carefully verified.

(4) Region-of-Interest Analysis.

The use of region-of-interest image analysis techniques are sometimes used for checks important to dose calculation QA, and so are also of interest here.

f. Anatomical Display:

Display of anatomical, beam, and dose information in 3-D is one of the more obvious differences between modern 3-D systems and older 2-D systems. It should verify the three dimensionality of the displays which are available, including 2-D CT scan type displays as well as 3-D displays like the Beam's Eye View (BEV) and other 3-D projections. Accurate coordinate information is of course necessary. Note that much of this information may be available in a number of different coordinate systems, so all must be checked. Related functions, like measuring distances and angles, or setting the size of the cursor to a specific diameter, may be important for geometric planning. Display functions, such as measuring tools, must be tested in all display types in which they are available. Although perhaps not as quantitative as some of the other functions, the way information is kept updated on each of the various types of displays must also be tested. In particular, when multiple display windows are available for viewing by the user, all information which is displayed must be continuously updated so that it remains consistent with the current status of the anatomical structures, beams, doses, sources, and any other objects used by the planning system.

g. Beams:

Definition and display of radiotherapy beams (or fields) is a very important part of external beam treatment planning. The beam description is the basis of all dose calculations, and is even more important from a geometrical point of view, since placing the beam or its aperture in the wrong place will potentially cause the target volume of the radiation treatment to be completely missed. A number of important aspects of the beam functionality must be carefully verified.

(1) Beam Display.

3-D planning makes use of many display types, including planar, 3-D, BEV, and others. The model of the beam and aperture (blocks, multileaf collimator) which system uses must be confirmed to correctly project all of the intersections between the beam and the anatomical information which is displayed. Note that for a 3-D system, these projections should be correct in 3-D. However, for systems with some 2-D limitations, the verification checks must take into account that the system will not project the beam edges as they actually are, but will perform the display with some limitations.

(2) BEV Projection of Anatomy.

The use of the Beam's Eye View (BEV) is one of the most powerful functions in 3-D planning system. The divergent beam geometry must be correctly calculated and displayed, or the design of beam and/or aperture may be incorrect.

(3) Machine Limits and Capabilities.

As 3-D plans use more and more of the capabilities of the treatment machine, an increasingly sophisticated description of the limits of those capabilities, for a particular machine, must be a part of the beam technique module of the planning system. For simple systems, the energies available, field size limits, and number and type of wedges may be significant. However, in more sophisticated 3-D systems, the naming conventions, machine angle conventions, limitations and resolution of readouts for each motion, the speed of those motions, and various other parameters may be included in the planning system capabilities, and in fact in how the plans are generated.

(4) Beam Aperture Definition.

The definition of the beam aperture, created with normal collimator jaws, blocks, and/or multileaf collimator, is one of the critical aspects of modern conformal therapy. Both geometric and dosimetric aspects of this definition are important, and must be verified. The most common approaches involve the use of BEV displays, and interactive drawing of the beam aperture which is desired. Specialized drawing aids, for example a circular cursor which helps the aperture be defined with a particular geometric margin around the target volume, should be checked for geometrical accuracy. The measurement geometry for any drawing done in that image, particularly the distance from the source at which the displayed "BEV plane" is located must be confirmed. Automatic algorithms are often used also, such as the autoblock methodology described by [13,14,41]. Here, a much more complex testing procedure is necessary, since the algorithm includes 3-D projection of the selected 3-D surface(s) onto the BEV plane, followed by an automatic routine which generates the correct aperture shape. Both of these algorithms can be sensitive to details of the anatomical or beam aperture representations, and should be carefully checked over a series of different situations.

(5) Multileaf Collimator Definition.

Much of the testing necessary to include the capabilities of a multileaf collimator system has been discussed above. However, some planning systems may include some fairly advanced capabilities which are specific to the use of the MLC. For example, it is often desirable to optimize the collimator angle along with the leaf shape determination, since rotating the head of the machine may improve the ability of the plan to align the MLC leaf ends along a critical normal structure.

h. Operational Aspects of Dose Calculations:

Although dose calculation algorithm verification has been discussed above, the operational aspects of the calculation methodology has not been discussed. The need for these checks is quite dependent on the planning system implementation. However, even if some of the details discussed below are not handled by the planning system, each institution should consider the relevance of the issue, since somewhere inside the planning process, these issues are being handled, either explicitly or implicitly.

(1) Calculation Grid Definition.

The way in which calculational grid points are chosen, and how that grid is maintained through changes in the anatomy or beam orientations on which the original choice was based, must be verified.

(2) Inhomogeneity Corrections.

The status of the inhomogeneity correction, and how the results of corrected and uncorrected calculations are stored and documented on hardcopy are of course important to how the physician uses the planning information.

(3) Plan Normalization.

All treatment plan dose distributions are based on a plan normalization method, whether it be implicit or explicit. A check of all the variations which are allowed within a particular implementation is critical, because it helps determine the absolute dose delivered to the patient.

(4) Calculation Validity Logic.

In conventional systems, there is often little flexibility in how dose distributions are calculated, saved, and displayed. In 3-D, however, the time and computer resources required for 3-D calculations can be extensive, and one would like to make efficient use of those resources to make planning as fast as possible. For our planning system, validity checks are used to assure that dose calculations which should be invalidated by some change (to the anatomy or beam configurations) are invalidated, while at the same time maintaining all of the valid calculations so that they are not unnecessarily redone. Tests of this kind of functionality depend on detailed knowledge of the way the process works.

(5) Reading Saved Dose Calculations.

A complex database and/or file system is typically used for 3-D planning systems. Testing of the functionality associated with reading stored anatomical, beam, dose, and source information is similar to that discussed above, since it is dependent on the storage mechanisms used by the planning system. Detailed tests of these functions, designed with detailed knowledge of the system so that relevant possible hazards are checked, should be a high priority.

i. Dose Display:

The display of the dose distribution, and particularly the display of isodose lines on CT or other image data, is a very important part of the planning system. Although often dose distributions are viewed qualitatively, isodose lines (and isodose surfaces in 3-D displays) can be used in quite quantitatively. The basic interpolation and display mechanisms of the system must be tested to assure an accurate representation of the location of the dose lines (or surfaces). Point dose displays, and interrogation of the dose displays using mouse/cursor -type display of the dose at particular points, can also change a physician impression of the plan, and so must be verified. Many of these functions, however, can be checked in a relatively simple manner, since one can do self-consistency checks among all the various kinds of dose displays, and then just check one of those display methods in a qualitative way. Note that checks of isodose surface creation and display contain many of the possible problems associated with complex algorithms such as surface rendering algorithms, and it is not possible to check all relevant possibilities or problems.

j. Dose Volume Histograms:

The use of dose volume histograms (DVHs) [42] is one of the more significant differences between conventional planning and 3-D planning [43]. Checks of DVH calculations should be of two different types. The proper functioning of the DVH calculations (and any associated Volume-region-of-interest (VROI) calculation) should be checked. In addition, one should investigate the robustness of the volume, VROI, and DVH results that one gets from the system as input data are changed over the range expected in clinical practice. DVHs may be fairly sensitive to grid sizes, contouring methodology, and other details of the implementation of the capability.

k. Evaluation Tools.

For 2-D planning systems, the sole plan evaluation tool typically involved looking at the displayed dose distribution for a particular plan. Modern planning systems often use models to calculate the normal tissue complication probability (NTCP) [44-47] and tumor control probability (TCP) [48] models, as well as other aids to optimize, rank, and score plans. If these capabilities are used for clinical planning, they should be included in the QA program. Note many of the parameters of NTCP and TCP models are not well-known and may be the subject of significant controversy [49]. The checks of these functions should verify that the calculation works correctly. One should not confuse lack of good data (for input parameters) with errors in the implementation of the model.

l. Plan Verification Tools

The use of 3-D planning requires quantitative plan and portal verification, and tools for this verification should exist within the 3-D planning system. In the system reported here, portal and/or simulator images are input into the system directly from digital imagers, or through the use of a laser digitizer system. To use these images, they must be accurately registered with the coordinate systems used for planning. Since the accuracy of the registration is often determined by the user, the clinical use of this feature must include QA which assures that the registration is confirmed each time. Image enhancement tools must also be checked since they can change the way the image information is used.

m. Composite Plans.

In order to generate the complete 3-D dose distribution that the patient was treated with, a composite plan is often generated which is the sum of all the individual plans which were used. QA for this mode includes checking all the perturbations of different plan parameters which can be added together, including plans with different dose calculation grids, plans of different plan normalization types, brachytherapy as well as external beam plans, plans with different dose units, and others.

n. Hard Copy Output:

The output of the description of the treatment plan, and the implementation of that information for use in treatment of the patient, is a critical area for quality assurance. All aspects of this documentation of the plan must be accurate, particularly the dose, monitor unit, and treatment technique parameters. Classes of information which should be verified include the text information on the beams, calculations, and anatomy, BEV displays, contour scaling, isodose displays, gray scale imaging, 3-D displays, calculation points, and plan normalization data.

Clinical System Tests

As a final check of non-dosimetric aspects of the planning system, a number of clinical system tests can be designed to test the most important functions of the system, using normal clinical use of the system. This test protocol can use several routine cases to run through the entire planning process, including dose prescription and monitor unit calculations. Measuring doses in phantom for treatments for these cases may act as a final verification of the entire system, as well as verifying the self-consistency of the treatment process. These test cases may be designed with a graded level of complexity. For example, the following tests might be considered: (1) Square manual contour with several blocked fields; (2) Tangential breast plan with manual contour; (3) CT-based phantom plan with density correction; (4) 3-D plan with CT phantom, non-axial and non-coplanar fields, conformal blocking, etc.

QA for the Entire Clinical Planning and Treatment Process

After all the planning system testing has been performed, there is another major segment of the QA process which must be implemented. One main conclusion of our many years of experience trying to perform comprehensive QA testing for our 3-D planning system is that the most essential part of that QA program is neither dosimetric or non-dosimetric QA tests. The most important part of the program is in fact the implementation of a sophisticated treatment planning/delivery process which integrates as much QA as possible into the normal routine planning process. This helps make the planning for each patient as safe as possible.

There are three distinct reasons for the conclusion above. First, a modern 3-D planning system may be the result of many tens of person-years of work, and may consist of as much as one million lines of code. It is clear even a well-designed and implemented software system with a large amount of testing will still contain errors [28]. Therefore, there will always be software bugs, some of which will be important in some situations.

Secondly, these systems consist of complex data structures, algorithms, and a great deal of flexibility in input data. It is not difficult to convince oneself that it is impossible to perform exhaustive testing on any section of a planning system, let alone the entire system. For example, consider the tiling algorithm used to create 3-D solid surface descriptions from a series of parallel contours. A very wide assortment of situations can be imagined, where atypical or very complex contour data can be entered into the surface rendering algorithm. It is clearly not possible to perform an exhaustive test of all possible situations. Therefore, another type of quality assurance tool must be used to help assure the correct behavior of the algorithm. In this example, the necessary QA may just involve the visual inspection of the critical surfaces (the external surface, etc.) from several viewing angles, to assure that there is no catastrophic breakdown in the algorithm. In addition, routine cutting of contours from the relevant structures onto slices orthogonal to those used for contour entry (for example, onto sagittal and/or coronal cuts) can help demonstrate the integrity of the surfaces for each patient.

The third reason for building QA into the planning process is that the planning/delivery process involves a complex series of procedures and decisions. One of the most powerful aspects of 3-D planning systems is their flexibility. Use of self-consistency checks and other kinds of QA procedures can help prevent incorrect application of planning system features, or other problems caused by inappropriate use of the software or data. It is essential to develop a planning/delivery process which includes checks of patient and plan -specific decisions which have been made during the process.

Some examples of procedures which can fulfill this aim are listed below:

a. Routine Calculation Checks:

Inspection of the dosimetric aspects of each plan and its prescription and monitor unit calculation are of course essential. In the end, assuring that the dose delivered to the prescription point of each beam is correct is one of the most essential checks of the planning process.

b. Verification of Image Registration:

The use of multiple imaging modalities is becoming much more common in 3-D planning. While this typically means the use of CT and MR, it can also include much simpler issues, such as registering the treatment planning CT scan with the localization simulation coordinate system, which is based on orthogonal films and skin marks (for alignment with lasers). Checks on the alignment accuracy between different datasets is essential for accurate implementation of the CT-based plan on the real patient.

c. Sagittal and Coronal CT Reconstructions:

The use of CT reconstructions made in sagittal, coronal, or oblique planes can highlight numerous potential problems, while at the same time being a useful way to show 3-D characteristics of the plan. Problems with inconsistencies in the CT data due to table motion, patient movement, field-of-view changes, mislabeling or misreading of slice location information, etc. will be demonstrated by problems or artifacts in the reconstructed images.

d. 3-D surface Displays:

To create the 3-D structures which are used for planning, contours are typically drawn on serial axial CT slices. It is extremely difficult to envision the 3-D extent of these structures as one draws contours on one slice at a time, and there are volume averaging and other effects which can make contouring structures difficult. Viewing the 3-D surfaces created from these contours is essential to verifying that the contours are all consistent and realistic. Viewing a solid surface display of the target volume will quite often show several places where the surface looks unrealistic, and where inspection and perhaps editing of the contours used on a particular slice will make the volume more realistic and self-consistent. "Cutting" a contour from the 3-D surface onto orthogonal image(s) (CT sagittal and/or coronal) can also illustrate problems. Review of the 3-D surface and the "sculpting" of that surface which must be performed if there is a problem, help distinguish 2-D from 3-D planning.

e. Oblique CT image in thePplane of the Beam:

In 3-D, there are numerous aids that can be used to verify that plans are being performed correctly. For example, it is often difficult to determine how wedges should be oriented when fields are non-axial. Since many non-axial plans are just relatively standard wedge pair or 3-field plans, except that they are not in an axial plane, generation of an oblique CT image in the plane of the beams can make the determination and/or checking of wedge orientations very straightforward.

f. Patient Alignment Consistency Checks:

Verification that the patient is correctly positioned with respect to the treatment plan should be performed whenever possible, for example at the verification simulation, and when the patient begins treatment. This check uses comparison of BEV plots (with bony anatomy) or DRRs with the orthogonal simulator (or treatment) films taken to verify the isocenter of the plan. After the patient position and isocenter are verified, the field ports should also be verified. These checks require a good understanding of which anatomy to draw into the planning system, and how that anatomy projects onto films and BEV displays. The use of DRR displays rather than simple BEV plots can make this technique somewhat more straightforward, although it requires more technology (networking, digital imaging) to implement quantitatively.

g. Target Volume Checks:

As institutions begin to use CT-target volume definition rather than targets drawn on simulator films, the projection of the CT target volume onto BEV displays, and then onto the simulator films themselves, may help the physicians and other staff make the logical connection between the way targets are drawn with both the old and new techniques, improving the confidence of the staff in the newer techniques.

h. Point Dose Calculations:

Where possible, it is very helpful if the point to which the dose is prescribed, or the plan normalization point, are situated so that a hand calculation of the dose delivered to that point is possible. If that is the case, then one can verify that the total dose prescribed by the plan is actually being delivered, at least to one point inside the patient. This will help remove the possibility of any major dosimetric problems involving the wrong total dose to the patient.

i. SSD Checks:

It is possible, in the simulator and/or treatment machine, to measure the SSD to the central axis of each treatment field. This routine check measurement, when compared to the SSDs expected by the planning system, are a reasonably good check for large setup errors or other inconsistencies in the planning process. In a similar fashion, checks of the table coordinate which is required to set the isocenter at the correct spot inside the patient is a similar candidate for a consistency check that will show possible errors in SSD indicator or other machine-related or planning system-related problems that might affect the correctness of the treatment.

Summary

This work describes a framework which can be used to organize the clinical quality assurance testing which is appropriate for a modern 3-D treatment planning system, and the planning/delivery process with which it is used.. A detailed description of this approach is presented 1) to highlight the kind of detail which must often be considered, and 2) to broaden the scope of quality assurance as it should be applied to treatment planning. The broad scope of testing required for 3-D systems has not been discussed in the literature, and is in direct contradiction to much earlier literature on planning system QA in which dose calculation verification is the main (and sometimes only) type of testing which is suggested. Clearly, the expansion in the scope of the entire treatment planning process is responsible for the analogous expansion in QA requirements.

The extent of possible tests which are described here will likely be daunting to most workers in the field. However, the very sophistication which requires so much attention to QA concerns also makes those QA tasks easier. First, from a clinical physics point of view, the most critical planning system testing and documentation is that which is related to functions which are used in clinical practice. Therefore, it is possible to develop a QA program which concentrates on those capabilities of the system which are clinically used. As desire for new clinical capabilities grows, then the QA work on those functions can then be performed. The QA program thus evolves along with the clinical use of the system.

Another aspect of 3-D planning systems which makes the QA tractable is that system capabilities can be used to help self-test various functions. Attention to design and implementation of the clinical planning/delivery process cam allow most critical aspects of the system to be checked while performing each plan. This is facilitated if the entire process is designed with detailed knowledge of the planning system design. Implementation of this process-based QA thus is the responsibility of all members of the radiotherapy department, and can lead to considerable awareness of the capabilities and limitations of the entire process with which we treat our patients.

Acknowledgments

The authors would like to thank Robin Stern, Ph.D., Lon Marsh, CMD, Paul Archer, CMD, Beth Yanke, CMD, Peter Roberson, Ph.D., Randall Ten Haken, Ph.D., Marc Kessler, Ph.D. and many other members of the department for their helpful comments and suggestions.

References

1.   Kutcher GJ et al.: Report of Task Group 40 of the Radiation Therapy Committee of the AAPM, 1993.

2.   McCullough EC, Krueger AM: Performance evaluation of computerized treatment planning systems for radiotherapy: external photon beams. Int J Radiat Oncol Biol Phys 6:1599-1605, 1980.

3.   Westmann CF, Mijnheer BJ, van Kleffens HJ: Determination of the accuracy of different computer planning systems for treatment with external photon beams. Radiother and Oncol 1:339-347, 1984.

4.   Sauer O, Nowak G, Richter J: Accuracy of dose calculations of the Philips treatment planning system OSS for blocked fields. in The Use of Computers In Radiation Therapy, eds. Bruinvis IAD, van der Giessen PH, van Kleffens HJ, Wittkamper FW, (eds) Elsevier Science Publishers BV, North-Holland, 1987 p 57-60.

5.   Rosenow UF, Dannhausen H-W, Lu(e)bbert K, Nu(e)sslin F, Richter J, Robrandt B, Seelentag W-W, Wendhausen H: Quality assurance in treatment planning. Report from the German Task Group. in The Use of Computers In Radiation Therapy, eds. Bruinvis IAD, van der Giessen PH, van Kleffens HJ, Wittkamper FW, (eds) Elsevier Science Publishers BV, North-Holland, 1987, p 45-58.

6.   Curran B, Starkschall G: A program for quality assurance of dose planning computers. In Starkschall G, Horton JL (eds) Quality Assurance in Radiotherapy Physics, Med Phys Publishing, Madison Wisc, p 207-228, 1991.

7.   Ten Haken RK, Kessler ML, Stern RL, Ellis JH, Niklason LT: Quality assurance of CT and MRI for radiation therapy treatment planning. In Starkschall G, Horton JL (eds) Quality Assurance in Radiotherapy Physics, Med Phys Publishing, Madison Wisc, p 73-103, 1991.

8.   Fraass BA, McShan DL: 3-D Treatment Planning: I. Overview of a clinical planning system. In: Bruinvis IAD, van der Giessen PH, van Kleffens HJ, Wittkamper FW (eds) The Use of Computers In Radiation Therapy. Elsevier Science Publishers BV, North-Holland, p 273-276, 1987.

9.   Fraass BA, McShan DL, Ten Haken RK, Hutchins KM: 3-D treatment planning: V. A fast 3-D photon calculation model. The Use of Computers in Radiation Therapy, ed., IAD Bruinvis, et al. Elsevier Science Publishers BV, (North-Holland), 521-525, 1987.

10. Fraass BA: Clinical application of 3-D treatment planning, in Advances in Radiation Oncology Physics: Dosimetry, Treatment Planning, and Brachytherapy. Ed. JA Purdy. American Institute of Physics, Woodbury NY, 1992. pp. 967-997.

11. Fraass BA, McShan DL, Diaz RF, Ten Haken RK, Aisen A, Gebarski S, Glazer G, Lichter AS: Integration of MRI into radiation therapy treatment planning. Int J Rad Oncol Biol Phys 13:1897-1908, 1987.

12. Fraass BA, McShan DL, Weeks KJ: 3-D treatment planning: III. Complete beam's-eye-view planning capabilities", in The Use of Computers In Radiation Therapy, eds. Bruinvis IAD, van der Giessen PH, van Kleffens HJ, Wittkamper FW, (eds) Elsevier Science Publishers BV, North-Holland, p 193-196, 1987.

13. Fraass BA, McShan DL, Weeks KJ: Computerized beam shaping, in Computers in Medical Physics, (Med. Physics Monograph 17), ed. Benedetto AR, Huang HK, Ragan DP (eds) publ. by Amer Inst Physics, Woodbury NY, p 333-340, 1990.

14. McShan DL, Fraass BA, Lichter AS: Full integration of the beam's eye view concept into computerized treatment planning. Int J Rad Oncol Biol Phys, 18:1485-1494, 1990.

15. McShan DL, Fraass BA: 3-D treatment planning: II. Integration of gray scale images and solid surface graphics, in The Use of Computers In Radiation Therapy, eds. I.A.D. Bruinvis, P.H. van der Giessen, H.J. van Kleffens, F.W. Wittkamper. Elsevier Science Publishers B.V., (North-Holland), pp 41-44, 1987.

16. McShan DL, Fraass BA: Use of an octree-like geometry for 3-D dose calculations. Med Phys 20: 1219-1228, 1993.

17. McShan DL, Fraass BA, Ten Haken RK: Dosimetric verification of a 3-D electron pencil beam dose calculation algorithm. Med Phys, in press, 1993.

18. McShan DL, Ten Haken RK, Fraass BA: 3-D treatment planning: IV. Integrated brachytherapy treatment planning, in The Use of Computers In Radiation Therapy, eds. I.A.D. Bruinvis, P.H. van der Giessen, H.J. van Kleffens, F.W. Wittkamper. Elsevier Science Publishers B.V., (North-Holland), pp 249-252, 1987.

19. McShan DL, Matrone G, Fraass BA, Lichter AS: A large screen digitizer system for radiation therapy treatment planning. In press, Int J Radiat Oncol Biol Phys, 1992.

20. Ten Haken RK, Diaz RF, McShan DL, Fraass BA, Taren JA, Hood TW: From manual to 3-D computerized treatment planning for 125-I stereotactic brain implants. Int J Radiat Oncol Biol Phys 15:467-480, 1988.

21. Lichter AS, Sandler HM, Robertson JR, Lawrence TS, Ten Haken RK, McShan DL, Fraass BA: Clinical Experience with Three-Dimensional Treatment Planning. Sem Rad Onc 2: 257-266, 1992.

22. Stern RL, Fraass BA, Gerhardsson A, McShan DL, Lam KL: Generation and use of measurement-based 3-D dose distributions for 3-D dose calculation verification. Med Phys 19:165-174, 1992.

23. Shiu AS, Tung S, Hogstrom KR, Wong JW, Gerber RL, Harms WB, Purdy JA, Ten Haken RK, McShan DL, Fraass BA: Verification data for electron beam dose calculation algorithms. Med PHys 19: 623-636, 1992.

24. Ten Haken RK, Fraass BA, Jost RJ: Practical methods of electron depth-dose measurement comapred to use of the NACP design chamber in water. Med Phys 14: 1060-1066, 1987.

25. Purdy JA, Biggs PJ, Bowers C, Dally E, Downs W, Fraass BA, Karzmark CJ, Khan F, Morgan P, Morton R, Palta J, Rosen II, Thorson T, Svensson G, Ting J: Medical accelerator safety considerations: Report of AAPM Radiation Therapy Committee Task Group 35, Med Phys 20: 1261-1275, 1993.

26. Bezier B: Software System Testing and Quality Assurance. Van Nostrand Reinhold, New York, 1984.

27. Meyers GJ: The art of software testing. John Wiley and Sons, New York, 1979.

28. Jacky J, White CP: Testing a 3-D radiation therapy planning program, Int J Rad Oncol Biol Phys 17:253-261, 1990.

29. Wittkamper RW, Mijnheer BJ, van Kleffens HJ: Dose intercomparison at the radiotherpy centers in The Netherlands. 2. Accuracy of locally applied computer planning systems for external photon beams. Radiother and Oncol 11:405-414, 1988.

30. Lepinoy D, Aletti P, Boisserie G, Bouhnick H, Estrade G, Hoornaert MT, Horiot JC, Piret P, Piron A, Redon C, Rosenwald JC: (SFPH) Quality assurance program for computers in radiotherapy: progress report. IEEE, p 322-327, 1984.

31. Thomas SJ, Wilkinson ID, Dixon AK, Dendy PP: Magnetic resonance imaging of Fricke-doped agarose gels for the visualization of radiotherapy dose distributions in a lung phantom. Br J Radiol, 65(770):167-9, 1992.

32. van de Geijn J, Fraass BA: The net fractional depth dose: a basis for a unified analytical description of FDD, TAR, TMR, and TPR. Med Phys 11: 784-793, 1984.

33. Photon Treatment Planning Working Group: Three Dimensional Dose Calculations for Radiation Therapy Treatment Planning. Int J Rad Oncol Biol Phys 21: 25-36, 1991.

34. Mackie TR, Bielajew AF, Rogers DWO, Battista JJ: Generation of photon energy deposition kernels using the EGS Monte Carlo code. Phys Med Biol 33:1-20, 1988.

35. Ahnesjo A: Collapsed cone convolution of radiant energy for photon dose calculation in heterogeneous media. Med Phys 16:577-592, 1989.

36. Burman C, Kutcher GJ, Hunt M, Brewster L: Acceptance testing criteria for a CT based 3-D treatment planning system. Med Phys 16:465, 1989 [Abstract].

37. Kessler ML, McShan DL, Fraass BA: Displays for Three-Dimensional Treatment Planning. Sem Rad Onc 2: 226-234, 1992.

38. Chen GTY, Pelizzari CA: Image correlation techniques in radiation therapy treatment planning. Comp Med Imaging and Graphics 13:235-240, 1989.

39. Kessler ML, Pitluck S, Petti P, Castro JR: Integration of multimodality imaging data for radiotherapy treatment planning. Int J Rad Oncol Biol Phys 21:1653-1667, 1991.

40. Pelizzari CA, Chen GTY: Registration of multiple diagnostic imaging scans using surface fitting. In: Bruinvis IAD, van der Giessen PH, van Kleffens HJ, Wittkamper FW (eds) The Use of Computers In Radiation Therapy. Elsevier Science Publishers BV, North-Holland, p 437-440, 1987.

41. Brewster L, Mageras GS, Mohan R: Automatic generation of beam apertures: Med Phys 20: 1337-1342, 1993.

42. Drzymala RE, Mohan R, Brewster L, Chu J, Goitein M, Harms W, Urie M: Dose volume histograms. Int J Rad Oncol Biol Phys 21:71-78, 1991.

43. Lawrence TS, Tesser RJ, Ten Haken RK: An application of dosevolume histograms to treatment of intrahepatic malignancies with radiation therapy. Int J Radiat Oncol Biol Phys 19:1041-1047, 1990.

44. Lyman JT: Complication probability as assessed from dose volume histograms. Rad Res 104:5-13-S-19, 1985.

45. Lyman JT, Wolbarst AB: Optimization of radiation therapy III: A method of assessing complication probabilities from dose volume histograms. Int J Radiat Oncol Biol Phys 13:103-109, 1987.

46. Lyman JT, Wolbarst AB: Optimization of radiation therapy IV: A dose volume histogram reduction method. Int J Radiat Oncol Biol Phys 17:433-436, 1989.

47. Burman C, Kutcher GJ, Emami B, Goitein M: Fitting of normal tissue tolerance data to an analytical function. Int J Rad Oncol Biol Phys 21:123-135, 1991.

48. Goitein M, Schulthesis TE: Strategies for treating possible tumor extension: some theoretical considerations. Int J Rad Oncol Biol Phys 11:1519, 1985.

49. Lawrence TS, Ten Haken RK, Kessler ML, Robertson JM, Lyman JT Lavigne ML, DuRoss DJ, Brown MB, Andrews JC, Ensminger WD, Lichter AS: The use of dose-volume analysis to predict radiation hepatitis. Int J Oncol Bio Phys 23:781-788, 1992.

Chapter 9

Clinical Experience with 3-D Radiotherapy: The University of Michigan Experience

Theodore S. Lawrence, M.D., Ph.D., Randall K. Ten Haken, Ph.D., Howard M. Sandler, M.D., Mark B. Hazuka, M.D., John M. Robertson, M.D., Mary K. Martel, Ph.D., Marc L. Kessler, Ph.D., Andrew T. Turrisi, M.D, Benedick A. Fraass, Ph.D., Allen S. Lichter, M.D.

Department of Radiation Oncology, University of Michigan Medical Center, Ann Arbor, Michigan

Since three dimensional radiation treatment planning (3-D RTP) was initiated at the University of Michigan in 1985, sufficient experience has accumulated that it is possible to begin to evaluate the toxicity and efficacy of treatment. In this paper, we will summarize our maturing results concerning intrahepatic, lung, and prostate cancer, as well as our preliminary results concerning high grade gliomas and parotid sparing techniques in the treatment of head and neck cancer. Reviews focusing on the conceptual framework and technical aspects of 3-D RTP at the University of Michigan have been published recently (7,11).

Before describing treatment results, it is worthwhile to begin with brief a overview of the general concepts of protocol design using 3-D RTP. Our long term goal of 3-D RTP has been to escalate target dose without producing unacceptable toxicity. This goal is based on the hypothesis that an increase in dose will improve local control which, in appropriately chosen malignancies, would be anticipated to improve survival (18). For intrahepatic cancers, local control is virtually never achieved using conventional radiation doses. For lung cancer, local failure is a prominent factor in producing morbidity and mortality. For prostate cancer, recent evidence shows an alarmingly high rate of positive biopsies after treatment with conventional radiation doses. In all these cases, the ability to deliver high doses has been limited by toxicity of normal tissues which are unavoidably irradiated using convention RTP. Therefore, these appear to be promising sites for the application of 3-D RTP techniques.

The escalation of target dose can, in general, come about through three related aspects of a full 3-D treatment planning system (discussed in more detail below). First, integration of image-based anatomic data with beam's eye view (BEV) displays allows a 3-D appreciation of the relationship of conformal beam edges to both tumor and normal tissues. This helps ensure that the target is adequately treated while minimizing treatment of normal tissues. Second, 3-D RTP permits the use of beams of which are not confined to the axial plane (19). These non-axial beams often treat less critical normal tissue than traditional axial beams. Third, correlation of the 3-D dose distribution with patient anatomy can lead to a better understanding of the volume dependence of normal tissue toxicity. This improved understanding should permit increased target doses which approach, but not exceed, organ tolerance. Such knowledge is essential in the treatment of tumors within organs whose tolerance exhibits strong volume dependence, such as the lung and liver.

Although we have developed 3-D based clinical protocols in a variety of sites, it is possible to identify a general theme in dose escalation protocol development. We have begun with estimates of the whole and partial tolerance of the dose limiting normal structures based on the available clinical data and the judgment of experienced clinicians (for one such summary see (2)). These clinical estimates were used to determine starting points for dose escalation studies described below. 3-D RTP was used to design fields which delivered the highest possible target dose within the estimated constraints of critical normal tissue tolerance. Although preliminary results indicate that these higher doses have increased tumor control, treatment was associated with a low (but non-zero) frequency of complications. These complication data have been analyzed retrospectively to obtain a more accurate assessment for the volume and dose dependence of normal tissue toxicity.

The information derived from these analyses can be used in a NTCP model to design dose escalation protocols which would be anticipated to permit the safe delivery of higher doses of radiation than are currently possible using conventional techniques. In one approach (20), iso-NTCP contours are generated as a function of dose and partial volume using parameters derived from the retrospective analysis. To determine the dose escalation scheme, single step dose volume histograms (DVHs) are generated from the 3-D dose distributions using the effective volume (V_{eff}) method of histogram reduction (8). In this approach, V_{eff} is a function only of the relative dose distribution (% isocenter dose), rather than the dose itself (Gy). Therefore, bins containing a range of V_{eff} values can be constructed which will subject patients to a particular NTCP (with an arbitrarily small range) prior to the assignment of dose (Gy). The doses for each bin of V_{eff} values can then be escalated independently (Figure 9-1). This scheme is currently being used in our dose escalation study for patients with lung cancer and it is anticipated that it will be applied to patients with intrahepatic malignancies in the future.

Intrahepatic cancers

3-D RTP and Tumor Response

Surgeons have shown that parts of the liver can be safely resected as long as an adequate volume of normal liver is preserved. Likewise, although the tolerance of the whole liver to irradiation is quite low ($\approx$ 30-33 Gy), it is well known that parts of the liver can be treated with high doses without untoward effects as long as an adequate volume of normal liver is not incapacitated. There were two main difficulties in applying high dose radiation to the liver. First, the tolerance of the liver to partial organ tolerance could not be quantified. Second, standard techniques in which beams are confined to the axial plane often treat large volumes of normal liver, especially for deep tumors.

The introduction of 3-D RTP techniques changed this situation dramatically. We initially showed that the use of beams that are not in the axial plane could reduce the dose to the normal liver while encompassing the target volume with adequate homogeneity (19). We were then able to design a clinical protocol based on the volume of normal liver treated (10). In this protocol, the 3-D dose data for the most promising plans were expressed in terms of DVHs. The planning process placed patients into one of three categories: focal, high dose ($\geq$ 60 Gy); focal, moderate dose ($\approx$ 48 Gy); diffuse (whole liver only treated with 33 - 36 Gy). Treatment was delivered with concurrent intraarterial hepatic fluorodeoxyuridine as a radiation sensitizer.

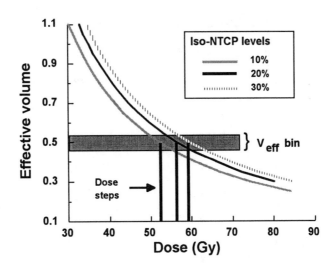

Figure 9-1. *Theoretical scheme for dose escalation for patients with intrahepatic cancer. Iso-NTCP curves, based on our recalculation of the parameters of the Lyman NTCP model (8), are overlaid on a plot of dose versus effective volume. For patients whose plan had an effective volume between 0.48 and 0.52 ("V$_{eff}$ bin:" stippled bar), the first step of this dose escalation protocol would be 52 Gy (10% iso-NTCP curve). After an adequate number of patients had been entered without evidence of toxicity, the dose would be escalated to 56 Gy (20% iso-NTCP curve) and then to 59 Gy (30% iso-NTCP curve). See text for details.*

We have recently published the results of treatment of unresectable primary hepatobiliary cancer (15). A total of 26 patients were treated, 20 of whom had focal disease. For patients with focal disease there was a 70% 2 year actuarial freedom from hepatic progression (Figure 9-2); the median survival in this group was 19.4 months, compared to 4-10 months usually found for similar patients. Thus, the application of 3-D RTP in this phase II study appeared to produce a substantial improvement compared to other non-surgical series; indeed, the median survival approaches that obtained by surgical resection (in what is probably a more favorable group of patients).

3-D RTP and Toxicity

We have also analyzed the toxicity of treatment in our entire series of patients (9). Of our first 79 patients treated, 9 developed radiation hepatitis (all of whom had a component of whole liver irradiation in their treatment). We attempted to apply the NTCP model developed by Lyman (12) (using the histogram reduction method of Kutcher and Burman (8)) with literature-based parameters (1) to our 3-D data and observed complications. We found that the model with the literature-based parameters accurately predicted the toxicity of whole liver irradiation. However, the risk of radiation hepatitis resulting from focal irradiation was greatly overestimated. We recalculated the parameters based on our data, and found that if the volume effect parameter (n) were increased from the literature based estimate of 0.32 to 0.69 an excellent fit of our clinical data could be obtained. These findings suggest that it will be possible to use NTCP models to predict complications in volume effect organs such as the liver (although it will take independent data to determine if the recalculated parameters have predictive value).

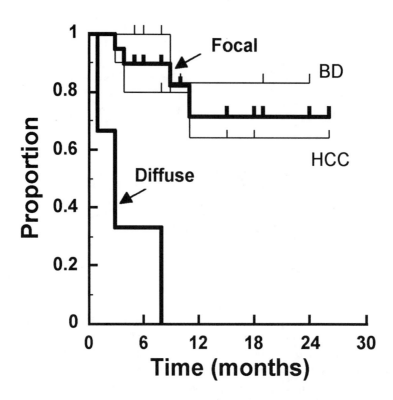

Figure 9-2.   *Hepatic progression free survival for patients with primary hepatobiliary cancer treated with 3-D planned radiation. Graph shows Kaplan-Meier plot of 20 patients with focal disease and 6 patients with diffuse disease treated with intraarterial hepatic fluorodeoxyuridine and radiation as described in the text. An event is defined as any evidence of recurrence in the liver (1 failure in field, 3 failures elsewhere in liver). (Reprinted with permission from reference 13.)*

Although we were encouraged by these results, we felt that a limitation to this approach was the need for reduction of the non-uniform dose-volume distribution to a single partial volume uniformly irradiated to a single dose. This extra step, which depends on n, makes it difficult to see the direct relationship between the actual (non-uniform) DVH and toxicity. Recently, comprehensive biologically based models have been developed which describe heterogeneous irradiation of organs exhibiting a parallel architecture (5,14). Along similar lines, we have been motivated to search for a simpler approach that permits a more direct visualization of the relationship between the DVH and the risk of radiation hepatitis.

This simplified approach is based on two assumptions. The first is that the fraction, f, of a macroscopic volume element of liver incapacitated by dose D can be described by a simple response function; for example, a sigmoid curve (logistic function):

$$f = \frac{1}{(1 + (D_{50}/D)^k)}$$ (1)

where D_{50} is the dose which incapacitates half of the volume and k describes the steepness of the sigmoid function. The fraction of the entire liver (F) incapacitated is, therefore, the sum of the incapacitated fractions from each bin of the differential dose volume histogram. The second assumption is that a complication occurs when F exceeds a critical value and that this fraction can be represented as another response function across the population; for example, another sigmoid curve:

$$NTCP = \frac{1}{(1 + (F_{50}/F)^j)}$$

(2)

where F_{50} is the fraction of liver incapacitated which would produce a 50% complication rate across the population and j describes the steepness of the sigmoid function. We have begun analyzing our previous complication data using this simple approach as well as with use of a more comprehensive model (6). Although we have not yet optimized the parameters of equation 1, reasonable values of D_{50} and k produce a realistic ordering of patients, with an increased complication rate among patients with a higher calculated F.

Lung

3-D RTP and Tumor Response

3-D RTP has permitted an aggressive approach in the primary treatment of non-small cell lung cancer patients who are not surgical candidates. The results of treatment were recently summarized for 88 consecutive patients diagnosed with either medically inoperable or locally advanced unresectable non-small cell lung cancer who were treated with thoracic irradiation with radical intent (4). The purpose of this review was to use our experience with high dose treatment to establish a starting point for a dose escalation study for the treatment of lung cancer. All of the high-dose patients save four underwent 3-D RTP. Patients received radiation alone in standard fractionation (uncorrected isocenter dose of 60-74 Gy (median 67.6 Gy)) and have been followed for 12 - 72 months (median follow-up > 24 months).

The study found that the median survival time for the entire group of patients was 15 months, which compares favorably to similar patients treated either with radiation alone or combined modality therapy. More importantly with respect to the underlying hypothesis of 3-D RTP, this relatively high dose treatment was well tolerated. There were no treatment related deaths and only 1 patient evidenced grade 4 radiation pneumonitis. However, local failure (either as sole first site or as component with distant failure) occurred in 62% of patients in whom first site of failure could be determined. The fact that patients with Stage III disease who received more than the median dose had significantly longer disease free survival and greater overall survival than patients who received less than the median dose suggests that a radiation dose response curve may exist in the clinically achievable range (Figure 9-3). Some patients were treated with large fields (including prophylactic lymph node irradiation) while others were treated with small fields addressing the tumor only; the survival and failure rate of these two groups were similar.

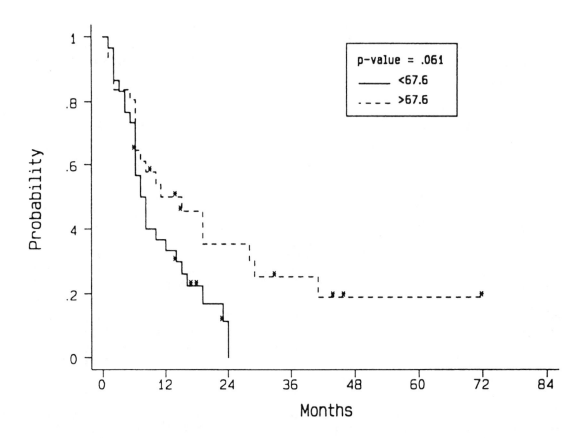

Figure 9-3. *Survival as a function of dose in patients with Stage III non-small cell lung cancer treated radically with 3-D planned radiation. Kaplan-Meier plot of 69 patients with unresectable or medically inoperable Stage III non-small cell lung cancer treated with radiation therapy as described in the text. Two groups were formed by using the median dose for all patients treated. (Reprinted with permission from reference 4.)*

The findings that: a) local failure remains a problem, b) there appears to be a dose response relationship, c) there were few complications with 3-D guided radiation and d) small fields produced similar results to large fields suggests that higher doses may be feasible and important. Therefore, a radiation dose escalation trial was initiated for patients with unresectable lung cancer. Patients are segregated by volume of normal lung treated, and dose will be systematically increased for each patient bin after safety is established at each level.

3-D RTP and Toxicity

In addition to this analysis of the outcome of patients treated with 3-D RTP, a detailed analysis of the dose and volume dependence of pulmonary toxicity has recently been carried out (13). In this study, radiation pneumonitis (any grade) was observed in 14 of 63 patients (5/21 patients with Hodgkin's disease; 9/42 patients with lung cancer) who had undergone 3-D RTP. Dose volume histograms were analyzed in a fashion similar to that used for the liver (see above) and NTCPs were calculated using literature-based parameters. It was found that the literature parameters gave a reasonable description of the data for patients with Hodgkin's disease (Figure 9-4). However, the results with the lung cancer patients were more variable. A likely explanation for the greater variability of the lung cancer data is that, in contrast to patients with Hodgkin's disease, patients with lung cancer typically have significant pulmonary compromise.

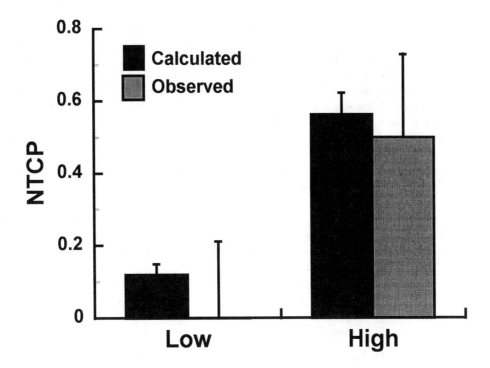

Figure 9-4.   *Prediction of radiation pneumonitis in patients with Hodgkin's disease. 21 patients with Hodgkin's disease (out of a total of approximately 120 patients with Hodgkin's disease treated at the University of Michigan during the same time period) were irradiated after 3-D RTP. The observed risk of complication (stippled bar) is compared to the calculated NTCP, based on the Lyman model with parameters from the literature (except that the TD_{50} was corrected for lung inhomogeneity ($n = 0.87$, $m = 0.18$; $TD_{50} = 28$ Gy.) The two groups were formed by using the median NTCP for all patients treated. Error bars: 80% confidence interval for observed NTCP; standard error for calculated NTCP.*

Prostate

In contrast to intrahepatic and lung cancer, in which median follow-up times of 24-36 months are adequate to begin to assess the impact of 3-D RTP on local control and survival, prostate cancer requires a significantly longer interval. Therefore, it is premature to attempt to analyze the clinical efficacy of treatment. However, the available 3-D RTP data does permit a toxicity analysis, which has recently been performed on 539 prostate cancer patients (treated at the University of Michigan and Providence Hospitals between 1987-92). All had a treatment planning CT scan, multiple structures contoured on the axial images, and BEV conformal beams edited to provide 3-D dose coverage. 389 patients had T1-T2 tumors, 102 had T3-T4 tumors, and 48 were treated post-prostatectomy. Pelvic lymph nodes were treated in 330 patients. Prostate boosts were delivered with 4-field axial, 6-field axial, or 4-field oblique, non-axial fields. The median isocenter dose was 68.4 Gy (range 59.4-80.4). Median follow-up is 16 months; 116 have been followed more than 3 years. Toxicity was graded using the RTOG system.

A total of 65 complications have been noted in this series. Most episodes of rectal morbidity have been mild: 55 grade 1 or 2. There have been only 10 more serious complications including eight grade 3 (6 have resolved) and two grade 4. The actual risk of a grade 3 or 4 complication is 3% at 3 and 5 years (16).

A subset of 38 patients in this group have been treated on a formal dose escalation trial. In this trial, which was initiated in 1987, patients with T3-T4 prostate cancer have been treated with escalating doses of 3-D planned radiation, beginning with 76 Gy (isocenter dose; minimal tumor dose $\geq$ 95% isocenter dose). When our initial results showed that this was tolerable (17), we escalated the dose to the current level of 80 Gy. Only one patient in this group has suffered a grade 4 complication (colostomy); there have been 2 mild grade 3 events. Thus, the 5 year actuarial risk of grade a 3 or 4 complication is approximately 10% (Figure 9-5), which is similar to the complication rate reported for conventional radiation doses (65 - 70 Gy) delivered using standard techniques. Therefore, it appears that 3-D RTP has permitted at least a 10 - 15% dose escalation above standard dose levels without a significant increase in complications, and dose limiting toxicity has not yet been reached.

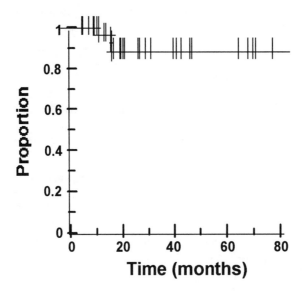

Figure 9-5. *Rectal complications from treatment of T3-T4 prostate cancer using a dose escalation protocol. Kaplan Meier plot of grade 3 or 4 rectal toxicity for 38 patients with T3-T4 prostate cancer who were treated under the dose escalation protocol described in the text.*

Preliminary Studies

High Grade Gliomas

We have begun a radiation dose escalation study to treat patients with high grade brain tumors. One feature of 3-D RTP, unique to the treatment of brain tumors thus far, is the ability to incorporate MR directly into the planning process by 3-D image registration of the MR data set with the CT data set (needed to supply density data) (21). Since the image data sets can be manipulated and registered to correct for differences in patient position during the acquisition of the CT and the MR, the MR need not be obtained in the radiotherapy treatment position. This facilitates the use of MR images obtained previously for diagnostic purposes and eliminates the expense and inconvenience of repeating an MR for RT-planning alone. Thirty three patients have been entered into the study. Twenty-one were treated to 70 Gy and, when no toxicity was observed, the 80 Gy dose level was opened. Since October 1992, 12 patients have been treated to 80 Gy without detectable toxic reaction. After additional patient accrual, if morbidity remains acceptable, further escalation is anticipated.

Parotid Sparing in the Treatment of Head and Neck Cancer

In addition to the organ-specific dose-escalation projects discussed above, 3-D RTP provides us the opportunity to reduce the toxicity associated with external beam irradiation. Xerostomia is a frequent complication and major cause of morbidity in patients receiving head and neck irradiation. We recently activated a parotid sparing protocol in which the contralateral normal parotid gland is completely spared using BEV technology. A feasibility study in the first 12 patients suggested that this approach was feasible in most cases (3). Resting and stimulated parotid salivary flow measurements are obtained and correlated with parotid DVHs. A preliminary analysis of this study suggests that patients are able to maintain salivation and complain less frequently of a dry mouth when treated with parotid sparing 3-D RTP.

Summary

We feel we have made substantial progress in the application of 3-DRTP to improve patient outcome. In the case of intrahepatic cancers, 3-D planned high dose radiation appears to improve both local control and, more importantly, survival. For patients with lung cancer and prostate cancer, 3-DRTP permits the safe delivery of high doses of radiation with acceptable complication rates. Dose escalation trials based on our previous 3-DRTP experience should permit us to determine if these higher doses of radiation can improve local control and survival in sites other than the liver. These trials should be facilitated by the recent acquisition of a computer-controlled Racetrack Microtron. It is anticipated that this device will permit us to increase target dose still further by permitting us to treat multiple field plans that produce dose distributions which conform to the target more precisely than is possible with a conventional linear accelerator.

Acknowledgements

This work was supported in part by P01-CA59827, an American Cancer Society Career Development Award (T.S.L), and an American Society for Clinical Oncology Career Development Award (J.M.R).

References

1. Burman, C.; Kutcher, G. J.; Emami, B.; Goitein, M. Fitting of normal tissue tolerance data to an analytic function. Int. J. Radiat. Oncol. Biol. Phys. 21:123-135;1991.

2. Emami, B.; Lyman, J.; Brown, A.; Coia, L.; Goitein, M.; Munzenrider, J. E.; Shank, B.; Solin, L. J.; Wesson, M. Tolerance of normal tissue to therapeutic irradiation. Int. J. Radiat. Oncol. Biol. Phys. 21:109-122;1991.

3. Hazuka, M. B.; Martel, M. K., Marsh, L., Lichter, A. S.; Wolf, G. T. Preservation of parotid function after external beam irradiation in head and neck cancer patients: a feasibility study using 3-dimensional treatment planning. Int J Radiat Oncol Biol Phys;(in press).

4. Hazuka, M. B.; Turrisi, A. T.; Lutz, S. T.; Martel, M. K.; Ten Haken, R. K.; Strawderman, M.; Borema, L.; Lichter, A. S. Results of high-dose thoracic irradiation incorporating beam's eye view display in non-small cell lung cancer: Int. J. Radiat. Oncol. Biol. Phys.;(in press).

5. Jackson, A.; Kutcher, G. J. Probability of radiation-induced complication for normal tissues with parallel architecture subject to non-uniform irradiation. Med. Phys. 20:613-625;1993.

6. Jackson, A.; Ten Haken, R. K.; Lawrence, T. S.; Kessler, M. L.; Kutcher, G. J. Analysis of clinical complication data from radiation hepatitis using a parallel architecture model. To be presented at the American Society for Therapeutic Radiology and Oncology, New Orleans, LA, October, 11-15, 1993. (Abst.)

7. Kessler, M. L.; McShan, D. L.; Fraass, B. A. Displays for three-dimensional treatment planning. Seminars in Radiation Oncology 2:226-234;1992.

8. Kutcher, G. J., Burman, C.; Brewster, L.; Goitein, M.; Mohan, R. Calculation of complication probability factors for nonuniform tissue irradiation: The effective volume method. Int. J. Radiat. Oncol. Biol. Phys. 16:1623-1630;1989.

9. Lawrence, T. S.; Ten Haken, R. K.; Kessler, M. L.; Robertson, J. M.; Lyman, M. T.; Lavigne, M. L.; Duross, D. J.; Brown, M. B.; Andrews, J. C.; Ensminger, W. D.; Lichter, A. S. The use of 3-D dose volume analysis to predict radiation hepatitis. Int. J. Radiat. Oncol. Biol. Phys., 23:781-788;1992.

10. Lawrence, T. S.; Tesser, R. J.; Ten Haken, R. K. An application of dose volume histograms to the treatment of intrahepatic malignancies with radiation therapy. Int. J. Radiat. Oncol. Biol. Phys., 19:1041-1047;1990.

11. Lichter, A. S.; Sandler, H. M.; Robertson, J. M.; Lawrence, T. S.; Ten Haken, R. K.; McShan, D. L.; Fraass, B. A. Clinical experience with three-dimensional treatment planning. Seminars in Radiation Oncology 2:257-266;1992.

12. Lyman, J. T. Complication probability as assessed from dose volume histograms. Radiat. Res. 8(Suppl.) 513-519;1985.

13. Martel, M. K.; Ten Haken, R. K.; Hazuka, M. B.; Turrisi, A. T.; Fraass, B. A.; Lichter, A. S. Dose-volume histogram and 3-D treatment planning evaluation of patients with pneumonitis. Int. J. Radiat. Oncol. Biol. Phys.;(in press).

14. Niemierko, A.; Goitein, M. Modeling of normal tissue response to radiation: the critical volume model. Int. J. Radiat. Oncol. Biol. Phys. 25:135-145;1992.

15. Robertson, J. M.; Lawrence, T. S.; Dworzanin, L. A.; Andrews, J. C.; Walker, S.; Kessler, M. L.; Ensminger, W. D. Treatment of primary hepatobiliary cancers with conformal radiation therapy and regional chemotherapy. J. Clin. Oncol., 11:1286-1293;1993.

16. Sandler, H. M.; McLaughlin, P. W.; Ten Haken, R.; Addison, H.; Forman, J.; Lichter, A. 3-D conformal radiotherapy for the treatment of prostate cancer: Low risk of chronic rectal morbidity observed in a large series of patients. To be presented at the American Society for Therapeutic Radiology and Oncology, New Orleans, LA, October, 11-15;1993. (Abst.).

17. Sandler, H. M.; Perez-Tomayo, C.; Ten Haken, R. K.; Lichter, A. S. Dose escalation for stage C (T3) prostate cancer: Minimal rectal toxicity observed using conformal therapy. Radiother. Oncol. 23:53-54;1992.

18. Suit H. The scope of the problem of primary tumor control. Cancer 61:2141-2147; 1988.

19. Ten Haken, R. K.; Lawrence, T. S.; McShan, D. L.; Tesser, R. J.; Fraass, B. A.; Lichter, A. S. Technical considerations in the use of 3-D beam arrangements in the abdomen. Radiother. Oncol., 22:19-28;1991.

20. Ten Haken, R. K.; Martel, M. K.; Kessler, M. L.; Hazuka, M. B.; Lawrence, T. S.; Robertson, J. M.; Turrisi, A. T.; Lichter, A. S. Use of V_{eff} and iso-NTCP in the implementation of dose escalation protocols. Int. J. Radiat. Onc. Biol. Phys.;(in press).

21. Thornton, A. F., Sandler, H. M.; Ten Haken, R. K.; McShan, D. L.; Fraass, B. A.; LaVigne, M. L.; Yanke, B. R. The clinical utility of magnetic resonance imaging in 3-dimensional treatment planning of brain neoplasms. Int. J. Radiat. Oncol. Biol. Phys. 24:767-775; 1992.

Chapter 10

Clinical Experience with Three-Dimensional Radiation Therapy at the Memorial Sloan-Kettering Cancer Center[1]

Steven A. Leibel, M.D.,[*] Gerald J. Kutcher, Ph.D.,[**] John G. Armstrong, MB,[*] Michael J. Zelefsky, M.D.,[*] Louis B. Harrison, M.D.,[*] Chandra M. Burman, Ph.D.,[**] Radhe Mohan, Ph.D.,[**] C. Clifton Ling, Ph.D.,[**] Zvi Fuks, M.D.[*]

Departments of Radiation Oncology[*] and Medical Physics,[**]
Memorial Sloan Kettering Cancer Center, New York, New York

Three-dimensional conformal radiation therapy (3-D CRT) was introduced into clinical practice at the Memorial Sloan-Kettering Cancer Center (MSKCC) in 1988, after the design and implementation of a first-generation 3-D treatment planning system (1). A second generation system, based on new graphics and new treatment planning tools, is being readied for clinical use. To facilitate 3-D CRT delivery, new treatment machines equipped with multileaf collimators (MLCs) for field-shaping and beam scanning capabilities for radiation intensity modulation have also been introduced. An algorithm for conformal treatment verification, delivery and recording (CTVDR) was developed and implemented to provide a computer-controlled interface system between the treatment planning systems and treatment machines (2). Under such control systems one of the treatment machines at MSKCC, the Scanditronix MM50 Racetrack Microtron (MM50) (Scanditronix Medical Systems AB, Uppsala, Sweden), is fully capable of delivering automated multiple static, shaped fields in succession rapidly under full computer control and without human intervention. Furthermore, two of our Varian 2100C and one of our Varian 6100C linear accelerators (Varian Associates, Palo Alto, CA) have been retrofitted with MLCs. On-line real time imaging systems are being used to monitor automated treatments and to document their accuracy.

3-D CRT systems have now been implemented at MSKCC for treatment of locally advanced tumors of the prostate, lung, and nasopharynx (3). These represent primary tumors in which local control is poor with conventional radiotherapeutic approaches. Furthermore, in each of these disease entities radiation dose-response relationships have been observed, and the impact of improved local control on outcome can be tested (4). The feasibility and potential of the 3-D approach for these tumors was demonstrated in a series of preliminary studies (5,6,7). The findings confirmed that, when compared to the 2-D approach, 3-D techniques improved target coverage, reduced the volume of normal tissue receiving high radiation doses, and in the treatment of prostate carcinoma, decreased acute normal tissue morbidity. Based on these observations, a series of dose-escalation studies were designed. The MSKCC 3-D treatment planning and delivery procedures and preliminary observations from our dose-escalation studies are summarized in this review.

Treatment Planning

Whereas all of the available imaging methods may contribute to the acquisition of the detailed anatomical information required for 3-D treatment planning, dose calculation formalisms necessitate that the anatomical information be presented in terms of electron density ratios, which

---

[1] Supported in part by Grant CA 54749 from the National Cancer Institute, Department of Health and Human Services, Bethesda, Maryland.

can be obtained only from computerized axial tomography (CT) images (8). Magnetic resonance imaging studies may provide complementary information on tumor volume and adjacent normal organ definitions, and currently image correlation programs are under development to directly integrate this information into the treatment planning image data set. However, at the present time, the MSKCC treatment planning system is essentially CT-based.

Simulation, Image Acquisition, and Beam Definition

The simulation process incorporates a combination of traditional simulation and CT imaging. Individually designed immobilization devices (i.e., thermoplastic body casts for prostate, alpha cradle body molds for lung, and thermoplastic facial masks for nasopharynx) are fabricated to ensure that the patient can be positioned for planning and treatment in a reproducible fashion. Conventional simulators are used to determine the treatment position of the patient, to define a provisional isocenter, and to produce reference localization skin marks. CT scans are subsequently obtained with the patient in the immobilization device. Alignment lasers in the scanner room are matched to the skin marks, and the correct positioning of the patient and location of the isocenter are reconfirmed using anterior and lateral radiographic scout views. To produce high resolution 3-D reconstructions, consecutive CT images with a 0.3-0.5 cm slice thickness are obtained from approximately 3.0 cm above to 3.0 cm below the target volume. Additional images with a slice thickness of 1.0 cm are obtained above and below these levels with the extent based upon the region to be treated and the treatment technique to be used.

Contours of the target volume and surrounding normal tissues are drawn manually from the simulation CT slices using a track ball, whereas the contours of the body surface, lungs, head and neck air cavities and of bony structures can be outlined automatically using an edge-detection algorithm. For the prostate, the planning target volume (PTV) (9) is identified on each relevant CT slice by drawing a 1.0 cm margin around the CT-identifiable prostate tissue (gross target volume [GTV]) extending from the prostatic apex to the superior tips of the seminal vesicles, except at the interface with the rectum where a 0.6 cm margin is used. A 1.0 cm margin is added in the cephalad and caudad directions of the target volume using an auto-copy mode on the treatment planning system. The bladder wall, rectal wall, and pelvic small bowel are also contoured. The PTV for lung carcinoma is made up of the primary tumor and known nodal disease with a 1.5 to 2.0 cm margin of tissue to allow for microscopic tumor extension, treatment set-up errors, organ motion, and other uncertainties. The lung surfaces, heart, esophagus, and spinal cord are contoured as well. For planning nasopharyngeal tumors, a 1.0 cm margin is added to the CT-defined GTV. A wider margin is used when the borders are poorly visualized to ensure adequate target coverage. Critical organs of interest include the spinal cord, brain stem, temporal lobes, optic chiasm, retinas, lenses, parotid glands mandible and temporomandibular joints.

Target and normal tissue structure contours are delineated using a VAX 8810 dual cluster computer system (Digital Equipment Corporation, Mynard, MA) equipped with Lexidata 3700 graphical image processors (Lexidata, Billerica, MA) and AP 500 array processors (Analogic, Peabody, MA). The target volume and the normal organ images required for treatment planning and plan evaluation are reconstructed in 3-D and displayed with the beam's eye view (BEV) technique (10,11), using wire-frame graphics to delineate surfaces and color to distinguish different anatomical structures. To enhance the recognition of the spatial orientation of the BEV, reference images are concomitantly displayed, including the intersection of the beam on axial, sagittal, and coronal CT images through the isocenter. In addition, the treatment machine configurations, including gantry, couch, and collimator angles and collimator jaw positions, are shown in the BEV as a three panel representation of the treatment machine viewed from three orthogonal perspectives (1,3).

Beam apertures for cerrobend blocks are automatically shaped by applying a continuously varying aperture with a margin of 0.5 cm around the outline of the tumor target as reconstructed in the BEV mode to account for beam penumbra. For MLC fields each leaf is positioned to transect the original (cerrobend) aperture such that an equal, although somewhat different, volume is treated. Using this positioning approach and taking into account the effects of scatter within the patient, the contributions from many fields to the dose at each point in the patient and the influence of patient set-up uncertainty, the dose distributions for cerrobend- and MLC-shaped fields are virtually identical (12).

Dose Calculations

Dose distributions are calculated in 3-D using a pencil beam convolution algorithm with pixel-by-pixel inhomogeneity corrections on a 0.5 cm grid (8,13,14). In this technique, the broad radiation beam is divided into a large number of narrow beams (called pencils), and the dose is computed by summation of the contributions from each of the individual pencil beams. The computation formalism uses the convolution of Monte Carlo-generated 2-D pencil beam profiles (called pencil beam kernels) with photon fluence distributions to calculate dose distributions for irregularly shaped fields (13,14). Surface curvature and internal inhomogeneity corrections are performed using the conventional radiological pathlength technique (15).

Qualitative Treatment Plan Evaluation

Target coverage and critical normal tissue doses are evaluated by examining isodose surface distributions on 2-D midplane axial, sagittal, and coronal CT images. Color wash techniques, in which the pixels within a given dose range are assigned a specific color are displayed as CT overlays, are used to assess the difference in dose distributions between rival plans and for images of regret, in which regions of overdose to normal critical structures or of underdose to the target volume may be identified. The target dose is prescribed to the maximum isodose surface that completely encompasses the PTV. Dose inhomogeneity within the target volume generally varies from 4-10% for the prostate and lung, whereas in nasopharynx boost plans a small 20-25% volume of inhomogeneity is considered to be acceptable, provided that it is contained within the target volume and that it is remote from critical dose-limiting structures.

Quantitative Treatment Plan Evaluation

Cumulative dose-volume histograms (DVHs) are at the present time the most useful numerical treatment plan evaluation method (16,17). DVHs are generated for the tumor and for each organ of interest depending on the site treated, and compilations of such curves are used for comparing treatment plans. Although this approach had several well recognized limitations (3), we have found DVHs to be useful for evaluating and comparing rival treatment plans and for making therapeutic decisions. For example, rectal wall, bladder wall, and small bowel DVHs are used to determine the need for neoadjuvant cytoreductive hormonal therapy in prostate cancer patients. When the volume of any of these structures receiving the prescription dose exceeds limits that place the patient at a presumed increased risk of treatment-related complications (> 30% for rectal wall, [3]50% for bladder wall, and [3]65% for small bowel), a three month course of androgen deprivation therapy is given before proceeding with radiation therapy. We have observed significant reductions in the respective volumes irradiated in 89% of such patients. Although to date we have not observed even a moderate grade late rectal, bladder, or bowel complication by adhering to this treatment policy, longer follow-up will be required to establish the likelihood of complications in hormone-primed patients (18).

The most useful quantitative indices are normal tissue complication probabilities (NTCPs) (19-27) and tumor control probabilities (TCPs) (28,29), that condense structure-specific dose distribution data to yield a single number for each tissue of interest. Unfortunately, NTCP and TCP indices are at present based upon somewhat rudimentary models normalized to clinical endpoints that are generally not well established. Thus, their predictions should be viewed with caution. Nevertheless, their potential predictive power makes their development important. We calculate NTCP for all conformal plans according to the effective volume method of Kutcher et al. (20,21) and TCP using an algorithm by Goitein (28) in order to evaluate the consistency and accuracy of the models.

Although in some cases we have found that the absolute value of the calculations do not at all agree with clinical experience, in others they appear to be clinically consistent. Nevertheless, the calculations are still useful for ranking rival treatment plans, since certain systematic errors may cancel out. New approaches to refine the computation of NTCP and make it more consistent with clinical observations are currently under development at MSKCC (3,30,31).

Field Shaping

Once the plan evaluation process is completed and the optimal beam arrangement is selected, digitally reconstructed radiographs (DRRs), produced from the CT image set, are used to transfer the treatment portal outline onto simulator films. The patient is set-up with a simulator according to the treatment parameters defined by the 3-D plan. Radiographs are obtained and compared with anterior and lateral "set-up" field DRRs to confirm that the alignment of the patient is correct. Subsequently, a radiograph is obtained for each of the treatment fields, and the beam aperture block outline for each treatment field on the DRR is transferred onto the simulator films which are used as templates for cerrobend block fabrication and for comparison to treatment portal and verification films. For prostate cancer patients, conventional cerrobend blocking has been replaced by automated computer-driven MLCs. To guide the individual leaf positioning of the MLC during treatment, data are transferred directly from the 3-D treatment planning computer via the CTVDR system to the MM50 control computer or via diskette to the Varian MLC computer. The MLC leaf positions for each treatment field are also transferred from DRRs to simulator films for comparison with portal images.

Treatment Delivery

Since a larger number of beams will in general improve the ratio of tumor dose to normal tissue dose, computer-optimized 3-D conformal plans are in the future expected to involve larger numbers of treatment fields than current conventional 3-D plans (32). Therefore, the practical application of 3-D CRT requires newly designed treatment machines that are able to rapidly deliver multiple arbitrarily shaped fields. Automated beam shaping is considered an essential component of 3-D CRT delivery systems. MLCs have been introduced to automatically shape treatment fields in rapid succession under computer control to conform to the specific shape of the tumor from the corresponding treatment direction. We have implemented two types of automated MLCs (Scanditronix and Varian) for 3-D CRT patients. A recent analysis compared the treatment session length over a 3 month period for patients with carcinoma of the prostate treated on a dedicated linear accelerator using a co-planar 6-field conformal technique with either cerrobend or MLC blocking. As shown in Table 10-1, the findings demonstrated that multisegment therapy can be delivered using MLCs within the same duration of time as traditional techniques and in considerably less time than multisegment treatments using cerrobend blocking for each treatment portal.

Dose-Escalation Studies

Dose-escalation studies are being conducted at MSKCC to establish the maximum tolerable doses of radiation that can be delivered with conformal techniques to patients with Stages B2 (T2c) and C (T3-T4) carcinoma of the prostate, T1-T4, N0-N2 non-small cell lung carcinoma, and T3 and T4 carcinoma of the nasopharynx. The current dose levels being tested are 81.0 Gy for the prostate, 70.2 Gy for the lung, and 75.6 Gy for the nasopharynx (in daily fractions of 1.8 Gy). According to the design of these studies, the dose is escalated in 5.4 Gy increments provided that the incidence of treatment-related morbidity does not exceed that observed with conventional techniques. The primary endpoint for the prostate and nasopharynx studies is late toxicity, and the dose is escalated if the incidence of grade 3 (prostate) or grade 4 (nasopharynx) late complications (Radiation Therapy Oncology Group ([RTOG] morbidity scoring scheme) does not exceed 10%. Both acute and late toxicity are endpoints in the lung study, because acute pneumonitis is life-threatening, and therefore, dose-limiting. Escalation in this study is permitted if the incidence of acute grade 3 pulmonary and esophageal toxicity remains below 20%, and grade 3 or higher late toxicity is less than 10%.

Table 10-1. *Duration of treatment session per patient on a dedicated linear accelerator for the treatment of carcinoma of the prostate with co-planar conformal 6-field technique*

	1992 (Cerrobend)		1993 (MLC)	
Month	**Pts/Day**	**Minutes***	**Pts/Day**	**Minutes***
March	12	27.2	31	15.9
April	14	24.3	25	15.9
May	15	24.0	24	16.2

*includes the time required for patient set-up, treatment delivery, and for production of one portal film per week for each treatment field

Abbreviations: Pts = patients; MLC = multileaf collimatior

Prostate

We are testing the feasibility of increasing the target dose with 3-D CRT in patients with prostate carcinoma (5). The treatment volume encompasses the entire prostate and seminal vesicles, but does not include the regional pelvic lymph nodes. Initially, a phase I study was instituted using conventional doses ranging from 64.8 to 70.2 Gy. When baselines for acute tolerance and 2-year late complications were established at these dose levels, the dose was increased to 75.6 Gy, implemented exclusively in bilobar Stage B2 (T2c) and C (T3-T4) patients. At the time of this analysis (June 1993) 254 patients were accrued to our studies. Twenty-two patients were classified as Stage A2, 36 as B1, 107 as B2, and 89 as Stage C. The median follow-up time was 15 months. The majority of patients (240/254) were treated using a co-planar 6-field conformal technique (5), whereas the remainder were treated with conformal 4- or 8-field plans. The minimum tumor dose was 64.8-66.6 Gy in 70 patients, 70.2 Gy, in 102, 75.6 Gy in 57, and 81 Gy in 25 patients.

A restriction imposed in designing the treatment plan for 81.0 Gy limits the rectal dose to no more than that received in patients given 75.6 Gy. This requires a separate treatment plan that begins after 72.0 Gy. A 6-field co-planar arrangement with beams oriented in lateral and posterior-lateral orientations is used with the rectum blocked in each field. The seminal vesicles are also excluded if they are not clinically involved by tumor.

Acute toxicity and late treatment complications were graded according to the RTOG scheme (5). Conformal therapy at these dose levels was well tolerated. Table 10-2 summarizes the acute rectal and urinary morbidity observed in the 254 treated patients. Overall, 68% of patients had either no or mild (grade 1) acute rectal or urinary toxicity, whereas only 32% had grade 2 or higher acute morbidity requiring therapeutic intervention. The incidence of grade 2 or higher acute toxicity was about one-half that expected with conventional approaches (33). The late complications of treatment observed up to the time of this analysis are summarized in Table 10-3. Only one patient (0.4%), who received 64.8 Gy, developed a grade 4 late rectal complication.

Table 10-2. Carcinoma of the prostate: Acute toxicity at 65-81 Gy

	Rectal	Urinary
None	121/254 (48%)	76/254 (29%)
Grade 1	95/254 (37%)	13/254 (44%)
Grade 2	38/254 (15%)	64/254 (26%)
Grade 3	0	1/254 (0.4%)
Grade 4	0	0

Table 10-3. Carcinoma of the prostate: Late toxicity at 65-81 Gy

	Rectal	Urinary
None	236/254 (93%)	237/254 (93%)
Grade 1	2/254 (5%)	12/254 (5%)
Grade 2	5/254 (2%)	5/254 (2%)
Grade 3	0	0
Grade 4	1/254 (0.4%)	0

The 18-month actuarial serum prostate specific antigen (PSA) normalization rate was 88%. The normalization rate by stage is shown in Table 10-4. The median time to PSA normalization in those patients with an initially elevated level (> 4.0 ng/ml) and who did not receive neoadjuvant androgen deprivation therapy was 4.5 months. Normalization of the prostate on digital rectal examination closely paralleled that of the PSA (5). Currently, 228 patients (90%) are free of disease, whereas 6 (2%) have relapsed locally only and 20 (8%) have developed distant metastatic dissemination. The 4-year actuarial survival rate is 91%.

Accrual to the 75.6 Gy arm of the dose-escalation study was completed in May, 1992. Forty patients were treated at this dose level. There have been no grade 3 or higher late complications observed with a median follow-up time of 26 months. Entry at the 81 Gy level began in October, 1992, and the required 40 patients have now been accrued. The length of follow-up is too short to make any comments regarding morbidity at this dose level. The 86.4 Gy arm will open in April 1994, provided that no severe adverse reactions are observed in the lower dose patient groups.

Table 10-4 18 Month actuarial normalization of PSA

Stage	No. Pts	% Normal PSA
A2	22	100%
B1	36	100%
B2	107	90%
C	89	72%

Lung

The potential of 3-D treatment planning was evaluated by comparing 2-D treatment plans with 3-D plans in 9 patients with non-small cell lung cancer. The goal of treatment planning in this analysis was to deliver 70.2 Gy to all known sites of disease and 50.4 Gy to elective nodal volumes. Whereas target volume coverage with the 2-D treatment plans was comparable to the 3-D plans, the 3-D approach in many cases significantly reduced the dose accrued to normal tissues outside of the target volume. The average volume of ipsilateral lung receiving [3] 25 Gy was reduced by 11% with 3-D treatment planning, whereas there was a 51% reduction in the contralateral lung volume receiving this dose. The volume of the esophagus receiving 60 Gy was reduced by an average of 25% with 3-D planning, while esophagus NTCPs were reduced from 33% with 2-D planning to 22% with 3-D. Using the doses delivered to normal tissues with traditional 2-D planning methods as constraints, these data suggested that escalation of the tumor dose by 20-30% may be feasible with the 3-D approach (6).

Eighteen patients, the majority of whom had locally advanced disease (Stage I-11%; II-11%; IIIa-44%; and IIIb-33%), received 70.2 Gy on the non-small cell lung carcinoma dose-escalation study. Areas of known disease and elective nodal areas were initially treated to 18 Gy through anterior-posterior opposed fields. A multifield 3-D plan was used deliver an additional 32.4 Gy to the same target volume (total of 50.4 Gy to elective nodal areas). Sites of known disease were then given an additional 19.8 Gy (total of 70.2 Gy). The median boost target volume was 203 cc (range, 30-550 cc). A summary of the acute toxicity observed at this dose level is shown in Table 10-5. Two patients (12%) experienced severe acute complications, one with grade 3 and a second with grade 5 (fatal) acute radiation pneumonitis. In the patient with the fatal complication approximately 50% of the total lung volume received $\geq$ 25 Gy, and the predicted NTCP was greater than 80%. While there were too few complications to draw firm conclusions, the data obtained thus far suggest that pulmonary toxicity increases with rising calculated NTCP and the percentage of the lung parenchyma receiving $\geq$ 25 Gy (34). Based on these observations, the protocol was modified and only patients with a pulmonary NTCP of $\geq$ 20% are eligible for dose-escalation. Furthermore, because prophylactic mediastinal radiation therapy may limit the feasibility of dose-escalation and in the absence of convincing data that such treatment is efficacious, the mediastinal lymph nodes are no longer electively irradiated.

Table 10-5. Carcinoma of the lung: Acute toxicity at 70.2 Gy

	Lung	Esophagus
None	4/18 (22%)	1/18 (6%)
Grade 1	10/18 (55%)	11/18 (61%)
Grade 2	2/18 (11%)	6/18 (33%)
Grade 3	1/18 (6%)	0
Grade 4	0	0
Grade 5	1/18 (6%)	0

Nasopharynx

We have previously reported the advantages of 3-D CRT in patients with carcinoma of the nasopharynx (7). Ten newly diagnosed patients and 5 previously irradiated patients with locally recurrent disease were studied. The new patients initially received 50.4 Gy through conventional bilateral parallel opposed fields to the primary tumor and the cervical lymph nodes, and the 3-D CRT component was limited to a boost of 19.8 Gy given to the region of the primary tumor. Patients with locally recurrent disease received their entire treatment (21.6-54 Gy; median 36 Gy) by 3-D CRT. Patients were planned independently by two teams of physicians and physicists. One team performed a conventional 2-D plan using bilateral opposed fields, while the other performed a 3-D plan to select the best field configurations and target volume apertures. All patients except one were treated with coplanar 3-D plans using 5-9 fields in posterior, lateral, and oblique orientations. The remaining patient was treated with a non-coplanar field arrangement. With few exceptions, the 3-D plans showed improved tumor coverage, such that the target volume underdosed (receiving < 95% of the prescription dose) was reduced by an average of 15%. Whereas there was no intentional effort to increase the dose beyond the prescription dose, nonetheless the mean tumor dose increased with the 3-D plan for all cases by an average of 13%. This was due mainly to improved target volume coverage and to regions of increased dose within the target volume, rather than in the surrounding normal tissues, as was the case in the traditional plans. At the same time the volume of normal tissue receiving high doses (≥ 80% of the prescription dose) was reduced by about one-half in the 3-D plans compared to the traditional 2-D plans. Even though 3-D CRT was used for the boost portion of the treatment only (2/7 of the total treatment), the 3-D approach provided a significant improvement in uncomplicated tumor control probability for each patient, with an average increase of 15%.

Twelve patients with T3-T4 primary tumors have been accrued to the 75.6 Gy arm of the nasopharynx dose-escalation study. There have been no grade 4 late complications observed to date with follow-up ranging from 3-22 months. However, the number of patients studied is too small and the length of follow-up is too short to make any conclusions regarding dose-escalation in carcinoma of the nasopharynx at this time.

Conclusions

The experience with early prototypes of 3-D treatment planning and delivery systems already indicates that 3-D CRT offers an enormous therapeutic potential. The routine application of 3-D CRT is expected to improve the accuracy of target definition and treatment delivery, and when applied at traditional dose levels, this approach will allow radiation therapy to be administered with substantially less normal tissue morbidity than is currently observed with traditional radiotherapeutic techniques. Furthermore, the risk of overlapping treatment-related toxicities may be reduced when 3-D CRT is used in conjunction with other cytotoxic agents. A reduction in both acute and late radiation morbidity with 3-D CRT has already been demonstrated in the treatment of prostate cancer. However, the true clinical advantages of 3-D CRT will not be determined until future studies are conducted to test whether improved local control can be achieved with dose-escalation, and whether it affects the outcome in properly selected patients with several different human cancers.

While clinical trials are in progress, more sophisticated 3-D treatment planning tools are also being developed at MSKCC. Because of the increasing complexity of three-dimensional treatment planning and the need to evaluate large numbers of competing plans, a critical development is the introduction of computer-aided optimization of treatment planning. We are developing a method of computer-aided optimization that incorporates biophysical models to quantify the clinical consequences of associated dose distributions (32). In this method a "domain of search," made up of a number beams and their characteristics, is initially defined. The optimization process is used to determine the subset of beams and their weights within the domain that will result in the maximum clinical benefit to the patient. The delivery of conformal radiotherapy is extraordinarily complex. To address this issue, we are considering the use of on-line verification systems that have feedback control loops to automatically correct set-up errors before treatment or even during treatment. We are also developing on-line collision reduction software as well as other patient safety devices that will reduce even further the probability of unsafe machine trajectories. The impact of treatment uncertainties related to rigid organ motion and the expansion and contraction of internal organs on dose distribution and target coverage is also being examined (35,36). Organ motion and set-up uncertainties that cannot be corrected will be incorporated into treatment plans (37). Two methods for incorporating uncertainties into treatment plans have been developed. For rapid calculations, the mean dose distribution is obtained via convolution (13). To incorporate confidence limits of the dose distribution, the spatial distribution of set-up errors is sampled (35). Each technique can also include organ motion and the net effect of set-up errors and organ motion on the dose distribution. These investigations may further elucidate whether the use of margins for the target volume and perhaps also for normal organs will correctly account for set-up errors and organ motion. Each of these developments is likely to improve the efficacy, accuracy and curative potential of 3-D CRT.

References

1. Mohan R, Barest G, Brewster LJ, et al. A comprehensive three-dimensional radiation treatment planning system. Int J Radiat Oncol Biol Phys 15:481-495, 1988.

2. Mageras GS, Podmaniczky KC, Mohan R: A model for computer-controlled delivery of 3-D conformal treatments. Med Phys (in press).

3. Leibel SA, Kutcher GJ, Mohan R, et al. Three-dimensional conformal radiation therapy at the Memorial Sloan-Kettering Cancer Center. Seminars in Radiat Oncol 2:274-289, 1992.

4. Leibel SA, Ling CC, Kutcher GJ, et al. The biological basis of conformal three-dimensional radiation therapy. Int J Radiat Oncol Biol Phys 21:805-811, 1991.

5. Leibel SA, Heimann R, Kutcher GJ, et al. Three-dimensional conformal radiation therapy in locally advanced carcinoma of the prostate: Preliminary results of a phase I dose-escalation study. Int J Radiat Oncol Biol Phys (in press).

6. Armstrong JG, Burman C, Leibel SA, et al. Three-dimensional conformal radiation therapy may improve the therapeutic ratio of high dose radiation therapy for lung cancer. Int J Radiat Oncol Bio Phys 26:685-689, 1993.

7. Leibel SA, Kutcher GJ, Harrison LB, et al. Improved dose distributions for 3-D conformal boost treatments in carcinoma of the nasopharynx. Int J Radiat Oncol Biol Phys 20:823-833, 1991.

8. Mohan R: Three-dimensional radiation treatment planning. Aust Phys Engin Sci Med 12:73-91, 1989.

9. Landberg T, Chavaudra J, Dobbs J, et al. ICRU report: Prescribing, recording, and reporting photon beam therapy. (in press).

10. Goitein M, Abrams M, Rowell D, Pollari H, Wiles J: Multi-dimensional treatment planning: II. Beam's eye-view, back projection, and projection through CT sections. Int J Rad Oncol Biol Phys 9:789-797, 1983.

11. McShan DL, Silverman A, Lanza DM, et al. A computerized three-dimensional treatment planning system utilizing interactive colour graphics. Br J Radiol 52:478-481, 1979.

12. LoSasso TJ, Chui CS, Kutcher GJ, et al. The use of multi-leaf collimator for conformal radiotherapy in carcinomas of the prostate and nasopharynx. Int J Radiat Oncol Biol Phys 25:161-170, 1993.

13. Mohan R, Chui CS: Use of Fourier transforms in calculating dose distributions for irregularly shaped fields for three dimensional treatment planning. Med Phys 14:70-77, 1987.

14. Chui CS, Mohan RM: Extraxtion of pencil beams by the deconvolution method. Med Phys 15:1338-144, 1988.

15. Photon Treatment Planning Collaborative Working Group: Three-dimensional dose calculations for radiation treatment planning. Int J Radiat Oncol Biol Phys 21:25-36, 1991.

16. Shipley WU, Tepper JE, Prout GR, et al. Proton radiation as boost therapy for localized prostatic carcinoma. JAMA 241:1912-1915, 1979.

17. Drzymala RE, Mohan R, Brewster L, et al. Dose-volume histograms. Int J Radiat Oncol Biol Phys 21:71-78, 1991.

18. Zelefsky MJ, Leibel SA, Burman CM, et al. Neoadjuvant hormonal therapy improves the therapeutic ratio in patients with bulky prostatic cancer treated with thee-dimensional conformal radiation therapy. Int J Radiat Oncol Biol Phys (submitted).

19. Emami B, Lyman J, Brown A, et al. Tolerance of normal tissue to therapeutic irradiation. 21:109-122, 1991.

20. Burman C, Kutcher GJ, Emami B, et al. Fitting of normal tissue tolerance data to an analytic function. Int J Radiat Oncol Biol Phys 21:123-135, 1991.

21. Kutcher GJ, Burman C, Brewster L, et al. Histogram reduction method for calculating complication probabilities for three-dimensional treatment planning evaluations. Int J Radiat Oncol Biol Phys 21:137-146, 1991.

22. Munzenrider JE, Brown AP, Chu JC, et al. Numerical scoring of treatment plans. Int J Radiat Oncol Biol Phys 21:147-163, 1991.

23. Bush M, Rosenow U: Dose volume relationships in computer applications, in Sternick E (ed): Radiation Oncology. Hanover, NH, University Press of New England, 1976, pp 279-285.

24. Dritschilo A, Chaffey JT, Bloomer WD, et al. The complication probability factor: A method of selection of treatment plans. Br J Radiol 51:370-374, 1978.

25. Lyman JT: Complication probability as assessed from dose volume histograns. Rad Res 104:S-13-S19, 1985.

26. Lyman JT, Wolbarst AB: Optimization of radiotherapy III: A method of assessing complication probabilities from dose volume histograms. Int J Radiat Oncol Biol Phys 13:103-109, 1987.

27. Wolbarst AB, Chin LM, Swenssen GL: Optimization of radiation therapy: Integral-response of a model biological system. Int J Radiat Oncol Biol Phys 8:1761-1769, 1982.

28. Goitein M: The probability of controlling an inhomogeneously irradiated tumor, in Zink S (ed): Evaluation of Treatment Planning for Particle Beam Radiotherapy, Bethesda, M.D., National Cancer Institute, 1987, pp 5.8.1-5.8.17.

29. Brahme A: Dosimetric precision requirements in radiation therapy. Acta Radiol Oncol 23:379-391, 1984.

30. Jackson A, Kutcher GJ, Yorke ED: Probability of radiation-induced complications for normal tissues with parallel architecture: II. Non-uniform irradiation. Med Phys 20:613-625, 1993.

31. Yorke ED, Kuthcher GJ, Jackson A: Probability of radiation-induced complications for normal tissues with parallel architecture: I. Uniform irradiation of whole and partial organs. Radiother Oncol 26:226-238, 1993.

32. Mohan R, Mageras GS, Baldwin MS, et al. Clinical relevant optimization of 3-D conformal treatments. Med Phys 19:933-944, 1992.

33. Soffen EM, Hanks GE, Hunt MA, Epstein BE: Conformal static field radiation therapy treatment of early prostate cancer versus non-conformal techniques: A reduction in acute morbidity. Int J Radiat Oncol Biol Phys 24:485-488, 1992.

34. Armstrong J, Zelefsky M, Burt M, et al. Acute toxicity of high dose 3-dimensional conformal radiation therapy (3-D CRT) for non small-cell lung cancer (NSCLC). Proc Am Soc Clin Oncol 12:348, 1993 (abstr).

35. Kutcher GJ, Chui C, LoSasso T: Incorporation of set-up uncertainties in treatment plan calculations. Int J Radiat Oncol Biol Phys 21:123, 1991 (abstr).

36. Melian E, Kutcher G, Leibel S, et al. Variation in prostate position: Quantitation and implications for three-dimensional conformal radiation therapy. Int J Radiat Oncol Biol Phys 27 (suppl 1):137, 1993 (abstr).

37. Goitein M, Calculation of the uncertainty in dose delivered during radiation therapy. Med Phys 12:608-612, 1985.

Chapter 11

Clinical Experience with 3-D Radiotherapy: The University of North Carolina Experience

Julian G. Rosenman, Ph.D., M.D.

University of North Carolina at Chapel Hill, Chapel Hill, North Carolina

Three dimensional radiation therapy treatment planning has been under development at the University of North Carolina for almost ten years. The first patient had a 3-D treatment plan performed in December, 1987. To date 406 patients have undergone 3-D radiation treatment planning, of these 235 had their entire treatment planned in 3-D, and 131 had their boosts 3-D planned. The data from these 366 patients is the basis of this report. For 27 other patients, the 3-D treatment plan was done to check the result of a previous 2-D plan, and in 13 patients (3%) the 3-D treatment plan could not be completed because of technical problems or patient non-compliance. Table 11-1 shows the break down by treatment site.

Table 11-1. Distribution by tumor type

Treatment Site	Numbers	(%)
prostate	106	(29%)
brain	75	(20%)
head and neck	66	(18%)
lung cancer	39	(11%)
others*	80	(22%)
TOTAL	366	(100%)

*includes gyn, other pelvic and abdominal tumors, sarcomas, and a small other of most other tumors

The predominance of prostate cancer in our study is due to a departmental decision that all curative prostate cancer patients should undergo 3-D treatment planning. The large number of brain tumor patients represented here probably represents the ease with which these patients can be 3-D planned. In general, except for prostate cancer patients, there is no department-wide formula for determining which patients are to undergo 3-D planning. All but a few of the patients chosen for 3-D planning are potentially curative, and have tumors that might be difficult to localize with only 2-D methods. Patients must be selected carefully, because our department has limited resources, and cannot 3-D plan more than 5 patients per week at the most.

Efficiency of 3-D Treatment Planning

In contrast to other treatment planning systems, Plan UNC allows the physician to be involved with nearly every aspect of the treatment planning process. As currently implemented, our system consists of four basic steps. First, the data must be acquired. Patient immobilization and definition of patient origin are carried out while on the Departmental CT scanner; typically 50-100 slices are taken. The physicians role is to specify the patient treatment position and the volume to be scanned. Typically it takes about 30 minutes to build the immobilization cast and another 30 to complete the CT scan, although in a few cases several hours were required for the entire process.

Second, objects of interest in the CT data must be defined. These objects include skin (necessary for the 3-D dose calculation), tumor target (usually gross tumor volume), and specified normal anatomy. Typically the skin and other normal structures are hand or automatically contoured by the dosimetrists and checked by the clinician. The gross tumor volume (GTV) and clinical tumor volume (CTV) must be specified by the clinician. Object segmentation typically requires about 45 minutes of clinician time, but some very elaborate cases have taken over 2 hours.

Third, the segmented data is then passed to the virtual simulator where radiation beams are defined. This process is usually done by the clinician, much as he or she would do a conventional simulation. 3-D radiation doses and dose volume histograms are calculated immediately following the virtual simulation to act as feedback. The dose distribution can be calculated for a single slice in 2-3 seconds, so the plan can be modified rapidly, if necessary. Clinician input at this juncture is important. Clinician time with virtual simulation is typically 45 minutes to an hour.

Finally, radiographs are computed for each port, and the patient undergoes "check films" on the physical simulator to be sure that these match the computed radiograph. Usually the clinician needs only to verify that the real films match the computed ones. Table 11-2 gives a summary of the time involved in the various steps of 3-D planning using our system.

Table 11-2. Timing for various parts of 3-D planning

Procedure	No.*	Average Time	Minimum Time	Maximum Time	Average Clinician Time†
Casting	274	27 minutes	10 minutes	4 hours	none
patient	110	30 minutes	10 minutes	2 hours	5-10 minutes
CT	223	45 minutes	15 minutes	2 1/2 hours	30 minutes
Object	205	50 minutes	10 minutes	4 hours	45 minutes
definition	146	70 minutes	35 minutes	3 1/2 hours	5-10 minutes
Virtual	---	3 1/2 hours	Å 1/12 hours	16 hours	Å1 1/2 hours
Simulation					
Verification					
of set up					
TOTAL					

* timing data does not exist for all categories for all patients
† estimated

It must be pointed out that these times are very approximate and are meant to provide "ball park" figures rather than the results of detailed time-motion studies. It is the current feeling of the technical staff that the average time for a 3-D treatment planning is now more like 2 hours (including verification) than the 3 hour average since 1988.

Specific Tumor Sites

More than 25% of all 3-D plans are done for prostate cancer, as all curative prostate cases undergo 3-D planning in our department. This rule was instituted as an earlier study in our department indicated that - of patients who were first simulated conventionally, and then with the 3-D system had their blocks changed in a clinically meaningful way. As a special preparation for prostate planning, a urethrogram is done along with the CT, or during "check films" or both. We have found that this procedure helps identify the lower border of the prostate which can often be confused on CT.

Approximately 20% of all 3-D plans are for head and neck cancers. We have found that the design of boost fields with the 3-D planning system is more rational than with conventional planning. Also, it is sometime possible to spare part of the parotid gland (which in our experience has a lot positional variation from patient to patient.)

Brain tumors also comprised about 20% of our 3-D treatment planning. Our in-house protocol calls for astrocytomas to be treated to 4500 cGy with a 4 cm margin around the tumor and edema, an addition 1440 cGy with a 2 cm margin around tumor and edema, and 720 cGy to a 1 cm margin around the tumor. Multiple shaped ports are now standard treatment.

Most of remaining 3-D plans are done on patients with lung cancer or abdominal tumors. In lung cancer patients 3-D planning allows increased confidence in treating mediastinal lymph nodes (especially in the boost fields) and in avoiding the spinal cord after the delivery of 4500 cGy. In the abdomen 3-D has been useful in limiting kidney and liver doses in the treatment of pancreatic cancer.

In addition to the 406 patients undergoing 3-D planning, we have retrospectively planned approximately 40 patients with breast cancer. The purpose of this planning was not for beam placement, but to use lung inhomogeneity corrections and to provide for proper beam modulation. We have determined that in many cases these adjuncts to 2-D breast planning are essential.

Summary

In summary, we have 3-D planned 366 patients with 3-D treatment planning in the last 5 years at the University of North Carolina. The increasing use of our system attests to the value that our clinicians find it has for many of our patients.

Bibliography of The UNC Clinical 3-D Experience

1. Rosenman J, Sherouse, GW, Chaney EL, Tepper, JE: Virtual Simulation: Initial Clinical Results. *Int J Radiat Oncol Biol Physics,* 20:843-851, 1991.

2. Sailer SL, Sherouse GW, Chaney EL, Rosenman JG, Tepper JE: A comparison of post-operative techniques for laryngo-hypopharyngeal carcinomas using 3-dimensional dose distributions. *Int J Radiat Oncol Biol Phys,* 21:767-777, 1991.

3. Sailer SL, Chaney EL, Rosenman JG, Sherouse, GW, Tepper JE: Treatment planning at the University of North Carolina at Chapel Hill. *Sem. in Rad. Onc.* 2:267-273, 1992.

4. Sailer SL, Rosenman JG, Symon JR, Cullip TJ, Chaney EL: The terad and hexad: Maximum beam separation as a starting point for noncoplanar 3-D treatment planning. *Int J Radiat Oncol Biol Phys,* 27:138, 1993.

Chapter 12

Clinical Experience with 3-D Radiotherapy: The Washington University Experience

B. Emami, M.D.,* J. Purdy, Ph.D.,* M. Graham, M.D.,* J. Michalski, M.D.,* W. Harms, B.S.,*
C. Perez, M.D.,* R. Gerber, M.S.,* W. Bosch, D.Sc.,* John Matthews, D.Sc.,* Henry Lee, M.D.,*
Joseph Simpson, M.D.,* Harvy Glazer, M.D.,** J. Franz Wippold, M.D.**

Radiation Oncology Center, * Dept of Radiology, **
Washington University. School of Medicine St. Louis, Missouri

Research at Washington University on 3-D radiation therapy planning (3-D RTP) started almost a decade ago, primarily by participation in the three multi-institutional research contracts sponsored by the National Cancer Institute (NCI) (7-9). During the 1980s, significant progress was made in two important areas: (1) development of various components of 3-D conformal radiation therapy (CRT), both hardware and software, that resulted in a true interactive 3-D RTP system, on-line portal imaging and a CT-simulator; (2) experience of physicians, physicists, dosimetrists, and therapy technologists in using these tools, and learning the potential advantages and challenges.

The first patient treatments utilizing 3-D CRT at the Radiation Oncology Center at Washington University were initiated in 1989. Before actual clinical use of the 3-D planning system, a comparative treatment planning analysis of two-dimensional (2-D) and 3-D treatment plans was completed for 20 patients (3). The objectives of this study were to test the feasibility of large-scale implementation of 3-D CRT technology in the actual treatment of patients and to further familiarize the staff with the clinical use of 3-D planning tools. Treatment plans for 10 patients with prostate cancer were performed according to our department's traditional treatment methodologies (bilateral 120-degree arc technique without access to full 3-D volumetric information). Concurrently, CT scans were done on these patients to obtain full volumetric image data, and treatment plans were created using 3-D tools, (e.g., beam's-eye view, rooms-view, multiple noncoplanar beams, dose volume histograms, dose surface). Room-views six-field beam arrangement technique was used (3). Results were quantitatively compared using 3-D plan evaluation tools. The conclusion of this study was that, in prostate cancer, 3-D treatment planning showed the advantage of better tumor coverage and reduced dose to critical normal structures; in patients with head and neck cancer the results were mixed, and no clear conclusion could be reached. The mixed results in the latter group were attributed to the difficulty of treating this area. In addition to significant potential for improving the technical aspects of radiation therapy, these preliminary studies brought two very important areas to the attention of researchers: (1) the potential of 3-D CRT in gaining information on volumetric normal tissue tolerances to radiation; information that we neither possessed nor previously had the tools to acquire, and (2) the difficulty of 3-D delineation of target volumes. Subsequent to these preliminary studies, a series of site-specific research projects and clinical protocols have been carried out. Ongoing projects are reviewed in the following sections.

Prostate Cancer

Initial planning studies were carried out in which treatment plans for 10 patients were performed using both 2-D and 3-D beam arrangements. This comparative treatment planning analysis showed that, although both techniques were capable of proper coverage of target volume, 3-D CRT significantly reduced the volume of rectum and bladder exposed to high-dose irradiation (3). Currently, patients with prostate cancer at our institution are enrolled in a prospective randomized trial (CA Perez, principal investigator) in which patients are randomized to be treated with either traditional 2-D technique of bilateral arcs or 3-D CRT using a six-field beam arrangement with each beam portal designed using beam's eye view. We are also the recipient of an NCI contract (RFA 92-05) to carry out dose-escalation studies in prostate cancer using 3-D CRT (B. Emami, principal investigator).

Bronchogenic Carcinoma

As mentioned earlier, working with first-generation 3-D RTP systems, as part of a National Cancer Institute contract, we performed 3-D treatment planning for two patients with advanced lung cancer. In comparing these plans with the 2-D conventional plans used to treat these patients, we were able to show the potential of this technology for better sparing of normal tissues (2). On initiation of clinical trials, we performed a comparative treatment planning analysis for 10 patients with bronchogenic carcinoma comparing 2-D and 3-D plans. Graham et al. (4) were able to increase the radiation dose to the target volume in all patients, up to 8000 cGy, while keeping dose to the normal tissues within the acceptable tolerance dose levels. With 2-D treatment planning and beam arrangements this was not possible. Experience with this project also demonstrated the potential difficulties of target volume delineation and the need for consensus in methodology in this regard.

Subsequently, 3-D CRT has been used in the actual treatment of patients with bronchogenic carcinoma. Graham et al. (5) have published a preliminary analysis of clinical experience in treating patients with lung cancer with 3-D CRT. In their clinical work, they used the ICRU Report No. 50 recommendations for defining and designating target volumes (5).

The conclusions from this preliminary analysis were: (1) dose escalation studies in lung cancer are feasible using 3-D CRT with the clinical aim of improved local control; (2) research and consensus on the margins around gross tumor for delineation of various target volumes as recommended by ICRU Report No. 50 is needed; (3) critical attention must be given to the volume of normal lung irradiated in every patient and threshold tolerance doses for various volumes must not be exceeded to avoid unacceptable pulmonary toxicity. This project is ongoing.

Head and Neck Cancers

Initial comparative planning studies in head and neck cancer revealed mixed results. Admittedly, this was the learning curve in treating this group of patients with 3-D CRT. The complex anatomy of the head and neck region with 4 major sites and 17 subsites, each giving rise to different cancers with their special routes of extension, made the task of this initial comparative planning study enormously complex and difficult. Because of technical and logistic considerations, patients with head and neck cancers whom we thought would benefit more from 3-D CRT were studied with this technique. In some patients 3-D CRT showed a significant advantage in normal tissue sparing as well as proper coverage of target volume; in others there was no improvement using 3-D CRT technology.

Subsequently, the decision was made that, in order to take full advantage of our resources, the 3-D CRT protocols in patients with head and neck cancer should focus on specific aims and well-defined endpoints. Accordingly, a protocol was designed with the specific aim of reducing the dose to normal tissue (major salivary glands) with the hope of avoiding xerostomia, an important short- and long-term complication of irradiation of head and neck cancers. As a part of this ongoing project, thus far, 18 patients have had 3-D treatment planning performed. All patients have been treated according to 3-D CRT plans. In addition, in all 18 patients, 2-D treatment planning has been carried out according to routine treatment policies of our department for a given site. Results of the two series of plans regarding coverage of target volume(s) and the dose and volume of salivary glands, temporal mandibular joint, and other normal structures were compared (1). In all patients, significant reduction of the volume of major salivary glands (mostly parotids) subjected to high doses of radiation has been demonstrated. All patients have retained a fair degree of saliva secretion without a significant degree of xerostomia, albeit the evaluation of xerostomia has been subjective. This project is ongoing.

Pediatric Tumors

3-D CRT has been used treating selected patients with pediatric head and neck sarcomas and retinoblastoma. The specific aim of this project is reduction of dose to normal tissue structures. Young patient age and growing stage of normal tissue in the pediatric age group, their limited tolerance to radiation, and potential for very serious cosmetic and functional sequelae from irradiation mandate special attention. Currently, five patients have been treated with 3-D CRT as part of the ongoing protocol. This rewarding experience has resulted in two significant conclusions: (1) in a number of cases, proper coverage of target volume was not possible with conventional 2-D technologies, whereas with 3-D CRT full coverage of the intended target volume by the prescribed dose became a reality and, (2) in all patients, a significant reduction in the volume of normal tissue receiving the prescribed dose of radiation was possible in all patients, compared with conventional methods of treatment (6).

Liver Tumors

A few selected patients with liver metastasis have been treated with 3-D radiation therapy. The intent of this treatment has been to deliver higher doses, up to 7000 cGy, to a small volume encompassing the liver metastasis with a reasonably small margin. In a few patients treated as such, the tolerance has been excellent, and in one patient with liver metastasis from a primary colon tumor, significant reduction in the carcinoembryogenic antigen (CEA) level has been documented. This study is still in the early stages of development.

Conclusion

Modern image technology and the affordability of high performance computer technology has led us to the development of a powerful 3-D treatment planning system. This system has been used for planning treatment for several different sites. Improved target volume delineation, increased dose to target volume and reduced dose to normal structures have all been demonstrated as our clinic moves to becoming fully 3-D based.

References

1. Emami, B.; Harms, W.; Purdy, J.A.; Simpson, J.R.; Gerber, R.L.; Wippold, J.F. 3-D conformal radiotherapy in head and neck cancers: Significant reduction in dose to salivary glands and incidence of xerostomia. (in preparation).

2. Emami, B.; Purdy, J.; Harms, W.; Manolis, J.; Wong, J.; Drzymala, R.; Simpson, J. Three dimensional treatment planning for lung cancer. Int. J. Radiat. Oncol. Biol. Phys. 21: 217-227; 1991.

3. Emami, B., Purdy, J.A., Manolis, J.M., Gerber, R.L., Harms, W.B., Simpson, J.R., Wippold, F.J., Perez, C.A.: 3-D Static Conformal Radiotherapy: Preliminary Results of a Prospective Clinical Trial (Abstract), Int. J. Radiat. Oncol. Biol. Phys. 21(1):147, 1991.

4. Graham, M.L., Matthews, J.W., Harms, W.B., Emami, B. and Purdy, J.A.: 3-D Radiation Treatment Planning Study for Patients with Carcinoma of the Lung (Abstract), Int. J. Radiat. Oncol. Biol. Phys. 24(1):174-175, 1992.

5. Graham, M., Purdy, J., Emami, B., Matthews, J., Harms, W. Preliminary results of a prospective trial using 3-D radiotherapy for patients with lung cancer. Int. J. Radiat. Oncol. Biol. Phys. (submitted to Int. J. Radiat. Oncol. Biol. Phys.)

6. Michalski, J.M.; Sur, R.D.; Harms, W.B.; Purdy, J.A. Advantage of 3-dimensional conformal radiotherapy in pediatric parameningeal rhabdomyosarcomas. Int. J. Radiat. Oncol. Biol. Phys. (In Press).

7. NCI High Energy Electron Contract. N01-CM-67915.

8. NCI High Energy Photon Contract. RP #N01-CM-47696.

9. NCI Tools Contract. NCI-CM-97564-23.

Chapter 13

Clinical Experience with 3-D Radiotherapy: The German Experience

Günther F.E. Gademann M.D., Ph.D* and Wolfgang Schlegel, Ph.D.

Radiol. Department, University of Heidelberg and German Cancer Research Center, Heidelberg, Germany

The clinical application of three dimensional radiotherapy planning is currently very limited in Germany. The reason is that software suitable for clinical use was not available with the exception of some self-made programs, the computer hardware was too slow for those tools or too expensive and the usefulness of the software was not appropriate for fast clinical routine. There was only one institute in Germany, the German Cancer Research Center (DKFZ) that could develop a planning software for research purpose since 1978 (12). This program was gradually, step by step introduced into clinical application, starting with more stereotactical procedures (3) up to now covering any clinical condition of modern radiotherapy (5).

This program system is the major base for the cooperation between the DKFZ and the Radiological Department, University of Heidelberg. These two institutes have gained the most valuable experience with clinical 3-D planning in Germany since they started with stereotactical high precision radiotherapy in 1988. Their activities on the field of 3-D planned radiotherapy will be discussed in detail in the following. The general situation in Germany is very different to that in Heidelberg and can only be demonstrated as overview.

General Situation in Germany

Despite generally high interest in three dimensional radiotherapy planning the clinical application is restricted to some few institutes because of the above mentioned technical reasons. Currently there is no national working group for this problem or any interinstitutional clinical trials. In order to get a general view of the German situation we started a questionnaire to 150 radiotherapy departments in Germany and the German-speaking neighboring countries Austria and Switzerland. This survey included questions reg. the size of the institute (yearly new patients), machinery and personnel, the currently used planning software, and finally the future plans about 3-D treatment planning.

Ninety-seven institutes responded (61%). The majority of German institutes in Germany treat yearly between 1000 and 1600 patients. Single plane treatment planning is performed in 43,3%, multi-planar planning in 49.5 % of the responding institutes. Only 5(5.4)% institutes could handle real 3-D planning, however using old programs and hardware in 3 departments. Two had no computerized treatment planning at all. This is demonstrated in Figure 13-1a.

The distribution of the answers regarding the future plans shows up differently (Figure 13-1b). 70% wished to have 3-D planning within the next 2 years, 13% in addition had such plans for the next 5 years. Four institutes did not answer this question, only 6 gave a definite negative answer because of exclusively palliative treatments.

---

* New address of first author: Radiotherapy Clinic, Otto-von-Guericke-University, Leipziger Str. 44, D-39120 Magdeburg.

The implementation of 3-D treatment planning into clinical routine is open to fast changes. The survey gives an image of spring 1993 and has already changed by the installation of modern programs in at least three institutes. German publications about clinical use of 3-D treatment planning are still rare. Most of them are listed in the reference section (13).

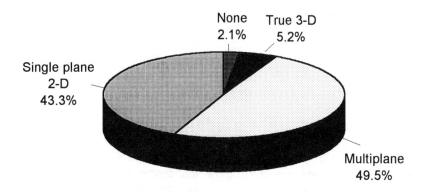

Figure 13-1a. Current Distribution of Used Planning Procedure

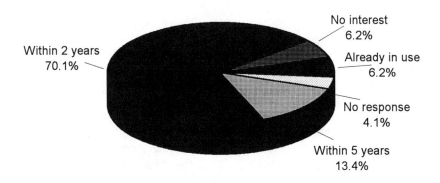

Figure 13-1b. Future Plans

Figure 13-1a/b. A survey about 3-D treatment planning, March 1993.

Specific Situation in Heidelberg

As already mentioned the Heidelberg institutes have gained pretty early clinical experience in 3-D treatment planning by using the self-made program VOXELPLAN HEIDELBERG. It provides a fully threedimensional voxel based dose calculation and any kind of modern tools like MR fully threedimensional voxel based dose calculation and any kind of modern tools like MR correlation interactive beam's-eye-view, 3-D dose display, dose-volume-histograms, non-coplanar treatment techniques, inverse dose calculations etc. (1).

The software is not commercially available and only released for research to cooperation partners. Thus, the program is available in other German institutes, i.e. in Wurzburg and Hamburg, however it is not used for clinical routine. This is possible in Heidelberg within two clinical investigations under the close control of the developers.

Stereotactically Guided High Precision Radiotherapy of Head and Neck Tumors at the German Cancer Research Center

The program VOXELPLAN supports stereotactically guided radiotherapy as software part of an integrated stereotactical system for high precision radiotherapy (11). It includes individual reversible mask fixation in a stereotactical frame, CT/MR image correlation, 3-dimensional treatment planning, beam shaping by a thin-leaf-collimator (2), and stereotactical localization.

The typical course of treatment preparation begins with production of a head mask that is screwed to a wooden stereotactical frame. The geometrical accuracy of this fixation is measured to 1 to 2 mm (9). CT with intravenous contrast medium and MRI with tumor adjusted sequences are performed having the patient fixed in his mask. During both imaging procedures a stereotactical marker system attached to the frame produces 12 little landmarks in the transversal CT and MR images.

The planning target volume is usually defined in the MR images that are correlated to the CT images by means of the stereotactical markers after software correction of image distortions (10). By using a virtual simulator (beam's-eye-view) in VOXELPLAN HEIDELBERG an isocentric configuration of usually 3 to 5 irregular non-coplanar fields is optimized regarding avoidance of damage to organs at risk, smallest target projection and homogenous dose distribution. (See color Plate 10.) The irregular field contour is drawn in the beam's-eye-view display, plotted and brought to a wooden template that again forms the manually driven MLC.

The program VOXELPLAN calculates cartesian stereotactical coordinates of the target points based on the imaged landmarks. A stereotactical localizer allows precise positioning to the isocenter of the treatment unit. The laser cross and the illumination of the field shapes are marked on the patient's mask in order to realign rapidly the patient in every single treatment and control the beam configuration. A port film in 0 and 90-degree gantry position with open leafs is obtained after the first irradiation. The center of the field is indicated by an metal dot and compared according to anatomical landmarks.

We started in 1988 with stereotactically guided conformal radiotherapy to low grade brain tumors, like gliomas, meningiomas, chordomas, neurinomas etc. The indications for this technique were extended to boost treatment, i.e. nasopharynx carcinoma, and preirradiated recurrences, i.e. nasopharynx carcinoma, high grade astrocytomas etc. (8). The clinical trials are performed as nonrandomized phase III studies and in part historically compared (6). The clinical use of the system in now more than 250 patients show that the time consumption is comparable to conventional external beam methods and the application can be handled as safely and reliably as in other routine procedures. A first preliminary evaluation shows a local control in 95% after a median follow-up of 25 months in the largest group of primary high precision irradiation with a very low incidence of delayed side-effects and no late complications.

A deeper evaluation is performed for low grade meningiomas (7). It compares the remission and late complication rate of conformal radiotherapy versus single dose linac based radiosurgery that was performed in Heidelberg. We observe significant improvement in tumor response for the fractionated radiotherapy combined with absence of complications in 64 patients. The patient group treated by radiosurgery (n=20) developed early delayed side-effects in 50% and late complications grade II to IV in 40%.

Although the median follow-up time of now about 30 months is certainly too short to draw final conclusions for these slowly growing low grade tumors, the method of fractionated conformal high precision radiotherapy that includes the geometrical accuracy of stereotaxy has good chances to become first choice for patients with a long life expectancy.

In another patient group of 11 patients with clivus chordomas the median follow up time is now 26 months. One local recurrence occurred 18 months after radiotherapy. The other chordomas showed stable disease after a maximal follow-up of 58 months. Despite maximal target doses of 72 Gy complications, especially to the optic system, were not observed in that patient group.

3-D Treatment Planning in the Clinical Routine of the Radiological Department, University of Heidelberg

In 1991 a clinically guided project was supported by the German Cancer Aid concerning questions for clinical implementation of 3-D treatment planning. This project was planned for receiving information about organization forms, time consumption, personnel, indications and 2-D/3-D comparisons in order to increase the clinical interest and decrease the reservations (5).

The program VOXELPLAN HEIDELBERG was installed at a VAX-station 3600, adapted to the specifics of the treatment unit of the clinic and in part modified for routine clinical use, i.e. the print options (protocol, dose display, irregular field contours etc.). The first patient with a cervical chordoma was treated with central blocking in August of 1991. End of March 1993 after 20 months 263 patients have been treated according to a 3-D treatment plan. The project is not limited to specific indications in order to be free for unexpected and complicated cases. Figure 13-2 shows the distribution of the treated body region with a strong weighting of the thoracic region. The distribution represents roughly the patient load at the clinic. Tumors of the head and neck are relatively rare because they were transferred to the program at the DKFZ as described above.

Meanwhile about 70% of all computer assisted treatment planning is performed 3-dimensionally at VOXELPLAN. This became possible because of a substantial decrease in time consumption within the last 18 months. Starting with a median of more than 10 hours for a complete 3-D plan, the same is now possible within less than 4 hours. Differentiation of time consumption concerning the body region and the different steps of the planning procedure shows shortest values for the mediastinum and the pelvis and longest for the retroperitoneum and head and neck (Figure 13-3). The medical part, the target contouring, usually needs about 30 minutes. This is completely accepted by the physicians. Target definition is performed at the computer display by the physician who is responsible for the treated patient. Currently about 10 to 15 3-D plans can be completed per week.

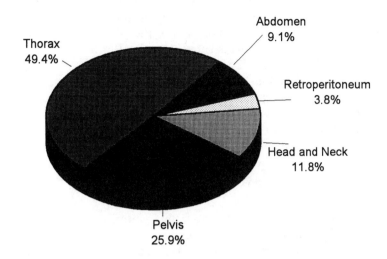

Figure 13-2. Distribution of the body region (targets) of first 268 patients who were treated according a 3-D plan

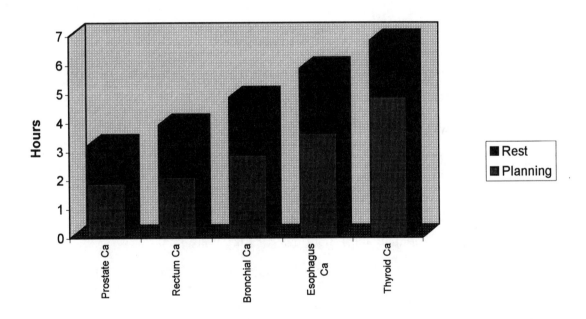

Figure 13-3. Differential time consumption for 3-D planning according to body regions

We performed controlled comparison of 2-D and 3-D plans and found larger target volumes in the 3-D versions. Despite this fact, the dose-volume histogram showed better target dosage and equal or improved protection of the organs at risk in the 3-D plans. The example of a larger mediastinal tumor (penetrating esophageal tumor) is shown in color Plate 11.

All patients treated with the system will be followed at our clinic. Case observation studies are running for a first evaluation of the clinical use, especially regarding complication and quality of life. The best defined trial concerns bronchial carcinomas after pneumonectomy and mediastinal irradiation, prostate carcinomas (without dose escalation) and rectal carcinomas. Retrospective comparison between biological modeling programs and clinical observations are performed in addition (4).

Summary

Clinical application of threedimensional treatment planning in Germany finds high interest, but is still very limited and focused to some few institutes. Interinstitutional clinical trials are not yet defined. With the commercial availability of suitable software this will certainly change very rapidly as it can be expected from the survey about 3-D treatment planning performed in March 1993.

Two 3-D activities at Heidelberg have been active since 1988 and 1991, respectively. One works with stereotactical high precision techniques in the head and neck region, the other with the routinely performed external radiotherapy of a large department. Both could demonstrate the easy clinical applicability and the usefulness for the patient and the potential for general improvement in radiotherapy.

References

1. Bauer, B., Schlegel, W., Boesecke, R., Doll, J., Hartmann, G.H. and Lorenz, W.J.: Three-Dimensional Treatment Planning of Conformation Therapy. In: Computer Assisted Radiology 85 (H.U.Lemke, M.L. Rhodes, C.C.Jaffee und R.Felix, eds.), 388394, Springer, Berlin, Heidelberg, NewYork, Tokyo, 1985.

2. Boesecke, R., Doll, J., Schlegel, W., Lorenz, W.J.: A multi-leaf collimator. Strahlentherapie und Onkologie 164, 151- 154; 1988.

3. Engenhart, R.; Kimmig, B.N.; Hover, K.H.; Wowra, B.; Sturm, V.; van Kaick, G.; Wannenmacher, M. Stereotactic single high dose radiation therapy of benign intracranial meningiomas. Int.J.Radiat.Oncol.Biol.Phys. 19:1021-1026; 1990.

4. Flentje M., Hensley F., Gademann G., Menke m:, Wannenmacher M. Renal tolerance to nonhomogeneous irradiation: Comparison of observed effects to predictions of normal tissue compliccation probablity from different biophysical models Int.J.Radiat.Oncol.Biol.Phys. 27:25-30;1993.

5. Gademann G., Schlegel W., Burkelbach J., Laier C., Behrens S., Brieger S. Threedimensional treatment planning: evaluations for clinical integration. Strahlentherapie und Onkologie 169: 159-167; 1993.

6. Gademann G., W.Schlegel, J.Debus, L.R.Schad, Th.Bortfeld, K.H.Hover, W.J.Lorenz, and M.Wannenmacher (1993) Fractionated stereotactically guided radiotherapy of head and neck tumors: a report on clinical use of a new system in 195 cases. Radiotherapy & Oncology, in press.

7. Gademann, G., Engenhart, R.; Schlegel, W.; Witton, T.;Hover, K.-H.; Kimmig, B.; Lorenz, W.J.; Wannenmacher, M. Results and historical comparison of single dose and fractionated stereotactic Radiotherapy in 85 low grade meningiomas. Int. J. Radiat. Oncol. Biol. Phys, submitted.

8. Gademann, G.; Schlegel, W.; Becker, G.; Romahn, J.; Hover, K.-H., Pastyr, O.; van Kaick, G. Wannenmacher, M. High precision radiotherapy of head and neck tumors by means of an integrated stereotactic and 3-D planning system. Int.J.Radiat. Oncol. Biol. Phys. 19 (Suppl.l): 135; 1990.

9. Menke, M.; Mack, T.; Schlegel, W. Modification of planned 3-D dose distributions by patient set-up errors. In: Minet, P.(ed.) Three dimensional treatment planning, European Assoc. of Radiology, Liege; 1993: 323-334.

10. Schad L., Gademann G., Knopp M., Zabel H.-J., Schlegel W., Lorenz W.J. Radiotherapy treatment planning of basal meningiomas: Improved tumor localisation by correlation of CT and MR imaging data. Radiotherapy and Oncology, 25:56-62, 1992.

11. Schlegel W., Pastyr O., Boesecke R., Bortfeld Th., Becker G., Schad L., Gademann G., Lorenz W.J. Computer systems and mechanical tools for stereotactical guided conformation therapy with linear accelerators. Int. J. Radiat. Oncol. Biol. Phys 24:781-787, 1992.

12. Schlegel W., Scharfenberg H., Doll J., Hartmann G.H., Sturm V., Lorenz W.J.Three dimensional dose planning using tomographic data. In: Proc.of the Eight Int. Conference on the Use of Computers in Radiation Therapy IEEEE Comp. Society. Silver Spring, MD:IEEE Comp Soc.Press: 191-196,1984.

13. Wiegel T., Schmidt R., Krull A., Schwarz R., Sommer K., Hubener K.-H. (1992) Advantage of three-dimensional treatment planning for localaitzed radiotherapy of early stage prostatic cancer. Strahlentherapie und Onkologie 168: 692-697.

Chapter 14

Clinical Experience With 3-D Radiotherapy: Treating Prostate Cancer

Gerald E. Hanks, M.D., Timothy E. Schultheiss, Ph.D. and Margie Hunt, M.S.

Department of Radiation Oncology, Fox Chase Cancer Center, Philadelphia, Pennsylvania

The conformal treatment of prostate cancer at Fox Chase Cancer Center began in March, 1989 in an effort to improve the technical execution of treatment, minimize dose to normal tissue, and assure that the entire target volume was irradiated each day. A number of physicians and physicists have been involved in this project and are listed in Table 14-1.

Table 14-2 contains some characteristics of our clinical program as it has developed. During the first 15 months only patients appropriate for treatment directed at their prostates alone were included. Since July, 1990 all new patients have been included in the conformal radiation program although the whole pelvis component of the radiation is not truly conformal.

Immobilization

In the Spring of 1989, we conducted a study of daily set-up variation.[1] The isocenter was located on the portal films of patients treated with conformal radiation therapy who were immobilized in a posterior Alpha Cradle* cast that extended from mid-thigh to mid-thorax. The variation in the location of the isocenter was measured and compared to a stage-matched group treated with conventional techniques without immobilization. This study demonstrated a reduction in isocenter variation with immobilization that is summarized in Table 14-3. Since that time, all patients have been immobilized in this fashion for all treatments.

This study provided the logical basis for determining the margin around the Clinical Target Volume (CTV). We define the CTV on CT images as the prostate or the prostate plus seminal vesicles, as appropriate. A retrograde urethrogram is used to define the inferior border of the prostate.[2] The Planning Target Volume (PTV) is the CTV plus the margin sufficient to give a high confidence of treating all of the CTV every day. Based on the results presented in Table 14-3, we have utilized a 1 cm margin around the CTV to define the PTV. The apertures (defining the Irradiated Volume) for a four field plan are determined from Beams Eye View (BEV) planning by adding sufficient margin to encompass the PTV within the 95°h isodose contour (Treated Volume). The aperture margin is generally 1.5 cm around the CTV. It is the matching of the Treated Volume to the PTV that characterizes conformal radiation therapy. Typical treatment fields for prostate only and whole pelvis irradiation are shown in Figures 14-1 & 14-2 and 14-3 & 14-4. Each institution must determine their own suitable margins and definitions of volumes in their practice.

---

* Smithers Corporation, Akron, OH.

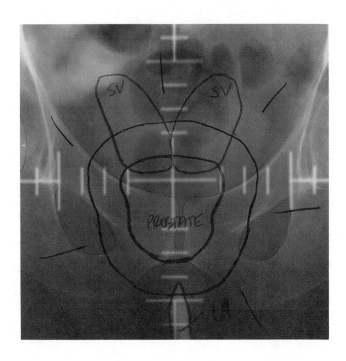

Figure 14-1. *Anterior prostate only conformal treatment field showing prostate, seminal vesicles and field aperture.*

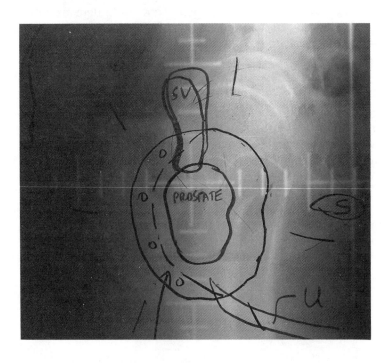

Figure 14-2. *Lateral prostate only conformal treatment field showing prostate, seminal vesicles and initial field aperture with increased rectal blocking.*

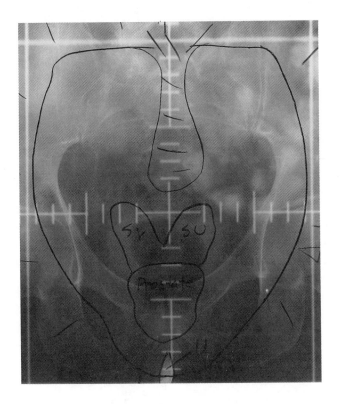

Figure 14-3. *Anterior whole pelvis treatment field showing prostate, seminal vesicles and field aperture*

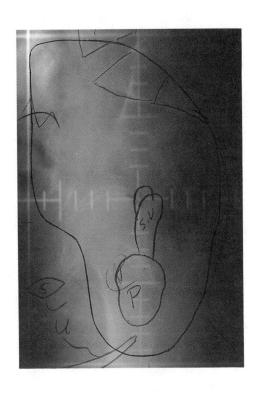

Figure 14-4. *Lateral whole pelvis treatment field showing prostate, seminal vesicles and field aperture.*

Table 14-1. Fox Chase Cancer Center Conformal Program in Prostate Cancer

Staff Physicians	Physicists	Residents/Fellows
Hanks	Schultheiss	Hunter*
Epstein*	Hunt	Ames*
Soffen*	Desobry	Berk*
Corn	McGee	D'Amico*
Lee	Gazda	Kaplan
Chu*		

* no longer at FCCC

Table 14-2. Fox Chase Cancer Center Conformal Program in Prostate Cancer

March 1989—July 1990 – Prostate Only Target Volume
July 1990—Present – All New Patients
4 Field Technique
200 cGy To PTV Daily
Dose Escalation From 66 Gy To 75 Gy
Integrated With LAN and PACS
March 1993—Dedicated CT Simulator

Table 14-3. Comparison of Port Films with Patients Casted and Not Casted

	Cast*	No Cast**
Average range daily error (mm)	3.3	8.0
Median daily error (mm)	1	3
Exact agreement with simulation (%)	43	22
Greatest error (mm)		
Superior/Inferior	6	10
Anterior/Posterior	6	15
Lateral	7	13

* total number observations 280
** total number observations 216

Reduction of Acute Morbidity

In 1990, we compared the acute RTOG grade 11 (medication required) morbidity for standard and conformal technique in our department.[3,4] Table 14-4 illustrates that patients treated with conformal fields experienced roughly half the acute symptoms of those with standard fields in this first report.

Dose volume histograms then showed that with prostate only irradiation, the conformal portals reduced the dose to the bladder and the rectum by an average of 14°h and suggested that this volume reduction resulted in fewer acute symptoms (Figures 14-5 and 14-6). This observation has subsequently been confirmed at other institutions.[5]

A recent multivariate analysis of 408 consecutive patients (Table 14-5) has shown that technique and volume are independent variables in acute reactions.[4] The study also makes the interesting observation that elderly patients appear to tolerate conformal radiation better than they do standard techniques.

Table 14-4. Acute Morbidity

	GROUP 1 (CG) (N=26)	GROUP 2 (NCG) (N=20)
Urinary Symptoms		
Present	17 (65%)	16 (80%)
Required medication	4 (15%)	10 (50%)
Required break	0	2 (10%)
Average duration (days)	17	24
(Range)	(14-21)	(7-35)
Rectal Symptoms		
Present	11 (42%)	11 (55%)
Required medication	6 (23%)	8 (40%)
Required break	0	0
Average duration (days)	10	14
(Range)	(7-17)	(7-21)
Urinary and Rectal Symptoms		
Present	7 (27%)	11 (55%)
Required medication for both	2 (8%)	5 (25%)
Urinary or Rectal Symptoms		
Present	20 (77%)	16 (80%)
Required medication	8 (31%)	12 (60%)
Required break	0	2 (5%)
Symptoms Persisting >1 month		
Post-therapy	3 (11%)	4 (20%)
Average duration (days)	45	70

CG=Conformal Group
NCG=Non-conformal Group

Late Morbidity with Conformal Treatment

Sandler first published a low frequency of late morbidity with conformal technique in prostate cancer.[7] In 1992 we reported grade 3 and 4 late morbidity in our first 108 patients.[8] Despite an increase in dose in the range of 5%-8% and an increase in daily increment from 180-200 cGy, late morbidity was still below our standard technique baseline of <2% and continues at that low frequency.

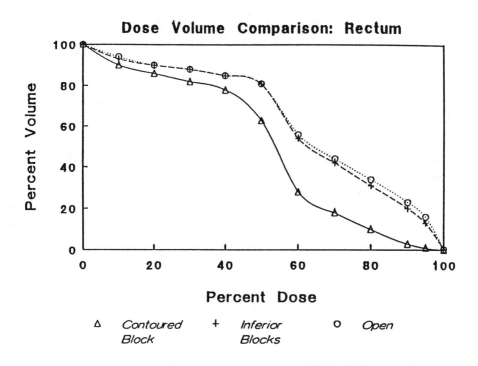

Figure 14-5. Integral dose-volume histogram of rectum averaged for five patients.

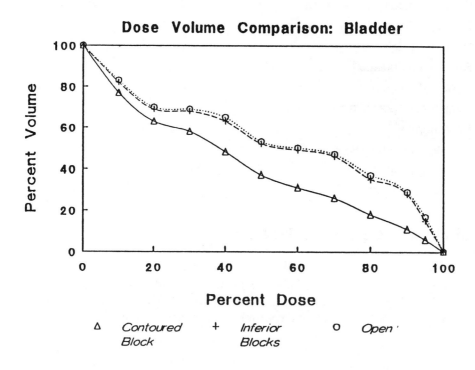

Figure 14-6. Integral dose-volume histogram of bladder averaged for five patients.

Integration with LAN and PACS

Four years ago we began to develop a local area network (LAN) and picture archiving system (PACS) with the goal of becoming fully digital.[8] Prostate cancer is the ideal site for integration into that effort and we are now fully digital in treatment simulation, treatment planning, conformal block fabrication, and portal film verification in that site. We believe that digital technology is one of the future directions for radiation oncology.

Table 14-5. *Factors Influencing Incidence of Acute Grade II Morbidity in Conformal and Standard Radiation Treatment of Prostate Cancer*

Univariate and Multivariate Analysis				
Factor/Selection Criterion	Conformal	Standard	Conformal vs. Standard	P Value on Logistic Regression
All Patients	84/247	93/162	P<0.00001	------
Age				
>65 Years	60/189	74/121	P<0.00001	N.S.
<65 Years	24/58 N.S.	19/41 P<0.1	N.S.	N.S.
Stage				
T-1	10/37	10/14	P<0.005	
T-2	47/152 N.S.	51/86 N.S.	P<0.00005	N.S.
T-3	24/54		27/51	N.S.
Volume:				
Prostate only	34/137	28/54	P<0.0005	P<0.001
Prostate + Pelvis	50/110 P<0.001	65/108 N.S.	P<0.03	P<0.001
Dose:				
>70 Gy	49/132	27/52	N.S.	N.S.
<70 Gy	35/115 N.S.	66/110 N.S.	P<0.00002	N.S.
Conformal vs. Standard:				P<0.001

Dose Escalation and Current Policies

We have cautiously proceeded with dose escalation, first by increasing our daily increment from 180 cGy to 200 cGy and by prescribing to the isodose encompassing the PTV. The second phase of dose escalation was an increase in the PTV dose from 66 Gy to 75 Gy in 2 Gy increments. We have also increased the volume irradiated to include patients with whole pelvis and patients with part or all of their conformal boost given to the seminal vesicles. We now have one group of 20 patients treated with 45 Gy to the whole pelvis and conformal prostate irradiation to 74 Gy and one group of 20 treated to 45 Gy to the whole pelvis with prostate and seminal vesicles carried to 75 Gy. Our current policy is described in Table 14-6 where one can see we have reduced our total dose to 68-72 Gy to the PTV while we assess any late effects from the earlier dose escalation. We do not anticipate increasing dose beyond these levels except as part of a multi-institution dose escalation study.

Table 14-6. Fox Chase Cancer Center Prostate Cancer Treatment Guidelines

T1a, T1b	GL≤5	Prostate+1.5	6000/200's
		Prostate (new blocks)**	800/200's
			6800
T1a, T1b	GL≥6	Pelvis*	4500/180's
		Prostate+1.5	1600/200's
		Prostate (new blocks)**	1000/200's
			7100
T1c, T2a, T2b	GL<7	Prostate+1.5	6000/200's
		Prostate (new blocks)**	1200/200's
			7200
T1c, T2a, T2b	GL≥7	Pelvis*	4500/180's
		Prostate+1.5	1400/200's
		Prostate (new blocks)**	1200/200's
			7100
T2c, T3a, T3b	Any GL	Pelvis*	4500/180's
		Prostate+SV+1.5	1200/200's
		Prostate+1.5+(new blocks)**	1400/200's
			7100
T3c	Any GL	Pelvis*	4500/180's
		Prostate+SV+1.5	1200/200's
		Prostate +SV***+1.5(new blocks)**	1400/200's
			7100

*pelvic Field: Mid S1 to 1 cm below urethrogram cone S2/S3 posterior, front of pubic symphysis anterior; use barium per rectum to protect posterior half of rectum, providing this does not block more rectum than conformal field

**prostate (new blocks): 1.5 cm margin around entire prostate except posterior aspect (lateral films) which have 0.5 cm margin round prostate

***involved SV only (if any)

The Future of Conformal Treatment

Prostate cancer has proven to be the ideal disease for the initial exploration of advancing technology of conformal irradiation. It has already clearly shown a reduction in acute side effects and a late side effect tolerance to doses that exceed those commonly given. A 10% increase in dose will almost certainly result in an increase in local control. It remains to be seen if that difference will be measurable.

The challenge to physicists and to radiation oncologists is to evaluate more cancer sites for the application of conformal technologies. This experience has reinforced the need to adequately immobilize all patients, to re-orient our thinking from apertures to targets and to not be confined by the treatment dogma of the past.

References

1. Soffen EM, Hanks GE, Hwang CC, Chu JCH: Conformal static field therapy for low volume low grade prostate cancer with rigid immobilization. Int J Radiat Oncol Biol Phys 20:142-146, 1991.

2. Ames JW, Epstein BE, Hartz W, Litwin S, Hanks GE: Comparison of urethrogram and pelvic cat scan in determining the caudal extent of the prostate. (Abstr.) Int J Radiat Oncol Biol Phys (in press).

3. Soffen EM, Hanks GE, Hunt MA, Epstein BE: Conformal static field radiation therapy treatment of early prostate cancer versus non-conformal techniques: a reduction in acute morbidity. Int J Radiat Oncol Biol Phys 24:485-488, 1992.

4. Schultheiss TE, Hanks GE, Hunt MA, Epstein BE, Peter R: Factors influencing incidence of acute grade II morbidity in conformal and standard radiation treatment of prostate cancer: univariate and multivariate analysis. Int J Radiat Oncol Biol Phys (in press).

5. Emami B, Purdy JA, Manolis JM, Gerber RL, Harms WB, Simpson JR, Wippold FJ, Perez CA: 3-D static conformal radiotherapy: preliminary results of a prospective clinical trial. (Abstr.) Int J Radiat Oncol Biol Phys 21:147, 1991.

6. Sandler HM, Perez-Tamayo C, Ten-Haken RK, Lichter AS: Dose escalation for stage C (T3) prostate cancer: minimal rectal toxicity observed using conformal therapy. Radiother Oncol 23:53-54, 1992.

7. Epstein BE, Peter R, Martin E, Hunt M, Hanks GE: Low complication rate with conformal radiotherapy for cancer of the prostate. (Abstr.) Radiother Oncol 24:394, 1992.

8. Stafford PM, Martin EE, Chu JCH, Davidson BA, Hanks GE: Digital imaging in the radiation oncology environment: a personal computer local area network solution. J Digit Imaging 4:177-184, 1991.

Chapter 15

What is a Fully Integrated CT Simulator?

Carlos A. Perez, M.D., James A. Purdy, Ph.D., Bahman N. Emami, M.D., Russell Gerber, M.S., and William B. Harms, B.S.

Radiation Oncology Center, Mallinckrodt Institute of Radiology,
Washington University School of Medicine, St. Louis, Missouri

Major changes have taken place in treatment planning and, to a lesser extent, in delivery of radiation therapy in the past 20 years. Over the past 25 years, computed tomography (CT) was increasingly used in two-dimensional treatment planning for radiation therapy; also, since the mid-1960s, simulators have been extensively used to design portals and verify the volumes treated (6). Computer capabilities have enhanced the practical application of three-dimensional (3-D) treatment planning in the management of patients with cancer. Several systems have been developed that incorporate CT information directly into the 3-D virtual simulation and treatment planning process (1,3-6,8,10,12,13,15). Some commercial devices including several of these features are available. In 1990, Nishidai et al. (11) described a CT simulator composed of a CT scanner, multi-image display console with data recording devices, treatment planning console with CT image processor, and a laser beam projecting device.

We describe the basic components of a fully integrated CT simulator, identify some problems, and offer solutions for optimal clinical application of this device.

Methods and Materials

A commercial CT scanner with a 70 cm ring was connected to a computer-based virtual simulation and 3-D planning system. With assistance from a commercial company[1] and support from Siemens Corporation,[2] a laser beam projector was incorporated into the gantry of the CT scanner to delineate portals on the patients; design accuracy of the beam aperture projection is 2 mm.

A fully integrated CT simulator will be of great assistance to radiation oncologists, physicists, and dosimetrists to accomplish the entire treatment planning process. Table 15-1 outlines the basic components and functions of what we initially envisioned as a fully integrated CT simulator. When a patient is treated with radiation therapy, the first step in treatment planning, after appropriate evaluation of the patient and formulation of therapeutic strategy, is accurate delineation of the gross (GTV) or microscopic (CTV) tumor volume and identification of radiation-sensitive normal structures (according to ICRU Report #50) (7). The second step is virtual simulation, which requires the ability to transfer the planned volumetric patient data and setup geometry to the 3-D-planning computer. Once the treatment geometry has been defined, the information is transferred to the patient. Sherouse et al. (14) considered immobilization of the patient, establishment and alignment of a coordinate system for the patient/couch system, and set up of the patient/couch system and the treatment machine as part of the virtual simulation. We incorporate these procedures in both the virtual and the physical simulation of the patient; the latter is carried out after the virtual simulation and the 3-D treatment planning have been completed. Once the most desirable dose distributions are obtained, the geometric information from the treatment

[1] Medical Knowledge Systems, Detroit, MI.
[2] Siemens DRH CT-Scanner, NJ.

plan is transferred to a patient marking device, and a portal outline is projected and marked on the patient. This can be accomplished with either the laser projection or a light field system. Subsequently, a radiographic verification of the patient volume encompassed by the treatment portals (geometric verification) is documented by comparing simulator radiographs with digitally reconstructed radiographs (DRR). With a better understanding of the treatment planning process, as we applied these concepts to our patients, a more detailed list of the elements constituting the CT simulator was identified (Table 15-2).

Table 15-1. Structure and Functions of Fully Integrated CT Simulator

Structure		Function
CT scan	•	Definition of anatomy/geometry (patient contour/patient outline)
Virtual simulation	•	Beam design/RX setup
		Digitally reconstructed radiographs
3-D treatment planning	•	Volumetric dose distribution and plan evaluation
Patient marking device	•	Portal outline on patient's skin
Radiographic capability	•	Portal placement verification

Table 15-2. CT Simulator Elements

Volumetric CT data-transfer to RTP System
Virtual simulation-contouring
Target volume
Normal tissues
Initial beam arrangement
3-D dose calculations and display
Plan evaluation-optimization
Standard beam
3-D beam arrangement
Digital reconstructed radiograph
Block template
Physical simulation
Identification of portals
Marking of patient
Radiographic verification
Blockmaking
Block check

Results

As we have worked with the prototype CT simulator and 3-D treatment planning system for the past year, we have identified a number of problems and, based on existing technology, offer some solutions to enhance the clinical application of this device. The following is an outline of problems identified and potential solutions:

I. Volumetric CT Data
   A. Problems
      1. CT ring size (large patients, asymmetric setups)
      2. Transfer of volumetric images to RTP system (time consuming: 20 to 30 minutes with DRH, 4 to 5 minutes with new scanner)
   B. Solutions
      1. Larger CT scanner ring size (100 cm)
      2. Faster scan data transfer. Implement DiCOM 3.0 data transfer.
II. Virtual Simulation (Physician Time and Contouring)
   A. Contouring Problems
      1. Target volume (1 hour)
      2. Normal structures (1.5 hours)
      3. Image analysis (diagnostic expertise)
      4. Software not user-friendly
   B. Solutions
      1. Improved automated contouring tools
      2. Training in diagnostic radiology
      3. Improved user interface (user-friendly software)
III. Dose Computation, Display, and Plan Evaluation
   A. Problems
      1. Slow (full scattered) dose algorithms
      2. Fast dose algorithms not accurate in some regions
      3. 3-D dose compensation algorithms (contours, tissue heterogeneity)
      4. 3-D beam modulation algorithms
      5. 3-D dose optimization algorithms
      6. Quantitative plan evaluation
   B. Solutions
      1. Faster computers
      2. Improved dose calculation algorithms
      3. Develop/improve dose modulation/optimization systems
      4. Develop/test quantitative evaluation systems
IV. Physical Simulation
   A. Problems
      1. Slow digitally reconstructed radiograph (DRR)
      2. Patient portal marking (laser system)
      3. On-site radiographic verification
   B. Solutions
      1. Faster hardware/software for DRR
      2. Integrate CT scanner/treatment planning with patient portal marking and radiographic verification
      3. Couch enhancement

Discussion

Numerous clinical reports strongly suggest that higher doses of irradiation delivered to appropriate target volumes result in better tumor control and disease-free survival. Furthermore, in some tumors, such as carcinoma of the uterine cervix, prostate, and lung, higher local tumor control has been correlated with a lower incidence of distant metastasis and higher survival. The advent of new technology has greatly improved the precision with which radiation therapy is planned and delivered. The described fully integrated CT simulator will substantially enhance our capability to consolidate and unify the treatment planning process, from the delineation of the tumor and normal, sensitive structures to the preparation of the patient for the actual treatment and verification of the volume to be treated. In the future, we may achieve computer-aided integration of the data generated by the CT simulation process with parameters to be used on the treatment machine, thus decreasing marginal error and enhancing the efficiency with which irradiation will be administered. New approaches to the delivery of irradiation, with modulation of beams to multiple portals and dynamic beam modifiers (multileaf collimator, wedges, etc.), as described by Carol et al. (2), will benefit considerably from the availability of a practical, fully integrated CT simulator device. We plan to continue to optimize the use of this device. Major steps in the near future include improvement of the patient-marking mode and possible incorporation of a radiographic unit in the CT simulator specifically for portal verification purpose.

References

1. Bruinvis IAD, van der Giessen PH, van Kleffens HJ, Wittkamper FW (eds): The use of computers in radiation therapy. Proceedings of Ninth International Conference on the Use of Computers in Radiation Therapy, Scheveningen, June 22-25. The Netherlands: Elsevier Science Publishers BV, 1987.

2. Carol MP, Targovnik H, Smith D, Cahill D: 3-D planning and delivery system for optimized conformal therapy. Int J Radiat Oncol Biol Phys 24(1):158, 1992.

3. Fraass BA, McShan DL: 3-D treatment planning. I. Overview of a clinical planning system. In Bruinvis IAD, van der Giessen PH, van Kleffens HJ, Wittkamper FW (eds): The use of computers in radiation therapy, pp 273-276. The Netherlands: Elsevier Science Publishers BV, 1987.

4. Goitein M, Abrams M, Rowell D, Pollari H, Wiles J: Multi-dimensional treatment planning. II. Beam's eye view back projection and projection through CT sections. Int J Radiat Oncol Biol Phys 9:789-797, 1983.

5. Goitein M, Mark A: Multi-dimensional treatment planning. I. Delineation of anatomy. Int J Radiat Oncol Biol Phys 9:777-787, 1983.

6. Heidtman CM: Clinical application of a CT-simulator: Precision treatment planning and portal marking in breast cancer. Med Dosim 15:113-117, 1990.

7. ICRU: Report No. 50, Prescribing, recording, and reporting photon beam therapy. International Commission on Radiation Units and Measurements, Washington, DC, 1993 (to be published).

8. Lamm IL: CART: Report on the Nordic Co-operation Programme. In Bruinvis IAD, van der Giessen PH, van Kleffens HJ, Wittkamper FW (eds): The use of computers in radiation therapy, pp 257-260. The Netherlands: Elsevier Science Publishers BV, 1987.

9. Mallik R, Hunt P: The Royal North Shore Hospital experience with the Varian Ximatron/CT option. Proceedings of the Varian 14th User's Meeting, Waikola, Hawaii, 1992.

10. Nagata Y, Nishidai T, Yukawa Y, Nohara H, Takahashi M, Abe M: Clinical application of CT simulator. In Bruinvis IAD, et al. (eds): Ninth International Conference on the Use of Computers in Radiation Therapy, Scheveningen, The Netherlands, pp 335-338. Amsterdam, Elsevier Science Publishers, 1987.

11. Nishidai T, Nagata Y, Takahashi M, Abe M, Yamaoka N, Ishihara H, Kubo Y, Ohta H, Kazusa C: CT simulator: A new 3-D planning and simulation system for radiotherapy. I. Description of system. Int J Radiat Oncol Biol Phys 18:499-504, 1990.

12. Ogino T, Hanai K, Egawa S, Takano H: Computed simulationgraphy: Concept and method of clinical application. Radiat Med 8(1):29-33, 1990.

13. Purdy JA, Wong JW, Harms WB, Drzymala RE, Emami B, Matthews JW, Krippner K, Ramchandar PK: Three dimensional radiation treatment planning system. In Bruinvis IAD, van der Giessen PH, van Kleffens HJ, Wittkamper FW (eds): The use of computers in radiation therapy, pp 277-279. The Netherlands: Elsevier Science Publishers BV, 1987.

14. Sherouse GW, Bourland JD, Reynolds K, McMurry HL, Mitchell TP, Chaney EL: Virtual simulation in the clinical setting: Some practical considerations. Int J Radiat Oncol Biol Phys 19:1059-1065, 1990.

15. Sherouse GW, Mosher CE, Novins K, Roseman J, Chaney EW: Virtual simulation: Concept and implementation. In Bruinvis IAD, van der Giessen PH, van Kleffens HJ, Wittkamper FW (eds): The use of computers in radiation therapy, pp 433-436. The Netherlands: Elsevier Science Publishers BV, 1987.

Chapter 16

CT-Based Simulation with Laser Patient Marking[1]

Don P. Ragan, Ph.D., Tongming He, M.S., Carmen F. Mesina, M.S.,
Vaneerat Ratanatharathorn, M.D.

Radiation Oncology Department, Wayne State University, Detroit, Michigan

Radiation Oncology treatment planning is an important component of successful radiotherapy. The treatment planning process is much more than isodose computation. It begins with appropriate patient diagnostic workup and physician assessment. Simulation, dose estimation and possible resimulation result in treatment portals which must be identified correctly on successive days of treatment. CT-Simulation, 3-D planning and real-time portal imaging are all areas of active research and development; all address improving radiation portal design and treatment.

CT scanning and 3-D dose computation offers significant advantages over conventional simulation and 2-D dose computation. Unfortunately, CT scanners do not offer the possibility of marking the central axis of the proposed treatment portal.

In order to more accurately transfer CT-based simulation and planning information to patient treatments, the authors have developed a laser beam projector mounted on a CT gantry, the purpose of which is to accurately transfer the patient plan onto the patient's skin for positioning and repositioning. This paper describes our initial experience using this laser beam projector for patient/portal localization.

Background

Room lasers are the accepted way to mark a patient in the simulator; corresponding lasers in the treatment room allow patient repositioning in approximately the same position. The central axis of each portal is marked on the simulator and checked with port films. During the mid 1980s, the concept of CT-Simulation became popular. Sherouse et al.[1], developed a package which replaced the simulator with a CT study in the treatment position followed by "Virtual Simulation" on a computer. This "simulation" plus 3-D planning affords the physician <u>significantly</u> more information with which to plan patient treatment than the conventional 2-D alternative. Unfortunately, the CT is not equipped with cross hair, field defining wires, etc., necessary for patient marking. Sherouse proposed immobilizing the patient prior to CT scanning and to rely on registration of this object on the therapy machine. This has not proven popular nor universally possible and may be less accurate than the combination of immobilization and patient marking proposed in this paper.[2]

A dedicated CT for simulation was developed in the mid 1980s.[3] This CT Sim device provides CT mounted lasers which can be made to point to the isocenter or field corners through appropriate movements of the scanner couch. This device was the first to recognize the need to couple patient marking with CT scans.

[1] This work was supported in part by a grant from Siemens Medical Systems, Inc.

In 1982, Goitein[4] proposed mounting a laser marking device on a ring concentric to the CT gantry. This device could take the portal design (based on CT data) and project it on the patient's skin potentially preserving the accuracy of the CT and computer planning calculations. Such a system has been implemented in Japan. Nagata, et al.[5] reported accuracies from ± 3 to 5 mm; somewhat less than optimal. They did demonstrate that it was effective on approximately 70% of their patients and that CT-Simulation (including target localization, portal design and patient marking) could often be accomplished in less than an hour (Personal Communication).

The C-arm design of Goitein and Nagata has three fundamental problems. First, the device must be rigidly and perfectly aligned with the CT geometry. Second, because it is a separate device, it is inherently more expensive to make compared to a device that might mount on a CT gantry. And third, it is cumbersome to use since it is at 100 cm SAD and the isocenter of the device must be moved to correspond to the isocenter of treatment.

The authors have developed a similar device but mounted on the CT gantry[6] (color Plate 12). Because of its physical location (on the CT gantry), it remains registered to the CT. It is relatively inexpensive since it uses the CT gantry for its mechanical base. Computer programs have been written to correct for small mechanical misalignments, lenses used to expand the scanning field size and to correct for a device to patient distance of much less than 100 cm. This later feature makes patient marking for 80 cm cobalt or approximately 180 cm neutron therapy devices trivial. A complete technical description is given in a previous paper.[7]

Methods

A clinical protocol has been established for the CT simulation with laser patient marking. The exact protocol is an evolving process and varies slightly by case. The generic CT simulation process consists of the following seven phases:

Patient Setup:
Patient is placed on the CT table, properly aligned and immobilized (approximately 10 minutes).

Reposition Marking:
The lateral positions are marked on the patient through two side alignment lasers near the CT scanner. The AP position is marked utilizing the laser marking device on the CT gantry. These marks are for the purpose of position verification and repositioning of patient with respect to the CT if the patient moves or has to leave the CT table (approximately 5 minutes).

CT Scanning:
The patient is scanned across the region of treatment planning by the appropriate number of slices (usually 40 to 50 slices; approximately 20 minutes).

Image Transfer and Skin Contouring:
CT slices are transferred to the treatment simulation/planning computer through the network as soon as scanned. Skin surface and other structures are contoured on these slices concurrently with scanning (approximately 25 minutes).

Target Contouring:
Physician participates to contour the target volume on CT slices (approximately 15 minutes).

Treatment Field Design:

The 3-D patient model is displayed on the Virtual Simulator[2] which provides Beam's Eye View of the contoured structures. Physician designs the fields on this Virtual Simulator (approximately 15 minutes).

Field Geometry Projection and Marking:

The geometry (i.e. the field axis cross and block contour) or the isocenter setup positions of the designed fields are projected on the patient's skin surface through the laser device on the CT gantry (color Plate 13) and marked for treatment setup on the therapy unit (approximately 10 minutes).

Results

We have performed this CT simulation with laser portal marking on several selected brain and prostate cases. In most of the cases, the simulation and the portal marking were finished in one session from Phase #1 to #7 within about one hour (less compliant patients took longer). The length of time spent on each phase varies with the patient's condition, computer speed at the time, number of CT slices scanned and the experience of participants. The approximate time for each phase is given above; phase #3, #4, and #5 are usually done concurrently. The total length of time to finish the CT simulation is about one hour (Table 16-1). The physician participates in only Phase #5 and #6; the total physician time is about 25 minutes.

Table 16-1. VRS Preliminary Data Summary of Simulation Time

Patient Name	DOC	Diagnosis	Total Time	Staff Tech	Staff Phys
CN	VR	Prostate, Adenoca	60	2	
FC	VR	Prostate, Adenoca	50		
MC	VR	Bladder, Transitional	100		
PL	ATP	Prostate, Adenoca			
LM	JDF	Prostate, Adenoca	80	3	
WS	JDF	Prostate, Adenoca	45	3	
WM	JDF	Prostate, Adenoca	50	2	2
HD	VR	Pituitary Adenoma	55	4	2
JW	VR	Pituitary Adenoma	65	2	2
		Average	**63.1**	**2.7**	**1.5**

The field projection and marking (Phase #7) on typically three or four fields took about 10 minutes. The inherent time spent on field projection by the device is about 10 seconds per field. The field projection accuracy was initially measured by using a conventional simulator following CT simulation. The data match very well and show no evidence that the conventional simulation gives better accuracy than the CT simulation.

Because of the uncertainty inherent in conventional simulation, the clinical accuracy of the laser device has also been assessed using a different approach. A thin wire (of 1 mm diameter) is attached

---

[2] G.W. Sherouse, "Virtual Simulator," Release 2, (1989). Personal Communication.

on the patient's skin at the position of the proposed treatment field isocenter projected by the device. The patient is then given a single scan through this isocenter. On the CT slices, the wire shows the projected field positions. On the computer, the previously designed fields are projected on these slices and one can measure how the field projection lines match with respect to the wire image. This positional uncertainty accounts for the overall simulation performance which includes patient movement, skin movement, CT imaging error, CT table position error and skin contouring error. The projection accuracy of the device was measured to be better than $\pm$ 1.4 mm (Table 16-2).

Conclusion

CT simulation with laser portal marking has been performed on several brain and prostate cases. In most cases, the simulation was finished in one session without the need for conventional simulation. The total simulation time ranged from 45 to 100 minutes. Most of the cases were simulated and the port marked within about one hour. The clinical accuracy of this CT simulation using the laser marking device has been measured to be better than 1.4 mm. The laser portal marking device transfers treatment field geometry efficiently; within 10 minutes for four fields. It is expected that this CT simulation with laser portal marking can be performed in most disease sites, can be completed in a time equivalent to conventional simulation time, with an accuracy better than 1.4 mm and without the need for conventional simulation. Simulation time averaged slightly over one hour.

Table 16-2. VRS Prelinary Data Summary of Simulation Accuracy

Patient Name	DOC	Diagnosis	Total Time	Staff Tech	Accuracy Phys	PA	LAT	Comment
CN	VR	Prostate, Adenoca	60	2	1	1.5	5	Patient moved
FC	VR	Prostate, Adenoca	50			1	2	
MC	VR	Bladder, Transitional	100					
PL	ATP	Prostate, Adenoca				0	0	
LM	JDF	Prostate, Adenoca	80	3				
WS	JDF	Prostate, Adenoca	45	3				
WM	JDF	Prostate, Adenoca	50	2	2	0		
WM	JDF	Prostate, Adenoca						Laser link down
JC	JDF	Prostate, Adenoca						Laser link down
HD	VR	Pituitary Adenoma	55	4	2			
JW	VR	Pituitary Adenoma	65	2	2	1	5	Patient moved
		Average	**63.1**	**2.7**	**1.5**	**0.8**	**1.9**	

References

1. G.W. Sherouse, E.L. Chaney, "The Portable Virtual Simulator," Int. J. Radiat. Oncol. Biol. Phys. **21**, 475-482 (1991).

2. G.W. Sherouse, J.D. Bourland, K. Reynolds, H.L. McMurry, T.P. Mitchell, E.L. Chaney, "Virtual Simulator in the Clinical Setting: Some Practical Considerations," Int. J. Radiat. Oncol. Biol. Phys. **19**, 1059-1065 (1990).

3. R.M. Smith, L.J. Sanfilippo, K.D. Steidley, H.T. Kohut, "Clinical Patterns of Use of a CT-Based Simulator." Med. Dos. **12**(2), pp. 17-22, 1987.

4. M. Goitein, D. Mento, "An Optical Scanner as Aid in Simulating Treatment with CT Data," Journal of Computer Assisted Tomography. 6(6), 1201-1204 (1982).

5. T. Nishidai, Y. Nagata, M. Takahashi, M. Abe, N. Yamaoka, H. Ishihara, H. Kubo, H. Ohta, C. Kazusa, "CT Simulator: A New 3-D Planning and Simulating System for Radiotherapy: Part 1. Description of System," Int. J. Radiat. Oncol. Biol. Phys. **18**, 499-504 (1990).

6. X. Liu, D.P. Ragan, "Contour Transfer using a Microprocessor Controlled Laser Scanner", Proceedings of SPIE on Application of Digital Image Processing XII. **1153,** 350-362 (1989).

7. D.P. Ragan, T. He, X. Liu, "Correction for Distortion in a Beam Outline Transfer Device in Radiotherapy CT-based Simulation." Med. Phy. (20) 1, pp. 179-185, 1993.

Chapter 17

Experience with CT Simulation at the University of Iowa

David H. Hussey, M.D., Edward C. Pennington, M.S., Womah S. Neeranjun, M.S., B-Chen Wen, M.D.,Fred J. Doornbos, M.D., Nina A. Mayr, M.D.

Division of Radiation Oncology, Department of Radiology, University of Iowa, Iowa

In January 1990, the University of Iowa Hospitals and Clinics (UIHC) acquired a Medical High Technology International (MHTI) CT-simulator (Model 0600). This equipment was purchased as part of a program to develop "high precision" radiation therapy treatment techniques, e.g., brachyradiotherapy, non-coplanar field arrangements, stereotactic radiosurgery, and conformal radiation therapy. A variety of imaging devices and treatment planning computers were already available in the department. These included an Imatron cine CT scanner, four conventional diagnostic computerized tomography units, a cyclotron for short-lived isotope production, a positron emission tomography (PET) scanner, two treatment planning computers, and a Silicon Graphics workstation for 3-dimensional treatment planning.

The purpose of this paper is to review the University of Iowa's experience with CT-simulation and to assess its role in the management of cancer patients in an academic setting. In the following pages, we will review: 1) how the CT-simulator has been used at the University of Iowa, 2) whether it has been a financially sound investment, and 3) what the users think of it.

The CT-Simulator

The MHTI CT-simulator is an integrated radiation therapy planning system. It combines in a single unit a whole body CT scanner, a treatment planning computer, and a laser system to delineate treatment portals. The CT scanner and the treatment planning computer can be used independently or as a single unit. When used together, the system is a true simulator since it can be used to plan the field arrangement and to outline treatment portals directly on the patient.[1]

The CT scanner is a fourth generation whole body scanner which utilizes 600 cadmium tungstate detectors. These are connected to a series of solid-state photodiodes. The detector system is arranged around a 69 cm diameter opening. The reconstruction area measures 48 cm in diameter for body scans and 24 cm in diameter for head CT scans. A variety of modifications have been made for radiation therapy purposes. The couch has been widened to simulate a standard radiotherapy treatment couch, and a laser cross-hair system has been incorporated for patient alignment. A second laser system has been added to delineate the treatment portals. This is located within the detector ring, pointing to the center of the aperture from any angle in that plane.

The treatment planning computer is a Theraplan TP-11 computer system. It uses a DEC PDP 11/73 computer, a 375 Mbyte Winchester storage module, a high resolution color monitor, an array processor, a printer, and a plotter. It can perform 3-dimensional calibrations, and can display beams-eye views which are useful for designing field shaping blocks and templates. The computer system allows one to automatically outline the external body surface and internal organ contours. It can be used to compute dose distributions for external beam field arrangements, brachyradiotherapy implants, or combinations of external beam portals and brachyradiotherapy implants. Dose distributions can be calculated for rectangular or irregularly shaped external beam fixed fields, or for moving fields using either SSD or isocentric (SAD) geometry.

The distinguishing feature of the CT-simulator is that it can be used to outline the treatment portals directly on the patient once the treatment plan has been selected. To accomplish this, the CT-simulator automatically positions the CT-simulator couch and the laser system located within the detector ring to illuminate critical points, e.g., the central axis or each corner of the treatment field.[1]

How Has It Been Used?

We have found the CT-simulator to have a wide variety of uses in our department.[2,3] Some of these would have been accomplished in other ways if the CT-simulator had not been available in our division. However, there are some uses for this machine which can be accomplished easily only with a CT-simulator (Table 17-1). These involve its function as a virtual simulator.

Table 17-1. Ways the CT-simulator has been used at the University of Iowa at UIHC

Uses for a CT-Simulator	% of CT-Simulator Cases
For virtual simulation	~20%
For dose distribution after conventional simulation	~40%
To check margins of portals	~5%
To measure tissue thicknesses	~10%
To follow tumor regression	~5%
For interstitial implant dosimetry	~15%
For stereotactic radiosurgery	~1-2%
To evaluate standard treatment techniques	~3%
Total	**100%**

Virtual Simulation

Simulation is a process in which a diagnostic imaging device is used to set up the radiotherapy treatment portals on a patient. It is a process which involves 1) the delineation of a target volume, 2) the selection of beam parameters i.e., gantry and collimator angles, field size and shape, and 3) the transfer of the treatment plan to the patient. The transfer of the treatment plan to the patient is usually accomplished by marking the field outline and central axis directly on the patient's skin. This process is termed "simulation" because it is usually performed with an apparatus which incorporates a diagnostic x-ray tube and is constructed in such a way as to simulate a radiation therapy treatment unit with respect to its geometrical, mechanical, and optical properties.

With a conventional simulator, the target volume is defined on the basis of information obtained by fluoroscopy or simulator radiographs. The beam parameters are obtained from the simulator gantry and collimator settings, and the fields are marked using the simulator light localizer. The dose distribution is usually determined as a subsequent process. Occasionally the simulation must be repeated after the dosimetry has been performed in order to obtain a satisfactory treatment plan.

With virtual simulation, all of the radiographic information is gathered prior to any decision regarding field arrangement. CT scans are obtained through the region of interest, and the tumor, skin surface, and specific organ contours are delineated on the CT images. This information is transferred directly to the treatment planning computer where dose distributions are calculated for a variety of field arrangements. Once a treatment plan has been selected, this information is transferred back to the patient for skin marking. With the MHTI CT-simulator, this is accomplished using the laser cross-hair system which is located in the detector ring. The CT-simulator automatically positions the treatment couch and the laser system to illuminate designated points, e.g., the central axis and the corners of each treatment field (Figure 17-1).

The virtual simulation process gives the radiation oncologist more freedom to design portal arrangements and to modify the treatment plan prior to marking the patient. It should result in a better dose distribution in certain clinical situations, but it is not needed for all cases. We have found it to be particularly useful in cases where oblique treatment portals are being employed next to critical normal structures, e.g., the spinal cord (Figure 17-2). In this situation, conventional simulator radiographs and portal films may be difficult to interpret. Approximately 20% of the cases studied with the CT-simulator at the University of Iowa have involved virtual simulation.

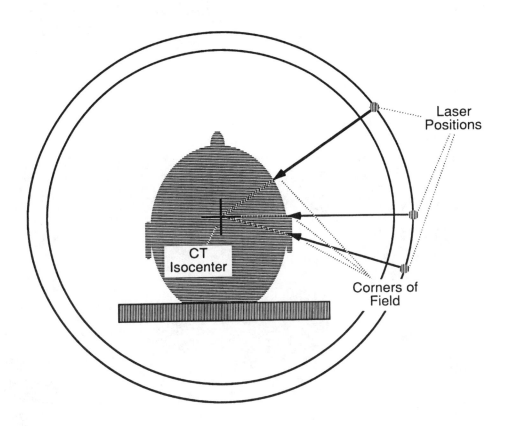

Figure 17-1a.

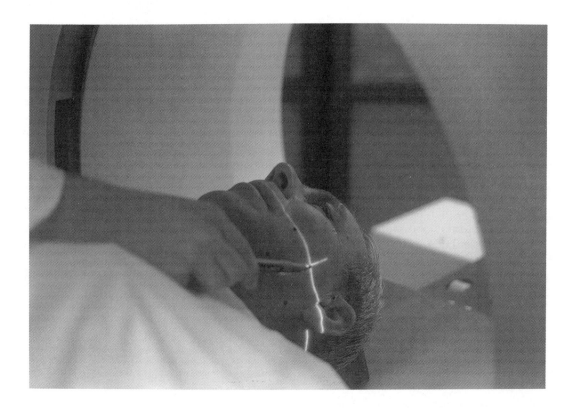

Figure 17-1b.

Figure 17-1a & b. *The laser in the detector ring points toward the CT isocenter intersecting the skin at specified points.*

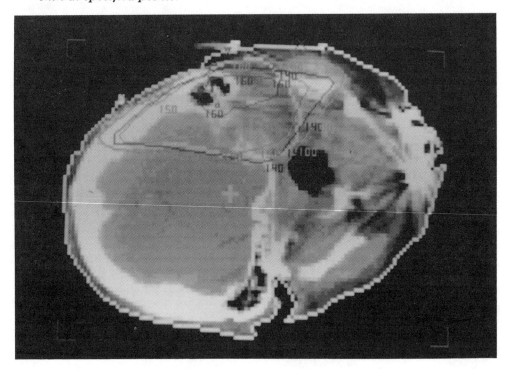

Figure 17-2. *Virtual simulation is useful in situations where oblique portals are being used next to critical normal structures.*

To Determine the Dose Distribution after Conventional Simulation.

Many radiation oncology patients are treated using a standard portal arrangement through fields designed to encompass the clinically detectable tumor with an ample margin and the first echelon of regional lymphatics. In this situation, it is often easier to set up the portals using external landmarks or a conventional simulator than it is to use a CT-simulator. However, many of these patients need CT-based dose distributions, and the CT-simulator is an effective way of accomplishing this (Figure 17-3). CT-based dosimetry is more accurate than dosimetry obtained using solder wire contours. It enables one to better assess the dose to the tumor and specific organs and to take tissue inhomogeneities into account. Approximately 40% of the CT-simulator cases at Iowa were performed to facilitate dosimetry after the portals were set up by other means.

To Check the Margins of the Portals.

We have also used the CT-simulator to check the margins of the fields after the portals have been set up and the dosimetry has been performed by conventional methods. Here, the CT scanner is simply used to determine whether the tumor is being encompassed in the treatment portals. Approximately 5 % of the CT-simulator studies at our institution were performed to evaluate the margins of the fields.

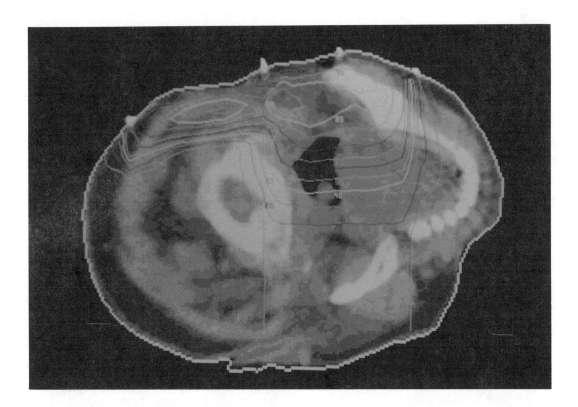

Figure 17-3.   *The CT-simulator is often used to aid in dosimetry after the treatment portals have been setup by other means. It is also useful for determining the depth of critical normal structures such as the spinal cord in patients receiving posterior cervical electron beam irradiation. This patient is being treated with combined x-ray and electron beams to the parotid bed and electrons to the posterior cervical nodes.*

To Measure Tissue Thicknesses.

The CT-simulator has also been used to determine the depth of the tumor or critical normal structures. In the past, this was accomplished using CT scanners in diagnostic radiology. Typical examples are the use of a CT-simulator to measure the depth of the spinal cord in a patient receiving posterior cervical electron beam therapy or to measure the thickness of the chest wall in bone marrow transplant patients receiving chest wall electron beam irradiation (Figure 17-3). Approximately 10% of the CT-simulator cases have been performed to determine tumor depth or the thickness of normal tissues.

To Follow Tumor Regression.

The CT-simulator is very useful for following tumor response during the course of treatment or at follow-up visits. This is analogous to taking weekly tumor measurements or photographs of superficial tumors during the course of treatment. However, these measurements can be made for deep-seated tumors if a CT scanner is available within the department. This information is often useful for planning boost treatments or for determining the total dose to be delivered (Figure 17-4). When serial measurements are planned, the tomographic plane of interest is marked on the patient's skin so that it can be scanned at designated intervals. This represents ~5% of the CT-simulator cases at Iowa.

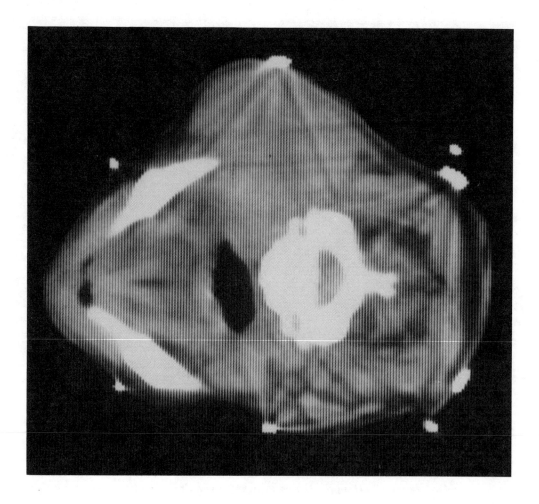

Figure 17-4a.

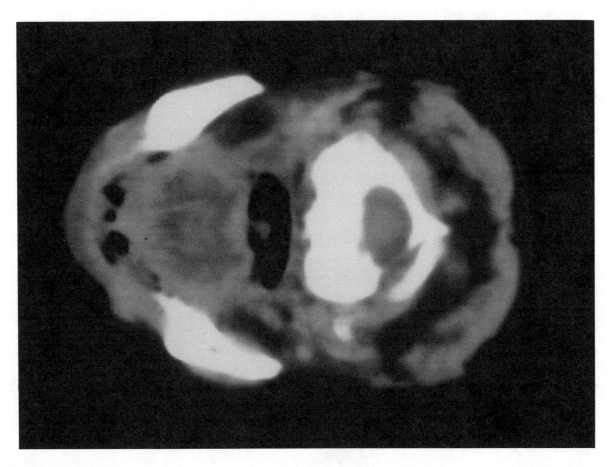

Figure 17-4b.

Figure 17-4a & b. *The CT-simulator is useful for following tumor response during the course of treatment and at follow-up visits. This is a patient with an adenoid cystic carcinoma of the parotid gland a) before treatment and b) after treatment with radiation therapy only.*

For Interstitial Implant Dosimetry.

The CT-simulator has also been used in the computation of dose distributions around radioactive implants. These include Au-198 seed implants for prostate cancer, I-125 implants for glioblastoma multiforme, and Ir-192 implants for head and neck cancers. The CT-simulator is useful for determining dose distributions around radioactive seeds, but not for dose distributions around radioactive needles or tubes because the metal in these sources produces artifacts which make it difficult to accurately compute the dose distribution. Approximately 15% of the patients studied with the CT-simulator at Iowa have been performed for interstitial implant dosimetry.

For Stereotactic RadioSurgery.

The CT-simulator has been very useful in treatment planning for stereotactic radiosurgery. With this technique, a stereotactic frame is fixed to the patient's head. A CT scan is then obtained with the CT-simulator and the target volume is delineated. After the tumor has been localized relative to the frame, the dose distribution is computed using both a Macintosh IIfx computer and a Silicon Graphics workstation wich allows us to do 3-D treatment planning. Stereotactic radiosurgery at Iowa is delivered with a 6 MV x-ray beam using multiple arcs in a non-coplanar field arrangement. Approximately 1-2% of the patients undergoing CT-simulation have been stereotactic radiosurgery cases.

To Evaluate Standard Treatment Techniques.

The CT-simulator has been used to evaluate a variety of standard treatment policies. One example is its use to evaluate prostatic cancer treatment techniques. At our institution, prostate cancer patients are typically treated a full bladder using a 4-field portal arrangement. However, little consideration has been given to the extent of rectal distension. A study was performed using the CT-simulator to determine whether treating the patient with the bladder empty or full, or with the rectum empty or full, significantly affects the dose distribution. Scans taken with the bladder empty and full showed that the position of the prostate and the seminal vesicles does not change significantly with bladder distension, although a full bladder is effective in displacing the small bowel out of the treatment beam. Scans taken with the rectum empty and full, however, showed that the prostate can be displaced anteriorly by as much as 2 cm with rectal distension (Figure 17-5). Prostate cancer patients are now asked to have a full bladder at the time of treatment, but to be sure that their rectum is empty.

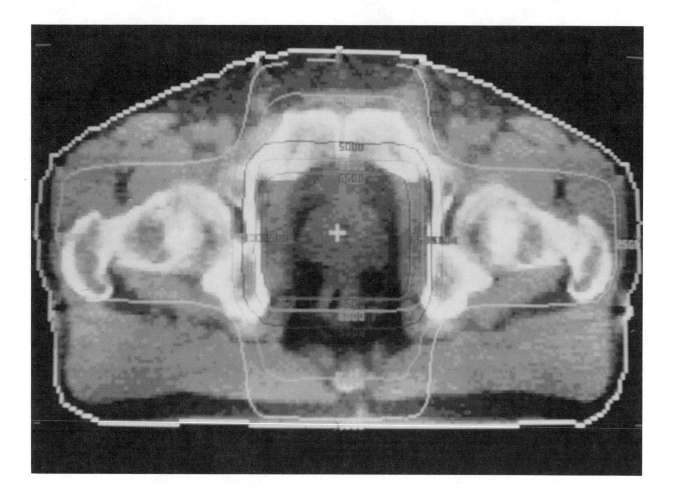

Figure 17-5a.

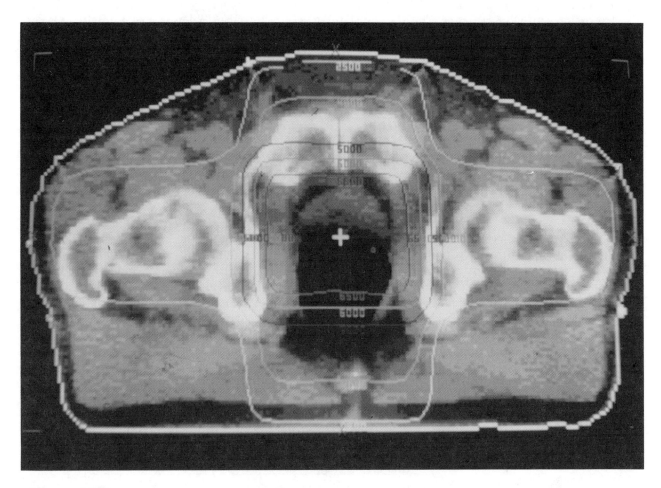

Figure 17-5b.

Figure 17-5a & b.A study was performed to show the effect of rectal distension on the position of the prostate. In this example, the prostate moves ~2 cm anteriorly when the rectum is filled with gas or fecal material. 17-5a. Initial treatment planning. 17-5b. Same patient 24 hours later.

Has It Lost Money?

A fiscal analysis was performed to determine whether the CT-simulator is a financially viable operation. The initial cost of the CT-simulator (exclusive of the treatment planning computer) was $340,000. This represents an annual cost of ~$75,000 if amortized over five years. The Theraplan TP-11 treatment planning computer had previously been purchased at a cost of $97,000. It was not included in the following analysis because it is used for other purposes and is supported in other ways.

Between March 1990 and January 1993, 1,078 patients were studied using the CT-simulator. During this time, it generated almost $550,000 ($396,000 in technical charges and $152,000 in professional fees). This represents an annual income of ~$200,000, including ~$145,000 in technical charges and ~$55,000 in professional fees. The annual cost of running the CT-simulator operation (exclusive of professional services) was estimated to be ~$135,000, including $75,000 for equipment depreciation, $20,000 for maintenance, $30,000 for a CT-simulator technologist, and $10,000 for film and supplies.

The fiscal analysis shows that the CT-simulator operation is a financially viable effort, although it is not a major source of revenue. The CT-simulator was purchased at a lower cost than its current price. However a yearly cost of $75,000 is probably a realistic figure since it was amortized over only 5 years, the time used to depreciate diagnostic CT scanners in our institution. The CT simulator should have a longer life span than diagnostic CT scanners which are replaced more frequently because improvements in image quality make them outmoded every few years.

What Do The Users Think of It?

A survey was performed to evaluate the usefulness of the CT-simulator at the University of Iowa. The survey team included five faculty radiation oncologists, nine residents (including five current residents and four former residents), and three physicists. All members of the survey team had had at least one year of experience using the CT-simulator.

The survey team was first asked to rank 17 modalities (i.e., equipment or techniques) that are available at the University of Iowa. They were asked to evaluate them with regard to their usefulness to a radiation oncology department (but not specifically to an academic radiation oncology department). Each modality was scored on a scale of 1-20, with 20 being the highest score. The CT-simulator came in eighth in this survey, just behind twice daily fractionation and ahead of stereotactic radiosurgery. However, almost all of the items scoring higher than the CT-simulator were modalities that are standard in most modern-day radiation oncology departments. The only recently introduced techniques scoring higher than the CT-simulator were total body irradiation for bone marrow transplantation and twice daily fractionation (Figure 17- 6).

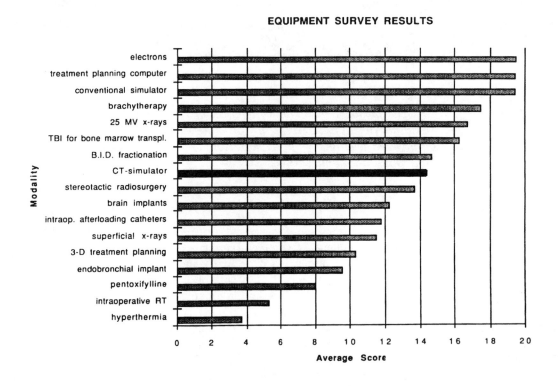

EQUIPMENT SURVEY RESULTS

Figure 17-6. *Survey results for modalities available at the University of Iowa.*

The survey team was then asked to rank 31 modalities that are available in the field. This included 14 modalities that are not available at the University of Iowa. The CT-simulator ranked eighth in this list of 31 techniques and 3-D treatment planning was 16th, ahead of most of the investigational modalities (Table 17-2).

*Table 17-2. Survey Results: The modalities are listed in terms of priority**

Avg. Score	Modality/Technique
19.5	ELECTRONS
19.5	TREATMENT PLANNING COMPUTER
19.5	CONVENTIONAL SIMULATOR
17.5	BRACHYTHERAPY
16.8	24 MV X-RAYS
16.3	TOTAL BODY IRRADIATION (BMT)
14.7	B.I.D. FRACTIONATION
14.4	**CT-SIMULATOR**
13.7	STEREOTACTIC RADIOSURGERY
12.4	*Lo dose-rate remote afterloading**
12.3	BRAIN IMPLANTS
11.9	*Multileaf collimator**
11.8	INTRAOPERATIVE CATHETERS
11.5	*Conformal therapy**
11.5	SUPERFICIAL X-RAYS
10.3	3-D TREATMENT PLANNING
10.5	*Hi dose-rate remote afterloading**
10.3	*Total body electrons**
9.5	ENDOBRONCHIAL BRACHYTHERAPY
8.3	*On-line portal imaging**
8.1	PENTOXIFYLLINE
5.3	INTRAOPERATIVE RADIOTHERAPY
5.2	*Hyperbaric Oxygen*
4.8	*Radioprotectors**
4.8	*Hypoxic cell sensitizers**
4.3	*Protons**
4.1	*Fast neutrons**
3.7	LOCAL-REGIONAL HYPERTHERMIA
3.2	*Total body hyperthermia**
2.4	*Heavy ions**
2.3	*Pions**

*the items in italics are not available at the University of Iowa

Discussion

We have found the CT-simulator to be a very useful tool. Although it ranked only eighth in a list of 17 modalities available in our institution, the majority of the techniques that ranked higher than the CT-simulator are standard treatment modalities available in most well equipped radiation oncology departments. The standard modalities ranking higher than the CT-simulator included electrons, conventional treatment planning computers, conventional simulators, brachyradiotherapy, and 24 MV x-rays. The only nonstandard treatment techniques that ranked higher than the CT-simulator were total body irradiation for bone marrow transplantation and b.i.d. fractionation.

The CT-simulator has a number of practical uses in an academic radiation oncology department. Some of these simply represent quicker, easier, or more accurate ways of doing what is already being accomplished using other methods. Examples of this would be the use of a CT-simulator for dosimetry after the portals have been setup by other means, or to perform dosimetry for interstitial implants or stereotactic radiosurgery. Without the CT-simulator, this dosimetry would have been performed using solder wire contours and orthogonal x-rays, or diagnostic CT scans.

Other uses for the CT-simulator have come from having a CT scanner available in the department. These are procedures that could be performed with diagnostic CT scanners, but are not routinely obtained in most departments because a CT scanner is not readily available. Examples of this would be the use of the CT-simulator to follow tumor regression during treatment or at follow-up visits, to plan boost treatments, or to check the margins of the fields. Information obtained with computerized tomography in these situations is often helpful in patient management, but it is usually not obtained because of cost or inconvenience.

The principal reason for acquiring the CT-simulator at our institution was its ability to perform virtual simulation. Virtual simulation is not easily accomplished with other machines. We have found it particularly useful in treating patients with oblique fields or non-coplanar field arrangements. Our goal is to use it to define the tumor volume for "high precision" treatment techniques, such as conformal radiation therapy.

In the past, radiation oncologists were reluctant to use narrow margins around the tumor because they were unable to determine the exact extent of the cancer, and they were unable to deliver treatment to such precise target volumes consistently. With improvements in diagnostic imaging, in treatment planning computers, and in linear accelerators, it is now possible to deliver radiation therapy much more precisely and consistently that we have in the past. Thus, it seems appropriate to reconsider the margins that need to be placed around the clinically detectable cancer.

However, even with the best imaging devices, there may be microscopic extensions of cancer beyond the clinically detectable disease. There is also a significant risk of regional lymph node metastasis with many cancers, and these nodes often need to be irradiated electively. In our opinion, "high precision" radiation therapy techniques will be useful only as a boost technique in most clinical situations. There is a danger that conformal radiation therapy will fail in clinical trials if radiation oncologists expect it to enable them to use extremely narrow margins throughout the course of treatment.

References

1. Pennington EC, Jani SK: Quality Assurance Aspects of a CT-simulator. In: <u>CT Simulation for Radiotherapy</u>. Jani SK (editor). Madison, Wisconsin: Medical Physics Publishing Co. 1993, p. 147-160.

2. Wen B-C, Jani SK, Pennington EC: Clinical Applications of a CT Simulator in Unconventional Radiation Therapy Techniques. In: <u>CT Simulation for Radiotherapy</u>. Jani SK (editor). Madison, Wisconsin: Medical Physics Publishing Co. 1993, p. 129-145.

3. Hussey DH: Clinical Assessment of CT Simulation. In: <u>CT Simulation for Radiotherapy</u>. Jani SK (editor). Madison, Wisconsin: Medical Physics Publishing Co., 1993. p. 57-72.

Chapter 18

CT Simulator: The Kyoto University Experience[1]

Yasushi Nagata, M.D., Kaoru Okajima, M.D., Rumi Murata, M.D., Mitihide Mitsumori, M.D., Takashi Ishigaki, M.D., Shoji Mizowaki, M.D., Masahiro Hiraoka, M.D., Koji Ono, M.D., Takehiro Nishidai, Ph. D., Masaji Takahashi, M.D., Mitsuyuki Abe, M.D.

Dept. of Radiology, Kyoto Univ. Hospital, Sakyo Kyoto, Japan

CT machines were originally developed for diagnostic use and thus were separate from treatment planning machines. However, CT is also a very useful modality for radiotherapy. Since 1987, we have developed a CT simulator system which is dedicated for radiotherapy. The CT simulator is defined here as a CT scanner with auxiliary equipment which allows rapid scanning in the treatment position, 3-D treatment planning, and laser field projection. The clinical value of this CT simulator during more than 5 years of use was assessed in the present study.

Materials and Methods

The original CT simulator was developed in 1987.[1-3] It consists of a CT scanner, two multi-image monitors, a 3-D treatment planning machine, and a laser field projector. A CT scanner designed for diagnostic use (SCT-2500, Shimadzu Corp., Kyoto, Japan) has been modified for radiotherapy use. Using 20-inch multi-image monitors, up to 12 CT slices with target outlines can be viewed at the same time and the radiation fields for multiple CT images can also be checked. The 3-D radiotherapy treatment planning machine (THERAC-2300, NEC Corp., Tokyo, Japan) makes use of visual optimization and the fast dose calculation method.[4] We have installed a practical 3-D dose calculation program, the modified equivalent tissue maximum ratio method. Simulated images (digitally reconstructed radiographs) and other special 3-D reconstructed images can also be viewed. The laser beam field projector is our own original system. Using this projector, the whole beam centers and radiation fields of any shape can be projected automatically over a radius of 180 degrees onto a patient lying on the CT couch.

CT simulation was carried out by the following procedure. At first, the patient was fixed in the treatment position on the CT table. Then scannograms were taken from the anterior and lateral directions. Over the scannograms, we defined the scanning range of the CT. CT scans were generally obtained with a 10-mm slice interval. During scanning, we could draw the outline of the targeted tumor and regions of interest (ROIs) on the previous CT images. Then the outlines of the target and the lenses were simultaneously superimposed on the CT slices and scannograms on the multi-image monitors. Thereafter, using the beam's eye view (BEV) computer facility, the most appropriate beam angle was selected to cover the whole tumor while sparing the ROIs. The shape of any block that was necessary could also be established using the BEV. In addition, the field established on the BEV could be simultaneously superimposed on multiple CT slices using beam indicators, after which 3-D dose distributions could be displayed on the same slices. After we finished planning, the fields established were projected onto the skin of the patient using a laser projector. As all the components of the system are on-line, the whole procedures from CT scanning to field projection could be completed within 30-40 min.

[1] This work was supported by a grant-in-aid for Cancer Research from the Ministry of Education. (01480273)

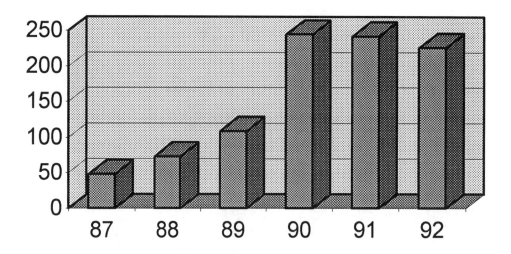

Figure 18-1. The number of the patients undergoing treatment planning with the CT simulator

Since June 1987, radiotherapy treatment plans have been developed for more than 900 patients using this system.[5] The number of patients receiving treatment planning with the CT simulator is increasing annually as shown in Figure 18-1. The simulator was used for determining the initial treatment and for shrinking the radiation field in 66% and in 34% of the patients, respectively. The types of patient whose treatment was planned with the CT simulator are summarized in Figure 18-2.

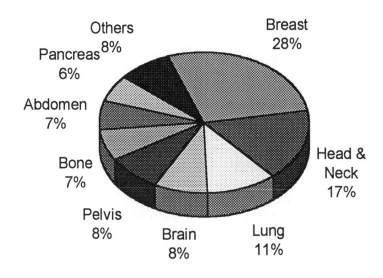

Figure 18-2. The diagnosis of patients undergoing treatment planning with the CT simulator

Results

Clinical value of the CT Simulator

Breast-Conserving Therapy

Radiation after lumpectomy is a very important part of breast-conserving therapy for patients with early breast cancer. After the patient is immobilized on the CT couch using a shell, multiple CT slices are scanned continuously. Using the beam's eye view, the most appropriate field size and beam angle are selected. Thereafter, 3-D dose distribution curves are calculated and the homogeneity of the dose within the target is confirmed. Since 1991, the dose has been compensated with various type of wedge filters, allowing the homogeneity of the dose to the breast to be maintained within 20%. In 1992, 36% of the patients were compensated with wedge filters. As a result, the patients with erosions of the nipple and axilla decreased to 5% in 1992 from 10% between 1989 and 1991 when wedge compensation was not used.

Maxillary Cancer

The 5-year survival rate of patients with maxillary cancer is over 50%, so accurate treatment planning to avoid irradiation to the lens is very important.[6-7] Using a beam's eye view, we could establish the most appropriate field size as well as the necessary blocks and the optimum beam direction.[8] Treatment planning was done in 25 patients using an x-ray simulator and plain x-ray films (1979-1982, group 1) in 34 patients using an x-ray simulator and CT films (1983-1987, group 2), and in 24 patients using the CT simulator (1988-1992, group 3). The number of patients with stage 4 disease increased in the order from group 1 to group 3, but the average radiation field was the smallest in group 3 (66.5 cm2) followed by group 2 (67.4 cm2) and group 1 (72.9 cm2). A radiation dose of more than 30 Gy to lens of the affected side was delivered to 13% of group 3, 44% of group 2, and 44% of group 1[9-13]. The dose to the lens on the unaffected side was zero in 56% of group 1, 74% of group 2, and 96% of group 3 (Table 18-1). A long-term decrease in visual activity on the affected side occurred in 11% of group 3, 32% of group 2, and 44% of group 1. However, a significant increase in survival was only noted in group 2 when compared with group 1, and no significant increase was achieved between groups 2 and 3 using the CT simulator. However, because the 3 population of patients were different, further evaluation of survival is necessary.

Table 18-1. *The radiation dose to the lens in the treatment of maxillary cancer. Group 1 is the patients whose treatment was planned using an x-ray simulator and plain x-ray films (1979-1982), Group 2 is the patients planned using an x-ray simulator and CT films (1983-1987), and Group 3 is the patients planned using a CT simulator (1988-1992).*

Table 18-1. Radiation Dose to Both Lenses

	Ipsilateral lens		Contralateral lens	
Group 1	>30 Gy	11/25 (44%)	>30 Gy	1/25 (4%)
	30 Gy>>0	0	30 Gy>>0	10/25 (40%)
	0	14/25 (56%)	0	14/25 (56%)
Group 2	>30 Gy	15/34 (44%)	>30 Gy	4/34 (12%)
	30 Gy>>0	1/34 (3%)	30 Gy>>0	5/34 (15%)
	0	18/34 (53%)	0	25/34 (74%)
Group 3	>30 Gy	3/24 (13%)	>30 Gy	0
	30 Gy>>0	7/24 (30%)	30 Gy>>0	1/24 (4%)
	0	14/24 (57%)	0	23/24 (96%)

Respiratory-Gated Intermittent Irradiation for Liver and Lung Cancer.

In patients with liver cancer and cancer of the lower lung fields, irradiation of the primary tumor is an important therapeutic modality. We have performed 3-D treatment planning in combination with a respiratory-gated intermittent irradiation system since 1989.

The system was developed in corporation with Mitsubishi Electronics (Osaka, Japan). Using this system, irradiation can be performed intermittently with the resting period preset. After a tape-recorded message, 7-10 seconds of irradiation is delivered during breath holding was performed and this process is repeated a number of times per session. The total number of patients treated with this system was 24 , including 17 with liver tumors and 7 with lung tumors.The mean age of the patients with liver and lung tumors was 57.6 years and 54.7 years, respectively, while the average radiation dose was 42.3 Gy and 46.5Gy. We used paired anteroposterior fields in 6 patients , paired oblique fields in 6 patients, paired rectangular fields in 2 patients, and other configurations in 3 patients with liver cancer. In the patients with lung tumors, the fields were anteroposterior in 4 cases, and rectangular in 3 . In the cases of primary liver cancer, we compared two groups treated before and after the introduction of our new system. The average irradiated field before and after the introduction of CT-S was respectively 109 cm2 and 85 cm2 , and the average radiation dose was 42.3 Gy and 43.3 Gy. In addition, the local control rate increased from 36% to 50%. Thus, use of the CT simulator and respiratory-gated irradiation system allowed the irradiated volume of normal liver to be markedly reduced and the local control rate to be increased. However, further study of survival study is needed.

Lung Cancer

In the case of lung cancer, we compared the results for patients who had treatment planning with the CT simulator between 1988 and 1991 and with an x-ray simulator between 1981 and 1991. Planning with the was done for 15, 3, 24,and 16 patients in Stage 1,2,3, and 4, respectively, while the numbers for the x-ray simulator were 3, 1, 26, and 12. Using the CT simulator, the field size was 30.2+7.8% in Stage 3 and 41.8+7.9 in Stage 4, while it was 25.7 +11.6 in Stage 3 and 40.2 +18.3 in Stage 4 with the conventional x-ray simulator. It mainly depended on the primary tumor size. The 1-year survival rates for Stage 3 and 4 patients were respectively 61.9% and 50.0% using the CT simulator compared with 43.8% and 28.6% using the x-ray simulator, but the increase was not statistically significant. However, our findings suggest that 3-D treatment planning with the CT simulator has the possibility of eventually improving the survival of lung cancer patients.

Bone and Soft Tissue Sarcoma

In patients with bone and soft tissue sarcomas, accurate evaluation of the tumor margin is important, so we generally use the CT simulator for planning the treatment of bone tumors. When the results of x-ray simulation were compared with CT simulation, the previously planned field was reduced in 38% of patients, enlarged in 31%, and unchanged in 31%. Currently, all bone tumor patients receive planning with the CT simulator except for those undergoing palliative irradiation.

Other Tumors

Patients with localized brain tumors, intraorbital tumors, and pancreatic cancer may also benefit from CT simulation.

Discussion

The usefulness of the CT simulator must be evaluated on the basis of the following considerations.

Survival

The survival rate can be increased by both better treatment planning and better treatment.[7] However, how far can we improve the survival rate of a disease? Although missing the target a few times will decrease the survival rate, the patients will not always die of locoregional recurrence. Therefore, we must continue our studies over the long term to assess whether 3-D treatment planning can prolong the survival of cancer patients. Lung cancer, liver cancer, and brain tumors are all areas where future study is necessary.

Complications

The following complications seem to be decreased by the CT simulator: radiation cataract in maxillary cancer, radiation pneumonitis in lung cancer and radiation hepatitis in liver cancer (simulator plus gating). Accordingly, studies to confirm the reduction of complications by the CT simulator are also necessary.

Practicality

The number of CT simulators in Japan is increasing, as shown in Figure 18-1, and a total of 23 machines have now been installed. However, the conventional x-ray simulator remains a useful modality. We think that both the CT simulator and the conventional simulator have an important place in clinical treatment planning. In the future, both simulators may be installed in many of the major radiotherapy institutions. However, in hospitals without enough space for both types of simulators, a combined system with a common patient couch may be useful (Figure 18-3).

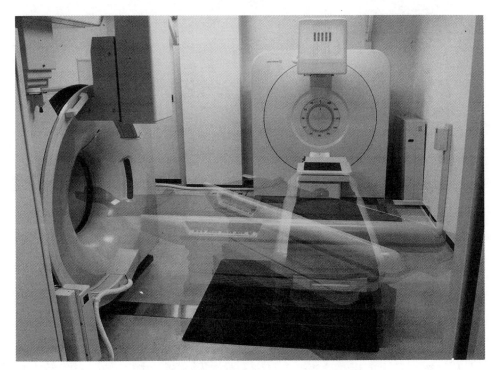

Figure 18-3. *A new system with a single couch for both a conventional x-ray simulator and a CT Simulator (Shimadzu, Kyoto, Japan).*

The original CT simulator has been completely replaced with a new simulator (the CTS-20 combined with the NEC-EWS-RTP), which is shown in Figure 18-4. As a result, the problems of the old system have mostly been resolved. The scanning time has been shorted(minimum scanning time is now 2 sec) and the gantry aperture has been widened to (65 cm in diameter). A network connection between the simulator and a multileaf collimator has been installed, allowing the rapid planning of conformal therapy. Even though there are still a few problems to be solved, this CT simulator appears to be a practical treatment planning system for radiotherapy.

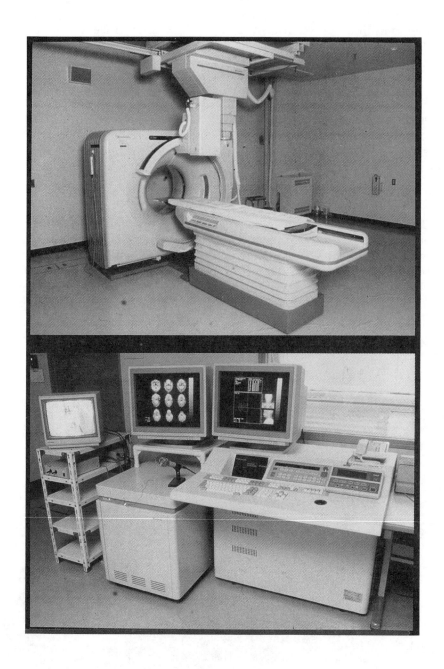

Figure 18-4. *Our new CT simulator system. The CTS-20 (Shimadzu Corp.) includes a CT scanner and a laser field projector. The NEC-EWS-RTP includes the 3-D treatment planner and a network connection with a CLINAC 2300 C/D.*

An integrated radiotherapy network has been developed at Kyoto University Hospital. We have devised a preliminary network incorporating a PAC(picture archiving and communicating) system, a CT simulator, and a linear accerelator.

The PAC system is a Shimadzu SAIPACS equipped with four 20-inch monitors (1,024 X 1,024 lines). Any x-ray film can be digitized within 20 sec by the digitizer. This system can be used for treatment planning as well as for patient data management. Our primary network incorporating the CT simulator, the PACS system, and a CLINAC2300C/D was completed in June 1993. The treatment planning of conformal therapy using the CT simulator is transported to the multileaf via a ethernet network with the TCP/IP protocol, and this should help us increase the accuracy of radiotherapy.

Finally, MRI is also a very important diagnostic modality and should be utilized for radiotherapy. We have installed a new MRI system (MRP 20EX, Hitachi, Japan) in the radiotherapy department and plan to use MRI images superimposed over CT images.

Conclusion

Studies need to be continued to determine the clinical value of the CT simulator. However, our preliminary results suggest that this system is both useful and practical for radiotherapy treatment planning.

References

1. Nishidai T, Nagata Y, Takahashi M. et al. CT simulator. A new 3-D treatment planning and simulating system for radiotherapy. Part 1. Description of the system. Int. J. Radiat. Oncol. Biol. Phys. 1990;18;499-504.

2. Nagata Y, Nishidai T, Abe M. et al. CT simulator. A new 3-D treatment planning and simulating system for radiotherapy. Part 2.Clinical application. Int. J. Radiat. Oncol. Biol. Phys. 1990;18;505-513.

3. Nagata Y, Nishidai T, Abe M. et al. Laser projection system for radiotherapy and CT-guided biopsy. L. of Computer Assisted Tomography. 1990;14:1046-1048.

4. Nakata M, Nishidai T, Nohara H, et al. New 3-D Dose calculation Using Modified Equivalent Tissue-Maximum Ratio Method -Dose Computation along the off-center axis.- Japanese Journal of Radiological Technology.10,23-34,1992.

5. Nagata Y, Abe M, Nishidai T. et al. Clinical application of CT simulator. Presented at the US-Japan Cooperative Cancer Research Program in radiation Oncology. 21-23 Nov. 1991, Ann Arbor, USA.

6. Nagata Y, Ono K, Nishidai T, et al. Clinical evaluation of 3-D treatment planning for maxillary cancer using the CT simulator. Int. J. Radiat. Oncol. Biol. Phys. 1991 21 Suppl1 231.

7. Leibel SA, Scott CB, Mohiuddin M et al. The effect of local-regional control on distant metastatic dissemination in carcinoma of the head and neck: result of an analysis from the RTOG head and neck database. Int. J. Radiation Oncology Biol. Phys.21,549-556,1991.

8. McShan DL,Fraass BA, Lichter AS. Full integration of the beam's eye view concept into computerized treatment planning.Int. J. Radiation Oncology Biol. Phys.18,1485-1494,1990.

9.   Nakissa N, Rubin P,Strohl R. et al. Ocular and orbital complications following radiation therapy of paranasal sinus malignancies and review of literature. Cancer 51;980-986,1983.

10. Parsons JT, Fitzgelrald CR, Hood CI, et al. The effects of irradiation on the eye and optic nerve. Int. J. Radiation Oncology Biol. Phys. 9,609-622,1983.

11. Shibuya H, Horiuti J, Suzuki S. et al. Maxillary sinus carcinoma: Result of radiation therapy. Int. J. Radiation Oncology Biol. Phys. 10,1021-1026,1984.

Tsujii H, Kamada T, Matsuoka Y et al. The value of treatment planning using CT and an immobilizing shell in radiotherapy for paranasal sinus carcinomas. Int. J. Radiation Oncology Biol. Phys. 16,243-249,1989.

Chapter 19

Simulator Based CT: 4 Years of Experience at the Royal North Shore Hospital, Sydney, Australia

Raj Mallik M.D .& Peter Hunt M.Sc.
E. Seppi Ph.D., J. Pavkovich Ph.D., E. Shapiro M.S., S. Henderson B.S.

Department of Radiation Oncology, Royal North Shore Hospital, Sydney, Australia
E.L. Ginzton Research Centre Varian Associates Palo Alto, California

In July 1989 a Varian CT attachment was installed at the Royal North Shore Hospital, Sydney, Australia. The original unit tested was the Alpha Prototype model, which was upgraded to the Pre Production model in November 1990; and the authors (1,2,3) have reported their preliminary development of the device. In the last three and a half years the device has scanned over 700 patients with an average of four cuts per patient, and the scans obtained have routinely been electronically transferred to our Theraplan treatment planning system for incorporation into the planning process. Since the Varian CT attachment became commercially available, about thirty units have been installed worldwide with seven units being installed in Australia. The image quality, while not that of diagnostic scanners, has been found to be of acceptable quality and has routinely been utilized in the planning process (Figure 19-1). CT numbers have been found to be accurate as have other tests to determine spatial linearity, image quality, contrast and resolution. The one minute acquisition time while leading to some minor degradation of images due to motion artifact has actually been found to be an advantage as the average position of all the targets and the average electron densities have been found to be indicative of what happ ens during treatment on a linear accelerator. The aperture of the scanner at 93 cm allows patients to be scanned in the traditional radiotherapy treatment positions with no compromise in patient set up or deterioration in image quality. This large patient aperture has been found to be of particular use in the management of patients receiving local irradiation to the breast (Figure 19-2). Significant errors in beam direction have been discovered when comparing CT's obtained on diagnostic CT's in different treatment positions from those routinely obtained on the Varian CT Simulator.

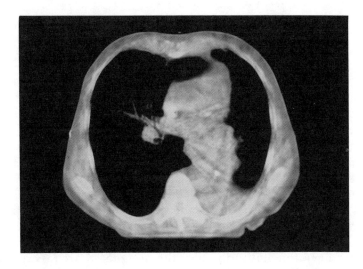

Figure 19-1. Scan through the Thorax demonstrates good image quality

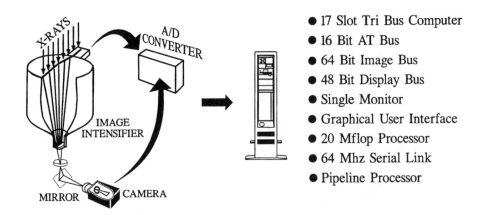

- 17 Slot Tri Bus Computer
- 16 Bit AT Bus
- 64 Bit Image Bus
- 48 Bit Display Bus
- Single Monitor
- Graphical User Interface
- 20 Mflop Processor
- 64 Mhz Serial Link
- Pipeline Processor

DIAGRAM OF SIMCT DETECTORS AND COMPUTER

Figure 19-2. Diagram of SIMCT DETECTORS

Early simulator based scanners suffered from poor spatial resolution and poor images; the Varian device however produces images of acceptable quality and in some sites of the body (head, neck and lung) close to diagnostic quality images can be obtained.

The generic term of non diagnostic CT scanners has been used by Webb(4) to describe these simulator based CT scanners but this term is accompanied by the connotation of poor quality images. We prefer to call these devices SIMULATORS CT's (SIMCT) and images produced have been judged by most of the users to be of very acceptable quality. On the Varian device a resolution of 1.5 mm is obtained with a density resolution of 1%, with a well tuned machine substantially better figures can be obtained.

Image Quality

The image quality seems most dependent on patient motion artifact and photon statistics. The slow acquisition time of one minute, while having a distinct advantage of accurately defining the average target volume, average lung density, average position of the organs, etc., does have the disadvantage of leading to a degradation of image from motion artifacts. This is most noticeable in scans taken around the diaphragm and upp er abdomen where motions have been measured in excess of a centimeter and a half. However, in images taken from the base of the brain to the diaphragm the quality of images is excellent, closely rivaling that of a diagnostic quality scanner. In the upp er abdomen the quality of images is still fairly adequate allowing the determination of positions of the kidney, spleen, liver, spinal cord, etc., to be easily determined. Down into the pelvis the quality of the image seems to be determined by photon statistics which in turn means the diameter of the patient. In very obese patients, the quality of the images can be poor while in patients who are thinner the quality of images can be extremely good. In the case of the bladder, prostate, esophagus, etc., contrast is used to help determine boundaries and volume. The treatment planning computer should have the ability to allow the designated area to receive correct density values so that the effect of artifacts on contrast and incorrect electron density figures can be corrected by feeding in app ropriate values. Some of the new generation treatment planning machines which deal with a large number of CT cuts seem unable to allow the physician to allocate the density value for treatment volumes and this can only lead to errors which would app ly to any CT scans taken either intravenous or intravesical contrast.

Some of the images suffer from ring artifacts that plague all third generation scanners, however these artifacts, while noticeable on some images do not detract from the overall value of the scanner and these scans are found to always offer valuable information on the patient and have been found to have a minimal effect on the CT numbers.

Hardware

Figure 19-3 shows the construction of the imaging chain which when fitted to a Ximatron Simulator allows CT scans to be performed. A hybrid detector system consisting of the image intensifier and a series of photo diodes in the edge detector are used as the primary radiation detector. The image intensifier output phosphor is viewed by a linear array of 512 detectors and an extension detector consisting of 32 photo detectors. The architecture of the image intensifier and extension detector effectively extends the scan circle to 50 cm. Systems that use an image intensifier as their only radiation detector suffer from a small scan circle generally of about 40 cm. Because of the limited size of the image detector a partial fan beam is used which results in a requirement for a full 360 degrees of rotation to be carried out in order to obtain an acceptable image. The outputs from the 512 channel linear array and the 32 channel extension detector are fed into an A-D converter and effectively a dynamic range of 1:500 000 is obtained which results in images of reasonably contrast and spatial resolution.

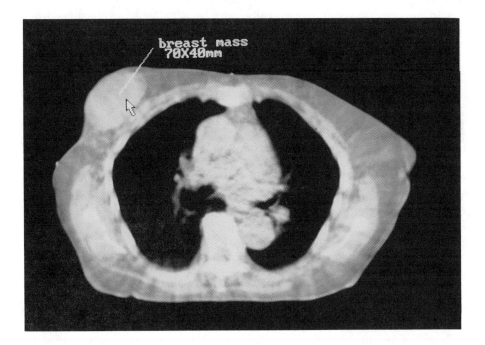

Figure 19-3. Breast scan obtained on the Varian device clearly shows a mass in the breast.

The computer system chosen was Virtual imaging 2000 system which essentially consists of three computer buses. A 16 bit AT (ISA bus), a 64 bit image bus and a 48 bit display bus. Images are displayed at a maximum resolution of 512 x 512 with a total of 12 images being displayed on the screen at a time. The main computing power is provided by a Sky Array Processor capable of performing 20 M flops. Image reconstruction occurs within about a minute and 20 seconds of completion of the scan. The familiar windows type interface has been chosen for interaction with the operator and most operators find it extremely easy to use with on screen help being provided that further improves user friendliness. Images are stored on a 600 megabyte optical disk which has the capacity to store over 3000 images and being a removable optical device with fairly rapid access allows the rapid retrieval of any of the images which can be CT images or images captured from the fluoroscope or other images imported into the system.

X-ray Output

The photon statistics determines the quality of the CT image. In the head and lungs it is possible to scan at 130 kV at 10 milliamps and obtain reasonable quality images. In the pelvis and abdomen the scan current often needs to be performed at 15 milliamps. This means that some consideration as to heat dissipation of the x-ray tube needs to be considered. On the prototype machine an electronic thermometer was connected to the housing of the tube and we constantly monitored the temperature. We found that it was possible to perform 9 scans before the temperature of the x-ray tube housing reached 55 degrees celsius. In spite of forced air cooling, the heat dissipation from the tube was fairly slow and as such a judicious selection of the kV in the mA was necessary to maximize the number of scans obtained. Recently Varian has developed a high heat output tube with an oil cooled heat exchanger and using this tube it is possible to perform 12 scans in a 30 minute period. In practice the average number of scans is 5 cuts for a 10 cm field which means that to all practical purposes continuous scanning is possible with a high heat output tube. On rare occasions when a large number of scans are required, i.e. when constructing a special purpose compensator then it is possible to reduce the current to around 7 milliamps and still obtain acceptable quality of scans where the outline, internal organs, lung, etc., can be readily defined. This variation in current however is generally unnecessary and in our department all scans are generated at a constant current of at 15 milliamps 130 kV with no over heating of the tube.

Advantages of Simulator Based CT Scanners

Large Patient Aperture

The advantage of Simulator based scanners, is that the procedure of simulation and scanning can be carried out in one session without the need to move the patient, in addition the large patient aperture of 93 cm ensures that most patients can be scanned in the actual treatment position. There is a compromise between the patient aperture and the scan circle, the prototype scanner which scanned at an FID (focus intensifier distance) of 147 cm had a scan circle of 81 cm, our model which can scan an FID of 150 obtains a patient aperture of 87 cm and a scan circle of 49 cm, the size of the scan circle being determined by the size of the image intensifier. Ximatron simulators with an isocenter height of 127 cm will be able to scan at a FID of 155 cm effectively delivering an aperture of close to 100 cm.

Accurate Dose Calculation and Electron Density Values

In breast treatments where the normal arm position for the tangential fields precludes scanning on standard CT the large patient aperture is crucial. Various studies by Webb (5) and Dieter (6) have shown a variation of up to 10% in dose distribution between patients scanned on conventional scanners in the non treatment position and scanning in the treatment position. However, in these studies the simulator based device was used to provide external contours and internal contours with an arbitrary density value assigned to the lung. The Varian device however is able to produce true CT numbers and thus leads to even more accurate dose distribution considering that variations of over 20% in density values have been reported by Van Dyck (7) in the lung between deep inspiration and deep expiration. These variations in CT numbers in turn have resulted in variations of dose delivery by as much as 25% for a single cobalt field and 10% for a multi field treatment for an esophagus. The SIMCT is also able to provide a sufficient number of cuts (6-7) to enable compensators to be constructed further improving the accuracy of beam delivery.

Slow Scan Acqusition Time

A further advantage of scanning on a SIMCT is that data is acquired over a minute and this data acquisition time closely mimics the treatment time as such scans obtained show a true average position of the target and organs taking into account respiration movements and vascular pulsations. While it is true that these movements do result in motion artifacts that degrade the picture the more accurate target localization is of prime importance. Ross (8) using ultra fast CT scanning has shown that significant errors in localization can occur from respiration, cardiac and aortic motions with geographic errors occurring in 30% of the cases.

Accurate Dose Delivery to a Moving Target

Most proponents of conventional CT scanners seem to ignore these errors and claim, we believe, unachievable levels of accuracy in targeting. While it may be possible to obtain great accuracy in sterotaxic radiotherapy in the skull even in this area errors of a few millimeters will occur from vascular pulsation. The Japanese (9) make some attempt to correct for target positioning errors brought on be respiration by asking the patient to cease breathing while scanning the patient, and then asking the patient to cease breathing for short periods of time while the treatment machine is gated on. Pertola reported the use of respiration gated radiotherapy on a series of patients treated in the 1980s. We chose to use the target averaging method where the long scan time gives a truer indication of the target position, this technique does result in a larger field but this is in keeping with most studies using CT that found that field sizes were increased rather than reduced when using CTs for planning.

The importance of simulators in radiotherapy can not be over stressed and is a regular part of most radiotherapist armory, at the same time CT scanners and MRI have enabled more accurate localization of target volumes. In most departments CT's are used in a fair proportion of patients, though dedicated CT scanners installed in radiotherapy departments are rare. The advantage of scanning the patient during the simulation process are well recognized, accuracy and treatment positions are seldom compromised by SIMCTs; on the other hand scanning on CT scanners will give good scans but may lead to poor accuracy because of the limited patient aperture generally less than 70 cm. In addition a simulator allows a true beams eye view to be obtained.

Figure 19-4 shows the steps in simulation planning and the delivery of treatment with the Varian SIMCT. Simulation, scanning and resimulation with beams eye view can all be done on one dedicated unit specifically designed for radiotherapy. As treatment planning units increase in speed and accuracy it should be possible to interactively plan the patient in a single session and display the treatment plan in real time. In conformal therapy where high dose deliveries are the norm the whole chain becomes critical with the weakest link in the chain determining the end result obtained. Furthermore as these planning and delivery chains are populated by widely dissimilar devices communications between them becomes a veritable Tower of Babel.

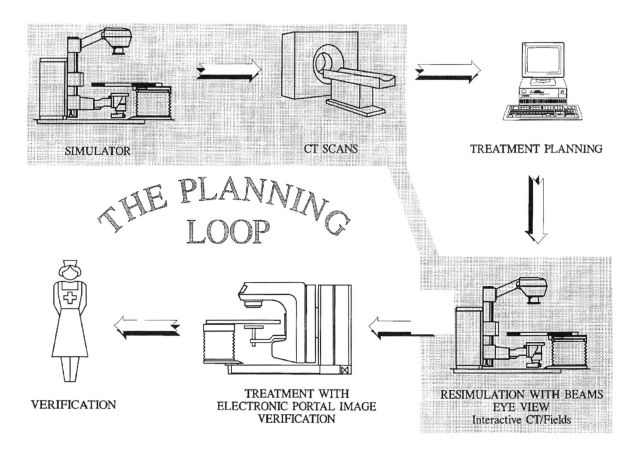

SIMULATOR **CT SCANS** **TREATMENT PLANNING**

THE PLANNING LOOP

VERIFICATION **TREATMENT WITH ELECTRONIC PORTAL IMAGE VERIFICATION** **RESIMULATION WITH BEAMS EYE VIEW** Interactive CT/Fields

Figure 19-4. The planning loop incorporating Simulation, CT scanning, Beam Summation and treatment delivery.

The advantage of the Varian SIMCT is that the simulation, CT scanning, resimulation with beam direction and beams eye view are performed on one integrated unit the simulator.

Planning still needs to be performed on a separate unit, however once the planning has been performed the SIMCT allows the physician to view the effect of changing the beams size and position interactively with the CT scan being displayed and the associated beams eye view including beam blocking shown on the Simulator. At present the field sizes and gantry and collimator angles need to be manually entered, however an interactive link to the Ximatron Simulator has been developed that enables the fields to be viewed on the CT images as the Ximatron is rotated around the patient.

The Ximatron Simulator attachment only requires the operator to superimpose the beam position on the central axis slice (Figure 19-5). The computer then displays the beam on all other slices automatically computing the position of the beam taking into account the beam offset (Figure 19-6). This we have found to be particularly useful in determining the length of the beam ensuring that the beam is long enough to target the structures that need to be irradiated but reducing unnecessary irradiation. At the same time it is possible to turn on the x-rays and obtain a beams eye view of the simulator ports and capture them in the patients electronic image file.

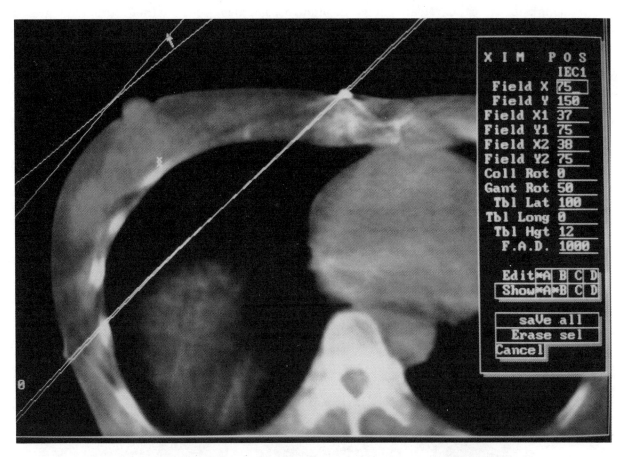

Figure 19-5. An example of a pair of opposing beams, used on a tangential breast treatment

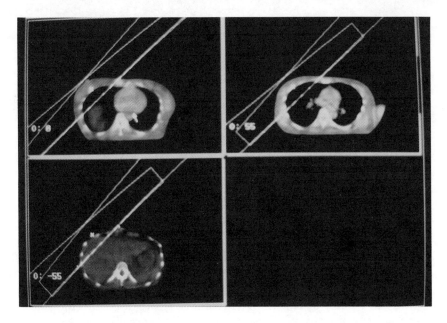

Figure 19-6. An example of multiple slices being displayed with the beam position being accurately shown

The final link in the chain, treatment verification, is obtained from another Varian integrated product the Electronic Portal Imager fitted to the treatment accelerator. By staying with one vendor with a common file structure and communication protocol the dream of a fully integrated system becomes a reality, with the only requirement being that the vendor of the treatment planning unit provide an interface to the Varian RMS network. Once the multileaf collimators become the norm for treatments the interchange of set up parameters and verification that correct treatments have been implemented will become crucial if conformal therapy is to succeed. We have been able to import images from other devices such as MRI electronic portal images scanned x-ray films and port films (Figure 19-7). These images together with Text will form part of the patients total files and work is being undertaken to incorporate them in an image and text data base networked to the RMS 2000 and other hospital data bases.

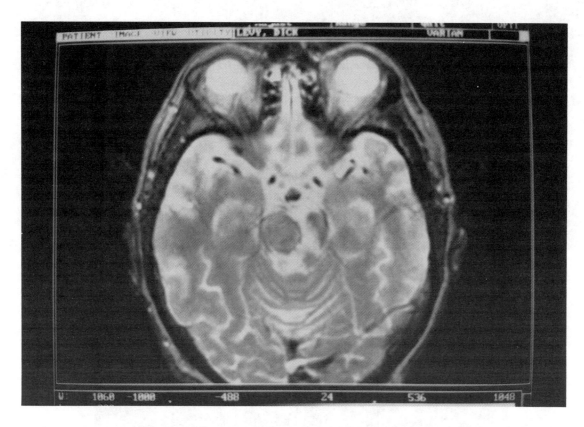

Figure 19-7. The figure shows an MRI image imported via 9 track mag tape from the Theraplan treatment planning computer.

Summary

In conclusion the Varian SIMCT has shown itself to be a useful and practical device able to allow simulation scanning and beams eye views to be obtained at one localization. The large patient aperture reasonable image quality and interfacing to treatment planning computers has made the device an integral part of our radiotherapy planning process. Most simulators based CT devices constructed in the past have been designed in University departments. The Varian device is a commercially built device and the sales of 60 world wide with over 30 installations have indicated that in many departments it plays a valuable role. Until a dedicated CT Scanner specifically designed for radiotherapy becomes available the SIMCT will continue to gain acceptance and we hope will become a routine addition to most simulators in radiation oncology departments.

References

1. Raj Mallik M.D., Peter Hunt M.Sc. "The Varian Ximatron/CT Option: One Year's Experience." The Varian Centerline Magazine. October 1990, pp 1-4.

2. Raj Mallik M.D., Peter Hunt M.Sc. "The Royal North Shore Hospital Clinical Experience with the Varian CT Option." Varian Proceedings, Second Asian Users Meeting. pp 61-68.

3. Raj Mallik M.D., Peter Hunt M.Sc. "The Royal North Shore Hospital Experience with the Varian Ximatron/CT Option." Varian Proceedings, 14th Users Meeting. pp 53-60.

4. S Webb. "Non-Standard CT Scanners: Their role in Radiotherapy." Int J Radiation Oncology Biol Phys., 1990. Vol.19, pp 1589-1607.

5. S Webb, et al. "Clinical dosimetry for radiotherapy to the radiotherapy to the breast based on imaging with prototype Royal Marsden Hospital CT simulator." Phys. Med. Biol., 1987, Vol. 32, No. 7, 835-845.

6. H Dieter Kogelnik, M.D., Marie-Gabrielle Brandis, M.D., Hassan Rahim, M.Sc. and Herwig Mandl, M.Sc. "Inadequacy of Conventional Computerized Tomography Scans for Treatment Planning of Tangential Breast (Chest Wall) Fields." Int J Radiation Oncology Biol Phys. 1988. Vol. 14 pp 721-727.

7. J. Van Dyk, M.Sc., F.C.C.P.M., * T.J.Keane, M.B., M.R.C.P.I., F.R.C.R.(C) and W.D. Rider, M.B., F.R.C.P.(C), F.R.C.R. "Lung Density as Measured By Computerized Tomography: Implications for Radiotherapy." Int. J. of Oncology Bio. Phys., Vol. 8. 1982, p.1363.

8. Ross C S, Hussey D H, Pennington E C, Stanford W, Doornbos JF. "Analysis of movement of intrathoracic neoplasms using ultrafast computerized tomography." Int J Radiation Oncology Biol. Phys., 1990. Mar. 18(3): 671-7.

9. Yasushi Nagata, M.D., Professor, Radiotherapy Division Kyoto University College of Medicine Kyoto, Japan (Personal Communication).

Chapter 20

The Reality of Virtual Simulation

George W. Sherouse, Ph.D.

Radiation Oncology Physics, Duke University Medical Center, Durham, North Carolina

In 1987 my colleagues at the University of North Carolina at Chapel Hill and I proposed that it should be possible to completely replace the conventional radiotherapy simulator with a computer-based simulation of the simulator.[1] In this scenario, the patient is replaced by a digital representation derived from 3-D tomographic image data, the simulator is replaced by custom radiotherapy design software, and the process is underpinned by a clinically sensible set of coordinate system conventions and patient repositioning techniques. The system, essentially as outlined in that 1987 manifesto, was subsequently implemented and went into clinical service in early 1988. In the years since then approximately 700 patients have been treated at UNC-CH and Duke University Medical Center using this system to design and deliver their therapy. This paper is a review of the mature technology that we call *virtual simulation*.

It is worthwhile to recall the context and motivation for the development of the virtual simulation technology. By the mid 1980s copious tomographic data were available for most patients presenting for radiotherapy, but there existed no satisfactory system for using those data directly in the design of therapy. Many investigators had solved pieces of the puzzle,[2-8] but most of these solutions represented extensions of traditional 2-D treatment planning rather than development of a new technology that fully leveraged the available 3-D information. This is an important philosophical point that bears further attention. Traditional treatment planning (RTP) was and still is almost exclusively concerned with the evaluation and modification of <u>dosimetry</u> once a set of beams has been set using a treatment simulator or clinical setup. In that setting, treatment planning means almost exclusively selection of wedges and weights. Only rarely is there any feedback in the system whereby treatment planning influences the choices of treatment <u>geometry</u>. This should be contrasted with the virtual simulation approach wherein the geometry of the treatment is also developed by use of appropriate computer tools. We and others have used the term <u>treatment design</u> or <u>RTD</u> to emphasize this important difference.

It was clear in the early 1980s that use of the relatively high-resolution digitization of the patient presented by CT and other tomographic data allows for greatly improved confidence in the localization of targets and other structures. What was less clear was how best to fully realize that advantage in a practical and efficient way. It was our assertion that the greatest advantage could be gained by performing a computer-aided design of the treatment directly from the image data. Not only does this approach improve confidence in localization, but it potentially allows for the trivially simple selection and implementation of non-traditional beam orientations. This in turn should significantly improve our ability to intelligently manage collateral damage. This line of thinking naturally leads to the realization that the evolution from RTP to RTD involves the migration of many tasks that were traditionally called simulation into the arena of computerized treatment planning. Our 1987 manifesto takes that point of view quite literally and proposes the development of a computer environment in which traditional simulation can be performed in the virtual world of the digital patient representation.

The concepts of virtual simulation presented here are not just meant as some clever play on words. I am quite literal and concrete when I speak of performing radiotherapy simulations in the virtual world of the computer. The virtual simulation metaphor has proven to be remarkably powerful both as a guide in engineering the details of the project and, more importantly, as a source of vocabulary and cultural framework for development of some complex new skills in physicians, physicists, dosimetrists, technologists and others. Clinical acceptance of any new technology is greatly enhanced if it can be packaged as compatibly as possible with existing practice rather than as a totally new procedure. The fact that the Virtual Simulator™ presents the functions of a conventional simulator in a way that feels like a simulator makes it immediately acceptable to anyone familiar with conventional simulators and treatment machines. At the same time, the functions of the Virtual Simulator™ which are in addition to those of a conventional simulator can be learned at the pace appropriate to the user's needs. Most importantly, though, the proper implementation of this metaphor allows the user to concentrate on the task rather than the arcane habits of the tool. This observation is offered here as a guide to both developers and consumers of RTD products.

System Concepts

The defining characteristic of virtual simulation, as we have defined it, is that the computer-based design process completely replaces the traditional process of treatment simulation. Virtual simulation has been characterized as the "SCAN, PLAN, TREAT" scenario. This should be contrasted with the more traditional 2-D or 3-D RTP-based process which is "SIMULATE, maybe SCAN, PLAN (dosimetry only), maybe ADJUST, TREAT." Note, in virtual simulation, no decisions regarding the geometry of the therapy are made prior to the computerized treatment design.

I would emphasize that the virtual simulation system is not just a piece of software. It is a comprehensive, interdependent set of mathematical descriptions and conventions, clinical practices and protocols, clinical engineering practices, and of course a lot of computer software. The software components which are described here are parts of the GRATIS™ 3-D radiotherapy treatment design system.

Conventional simulation and subsequent delivery of a radiotherapy treatment plan involves a number of specific functions. Table 20-1 presents a list of those functions and will serve as an outline to the rest of this paper. The reader is encouraged to critically assess this list of functions with attention to whether it represents a true and complete system analysis. I assert that each of the items listed has been successfully addressed by the virtual simulation project. Therefore, if the list is complete, then so-called CT-simulation is a solved problem.

One thing that is to some conspicuously absent from this table is computation and analysis of dose distributions. Dosimetry is, of course, an important part of the process of treatment design and must not be neglected. It is, however, not different in any fundamental way between RTP and RTD, nor has it ever been a function of a treatment simulator, and so is purposely omitted from the current discussion.

Table 20-1. The virtual simulation approach to the steps in conventional simulation

Function	Virtual simulation solution
localization of target and other structures	direct, spatially quantitative use of tomographic images
beam placement	Virtual Simulator™
portal design	Virtual Simulator™ and computer generated block templates
beam documentation	computer generated setup instructions
creation of reference image for QA	digitally reconstructed radiographs
patient marking	coordinate systems, patient fixation, cast marks

The sections which follow will describe each of the points of Table 20-1 in turn.

Structure Localization

Spatial localization of target, and anti-target[9] structures is, of course, the Big Win of image-based RTD. Even if therapy is planned in a wholly conventional way, physicians are obliged to by some means incorporate the geometric findings of diagnostic images into their treatment plans.

True spatially qualitative use of image data requires the establishment of at least one coordinate system. There are an infinitude of possible choices of coordinate system, all equally valid by some criteria. But, bearing in mind that the point of spatial quantification for RTD is to localize structures at the treatment machine, some care in selection of the coordinate systems can result in substantial simplification of the use of the data. This is no surprise to physicists who will have learned in Dynamics 101 (if not before) that selection of a good frame of reference can trivialize an otherwise very complex problem.

The virtual simulation project described here uses a Patient coordinate system which is a right-handed system referenced to the treatment couch.[10] As viewed from the foot of the couch the x axis is positive to the right, the y axis is positive up, and the z axis is positive toward the observer. Since the coordinate system is defined with respect to the treatment couch, the orientation of the axes with respect to the patient's principal axes are a function of the patient's position on the couch. If the patient is feet first and prone, the z axis will be toward the patient's head and the y axis toward the patient's back. This is consistent with the philosophy, further discussed below, that if due care is taken in fixing the patient to the table, then achieving the proper relative positions of patient and treatment machine to deliver a particular beam orientation is a simple matter of positioning the treatment machine appropriately.[11]

The origin of the Patient coordinate system is at the center of the couch top in x and y, and at a patient-specific level in z. This choice of origin is crucial in that it is clinically sensible. If, as we will do, we specify that the isocenter of the machine be at a specific coordinate in the Patient system to deliver a beam, we must have some mechanism for executing that instruction reliably in the treatment room. If the coordinate origin were defined by some accidental choice such as the center of reconstruction of some CT scan, a fairly complex mechanism could be required for localizing that point in the physical patient at treatment time. The choice of coordinate system referenced to the tabletop, however, avoids this problem. If, for instance, the y coordinate of isocenter is specified as 5.3 cm, I can execute that instruction by placing the end of a ruler on the tabletop and raising or lowering the table until the lateral laser shines on the ruler at 5.3. In practice we often use some surrogate for the tabletop reference such as the top of a fixation device for ease of access, but the argument holds.

Given a set of planning images and a coordinate system in which to operate, the spatial localization of structures amounts to identifying regions in the scan planes which constitute the structures of interest and then constructing a mathematical representation of those structures in the specified coordinate system. The most common abstraction used is a stack of planar polygons created as structure outlines on CT scans.

Beam Placement

The next step in development of a treatment design after the localization of important structures is the placement of treatment ports. In conventional practice this is done either by fluoroscopic localization on a treatment simulation or by simple clinical setup. It is instructive to consider for a moment the limitations which the use of fluoroscopic localization imposes on the system. The most obvious is that most target structures do not appear radiographically as different from their surround and are thus just not visualizable on fluoro. When beams are aimed at invisible targets under fluoro a complex and error-prone process must play out in the clinician's brain. This process starts with the mental development of an assumed 3-D geometry of the target based on reading of radiological studies, physical exam, etc. The clinician must then mentally visualize the 3-D shape and location of radiologically visible structures such as bone and airways with respect to the presumed 3-D target structure. Then those radiologically visualizable structures must be mentally radiographed and the resulting mental picture compared with the actual image presented by the fluorograph. It is to the credit of radiotherapy professionals that we manage this formidable task as well as we do.

Another limitation, more mundane but just as important, is that the range of possible motions of the simulator are more or less limited (depending on simulator design) by the very presence of the image intensifier tube that makes fluoroscopy possible. The set of combinations of table rotation and gantry rotation which can be physically realized may be severely limited, even compared to the limited motions of current treatment machines.

It is no surprise, then, that treatment ports have traditionally been generously sized and almost always oriented along axes of the patient's body. One extreme example of how these limitations have entered the collective consciousness is presented by a widely used technique for treatment of pituitary tumors. In this technique three fields are used; two lateral fields and a third field perpendicular to those two and entering from an angle about midway between anterior and vertex (A40S, for instance, in the UNC nomenclature[12]). This technique is usually implemented by *angling the patient's head* with a severe chin tuck and treating the semi-vertex field with the treatment machine in the nominal AP position. Even a trivial examination of the situation reveals that placing the patient's head in the neutral position, rotating the couch 90 degrees, and rotating the gantry by (in my example) 40 degrees achieves a treatment which irradiates almost exactly the same volume of tissue, is more comfortable for the patient and hence more reproducible, and is technically no more demanding to deliver. But, alas, couch rotation is one of the taboos of the prevailing radiotherapy culture.

The Virtual Simulator[TM] is a piece of software which implements a replica of a treatment simulator capable of accepting patients as modeled by digital images (see color Plate 14). Its capabilities and operation have been detailed elsewhere[13] and will not be repeated here. What is essential for the current discussion is that the Virtual Simulator[TM] can be used to set treatment beams in *exactly* the same way that a conventional treatment simulator is used. Both of the limitations discussed above are eliminated by this approach (perhaps too well as we shall see). Specifically, all of the mental gyrations described above are eliminated since the target volume is directly visualized as a graphical rendition of a geometric abstraction, viewed in the proper geometric projection at all times. It is possible to visualize *only* the target if that is of interest. Of course, since the Virtual Simulator[TM] has no physical existence, there are no physical limitations on its position and so *any* beam orientation can be visualized.

There are some losses in moving from the physical to the virtual world. Probably the most significant is that virtual patients do not (yet) breathe, pump blood, or transport food. Normal involuntary motion of anatomy which can be visualized to some extent radiographically cannot be seen at virtual simulation. In addition, freedom from the physical constraints of the physical simulator does not free one from the physical constraints of the physical treatment machine. Mathematical detection of undeliverable beams is a difficult but in principle solvable problem. In practice we rely on experience and dry runs.

Another incidental loss is that while the radiographic image does not visualize target directly, the bony and airway anatomy radiography presents are useful in beam placement and block placement. This is, to argue circularly, partly because the geometric rules physicians are taught for beam placement are steeped in the culture imposed by radiographic imaging. This problem happily has a straightforward technological solution, the calculation of simulated fluoro images, which is dependent only on the availability of sufficient computing horsepower.[14]

Portal Design

Portal design, or more specifically custom block design, is traditionally achieved by drawing the desired portal or blocks on a radiographic film acquired under strictly controlled geometric conditions. That film then goes to the block fabrication shop where it is used as a template for cutting the shielding block.

The virtual simulation analogy to this is straightforward. The portal can be drawn using the Virtual Simulator™ using one of many options including freehand drawing with an "electronic grease pencil" and/or automatic shaping of the field to the projected shape of a specified structure with a specified margin. The resulting digital outline of the desired port can then be used to cut a block by one of many mechanisms. The simplest is to plot the outline on a piece of paper with the proper magnification (see Figure 20-1) and send that template, labeled with its virtual TFD, to the block room as if it were a film. This is the approach currently in routine use at Duke. A more sophisticated approach is to electronically transfer the outline to a computer-controlled block cutting machine.

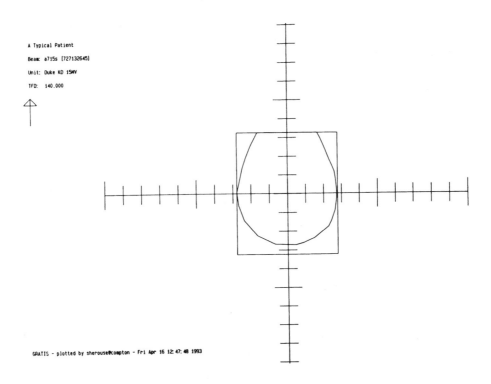

A Typical Patient

Beam: a715s (727132645)

Unit: Duke KD 15MV

TFD: 140.000

GRATIS - plotted by sherouse@compton - Fri Apr 16 12:47:48 1993

Figure 20-1. *A block template. This plotted outline, scaled to the designated TFD, is used in place of a simulator film for fabricating a custom shielding block. The arrow indicates the nominal direction of the gantry when the block is inserted.*

Beam Documentation

Once beams are placed using the physical simulator the specifics of the setup for each beam must be charted for use at the treatment machine and elsewhere. In the traditional setting this is accomplished by the simulator technologist making notations by hand in the patient's chart. This set of notes, again because of the limitations built into the current culture of radiotherapy, usually consists only of a very limited subset of the full specification. For instance, in many cases notation of SSD, gantry angle, and collimator setting, in combination with skin marks, is considered sufficient because those are the only things that ever vary patient to patient. Many radiotherapy charts do not even have a designated space for documenting table rotation. A more sophisticated approach is available on some current generation physical simulators which allow automatic electronic capture, storage, and printout of all setup parameters.

The Virtual Simulator™ requires a complete unambiguous description of each beam in order to function. By complete I mean that the value of every treatment machine parameter which influences beam placement is present, referenced to the Patient coordinate system described earlier. By unambiguous I mean that parameter values are specified in such a way that each set of values identifies a unique position of the treatment machine. These descriptions are stored and can be printed in any desired format. One particular format, used for setup documentation, is shown in Figure 20-2. These setup instruction pages are placed in the patient chart in the section reserved for simulation notes and so replace the notes conventionally made by the simulator operator.

```
A Typical Patient
Beam: a715s [727132645]
Unit: Duke KD 15MV
SAD: 100.0
predicted SSD: 92.6
tray: custom block tray
Collimator size: X: 5.6, Y: 6.5


Position table:
     12.5 cm down
      0.2 cm right (looking toward gantry)
      0.8 cm toward gantry
*OR*

Position isocenter:
     12.5 cm above tabletop reference
      0.2 cm left of midline reference (looking toward gantry)
      0.8 cm away from gantry


Set angles:
         Collimator: 90.0 degrees counterclockwise (looking into jaws)
         Gantry: 71.5 degrees clockwise
         Table: 90.0 degrees clockwise (looking down from above)

Machine                        Table     Gantry   Collimator
-------                        -----     ------   ----------

Duke KD 15MV                    90.0      71.5       270.0
Philips simulator              90.0      71.5       -90.0
Toshiba simulator              90.0      71.5       270.0
```

Figure 20-2. *A setup page for a virtually simulated beam. All parameters of the setup including three table translations, three machine rotations, collimator setting, and beam modifiers such as wedges are fully specified. These pages are inserted in the patient chart, one per field, in the section normally used for simulation notes.*

One particular item, another product of an historically constrained culture, deserves a moment's attention here. Note that the setup instructions of Figure 20-2 refer to the collimators as X and Y, not as width and height. Width and height are traditional designators for collimator jaws which refer to the jaw by its orientation with respect to the patient. In most clinics that use this designation, a 90 degree rotation of the collimator switches the meaning of width and height. The ambiguity of this convention is easily appreciated by considering a true lateral field for which a 45 degree collimator rotation is used. Which dimension of the collimator setting is width? In a setting where the beam may be entering from a compound oblique angle with respect to the patient and some collimator rotation may be required to orient a wedge filter properly, the concepts of width and length are nothing but dangerous. Consistent and unambiguous collimator designations should always be used. This becomes yet more important in the presence of asymmetric or multi-leaf collimators.

Creation of Reference Image

An important part of the residue from a physical simulation is the set of simulator films, one for each port to be treated and perhaps others for purposes such as isocenter localization. These films have a variety of uses, and in fact represent a very sophisticated mechanism for efficiently communicating a large amount of geometric and other data to a large number of people involved in the patient's care. Many of the roles served by the simulator film can be accomplished by other means as we have seen portal design can be. One role of the simulator film which is not readily usurped is that of gold standard against which subsequent portal films are to be judged for the purposes of continuing QA.

The strategy used in the virtual simulation system for acquiring simulator films is to compute an approximation of the simulator film by mathematically passing divergent rays through a CT dataset and acquiring x-ray attenuation information along the rays. Such a simulated or virtual radiograph is commonly referred to as a Digitally Reconstructed Radiograph or DRR. The method by which DRRs are calculated in GRATISTM is described in detail elsewhere.[15] The salient feature of that method for the present discussion is that it represents an attempt to create DRR images which are the best reasonable digital approximation of true simulation films in terms of both spatial resolution and subject contrast. This is crucial in a setting where virtual simulation completely replaces physical simulation and so the DRR must replace a physical film for QA purposes. A typical DRR is shown in color Plate 15. In the clinics at UNC-CH and Duke these DRR images are printed on film using laser cameras and are stored in the patient's film jacket just as if they were the physical radiographs they aspire to be. Again, the importance of the virtual simulation metaphor cannot be overemphasized.

Patient Marking

The traditional means by which patients and radiation beams are aligned on a day-to-day basis has been the use of marks on the patient's skin indicating the outline of the properly-aligned radiation beam. This, combined with other information such as expected SSD, has served the community reasonably well in the decades of relatively loose geometric tolerances and severely restricted treatment geometries. But it is a clearly flawed technology. Skin is a highly mobile structure, subject to significant and unavoidable random deformation as a patient assumes the treatment position. More to the point, for cases where a high degree of geometric precision is desired, as is typically the case for conformal radiotherapy, skin is in general significantly more mobile than is the underlying target volume.

The virtual simulation approach as my colleagues and I have described it rejects the use of skin marks altogether in favor of a more formal engineering approach based on the previously described coordinate systems. The assumptions of this approach are simply that:

1. The patient can to an acceptable tolerance be made to resemble a rigid body through the use of very aggressive custom immobilization casts. That is, patient shape can be reasonably reproduced.

2. The rigidified patient can be reliably positioned on the treatment couch such that the coordinate system of the patient is aligned with and registered to the coordinate system of the treatment unit.

3. Treatment of a specific beam geometry then reduces to simply positioning the treatment machine properly.

We have called this approach setup "by the numbers." In its most fully realized implementation <u>no marks at all</u> are required on the patient or on the patient's immobilization cast. In practice we use a variety of alignment marks on the cast in order to be assured of getting the patient/cast system properly repositioned on the treatment couch. We also continue to use skin marks, but as a secondary QA check rather than as a primary mechanism for beam alignment.

Color Plate 16 shows a patient in a cast typical of those used for prostate irradiation at Duke. The materials used in the fabrication of this cast are familiar ones in the radiotherapy community. The cast consists of a sheet of polyurethane foam insulation board to which a number of other pieces of foam have been attached. This form is placed inside a large plastic bag and filled with a two-component liquid foaming agent. The patient is quickly placed in position and polyurethane foam arising from the liquid is allowed to conform to the patient and set. Then some alignment marks are made on the cast using the sagittal and transverse lasers of the CT scanner and a set of planning CT images are acquired.

A few key features of the immobilization of prostate patients are noteworthy. The cast extends longitudinally from beyond the bottom of the feet to about the patient's waist, rising to about 2/3 of the patient's anterior-posterior thickness all the way along. The knees are elevated about 10.0 cm on foam wedges. It was our hope, now borne out by experience,[16] that the combination of foot immobilization and knee elevation would result in good reproducibility of pelvis position. In particular, knee elevation helps to prevent rotation of the pelvis.

Color Plate 17 shows a conceptually very similar technique used at Duke for head and neck patients. The immobilization consists of a custom foam pillow under the patient's head and neck and a thermal plastic mask over the patient's face. The two pieces are made in rapid succession without allowing the patient to move in between and so represent a custom fit with essentially zero tolerance. The cushion and mask lock into place in a head holder base, developed at the University of Michigan,[17] which in turn mates reproducibly to the CT and treatment couches. The use of a custom foam sponge, such as the ones we manufacture by putting two-component liquid foam in a Sunday newspaper wrapper, is in our view essential. So-called "standard" head sponges are not adequate for precision radiotherapy because of significant variation in manufacture and more importantly because they do not conform to the shape of the patient's head and so leave considerable room for error in head repositioning. For the same reason we prefer that patients not have unusually long or thick hair. We have on one occasion referred a patient for a stat haircut before building the head cast.

Casts and masks for other sites are produced in a similar manner. In all cases our goal is to make the casts big enough to provide adequate repositioning cues to both the patient and treatment staff. We counsel our patients to notice how the cast and/or mask feels to them and to try to make sure that the fit is the same each time they visit. In the case of the face masks patients can experience considerable discomfort from even relatively small variation in setup, for instance because of failure to remove a collared shirt. This is considered a good thing as it gives us valuable instant feedback as to the quality of the patient's setup. It is at first perhaps surprising that we encourage our patients to squirm into position but it is our experience that good patient compliance is as important as good casting technique in achieving reproducible setup and it is only the patient who can feel the fit from day to day.

Our 1987 manifesto included an endorsement of the use of a special device attached to the CT scanner to project virtually simulated beams onto the patient so that skin marks could be made. It is currently my strong conviction, given years of experience with the system described above, that skin marks on patients who have undergone virtual simulation are unnecessary and perhaps counterproductive. It has often been the case in our clinic that if a virtual simulation patient is not setting up well the problem can be remedied by ignoring any skin or cast marks that may have been made by the technologists to designate field positions and simply setting the patient up from scratch by the numbers.

Conclusion and Observations

CT-based radiotherapy treatment simulation is demonstrably a solved problem. All of the essential functions involved in designing, simulating, and delivering a set of radiation beams can be accomplished using 3-D tomographic image data and appropriate RTD software. Furthermore, the use of this technology is now truly routine at Duke University Medical Center and many other radiotherapy departments where it yields the dual advantage of increased confidence in tissue and beam localization for all cases and increased capacity to render unconventional treatment geometries where appropriate. Treatments such as the one illustrated in color Plate 18 are now designed and executed at Duke on a routine basis.

As the price/performance ratio of computer hardware continues to improve it is reasonable to expect that the realism of the virtual environment presented by virtual simulation software will similarly continue to improve. It is important to realize, however, that this continuing improvement represents incremental refinement of a process and set of tools that are already fully functional and widely available.

Commercial products are beginning to appear which make a variety of claims regarding their ability to perform virtual simulation or CT-simulation. The functionality described in this paper should be considered minimal for such a product. Consumers are well advised to evaluate products claiming to be virtual simulators by the same standards used for purchasing physical simulators. One would not normally purchase a treatment simulator that did not provide for couch rotation or which produced unreadable radiographs or which had an extremely complex control panel. The astute consumer will accept nothing less of a virtual simulator.

References

1. G.W. Sherouse, C.E. Mosher, K.L. Novins, J.G. Rosenman and E.L. Chaney, "Virtual Simulation: Concept and Implementation," in *Proceedings of Ninth International Conference on the Use of Computers in Radiation Therapy*, Scheveningen, The Netherlands, (North-Holland Publishing Co., 1987), pp. 433-436.

2. D.L. McShan, A. Silverman, D.M. Lanza, L.E. Reinstein and A.S. Glicksman, "A Computerized Three-dimensional Treatment Planning System Utilizing Interactive Color Graphics," Br. J. Radiol. **52**, 478-481 (1979).

3. R. Mohan, C. Chui, D. Miller and J. Laughlin, "Use of Computed Tomography in Dose Calculations for Radiation Treatment Planning," CT: The Journal of Computed Tomography 5, 273-282 (1981).

4. R.L. Siddon, "Solution to Treatment Planning Problems Using Coordinate Transformations," Med. Phys. **8**(6), 766-774 (1981).

5. I.J. Kalet and J.P. Jacky, "A Research-Oriented Treatment Planning Program System," Computer Programs in Biomedicine **14**, 85-98 (1982).

6. L.V. Verhey, M. Goitein, P. McNulty, J.E. Munzenrider and H.D. Suit, "Precise Positioning of Patients for Radiation Therapy," Int. J. Radiat. Oncol. Biol. Phys. **8**, 289-294 (1982).

7. M. Goitein, M. Abrams, D. Rowell, H. Pollari and J. Wiles, "Multi-dimensional Treatment Planning: II. Beam's Eye-view, Back Projection, and Projection Through CT sections," Int. J. Radiat. Oncol. Biol. Phys. **9**(6), 789-797 (1983).

8. G.T.Y. Chen and M. Goitein, "Treatment Planning for Heavy Charged Particles", in *Advances in Radiation Therapy Treatment Planning* (American Institute of Physics, 1983), pp. 514-541.

9. G.W. Sherouse, "Images and Treatment Simulation", in *Advances in Radiation Oncology Physics: Dosimetry, Treatment Planning and Brachytherapy* (American Institute of Physics, 1992), pp. 925-947.

10. G.W. Sherouse, "Coordinate Transformation as a Primary Representation of Radiotherapy Beam Geometry," Med. Phys. **19**, 175-179 (1992).

11. G.W. Sherouse, J.D. Bourland, K.L. Reynolds, H.L. McMurry, T.P. Mitchell and E.L. Chaney, "Virtual Simulation in the Clinical Setting: Some Practical Considerations," Int. J. Radiat. Oncol. Biol. Phys. **19**, 1059-1065 (1990).

12. S.L. Sailer, J.D. Bourland, J.G. Rosenman, G.W. Sherouse, E.L. Chaney and J.E. Tepper, "3-D Beams Need 3-D Names," Int. J. Radiat. Oncol. Biol. Phys. **19**, 797-798 (1990).

13. G.W. Sherouse and E.L. Chaney, "The Portable Virtual Simulator," Int. J. Radiat. Oncol. Biol. Phys. **21**, 475-482 (1991).

14. T.J. Cullip, J.R. Symon, J.G. Rosenman and E.L. Chaney, "Digitally Reconstructed Fluoroscopy and Other Interactive Volume Visualizations in 3-D Treatment Planning," Int. J. Radiat. Oncol. Biol. Phys. , (in press).

15. G.W. Sherouse, K.L. Novins and E.L. Chaney, "Computation of Digitally Reconstructed Radiographs for Use in Radiotherapy Treatment Design," Int. J. Radiat. Oncol. Biol. Phys. **18**, 651-658 (1990).

16. G.C. Bentel, L.B. Marks, G.W. Sherouse, D.P. Spencer and M.S. Anscher, "The Effectiveness of Immobilization During Prostate Irradiation," Int. J. Radiat. Oncol. Biol. Phys. , (submitted).

17. A.F. Thornton, R.K. Ten Haken, K.J. Weeks, A. Gerhardsson, M. Correll and K.A. Lask, "A Head Immobilization System for Radiation Simulation, CT, MRI, and PET imaging," Medical Dosimetry **16**, 51-56 (1991).

Chapter 21

3-D Treatment Planning at the University of North Carolina: Recent Progress

Julian G. Rosenman, Ph.D., M.D.

University of North Carolina at Chapel Hill, Chapel Hill, North Carolina

The original treatment planning system at the University of North Carolina has always differed from others because it was designed to be used by clinicians as well as dosimetrists. To that end we have relied heavily on cutting-edge display technology, rapid feedback mechanisms, and effective man-machine interfaces. In addition, the software was written to be as modular and portable as possible because it was recognized that 3-D treatment planning is an evolving science that will necessitate many additions and changes in the future. Finally, the fast paced improvements in computer hardware made it a certainty that there would be a need to continually port the software to newer computing platforms.

The initial version of our treatment planning software was completed by 1991. It has been well described in the literature (please see references). Thus a brief review of the process, will suffice:

3-D treatment planning at UNC begins with the acquisition of a CT volume data set. CT scanning is performed through the tumor containing volume with generous margins both above and below the tumor to allow for radiation beams that do not lie in the transverse plane. The patient is immobilized in the treatment position, and the CT data registered with the patient by marking the point of the first CT cut on the patient's cast. At the University of North Carolina we typically take 60-120 slices contiguous slices, with a 4 millimeter separation in the area of the tumor, and 8 millimeters above and below the tumor.

The next step is to segment the CT data set so that anatomic objects of interest and tumor volumes are identified. Perhaps the most important anatomic object of interest is the skin, which can usually be identified automatically by means of edge detection algorithms. Delineation of the skin/air boundary is the 3-D analog of the traditional 2-D skin contour measurement, often done with solder wire, pencil and paper. Like its 2-D counterpart, identification of the skin/air boundary is necessary for dose calculation. Other anatomic objects, such as kidneys, lungs, liver or other organs that whose dose tolerances will put constraints on the treatment planning process must also be identified. Although some of this segmentation can be done automatically, much of it currently must be done by hand; this is sometimes quite time consuming. Finally, the tumor volume must be identified. Actually, there are two distinct "tumor" volumes, the abnormality as seen on CT, or gross tumor volume (GTV), and the inferred or clinical tumor volume, CTV. The CTV, therefore, consists of the GTV plus local or regional volumes (such as lymph nodes) that the clinician feels are likely to harbor tumor. Typically we identify the GTV on CT and defer defining the CTV until later in the treatment planning process.

Once the CT data is satisfactorily segmented, the anatomic and tumor volumes are assembled to produce a 3-D model of the patient which then undergoes "virtual simulation," a concept due to George Sherouse, wherein a superset of the function of a physical radiation simulator is modeled in software. The virtual simulator is a true 3-D planning tool—all dimensions are treated equally in that the patient can be rotated to any desired compound angle. The virtual simulator calculates what positions of the table, gantry, and collimator are necessary to achieve this beam orientation, so that the physician can concentrate solely on what beam angles are best for the patient, and not on how to achieve them.

The output of the virtual simulator is a hard copy (on film) of a computed radiograph and set up instructions for each radiation beam. The patient then undergoes physical simulation as a quality control; if the simulation film matches the computed radiograph then the set up is correct. In this way the 3-D treatment planning system enforces precision in the setup. If the portal films match the simulation film (actually if they match the computed radiograph) then the radiation beams are certain to encompass the GTV as outlined on the CT data.

The New PLAN UNC

In February, 1993, we undertook to revise and rebuild our treatment planning system because new advances in computer hardware made many of the compromises adopted in the original software unnecessary. For example, the original virtual simulator could not be equipped with high quality graphics because at the time of its development such displays took too long to compute. Instead, wireloops were used to represent anatomy and tumor target as these had the virtue of near real-time update, even on modest computing platforms. Also memory limitations made it necessary to write the treatment planning software as a collection of modules of "tools" that could be invoked, run, and then closed. This meant that shifting back and forth between different parts of the planning system was cumbersome and time consuming. Finally, we had developed an entirely new set of capabilities during our work with collateral projects, and it was desired to bring them into the main treatment planning system. In this paper we will focus on the improvements to old capabilities, and the entirely new tools that have now been incorporated into the treatment planning system.

One of the most important new capabilities added to PLAN UNC is the upgrade of the virtual simulator to take advantage of faster hardware, parallel processing, and new display algorithms. The current version of the virtual simulator displays a computed radiograph with anatomic overlays in the beam's-eye view window. Therefore, the clinician can now design the treatment portal on an electronic version of a simulation film, an approach that is both natural and consistent with previous experience. In addition, the virtual simulator now displays a high quality view of the patient's surface anatomy with an overlaid light field, the so-called "observer's-eye" view of the patient. This combination of computed radiograph with overlays, CT scans with beam overlays, and surface anatomy view of the patient, all dynamically linked in near real time (approximately 1 frame/second), represents a powerful new approach to radiation beam placement. This upgrade is made possible by newer and more efficient techniques for computing radiographs, and because microprocessors are now faster and more efficient in the way they handle data.

PLAN UNC now uses a "document oriented" rather than tool oriented approach to treatment planning. In the past, one invoked a tool such as *imex* (used for CT object definition) and then wrote out a contour file, and closed the application. Today all these tools reside in memory and can be quickly invoked *around the patient document*. For dose calculations this means that radiation beams can be set up, and the resulting dose viewed immediately. One quickly switch back to the virtual simulator, change the beams, and recalculate the dose. Using some of the efficient algorithms developed in VISTAnet (see below) it is now possible to get the dose distribution on a single slice in 1-2 seconds.

Although getting the geometry correct is an important first step in radiation treatment planning, the ultimate goal must be the design of a good radiation dose distribution. 3-D treatment planning is frustrating because of the large number of possible treatments that can be delivered, the slow calculation time of a full 3-D dose distribution, and the difficulty in displaying the dose in a comprehensible way. Although many tools for examining dose distribution have been developed, including the dose-volume histogram, and NTCP models, it is still the case that the dose distribution must be understood by the clinician before trusting the patient to that treatment. In 1988 we began the VISTAnet project which linked a CRAY-YMP™ (the dose calculating engine) to

Pixel-Planes 5, arguably the world's fastest graphics engine, with an experimental gigabit network. The project, funded by NSF, DARPA, BellSouth and GTE, has resulted in a "metacomputer" (the CRAY and Pixel-Planes together) that has the capability of near real-time dose calculation and display. Using the virtual simulator as the interface, it is possible to move a radiation beam and see the change *in the entire 3-D dose distribution* in less than a second.

Recent work with VISTAnet has convinced us that many unexplored possibilities using static (fixed field) conformal technology still remain. Specifically, the use of non-coplanar, non-opposed radiation beams can result in very tight dose distributions, even for a four beam treatment plan.

PLAN UNC and VISTAnet (or other dose optimizing tools) effectively solve the problem of treatment planning precision (getting the radiation beams where they are desired) and developing conformational treatment plans. However, the problem of *treatment planning accuracy* (correctly defining the planning target volume) remains. We have come to the conclusion that multimodality imaging is going to be the next important advance in radiation treatment planning. For example, supposing a patient has a brain tumor that only shows up on MRI. We would now 1) contour the tumor as seen on MR 2) tile the contours into a volume file 3) register the MR with the planning CT 4) reslice the tiled contour file 5) display the resliced contours on the CT scans and then 6) continue treatment planning based on CT and the transferred MR contours. Of course we are not limited to MR and CT. In the future we expect that planning target volumes will be derived from a wide variety of imaging technologies including ultrasound, PET, antibody scans, and a whole range of SPECT immunoscintigraphies.

Summary

The 3-D treatment planning system at UNC, PLAN UNC enforces treatment planning precision and has some tools for developing conformal plans. We are just beginning to incorporated multimodal imaging into the system for purposes of improving treatment planning accuracy.

Reference

1. Rosenman J, Sherouse GW, Fuchs H, Pizer SM, Skinner AL, Mosher C, Novins K, Tepper JE: Three-dimensional display techniques in radiation therapy treatment planning. *Int J Radiat Oncol Biol Physics* **16**:263-269, 1989.

2. Fuchs H, Levoy M, Pizer SM, Rosenman JG: Interactive visualization and manipulation of 3-D medical image data. *Proceedings of the NCGA Conference* **1**:118-131, (April) 1989.

3. Pizer SM, Fuchs H, Levoy M, Rosenman JG, Renner J, Davis R: 3-D display with minimal predefinition. *Proceedings of the Computer Assisted Radiography* (CAR), Springer Verlag: Berlin, 1989, pages 723-736.

4. Pizer SM, Levoy M, Fuchs, H, Rosenman JG: Volume rendering for display of multiple organs, treatment objects and image intensities. *Science and Engineering of Medical Imaging, SPIE Proceedings* **1137**:92-97, 1989.

5. Mills PH, Fuchs H, Pizer SM, Rosenman JG: IMEX: A tool for image display and contour management in a windowing environment. Medical *Imaging 111: Image Capture and Display*, RH Schneider, S Dwyer ll, and RG Jost, eds, *Proceedings of the SPIE* **1091**:132-142, 1989.

6. Sherouse GW, Novins K, Chaney EL: Computation of digitally reconstructed radiographs for use in radiotherapy treatment design. *Int J Padiat Oncol Biol Phys* **18**:651-658, 1990.

7. Sailer S, Bourland D, Rosenman J, Sherouse G, Chaney E, Tepper J: 3-D beams need 3-D names. *Int J Radiat Oncol Biol Physics* **19**:797-798, 1990.

8. Levoy M, Fuchs H, Pizer SM, Rosenman J, Chaney EL, Sherouse GW, Interrante V, Kiel J: Volume rendering in radiation treatment planning *Proceedings of the First Conference on Visualization of Biomedical Computing* pp 4-10, IEEE Computer Society Press, Los Alamitos, California, May, 1990.

9. Rosenman JG, Chaney EL, Sailer S, Sherouse GW, Tepper JE: Recent advances in radiotherapy treatment planning. *Cancer Investigation* **9**:465-481, 1 991.

10. Fishman EK, Ney DR, Vannier M, Chaney EL, Pizer S, Rosenman J, Levin D, Magin D, Kulman J, Robertson D: Three-dimensional imaging: State of the art. Radiology 181:321-337, 1991.

11. Sherouse GW, Chaney EL: The portable virtual simulator. Int. J. Radiat. Oncol. Biol. Phys. **21**:475-482; 1991.

12. Rosenman J. 3-D modeling for radiation therapy treatment planing. *Contemporary Oncology.* **2** (March)53-57, 1992.

13. Sailer SL, Chaney EL, Rosenman JG, Sherouse, GW, Tepper JE: Treatment planning at the University of North Carolina at Chapel Hill. *Sem. in Rad. Onc.* **2**:267-273, 1992.

14. Cullip TJ, Symon JR, Rosenman JG, Chaney EL: Digitally reconstructed fluoroscopy and other interactive volume visualizations in 3-D treatment planning. *Int J Radiat Oncol Biol Physics,* **27**:145-151, 1993.

15. Rosenman, J: Future directions in 3-dimensional imaging and radiotherapy treatment planning. *Oncology,* **7**(11):97-107,1993.

Chapter 22

3-D Photon Beam Dose Algorithms

Thomas R. Mackie, Ph.D., Paul Reckwerdt B.S., and Nikos Papanikolaou, Ph.D.[*]

University of Wisconsin Medical School, Madison, Wisconsin

Considerable advances in radiotherapy dose planning can be made with the implementation of sophisticated three-dimensional dose algorithms. The progress of 3-D dose computation is closely coupled to computer performance and price. Lately the price/performance ratio of computer workstations have been dropping by a factor of 2 or 3 per year. This means that fully 3-D methods of dose computation, which would not be possible only a few years ago, are possible today. Today's impractical algorithms, such as the Monte Carlo method, will have a useful clinical role within a few years.

This paper will review dose computation in radiotherapy and explore two general approaches which are intrinsically three-dimensional. Correction-based methods modify dose distributions measured in a water phantom to account for beam modifiers, surface contours, and tissue heterogeneities. Model-based methods, such as the convolution/superposition method, attempt to compute the dose from first principles and use measurements to obtain a limited set of data to fit the model. The extension of the convolution/superposition method to optimized planning using solutions to the "inverse problem" will be summarized.

Dose Computation Based on Correcting Measured Dose

Dose calculation methods have traditionally been based on parametrizing dose distributions from a radiation detector probe measured in water phantoms. These algorithms have used these beam representations to correct the dose for patient and treatment specific changes such as:

- beam modifiers including blocks, wedges and compensators,
- the non-uniform surface contour of the patient or the obliquity of the beam,
- tissue heterogeneities.

Before describing the correction algorithms it is instructive to review typical procedures for parametrizing the homogeneous dose distributions.

Parametrizing Measured Dose Distributions

Except for beam calibration, dose measurements are rarely converted to absolute values but instead are normalized to relative values. The depth and lateral dependence of the dose distributions are usually dealt with separately even though they are not entirely separable. Relative central axis dose measurements as a function of depth may be obtained at a constant source-to-probe distance (SPD), as for example for tissue-air ratio (TAR), tissue-phantom ratio (TPR), or tissue-maximum ratio (TMR) measurements (Johns and Cunningham 1983, Khan 1984). Constant-SPD measurements have little variation with the distance from the source and are

---

[*] Present address: University of Kentucky, Lexington, Kentucky

therefore usually assumed to be totally independent of the source-to-surface distance (SSD). However, constant-SPD measurements are difficult to obtain using a water phantom and so depth-dose curves are usually obtained with the source-to-surface distance (SSD) constant and the dosimeter probe moving. These measurements are then corrected to the constant-SPD dose ratios (BJR Supplement 17, 1983) in order to remove most of the SSD dependence.

Scatter from the water phantom and the aperture of the radiation source results in the dose variation with depth being field size dependent. In general, the dose at a depth will depend slightly on the settings of each of the collimator pairs individually (e.g. a 5 cm x 20 cm field will not produce the same central axis dose when the settings of the upper and lower jaws are reversed to produce a 20 cm x 5 cm field) and moreover, for independent collimator jaws, the depth-dose will depend on the settings of each of the individual jaws. These distinctions are usually overlooked and the field size variation is tabulated for "equivalent square" or "equivalent circular" fields.

Many correction methods are based upon the separation of primary and scatter normalized dose contributions. The separation is based on the assumption that the primary dose, in full electronic equilibrium, does not change with field size. If the dependence of central axis dose versus field size is plotted the dose will decrease monotonically as the field size is reduced. As shown in Figure 22-1, the primary component of dose (called the zero-area tissue-air ratio (TAR_0) for TAR) is equal to the intercept of the extrapolated curved line. The scatter component of dose (called the scatter-air ratio (SAR) for TAR) is then the difference between the measured normalized dose and the primary dose. In order to satisfy the constraint of electronic equilibrium, the dose cannot be acquired at very small field sizes. This means that some extrapolation error is introduced.

The lateral variation in the dose distribution is mainly dependent on the field size. Most of the labor in commissioning a radiation source involves acquiring dose profiles along the beam's principal axes for a large variety of field sizes and depths. The lateral profiles are depth dependent because radiation beams are diverging and scattered radiation is mainly forward-directed. Dose profile values at depths between measured profiles are obtained by interpolation. The interpolation can be made with more fidelity by tabulating the profiles along diverging fan lines from the radiation source. The rapid variation in dose in the beam penumbra requires fine resolution in tabulated values. To make the profile representation more compact the penumbra is sometimes fit to appropriate functional forms.

It can be seen that there is a great deal of data processing intervening between the raw measured values and computed water dose distributions even before any patient-specific corrections are made. Several assumptions about the characteristics of the data is made in order to reduce it in size. Problems with the dose representation can occur if it is used in situations where some of the assumptions break down, as occurs for very narrow spinal fields, broad extended-SSD fields required for whole-body radiotherapy, or at points a large distance outside the field to evaluate radiation risk to a fetus or reproductive organs.

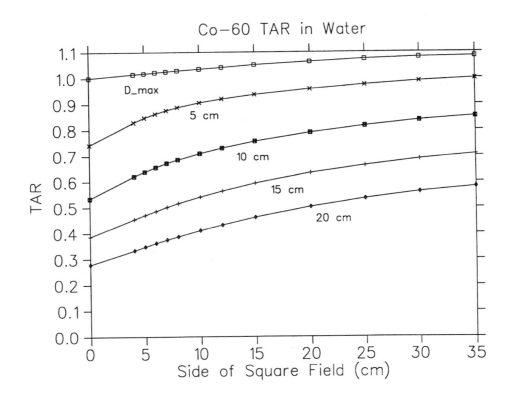

Figure 22-1. *Co-60 tissue-air ratio (TAR) in water as a function of side of square field at a variety of depths. The zero-area tissue-air ratio (TAR$_0$) is the extrapolated intercept of each of the lines. It represents the primary component of TAR and depends only on depth in the phantom. The scatter-air ratio (SAR) is the scatter component of the TAR and is the difference between the TAR and TAR$_0$. SAR depends on field size as well as depth.*

Corrections for Beam Modifiers

The usual method of correcting for irregularly shaped fields produced by custom blocks is attributed to Clarkson. This algorithm is similar in process to that of a planimeter finding the area contained within a complex boundary. The dose at a point is obtained by dividing the cross-section of the field into angular segments radiating from the point as shown in Figure 22-2. The angular segments can be defined by discrete points that define the edge of the boundary. The radius to the edge of the boundary for each segment is determined. Assuming that there is no transmission through the blocks, the correction factor to account for the tissue-air ratio (TAR)[1] for an irregular field within an equivalent square field of size W at a given depth d is found by a summation for each pair of sectors defined at the boundary:

$$CF = \frac{TAR(d, W')}{TAR(d, W)} = \frac{TAR_0(d) + \frac{1}{2\pi}\sum_i SAR(d, r_i)\Delta\phi_i}{TAR(d, W)} = \frac{\frac{1}{2\pi}\sum_i TAR(d, r_i)\Delta\phi_i}{TAR(d, W)} \tag{1}$$

---

[1] As usual, the use of TAR will be assumed but the development will be valid for any constant-SPD normalized dose such as TMR or TPR if they are corrected to account for phantom scatter at the depth of normalization.

where $\Delta\phi_i$ is the angular increment of the ith sector in radians. The above equations explicitly state that there is no need to separate the relative primary dose $TAR_0(d)$ from the scatter dose (here the scatter-air ratio (SAR)) (Thomadsen 1989). In effect, the calculation in the numerator is a way of determining the effective equivalent square field W' based on a sector-weighted average TAR.

Note that $\Delta\phi_i$ for counterclockwise angular intervals will be positive and clockwise will be negative. This allows concave regions or central blocks to be properly accounted for. The central block does not have to be connected by a "corridor" (as shown in Figure 22-2) because the contribution going inside the field will be canceled by the contribution going toward the outside of the field. The central block boundary need only be traced in the opposite rotation sense as the outside field.

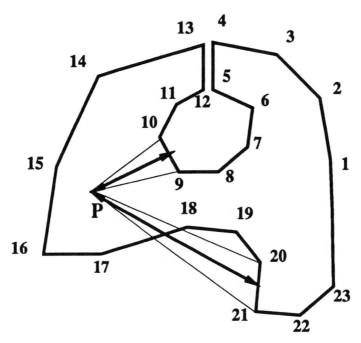

Figure 22-2. *Clarkson scatter summation to obtain the dose at a point P in an irregular field. Positive (counterclockwise) angular segments, such as the segment between vertices 9 and 10, result in adding scatter to the field. Negative (clockwise) angular segments, such as between vertices 20 and 21, remove a scatter contribution from the field. The contribution from the narrow corridor is nearly zero because positive contributions from the sector between 12 and 13 are almost canceled by the negative contribution between 4 and 5.*

The above irregular field correction does not include a factor to account for the attenuation of the tray holding the blocks, nor does it include a block transmission factor. The following generalization accounts for differential beam intensity across the field:

$$CF = \frac{TAR(d,W')}{TAR(d,W)} = \frac{\frac{1}{2\pi}\Sigma_i \frac{\Psi_i}{\Psi_0} TAR(d,r_i)\Delta\phi_i}{TAR(d,W)}$$

(2)

where $\frac{\Psi_i}{\Psi_0}$ is the relative energy fluence transmission factor when $\Delta\phi_i$ is negative and is equal to the tray factor when $\Delta\phi_i$ is positive.

The above irregular field correction equations are strictly correct only for a uniform surface contour which is normal to the central axis of the beam. The next section will illustrate a correction for the surface contour.

Correction for Patient Surface Contour

Patient contour corrections have usually been divided into separate primary and scatter corrections. A method employed in several commercial planning systems can be viewed as a generalization of the irregular field correction methodology. Figure 22-3 shows the n angular segments formed to account for scatter from each portion of the field boundary are further subdivided into N_i radial intervals. The contribution of each element is accounted for by finding the overlying thickness of tissue and looking up the amount of scatter that would contribute to the point of interest by summing over the beam area:

$$CF = \frac{TAR(d',W')}{TAR(d,W)} = \frac{\frac{1}{2\pi N}\Sigma_i^n \Sigma_{j=1}^{N_i} \frac{\Psi_{i,j}}{\Psi_0}[TAR(d_{i,j},r_{i,j}) - TAR(d_{i,j},r_{i,j-1})]|\Delta\phi_i|}{TAR(d,W)}$$

(3)

The inner summation, j is over the number of radial intervals dividing the angular segments, i. The use of the absolute value for $|\Delta\phi_i|$ stresses that the sector angular increment, in this formulation, always has a positive value. It will be shown later that the difference in TAR's is basic to scatter integration in correction-based heterogeneity correction methods. Now the ratio of energy fluence is generalized to include attenuation by any custom beam modifiers such as blocks, wedges or even compensators.

As illustrated in Figure 22-3, this procedure cannot properly account for missing tissue beyond the point of interest. In most cases backscatter perturbations change the dose by a very small amount. An exception is tangential irradiation of the breast where the backscattering thickness is very much smaller than what was used to acquire the data. Uncorrected perturbations in scatter greater than 5% are possible.

It is illustrative to formulate the above equation as an integral:

$$CF = \frac{\frac{1}{2\pi}\int \frac{\Psi(r',\phi')}{\Psi_0} \frac{dTAR(d(r',\phi'),r')}{dr} dr' d\phi'}{TAR(d,W)}$$

(4)

where the differential TAR with respect to radius is given by:

$$\frac{dTAR(d,r)}{dr} = \frac{TAR(d,r) - TAR(d,r - \Delta r)}{\Delta r}|\Delta r \rightarrow 0$$

(5)

In the next section this formulation will be generalized to account for patient heterogeneities.

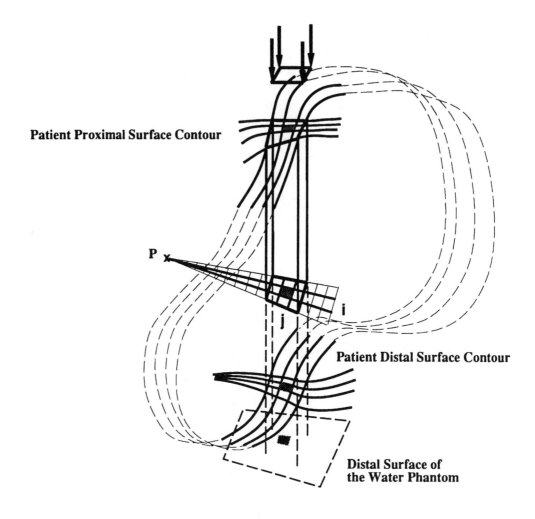

Patient Proximal Surface Contour

P

i

j

Patient Distal Surface Contour

**Distal Surface of
the Water Phantom**

Figure 22-3. *An illustration of the correction for the patient surface contour. The amount of beam intensity at point P is determined by summing through radial and angular intervals taking into account differing attenuation due to varying overlying tissue. Only the perturbation due to the patient's proximal surface contour is accounted for.*

Correction for Patient Tissue Heterogeneities

Heterogeneity corrections are more complex than other patient corrections. Low density tissue, such as lung, surrounding a point increases the fluence of primary photons which tends to increase both the primary and scatter dose. However, the scatter dose may in fact be reduced because of less scatter fluence arising from the low density region (Wong et al. 1981). Tissue interfaces may upset electronic equilibrium. For example, low densities near the edge of field boundaries results in more electrons leaving the field than in unit density tissue (Mackie et al. 1985). This results in lower dose inside the field and greater dose just outside. Greatly different atomic number tissue such as cortical bone may perturb the flux of electrons and their range (Mackie 1990). Corrections similar to those applied for dosimeter cavities should be applied to account for dose to small blood forming regions inside trabecular bone.

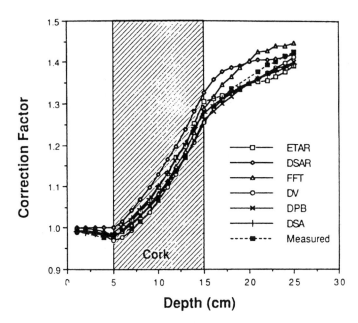

Figure 22-4. *Comparison of measurement and the results of a variety of heterogeneity correction methods obtained along the central axis with a constant 80 cm SSD Co-60 15 x 15 cm beam in a slab phantom with a 10 cm thick cork slab substituting for lung. The method labeled ETAR is the equivalent TAR method (Sontag and Cunningham 1978), DSAR is the differential scatter-air ratio method (Beaudoin 1968), and DV is the delta-volume method (Wong and Henkelman 1982). The methods labeled FFT (Boyer and Mok 1986), DPB (Mohan et al. 1986), and DSA (Mackie et al. 1985) are implementations of the convolution/superposition method. The electron density of the lung was measured to be 0.26 g/cm³. All of these methods agree within ±5%. The figure is courtesy of Wong and Purdy (1990).*

It is still a practice in some United States radiotherapy clinics and many facilities in the developing world to ignore heterogeneity corrections, even for thoracic radiotherapy. The justification is that clinical experience has been based on not correcting for heterogeneities and to do so would result in the need for modified dose prescriptions. The most often cited reasons are that CT-based planning is unavailable, inconvenient, or expensive at some centers and without CT there is very little justification for heterogeneity corrections. For example, older emphysematous patients may have lung densities as low as 0.15 g/cm³ and young well-perfused patients may have densities as high as 0.4 g/cm³. It is also argued, that since every heterogeneity correction algorithm gives a different answer it is better to do nothing. The degree of variation is larger than ideal but any correction is usually better than no correction at all. Comparisons between measurements and calculations from different algorithms in lung phantoms irradiated by Co-60 typically (such as shown in Figure 22-4) show variations between algorithms much smaller than the error that results from not performing heterogeneity corrections with densities obtained from CT. At low energies, corrections for lung can alter the homogeneous dose by relative amounts comparable to attenuation due to wedges. A partial exception to this is lung corrections for very small field sizes from high energy beams. In this case the correction factor can be less than unity <u>inside</u> <u>lung</u>, which means that failing to make the standard heterogeneity corrections would be worse than none at all, however, the dose on the <u>distal</u> <u>side</u> of the lung is elevated by a significant amount and all algorithms yield similar correction factors (this is illustrated in Figure 22-5). It should not be sufficient for oncologists to correct "in their head" for lung corrections just as it is unacceptable for them to approximate monitor set calculations. This is especially true for non-coplanar fields because the extent of the 3-D volume is more difficult to visualize.

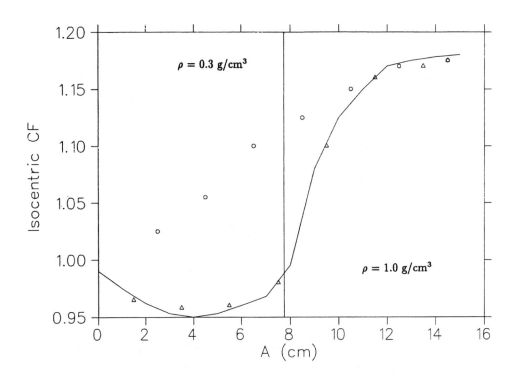

Figure 22-5. *Comparison of measurement and two dose computation algorithms to obtain the isocentric correction factor (TMR in a heterogeneous medium normalized to the TMR in a unit-density medium) along the central axis for a small high-energy field. The measuring probe was kept constant at 100 cm from the source and the thickness of overlying material was a constant 15.5 cm. The parameter A is the distance from the first cork interface to the probe. The field size was 5 x 5 cm and the beam energy was 15 MV. In this situation lateral electronic equilibrium is not established inside the cork heterogeneity along the central axis. The convolution/superposition result (triangles) agrees well with measurement inside and distal to the cork. The equivalent TAR method (open circles) is incorrect inside lung but is accurate distal to lung when lateral electronic equilibrium is established.*

Patient surface corrections can often be viewed as a specific type of heterogeneity correction wherein tissue is replaced by air outside the patient. The type of tissue heterogeneity correction method to be discussed next, differential scatter methods, will illustrate this principle more clearly.

Differential Scatter Methods

The differential scatter-air ratio (dSAR) method of Beaudoin and Cunningham (Beaudoin 1968, Cunningham 1972) was well ahead of its time. It can be viewed as a further generalization of the procedures discussed already for irregular fields and patient contours. The method performed 3-D scatter integration and took into account tissue heterogeneities by:

1. ray-tracing along the primary path, as shown by the vector labeled $\vec{r}' - \vec{r}'_o$ in Figure 22-6, to account for the perturbation of the transport of primary photons,

2. ray-tracing between the photon scatter site and the dose deposition site as shown by the vector $\vec{r} - \vec{r}'$ to account for the perturbation of the transport of scattered photons,

3. weighting the differential TAR at the photon scatter site by the relative electron density $\rho_e(\vec{r}') / \rho_e^{H_2O}$ at the primary interaction site.

Using an integral formulation, the differential scatter method is given by:

$$CF = \frac{\frac{1}{2\pi}\int \frac{\rho_e(\vec{r}')}{\rho_e^{H_2O}} \frac{\Psi_{r',\phi'}}{\Psi_0} \frac{d^2 TAR(|\vec{r}'-\vec{r}_0'|,r')}{drdd} e-(\overline{\mu}-\mu_0^{H_2O})|\vec{r}'-\vec{r}_0'|e-(\overline{\mu}_1-\mu_1^{H_2O})|\vec{r}-\vec{r}'|dr'\,d\phi'\,dd'}{TAR(d,W)}$$

(6)

where $\dfrac{d^2 TAR(d,r)}{drdd}$ is the doubly differential TAR that is computed from the differential TAR with respect to radius as follows:

$$\frac{d^2 TAR(d,r)}{drdd} = \frac{\dfrac{dTAR(d,r)}{dr} - \dfrac{dTAR(d-dd,r)}{dr}}{\Delta d}|\Delta d \to 0$$

(7)

The method was impractical to implement without modern fast computers and unnecessary because the extent of the tumor volume and its precise geometric relationship with respect to neighboring sensitive tissues or the patient's surface could not be ascertained from two-dimensional radiographic techniques.

O'Connors theorem states that the dose in a low density homogeneous phantom should be the same as the dose in a unit density phantom if all of the distances are scaled with respect to density such that the product of $\rho \cdot r$ is invariant. Sontag (1979) showed that the differential scatter method does not satisfy this principle.

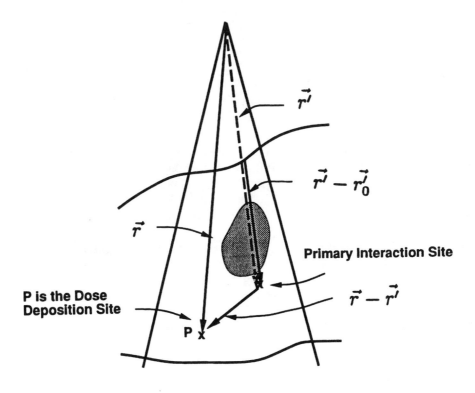

Figure 22-6. *A vector representation of the beam geometry of the primary ray-trace path and the ray-trace path between the site of the primary photon interaction and the dose deposition site labeled P.*

With the three-dimensional anatomy revealed by computer tomography (CT) in the late 1970's, there was renewed interest in fully 3-D dose algorithms. The equivalent TAR (EqTAR) method developed by Sontag and Cunningham accounted somewhat for the lateral perturbation of scatter transport that was not being accounted for by the dSAR method. The method guaranteed, in the limit of a homogeneous but non-unit density medium, that O'Connors theorem would apply by scaling the depth and the beam radius with the electron density.

The correction factor for the EqTAR method is given by:

$$CF = \frac{TAR(\bar{d}, \bar{r})}{TAR(d, W)}$$

(8)

where $\bar{d}$ is the radiological depth to the calculation point which is equal to the product of the depth and the average electron density relative to water along a ray to the calculation point. The effective beam radius $\bar{r}$ which is found from the product of the equivalent beam radius r' and an effective electron density:

$$\bar{r} = r' \cdot \bar{\varepsilon}$$

(9)

where the effective electron density is given by:

$$\bar{\varepsilon} = \frac{\int W(\vec{r}') \frac{\rho_e(\vec{r}')}{\rho_e^{H_2O}} d^3\vec{r}'}{\int W(\vec{r}') d^3\vec{r}'}$$

(10)

$W(i,j,k)$ is a position dependent factor which weights the contribution of the voxels to the effective electron density. The weighting factor distribution is ill-defined. Cunningham (1982) said that "there is no unique or correct set of weighting factors." He also stated that the weighting factor distribution is not spatially invariant.

When the EqTAR method was developed computer systems were fast enough to compute the primary dose contribution but not able to compute full 3-D scatter integration and heterogeneity corrections in a timely fashion. The method estimated the scatter from off-axis slices coalesced together into an effective slice, thus enabling dose planning throughout a volume to be possible (Sontag and Cunningham 1978). This "2 1/2 dimension" algorithm proves to be somewhat clumsy to implement for non-coplanar fields.

The delta-volume (DV) method (Wong and Henkelman 1983, Wong and Purdy 1990) was a direct descendent of the dSAR and EqTAR methods and differentiates between first and multiple photon scatter.

With the advent of fast inexpensive workstations, in the late 1980's, it is now possible to quickly visualize beam positioning of non-coplanar fields and for the first time to compute dose in 3-D taking into account tissue heterogeneity as accurately as possible.

Model-Based Dose Computation

The major operational difference between correction-based and model-based computations is that the goal of the latter is to compute the dose from first principles rather than correcting parametrized dose distributions obtained in a water phantom. Model-based methods still require some data to set up the model, and in some cases data which is not easy to measure. For example, the photon energy spectrum from a linear accelerator is difficult to measure because the flux used to treat patients would saturate particle counting systems and lowering the beam current will perturb the spectrum enough to render it unrepresentative of the treatment beam. The spectra of photon beams have been determined by transporting photons through representations of clinical accelerators using Monte Carlo simulation (Mohan et al. 1985). Fortunately, the dose distribution is not very sensitive to the energy spectrum because the mass attenuation coefficient is not rapidly varying with energy in the megavoltage range and so the spectrum need not be determined with great accuracy. In general, there is a smaller set of measurements in water required to set up the model-based methods. The distinction will be clearer after two model-based algorithms, the convolution/superposition method and the Monte Carlo method, are discussed.

The Convolution/Superposition Method

The convolution/superposition methods (Mackie et al. 1985, Boyer and Mok 1986, Mohan et al. 1986, Ahnesjö 1989) compute the dose from first principles and use a database usually derived from Monte Carlo simulation (Mackie et al. 1988, Mackie 1990). The method first computes the distribution of terma[2] in the patient due to photons generated in the accelerator. The accelerator-generated terma includes contributions from primary photons issuing from the target and scattered photons mainly produced in the field flattening filter and primary collimator (Jaffray et al. 1993) but it does not include scattered photons generated in the patient. This terma distribution is then convolved with a kernel, derived from Monte Carlo simulation, that accounts for the transport of charged particles as well as scattered photons.

(1) Convolution Kernels

Convolution energy deposition kernels describe the distribution of dose about a single primary photon interaction site. The convolution kernels are most often obtained by using the Monte Carlo method to interact monoenergetic primary photons at a single point in a phantom and to transport the charged particles and scattered and secondary photons that are set in motion. The energy that gets deposited about the primary photon interaction site is tabulated and stored for use in the convolution method. Figure 22-7 illustrates convolution kernels computed with the Monte Carlo method for water, bone, and lead at Co-60 (1.25 MeV) and 20 MeV energies (Papanikolaou, 1994).

In addition to describing how scattered photons contribute to dose absorbed at some distance away from the interaction site of primary photons, the convolution kernels take into account charged particle transport. This information can be used to compute dose in electronic disequilibrium situations such as occurs in the buildup region and in the beam penumbra.

(2) Modeling the Energy Fluence Incident on the Patient

Much of the computational burden and detail in the convolution/superposition method involves computing the energy fluence distribution incident on the patient. A linear accelerator is a very complex device producing a wide distribution of photon energies and directions. Any model of its output has to compromise between accuracy and complexity. A model will be presented here which will suffice to compute the energy fluence to within a few percent in a 3-D volume in times well under a minute on 20 MIPS workstations (e.g., a DECstation-5000).

---

[2] Terma which is "total energy released per unit mass," is a measure of the amount of photon energy interacting in matter per unit mass. For a monoenergetic beam it is the product of the mass energy attenuation coefficient and the energy fluence.

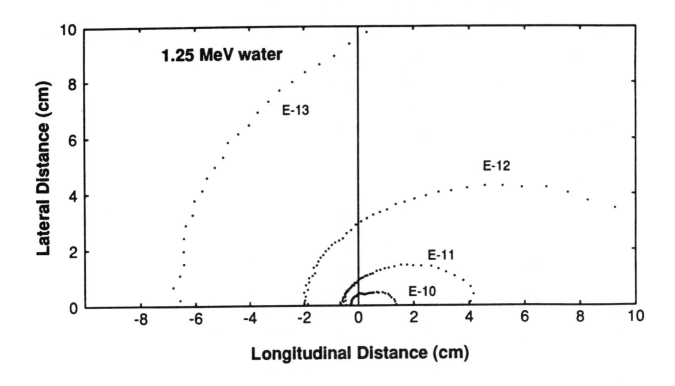

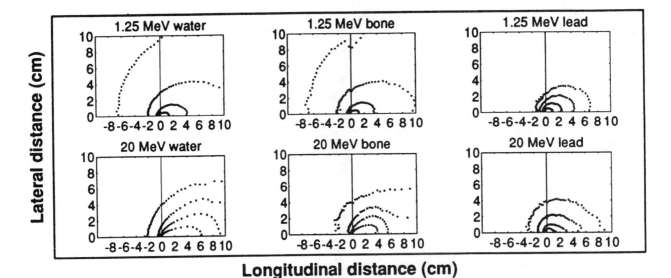

Figure 22-7. *An illustration of convolution kernels computed using the EGS4 Monte Carlo method. The upper panel is a kernel for water at 1.25 MeV. The lower panel contains kernels for water, bone, and lead at 1.25 MeV and 20 MeV. The kernels are more compact for dense, high-atomic number materials and more forward directed at high energies. The kernel isovalues in the lower panel, for all of the kernels, are the same as the upper panel; namely, 10^{-10}, 10^{-11}, 10^{-12}, and 10^{-13} in concentric lines with lower values at greater distances from the origin. The units of the kernels in both panels are $cGy/(MeV \cdot photon)$.*

The modeling begins before the beam interacts with the patient by computing the distribution of primary energy fluence $\Psi_0(\vec{r}_0)$ being emitted from the accelerator for the largest possible field size (typically 40 cm x 40 cm). This is not straightforward because, strictly speaking, energy fluence is not a measurable quantity. However, the energy fluence may be inferred from measured dose profiles in a water phantom by iterative deconvolution techniques (Chui and Mohan 1988). When this is done the primary energy fluence distribution has prominent "horns" away from the central axis as shown in Figure 22-8a.

Blocks can be taken into account by "masking" the primary energy fluence distribution such that outside the blocks the energy fluence has been reduced by the amount of attenuation produced by the tray used to fix the blocks in the beam and the amount of energy fluence underneath the blocks is reduced by the block transmission factor. This operation is shown in Figure 22-8b for an asymmetric field.

As schematically shown in Figure 22-8c the photon scatter produced in the upper collimator system, sometimes called "extrafocal" radiation, is also responsible for much of the scatter outside of the field and the variation in the machine output with field size at smaller field sizes. The scatter outside the field arises because the extrafocal source of radiation is closer to the isocenter than the target and so the collimator jaws do not completely shadow this source of radiation. Conversely, inside the field at small field sizes, the collimator jaws partially shadow the extrafocal radiation sources and increasing the collimator size increases the flux of scatter photons exiting the accelerator. A comprehensive model of extrafocal radiation would add scatter dose outside the field and under blocks as well as account for the machine-generated component of the output factor.

Figure 22-8c shows a Gaussian model of the extrafocal scatter radiation (the magnitude of which is exaggerated for illustration purposes). The central axis height of the Gaussian distribution is here set equal to the machine-generated component of the output factor[3] which will be discussed further in the next section.

Figure 22-8d illustrates the blurring of the incident energy fluence at the edge of the blocks and the collimator jaws because of the finite source size. The blurring is due to direct primary radiation from the finite-sized electron beam striking the target and photons scattered in the upper treatment head from the field flattening filter and primary collimators. The finite source of target-generated primary photons can be modeled by convolving the energy fluence distribution with an aperture function that represents the source distribution. Jaffray et al. (1993), using image reconstruction technology to map the source spot, have shown that the aperture function can be represented by a Gaussian distribution of a few millimeters width but this does not account for photons scattered high in the accelerator treatment head.

The beam filtration provided by compensators may be accounted for using exponential attenuation if the attenuation includes the effects of beam hardening. This approach may also be used to take wedges into account. Alternatively, the energy fluence profile for individual wedges could be dealt with as if they were separate photon beams in which case the deconvolution procedures described earlier would have to be done to establish the energy fluence distribution for the maximum possible wedged field size (typically less than 20 cm x 20 cm at the isocenter).

---

[3] This is in distinction to the phantom-generated component of the output factor which is well characterized by the convolution method.

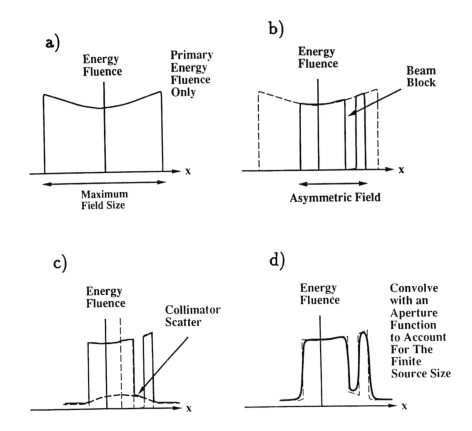

Figure 22-8. *Calculation of the energy fluence incident on the patient. a) illustrates the beam horns evident in the open field primary photon energy fluence profile. b) illustrates the effect of beam blocks on modulating the primary energy fluence for an asymmetric field. c) illustrates modeling the extrafocal radiation as a broad Gaussian distribution (the height of the distribution is exaggerated). This results in more energy fluence outside the field and underneath blocks. d) illustrates a blurring operation to account for the finite source size.*

(3) Computing the Terma Distribution in the Patient

Once the energy fluence distribution incident on the patient is known. It is ray-traced on divergent lines from the source through the patient representation taking into account inverse-square falloff, exponential attenuation and beam hardening. Referring to Figure 22-6), the terma in the patient is given by the following equation:

$$T(\vec{r} - \vec{r_0}) = \frac{|\vec{r_0}|^2}{|\vec{r}|^2} \int_0^{h\upsilon max} \frac{d\Psi(h\upsilon, \vec{r_0})}{dh\upsilon} \frac{\mu}{\rho}(h\upsilon) e^{-\int_{\vec{r_0}}^{\vec{r}} \frac{\mu}{\rho}(h\upsilon)\rho(\vec{r}-\vec{r_0})d|\vec{r}-\vec{r_0}|} \, dh\upsilon \tag{11}$$

where $\vec{r_0}$ is the distance vector to the point at which the energy fluence spectrum $\dfrac{d\Psi(h\upsilon, \vec{r_0})}{dh\upsilon}$ is referenced. The above energy integral can be computed in advance by summing over discrete energy bins. Most of the depth dependence can be removed by defining an effective mass attenuation coefficient $\frac{\mu_{eff}}{\rho}(\vec{r} - \vec{r}_0)$ which is computed from the relative change of terma with respect to distance in the phantom:

$$\frac{T(\vec{r} - \vec{r}_0)}{T(\vec{r} - \vec{r}_0 + \vec{\Delta r})} = e^{-\frac{\mu_{eff}}{\rho}(\vec{r} - \vec{r}_0)\rho(\vec{r} - \vec{r}_0)|\vec{\Delta r}|}$$

(12)

The above equation includes a dependence of the effective mass attenuation coefficient on position in the phantom. This dependence is due to hardening of the beam with depth (Papanikolaou et al. 1993) and "softening" of the beam as a function of angular displacement from the central axis (Mohan et al. 1985).

Since the source of extrafocal scatter radiation is mainly the primary collimator or field flattening filter, the inverse-square fall-off for this component should be downstream of the target. However, since the extrafocal contribution is only a few percent, originating the fall-off at the target for the entire energy fluence distribution causes little error.

(4) Convolving the Terma with the Kernel to Compute the Dose Distribution

In a homogeneous phantom, the kernel even for a polyenergetic beam is nearly spatially invariant. In this case, a convolution integral describes summing up contributions from homogeneous voxels in the phantom that intersects the beam as follows:

$$D(\vec{r}) = \int \frac{\mu}{\rho} \Psi(\vec{r}') A(\vec{r} - \vec{r}') dM$$

(13)

The convolution equation accounts for patient contours, including beam exit contours, irregular fields, and fields with non-uniform beam intensity. It <u>does not</u> take into account tissue heterogeneities. Papanikolaou et al. (1993) showed that kernel invariance due to beam hardening is a small effect that can be simply accounted for.

(5) Computing the Dose in Fourier Space

For homogeneous phantoms the convolution can be done more quickly in Fourier space (Boyer and Mok 1986). The convolution equation described by Eqn. 13 can be expressed in Fourier space if the kernel is spatially invariant:

$$F(D) = F(T) \times F(A)$$

(14)

The transformation to Fourier space can be done quickly using fast Fourier transforms (FFT). For example, for a phantom with 64^3 voxels the FFT-based convolution is about 600 times faster (Field and Battista 1987, Battista and Sharpe 1992) than a convolution approach where the contribution of scatter from all 64^3 primary photon interaction sites is spread to all 64^3 dose deposition sites. This comparison is misleading because the resolution in dose deposition at great distances need not be the same as at short distances. Real-space convolution can take advantage of the property whereas FFT-based methods cannot.

Fourier-based calculations are more difficult for heterogeneous phantoms and the more accurate (Wong and Purdy 1990) "superposition" approach, to be discussed next, keeps the calculation in real-space and density scales the kernel based on the radiological pathlength of the secondary radiation.

(6) The Superposition Method

In addition to performing heterogeneity corrections of the primary and scatter components, the superposition method is capable of accounting for electronic disequilibrium. This method is based on ray-tracing between primary photon interaction sites and dose deposition sites in addition to ray-tracing the path of primary photons. The kernel values are then indexed with respect to the radiological pathlength between these sites. The superposition equation is given by:

$$D(\vec{r}) = \int \frac{\mu}{\rho} \Psi(\rho_{\vec{r}'} \cdot \vec{r}') A(\rho_{\vec{r}-\vec{r}'} \cdot \vec{r} - \vec{r}') dM$$

(15)

where $\rho_{\vec{r}-\vec{r}'} \cdot \vec{r} - \vec{r}'$ is the radiological distance from the dose deposition site to the primary photon interaction site and $\rho_{\vec{r}'} \cdot \vec{r}'$ is the radiological distance to the photon interaction site from the source.

There are ways in which the superposition method can be sped up (Ahnesjö 1989, Mackie et al. 1990) so that these calculations are nearly as fast as Fourier-based methods. The kernel energy can be spread along rays emanating from the primary dose deposition site or converging toward a dose deposition site. The angular spacing can be quite coarse and yet achieve adequate accuracy, the radial spacing can become coarse at greater distance, calculations need only be done when the terma is varying, and ray trace calculations can be "reused" for many overlapping paths between different interaction and dose deposition sites.

Figure 22-9 illustrates a comparison of calculations and measurements from the fast 3-D superposition algorithm in a simulated "thorax phantom" which has been CT scanned and entered into a 3-D radiotherapy planning system. A 6 MV beam is entering the phantom normally which consists of Solid Water (RMI, Middleton WI) slabs sandwiching an acrylic phantom with two 5 cm high x 15 cm long x 4.5 cm thick cork inserts that have an average density of 0.22 g/cm^3 ($\pm$0.03 g/cm^3). The charged particles, in cork, are streaming out of the field which causes the isodose lines inside cork to be distorted due to lack of electronic equilibrium (Mackie et al. 1985b).

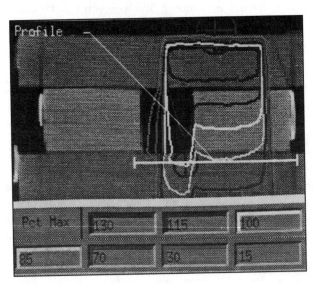
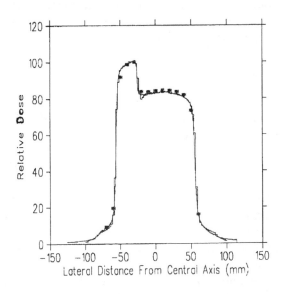

Figure 22-9. *The top figure is an axial view of the measurement phantom as imaged by a Siemens HiQ CT scanner and the bottom is a comparison of calculated dose profiles (histogram) and Kodak XV film (line) and 0.6 cc ion chamber (□) profiles under the distal end of the cork as marked by the line on the transverse image. The isocenter is marked by a circled cross at the surface of the phantom. A circled cross along the line underneath the cork marks the dose normalization point.*

Dose Optimization using Solutions to the Inverse Problem

Computational hardware is available which can rapidly perform solutions to the inverse problem of radiotherapy optimization. The convolution/superposition method offers a mathematical representation amenable to expressing dose optimization using solutions to the inverse problem (Webb 1993). Brahme (1988) used iterative deconvolution to predict the ideal beam pattern to produce an arbitrarily-shaped uniform dose distribution. Other methods use iterative filtered backprojection (Bortfeld et al. 1990, Holmes et al. 1991) and also employ the convolution/superposition method for the dose algorithm. Some solution strategies employ simulated annealing which involves a time-consuming stochastic search to find the optimal beam delivery (Webb 1989, 1991, 1992, Mohan et al. 1992). The inverse methods predict that conformal dose delivery can be obtained using non-uniform dose compensated beams. In general, the solution becomes "more optimal" with the increase in the number of beams (Webb 1992). The incorporation of biological "objective functions" into inverse planning algorithms is ongoing (Kallman et al. 1992, Mohan et al. 1992) and early results from these algorithms suggest that uniform dose prescriptions may not be optimal in all cases.

Delivery methodologies which can produce the highly modulated beams, suggested by these optimization methods, have been proposed. Convery and Rosenbloom (1992) and Galvin et al. (1992) detailed different ways that multileaved collimator could be made to provide compensation for fixed fields. Mackie et al. (1992, 1993) and Carol et al. (1993) have suggested using temporally-modulated set of multileaf collimators modulating a fan beam. Mackie et al. (1992, 1993) further suggested that the fan beams be delivered in a spiral pattern from a ring gantry much like that of spiral CT and that tomographic verification be integral with this delivery methodology that they have named "tomotherapy."

Modeling Radiotherapy Delivery and Verification

Dynamic dose delivery, discussed in the last section, requires real-time treatment verification. It is only possible to quantitatively verify beam dosimetry, in distinction to beam geometry, if the energy deposited in the portal verification system can be determined. Beam modulation systems produce more collimator scatter for a given primary beam intensity than open fields. Unlike wedge dosimetry, the beam intensity from a compensator or multileaf collimator are difficult to uniquely measure in advance because of the vast number of possible shapes and configurations.

The effect of beam modulation on dose to the patient (i.e. the beam output) and modeling the energy deposited in an imaging system requires "extending the phantom" from just outside the patient boundary as represented by CT to include the beam modulation system and the verification system. This will, in effect, elevate 3-D treatment planning to a computer simulation of the planning, delivery and verification process.

Figures 22-10 and 22-11 illustrate measurements and calculation of dose in extended phantoms using the convolution/superposition method. In Figure 22-10, 6 MV photons irradiate a 6 cm thick solid water partial attenuation block that has been placed at the block tray position of a Varian Clinac 2100C. The scatter to the phantom from the partial attenuation block is included in the calculation. The agreement was within 3%. In Figure 22-11 the megavoltage portal dose under a thorax phantom irradiated by a 6 MV beam is measured and calculated using the superposition/ convolution method. The calculated results for a 20 cm x 20 cm field is shown separated into total and scatter dose.

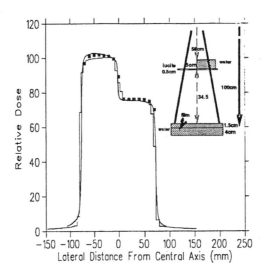

Figure 22-10. *Comparison of measured and computed dose in an extended phantom consisting of a partial attenuator placed on the block tray of a clinical accelerator and a plastic water phantom. The dose to the phantom was calculated (histogram) using the convolution/superposition method and measured with Kodak XV film (line) and a Victoreen 0.6 cc ion chamber (□).*

There are currently limitations to the use of the convolution/superposition method for simulating the radiotherapy process. The method does not presently include computations in media containing differing atomic compositions although efforts are underway to overcome this limitation (Sauer 1990, Papanikolaou 1994). In effect, the method has to be transformed into a cavity theory before accurate computational dosimetry is possible. The superposition/convolution method also does not exactly predict the perturbation in dose in disequilibrium situations because the method implicitly assumes that all secondary particles travel in straight lines from primary photon interaction sites whereas only the first scattered photon contribution does so. Currently, only the Monte Carlo method is able to compute the dose to high accuracy taking into account differing atomic numbers and non-linear transport of secondary particles.

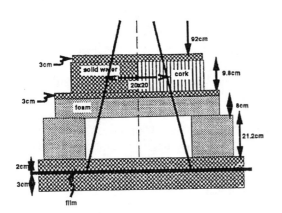

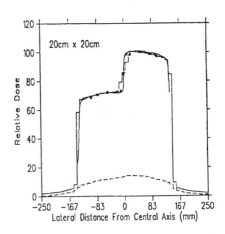

Figure 22-11. *Comparison of measured and computed dose for an extended phantom consisting of a thorax phantom and an "tissue-equivalent" imaging system placed distal to the phantom. Measured dose to film (solid continuous line) and an ion chamber (□) are obtained between solid water slabs to simulate a tissue-equivalent imaging system. The dashed line is the computed scatter dose.*

Monte Carlo Simulation

Direct Monte Carlo simulation of electron beam radiotherapy is currently fast enough to be useful clinically (Neuenschwander et al. 1995). However, photon beam dose distributions would currently require about one order of magnitude more computation time to simulate. For example, to compute the dose to 2% accuracy using the EGS4 Monte Carlo code for resolutions of 0.5 cm in a 10 cm x 10 cm field irradiating a 20 cm thick patient will require about 1 day on a 20 MIPS computer (e.g., DECstation-5000) if the electron secondary production and cut-off total energy is 800 keV. This time could be reduced by at least a factor of 10 using a number of variance reduction techniques (Mackie 1990, Rogers and Bielajew 1990) including:

- systematic sampling, which would interact primary photons relatively uniformly in the patient,

- splitting which increases the number of histories, at reduced statistical weight, where the information is more important (e.g., near the target volume and its neighboring sensitive tissues) and roulette which tends to reduce the number of histories through less interesting regions.

- correlated sampling which is most effective when used to compute a difference or a ratio (such as a heterogeneity correction factor).

There are several situations where Monte Carlo simulation may compete with analytic calculations. Only the Monte Carlo method is capable of computing the dose accurately near interfaces of very dissimilar atomic number materials, as for example, near metal prostheses. The method may be nearly as quick as analytic calculations for calculating multiple beam irradiation. This is because calculation times for analytic algorithms scale with number of beams, whereas for Monte Carlo simulation, the accuracy depends only on the number of histories through a region of interest, not where they were directed from.

Monte Carlo simulation of linear accelerators have already provided invaluable information about the energy and angular distribution of photon beams (Petti et al. 1983, Mohan et al. 1985). Much more effort is needed to understand the effect of beam modifiers and multileaf collimators.

The price/performance ratio of computer workstations have been decreasing by a factor of 2 to 3 each year in the late 1980's and early 1990's, and if this continues then the photon beam Monte Carlo simulation will be a practical alternative for radiotherapy dose computation by the year 2000.

Monitor Set Calculations

The calculations to determine the monitor units to deliver a given treatment for model-based algorithms can be different than traditional algorithms. Both the convolution/superposition and Monte Carlo methods can compute absolute dose to the patient per incident energy fluence. In order to do monitor set calculations the dose per monitor unit (MU) is required.

For a photon beam, the computed distribution of dose per energy fluence must be multiplied by the energy fluence at a reference point per unit MU to convert to dose per MU:

$$\frac{D}{MU}(\bar{r}, h\upsilon, W) = \frac{D}{\Psi}(\bar{r}, h\upsilon, W)\left[\frac{\Psi}{MU}(h\upsilon, W)\right]_{ref} \tag{16}$$

The reference energy fluence per MU is determined by a ratio of measurement to computation for the same reference conditions. The reference dose per MU, at a variety of field sizes, is first determined by measuring the dose in a phantom at a reference depth and distance from the source. The measurement includes both scatter in the phantom and accelerator-generated scatter. The dose per energy fluence is then computed at the same field sizes in a simulated phantom (same electron density and density) at the same reference depth, distance from the source as the measured phantom. The computation properly takes into account the increase in scatter dose in the phantom as the field size increases. The reference energy fluence per MU is then given by:

$$\left[\frac{\Psi}{MU}(h\upsilon, W) \right]_{ref} = \frac{[D/MU(h\upsilon, W)]_{ref}^{measured}}{[D/\Psi(h\upsilon, W)]_{ref}^{computed}}$$

(17)

The reference energy fluence per MU describes the machine-generated output of the accelerator. It differs from a traditional collimator scatter factor (Khan 1984) because it doesn't rely on a measurement of dose in a miniphantom or an equilibrium buildup cap in an attempt to remove the phantom scatter and it is not defined in relation to a reference field size but is an absolute quantity that depends on field size.

Discussion and Conclusions

All 3-D photon dose computation algorithms rely on measured beam data and radiation transport models to some extent. Correction-based models require significant labor to acquire sufficient beam data and are inherently accurate in conditions closely approximating the water phantom measurements. Many clinical situations are vastly different from the beam and geometry conditions as measured and so the magnitude of the corrections may be significantly different from unity.

Model-based algorithms require less measured data to set up the model, and may not replicate water phantom data as faithfully, but are more accurate than correction-based algorithms for complex clinical situations. They are also more amenable to describing optimization using the inverse treatment planning and the delivery and verification process. It is likely that convolution/superposition methods will come to dominate in dose calculation algorithms for 3-D treatment planning systems. Monte Carlo simulation will become increasingly useful for specialized dosimetric situations when they are nearly as accurate as measurement dosimetry and require comparable investment in time when compared with clinical measurements.

Acknowledgments

Fruitful discussions with Timothy Holmes, Cameron Sanders, Mark Gehring, and David Rogers are gratefully acknowledged. Funding was provided by NCI grant R01 CA48902 and R01 CA52692.

References

1. Ahnesjö A. (1989) Med. Phys. **16**, 577.

2. Battista J J and Sharpe M B. (1992) Aust. Phys. Eng. Sci. Med. **15**, 159.

3. Beaudoin L. (M.Sc. Thesis, University of Toronto, 1968).

4. Bortfeld Th, Bürkelbach J, Boesecke R, Schlegel W. (1990) Phys. Med. Biol. **35**, 1423.

5. Boyer A L and Mok E C. (1986) Med. Phys. **13**, 503.

6. Brahme A. (1988) Radiotherapy and Oncol **12**, 129.

7. BJR Supplement 17. (1983) (British Institute of Radiology, London).

8. Carol M, Targovnik H, Smith D, and Cahill D. (1992) Int. J. Radiat. Oncol. Biol. Phys. **24**, 158 (abstract).

9. Chui C-S and Mohan R. (1988) Med. Phys. **15**, 138.

10. Convery D J and Rosenbloom M E. (1992) Phys. Med. Biol. **37**, 1359.

11. Cunningham J R. (1972) Phys. Med. Biol. **7**, 45.

12. Cunningham J R. (1982) *"Tissue inhomogeneity corrections in photon-beam treatment planning"* In: *Progress in Medical Physics Volume 1,* Orton C.G. Ed., (Plenum, New York).

13. Field G C and Battista J J. (1987) Proceedings of the IXth International Conference on Computers in Radiation Therapy, Den Haag, The Netherlands, Elsevier p103.

14. Galvin J M, Chen X-G, and Smith R M. (1992) Int. J. Radiat. Oncol. Biol. Phys. **24**, 159 (abstract).

15. Holmes T, Mackie T R, Simpkin D, and Reckwerdt P. (1991) Int J. Radiat. Oncol. Biol. Phys. **20**, 859.

16. Jaffray D A, Battista J J, Fenster A, and Munro P. (1993) Med. Phys. **20**, 1417.

17. Johns H E, and Cunningham J R. (1993) *"The Physics of Radiology",* 4th ed., (Springfield Ill., C.C. Thomas).

18. Källman P, Lind B K, and Brahme A. (1992) Phys. Med. Biol. **37**, 871.

19. Khan F M. (1984) *"The Physics of Radiation Therapy",* (Williams and Wilkens, Baltimore MD).

20. Mackie T R, Scrimger J W and Battista J J. (1985) Med. Phys. **12**, 188.

21. Mackie T R, Reckwerdt P J, Gehring M A, Holmes T W, Kubsad S S, Thomadsell B R, Sanders C A, Paliwal B R, and Kinsella T J. (1990) Proceedings of the Tenth International Conference on the The Use of Computers in Radiation Therapy, Lucknow India, 322.

22. Mackie T R, Holmes T W, Reckwerdt P J, Swerdloff S, Paliwal B R, and Kinsella T J. (1992) Proceedings of the Third International Conference on Time, Dose and Fractionation, Madison WI, 300.

23. Mohan R, Chui C, and Lidofsky L. (1986) Med. Phys. **13**, 64.

24. Mohan R, Mageras G S, Baldwin B, Brewster L J, and Kutcher G J. (1992) Med. Phys. **19**, 933.

25. Neuenschwander H, Mackie T R, Reckwerdt P J. (1995) Phys. Med. Biol. **40**, 543.

26. Papanikolaou N, Mackie T R, Meger-Wells C, Gehring M, and Reckwerdt P. (1993) Med. Phys. **20**, 1327.

27. Papanikolaou N. (1994) Ph.D. Thesis (University of Wisconsin).

28. Petti P L, Goodman M S, Gabriel T A, and Mohan R. (1983) Med. Phys. **10**, 18.

29. Rogers DWO and Bielajew A F. (1990) *"Monte Carlo techniques of electron and photon transport for radiation dosimetry"* In: *The Dosimetry of Ionizing Radiation, Vol. III.* Kase K.R., Bjärngard B.E. and Attix F.H. Edu (Academic Press, San Diego.).

30. Sauer O A. (1990) Proceedings of the Tenth International Conference on the The Use of Computers in Radiation Therapy, Lucknow India, 329.

31. Sontag M R and Cunningham J R. (1978) Radiology **129**, 787.

32. Sontag M R (1979) Ph.D. Thesis (University of Toronto).

33. Thomadsen B R. (1989) Ph.D. Thesis (University of Wisconsin).

34. Webb S. (1989) Phys. Med. Biol. **34**, 1349.

35. Webb S. (1991) Phys. Med. Biol. **36**, 1227.

36. Webb S. (1992) Phys. Med. Biol. **37**, 1689.

37. Webb S. (1993) *The Physics of Three-Dimensional Radiation Therapy* (Institute of Physics Publishing, Bristol).

38. Wong J W, Henkelman R M, Andrew J W, Van Dyk J, and Johns H E (1981) Med. Phys. **8**,783.

39. Wong J W and Henkelman R M. (1982) Med. Phys. **9**, 521.

40. Wong J W and Purdy J A. (1990) Med. Phys. **17**, 807.

Chapter 23

Multileaf Collimation for 3-D Conformal Radiotherapy

Arthur L. Boyer, Ph.D., Thomas R. Bortfeld, Ph.D.***
Darren L. Kahler, Ph.D., Timothy J. Waldron, B.S.*

*Dept of Radiation Physics, The University of Texas, M. D. Anderson Cancer Center, Houston, Texas
**Deutsches Krebsforschungszentrum, Forschungsschwerpunkt Radiologische Diagnostik und Therapie, Im Neuenheimer Feld 280, Heidelberg, Germany

Conformal therapy is being investigated as a means of improving the efficacy of external beam radiotherapy. The aim of this technique is to produce a dose distribution that is adequately uniform in the tumor target, and at the same time spares normal tissue from unacceptable levels of complication. If this goal can be realized, it is hypothesized that in certain situations one may be able to escalate the tumor-targeted dose to levels that allow increased local control. This escalation would theoretically be pursued to the dose limit imposed by the normal tissue stroma within the target volume. Because the proposed schemes are complex, requiring multiple shaped fields, perhaps delivered at noncoplanar angles, the use of computer-controlled treatment machines is generally assumed (14, 15, 23,25).

Automated field shaping devices have been considered for many years as a means of improving radiotherapy delivery. In order to carry out field shaping for conformal therapy, multileaf collimators (MLCs) are being developed and implemented by the major manufacturers of medical linear accelerators. Takahashi (22) and Morita and Takahashi (18) have studied the use of the MLC for rotational conformal therapy. Computer control of an MLC is assumed to be essential for the multiple-leaf devices under development (20). Computer-controlled conformal therapy has been under investigation for four decades in England (4, 5, 10, 11). The concept has also been studied at the Joint Center for Radiation Therapy (JCRT) at the Harvard Medical School (13, 17), and, more recently, by Leavitt (16).

It now appears that the dose distributions delivered by multiple field irradiation techniques can be dramatically improved by modulating the in-field intensity of the individual fields (1, 4, 7, 12). The concept of in-field intensity modulation through the motion of an MLC was first introduced by Brahme (7). Källman et al. developed an algorithm to compute the irradiation density required to produce an arbitrary dose distribution. The intent was to realize the irradiation density by means of MLC-modulated beams (12). Model calculations that were performed for treatment volumes of both simple and clinically characteristic geometries were found to reproduce well the desired dose distributions.

Most recently, Convery and Rosenbloom have introduced an algorithm that calculates the MLC leaf motions necessary to produce an intensity-modulated field by dynamic collimation (8). The algorithm was developed to produce an arbitrary intensity profile by employing a continuous unidirectional sweep of the independently controlled MLC leaves while delivering the dose at a constant rate. However, as with the algorithm of Källman et al., the precision with which a given distribution was intended to be produced was not considered. Neither Convery and Rosenbloom, nor Källman have demonstrated the calculated distributions experimentally.

We have introduced an algorithm (3) that computes the MLC leaf movements necessary to produce an arbitrary distribution of dose. In contrast to the dynamic technique implemented by Convery and Rosenbloom, the present technique is similar to that proposed by Webb, in which the MLC leaves are moved through the delivery sequence in a series of discrete steps (24). The difference between our approach and that of Webb, however, is that many more steps are employed to generate the distribution, and a constant number of MUs are delivered at each step. It is assumed that one of the advantages of this technique, as compared to the dynamic technique, is that the MLC leaf positions are more easily controlled and verified than is continuous motion. An optimization technique is employed that allows the user to specify the precision with which the distribution is to be generated and that minimizes the total number of MUs required to produce the distribution for the selected precision. The leaf positions computed by the algorithm were used to perform experimental measurements of beam profiles and "beam's-eye-view" dose distributions obtained for 6-MV photons for several different cases.

Methods and Materials

Calculation of optimal fluence profiles

Calculation of the fluence modulation profiles is based on contours of the target and the organs at risk, as well as the patient's surface. For the present study the contour data was taken from an existing prostate treatment plan obtained from a 3-D treatment planning system developed at the M.D. Anderson Cancer Center (21). The prostate case was chosen for its clinical significance and because adequate dose conformation is difficult to achieve with conventional therapy techniques due to the concave shape of the target volume and the vicinity of the bladder and the rectum (see color Plate 19). The contours were entered into an optimization program that was developed at the German Cancer Research Center. This program is described previously in detail (1, 2). The program calculates the modulation profiles that minimize the least-square deviation of the 3-D dose distribution from a prescribed dose in the target, while allowing for thresholds to be set on the dose values in the organs at risk.

The coordinate systems used to describe this procedure are as defined by Siddon (19). Let (x,y,z) be the components of a vector in a coordinate system that is fixed in the treatment room (fixed system) with the z-axis pointing upward, the y-axis pointing toward the linear accelerator and the origin placed at isocenter (see Figure 23-1). (x',y',z') will denote the components of the same vector in the gantry system, that is derived from the fixed system by a rotation about the y-axis so that the z axis points toward the radiation source. Finally we let (x",y",z") denote the components of the vector in a fan-line coordinate system, that is derived from the gantry-system by a first order fan-line correction:

$$x" = x' \frac{\text{SAD}}{\text{SAD} - z'}$$

$$y" = y' \frac{\text{SAD}}{\text{SAD} - z'}$$

$$z" = z'$$

Now the entire optimization algorithm is based on fan-line projections and backprojections between dose defined in the three-dimensional (x,y,z) space and fluence defined in a two-dimensional projection space $(\hat{x}, \hat{y})$ defined in "projection planes" (see Figure 23-1) one plane for each treatment beam. The first step is the calculation of an initial estimate of the fluence profiles $\phi_\theta^{(0)} (\hat{x}, \hat{y})$ for beams delivered at discrete angles θ, using the method of projection filtering.

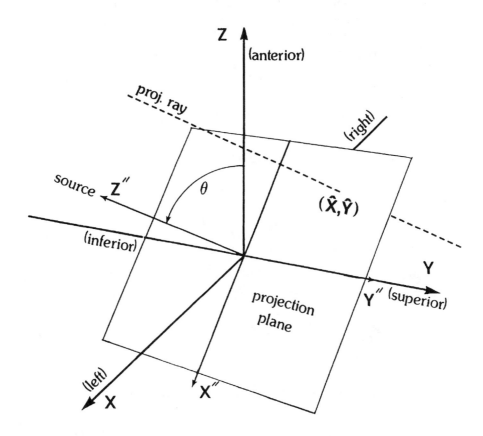

Figure 23-1. *The fixed coordinate system (x,y,z) and the fan-line system (x'',y'',z''). The terms in parentheses refer to orientations in a patient lying in the supine position on the treatment table. The "projection plane" is normal to the axis of rotation of the collimator and contains the axis of rotation of the gantry. A projection line intersects this plane at coordinates* $\hat{x}$ *and* $\hat{y}$.

Projection Filtering. This method applies a filter to the fan-line projections of the prescribed dose distribution $D_p(x,y,z)$. To facilitate the mathematical description, we define projection operators $P_\theta, \tilde{P}_\theta$ and a constraint operator $C+$ as follows.

Let $F(x,y,z)$ be any real-valued function of the coordinates (x,y,z). One may define f_θ, to be the geometric fan-line projection of F under gantry angle θ by the integrals,

$$f_\theta (\hat{x}, \hat{y}) = P_\theta \left\{ F(x,y,z) \right\} = \iiint_V F(x,y,z) \, \delta(\hat{x} - x'', \hat{y} - y'') \, dx \, dy \, dz$$

The use of integrals and delta-functions facilitates the mathematical description of the problem. However, in the implementation of the algorithm, summations over a discrete voxel-grid are used instead of integrations, and the delta-function is replaced by a nearest neighbor sampling function that equals one if the nearest neighbor of (x'',y'') is $(\hat{x}, \hat{y})$, and zero otherwise.

The dose projection $\tilde{f}_\theta$ is obtained by projecting F weighted with the depth dose profile T, so that points that are closer to the source are given a higher weight than are more distant points:

$$\tilde{f}_\theta\,(\hat{x},\hat{y}) = \tilde{P}_\theta\,\{F(x,y,z)\} = \iiint\limits_{v} F\,(x,y,z)\,T\,(x'',y'',z'')\,\delta\,(\hat{x}-x'',\hat{y}-y'')\,dx\,dy\,dz$$

T(x'',y'',z'') is approximated by the product of the tissue-maximum ratio (TMR) and the inverse square factor (ISF):

$$T(x'',y'',z'') = TMR(-z'' + SAD - SSD(x'',y'')) \cdot ISF(z'').$$

Furthermore, we use a positivity constraint operator C^+ defined by

$$C^+\,\{f(\hat{x},\hat{y})\} = \begin{cases} f(\hat{x},\hat{y}) & \text{if } f\,(\hat{x},\hat{y}) > 0 \\ 0 & \text{otherwise.} \end{cases}$$

Using the definitions given above, the method of projection filtering of $D_p(x,y,z)$ can be described mathematically as

$$\Phi_\theta^{(0)}\,(\hat{x},\hat{y}) = C^+\left\{\frac{P_\theta\,\{D_p(x,y,z)\}}{\tilde{P}_\theta\,\{Dp(x,y,z)\}}\,[P_\theta\,\{D_p\,(x,y,z)\} * h(\hat{x})]\right\}$$

where $h(\hat{x})$ is the (one-dimensional) filter function. In the numerical implementation of the algorithm, the filtering is performed by frequency domain multiplication. The frequency domain representation of the filter function is a modified ramp-function (1). The factor $P_\theta\{D_p(x,y,x)\}/\tilde{P}_\theta\{D_p(x,y,z)\}$ is used to partly correct for attenuation. It applies a higher weight to rays that pass through regions of the target with a larger average distance from the source, and vice versa. Thus it compensates for the fact that in general (below the buildup depth) a higher dose is delivered to points that are closer to the source than to more distant points.

Iterative Optimization. After the calculation of the initial guess, we apply an iterative optimization scheme to further improve the dose distribution. For this purpose, we first define the prescribed and tolerance dose distribution $D_{p,u}(x,y,z)$ as

$$D_{p,u}(x,y,z) = \begin{cases} D_p(x,y,z) & \text{if}(x,y,z) \in \text{target} \\ D_u(x,y,z) & \text{if}(x,y,z) \in \text{organ at risk} \\ 0 & \text{otherwise} \end{cases}$$

where D_p is the prescribed dose in the target and D_u is the tolerance dose in organs at risk. The value of D_u will generally be different for different organs at risk, and D_p as well as D_u may even vary within the target and the organs at risk.

Now we calculate the jth dose distribution $D^{(j)}$ resulting from the fluence distribution $\Phi_\theta^{(j)}$ by

$$D^{(j)}(x,y,z) = \sum_\theta \Phi_\theta^{(j)}(x'',y'')\,T(x'',y'',z''),$$

which can be considered as the sum of the dose-weighted backprojections of the $\Phi_\theta^{(j)}$. Thus the dose distribution is approximated by the simplified calculation model that was also used for the projections, i.e. neglection of inhomogeneities and side scatter. Subtraction of the prescribed/tolerance distribution $D_{p,u}$ from the actual distribution $D(j)$ at iteration step j results in the "error"-distribution:

$$\Delta^{(j)}(x, y, z) = D^{(j)}(x, y, z) - D_{p,u}(x, y, z).$$

Some further definitions are necessary before we will be able to write down the iteration scheme explicitly. We define a weighting distribution as

$$S^{(j)}(x, y, z = \begin{cases} 1 & if(x, y, z) \quad \in target \\ r & if(x, y, z) \quad \in \text{organ at risk and } D^{(j)}(x, y, z) \rangle D_u(x, y, z) \\ 0 & otherwise \end{cases}$$

The value of r controls the strength of the constraints in the organs at risk as compared to the objective in the target volume (1). Usually, r is in the range of [1. . . 10]. Again, r may be different for different target volumes. It is important to note that $S(j)(x,y,z)$ is greater than zero only in the target and in those points in the organs at risk where the dose is too high. Finally we need to define $\tilde{P}'_\theta$ another type of projection similar to the dose projection, but where the square of the depth dose at each point is used as a weighting factor. Applying this projection operator to $S(j)(x,y,z)$ yields

$$\tilde{P}'_\theta \left\{ S^{(j)}(x, y, z) \right\} = \iiint_V S^{(j)}(x, y, z) T^2(x'', y'', z'') \delta(\hat{x} - x'', \hat{y} - y'') \, dx \, dy \, dz.$$

Now, with N as the number of beams, we can write the iteration scheme as

$$\Phi_\theta^{(j+1)}(\hat{x}, \hat{y}) = C^+ \left\{ \Phi_\theta^{(j)}(\hat{x}, \hat{y}) - \frac{\tilde{P}_\theta\{\Delta^{(j)}(x, y, z) S^{(j)}(x, y, z)\}}{N \, \tilde{P}_\theta\{S^{(j)}(x, y, z)\}} \right\}$$

This equation basically says that the fluence profile at iteration step j+1 is obtained by subtracting the projection of the product of the error distribution and weighting distribution (numerator of the fraction on the right) from the former fluence profile. Note again that in the organs at risk only those points (x,y,z) are considered where the dose is above the tolerance limit. In other words, the algorithm never tends to increase the dose in an organ at risk to the tolerance level, but it decreases the dose, if it is too high. The term in the denominator merely scales the projection of the error distribution. This improves the convergence of the algorithm considerably, but it is not essential.

The program was run on a MicroVAX 3800 (Digital Equipment Corp.) and on a Sun SPARC 10 (Sun Micro Systems) in less than 15 min. Nine fixed fields were used with gantry angles set at 20° to 340° in steps of 40°. In order to avoid irradiation through the metal bar at the center of the table, the beam incident at 180° was inverted to 0°.

Calculation of the MLC Leaf-setting Sequences

Having planned beam modulations for each of the nine fields, each field area was divided into strips corresponding to the projection of each pair of opposing MLC leaves. The fluence modulation along each strip, $\Phi_\theta^{(j)}(\hat{x})$, was extracted from the iterative back-projection calculation. The argument $\hat{x}$ is the distance from the center of the field in the plane of isocenter, taken along the direction of travel of the leaves. The following section details the steps taken in developing the leaf-setting algorithm.

Interpolation of the Fluence Profile

Generally the desired fluence profile $\Phi^{(j)}\theta(\hat{x}_k)$ is obtained from discrete numerical data where the index k refers to calculation voxels along the projection of a MLC leaf trajectory. The first step is to perform an interpolation of the discrete profile to obtain, in principal, a continuous function of the position, $\Phi(x)$. In this case we assumed linear interpolation to be adequate. Figure 23-2 shows a discrete profile representation and the corresponding continuous profile. Since the fluence is to be delivered through a series of consecutive steps, it is desirable to have a function that is discrete in time (i.e. fluence), rather than in position. To accomplish this, a rebinning of the data is necessary.

Rebinning

In the second step, we want to represent the profile as a function of discrete fluence levels, $\Phi(i)$ from which the inverse, $x(\Phi_i)$, may be calculated. First, we establish the fluence levels as

$$\Phi_i = (i + i_0)\Delta\Phi, \quad i = 0, 1, ...,$$

where $\Delta\Phi$ is a preselected fluence interval (proportional to a MU interval) that determines the achievable resolution. It must be selected so that the dosimetry system being used to control the dose delivery can accurately deliver exposures of the selected size. Note that $\Delta\Phi$ is also the bin width of the discrete fluence (or time) bins. The index, i, labels the fluence level as illustrated on the right-hand axes of Figure 23-3. An offset value, i_0, of 0, 0.5, or 1 can be used to set the fluence levels at the lower, center, or upper boundary of the bins, respectively. We have used an offset of 0.5 in most of our work.

The obvious next step is to determine the intersections of $\Phi(x)$ with the fluence levels, $\Phi(i)$. In general, the desired fluence profile, $\Phi(x)$, is nonmonotonic and intersects each fluence level several times. The calculation of the intersection points yields a pseudoinversion of $\Phi(x)$ in the form

$$x_m(\Phi_i), \quad m = 1, ..., M_i,$$

where *m* denotes the *m*th point of intersection (from left to right), and M_i is the total number of intersection points for a given fluence level Φ_i. If there were positions within which $\partial\Phi/\partial x = 0$ and $\Phi(x) \equiv \Phi_i$, the number of intersection points, M_i, would become infinite. To avoid this, we set the additional constraint that the fluence profile must increase above Φ_i in the vicinity of the intersection points.

The results of the rebinning procedure are illustrated in Figure 23-3. In this example, the number of intersections is $M_i = 2$, for all fluence levels except i=1, for which $M_1 = 4$. The vertical error bars represent the fluence bins, $\Delta\Phi$.

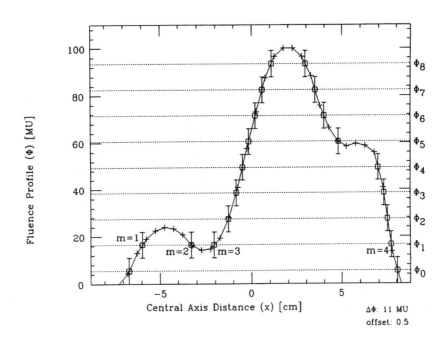

Figure 23-2. *Discrete profile representation (plus signs) and interpolated continuous profile (line). Rebinning is necessary to obtain a relation that is discrete in $\Phi_\theta^{(j)}$. Plus signs indicate original discrete calculated fluence values $\Phi_\theta^{(j)}(x_k)$. The solid line is the interpolated continuous fluence profile. The horizontal dotted lines are drawn at the centers of the fluence intervals of width $\Delta\Phi$. The squares indicate the locations of the points $x_m(\Phi_i)$ found by the rebinning procedure. The error bars indicate the boundaries of the fluence bins.*

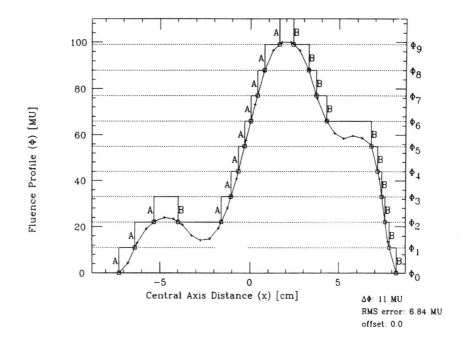

Figure 23-3a.

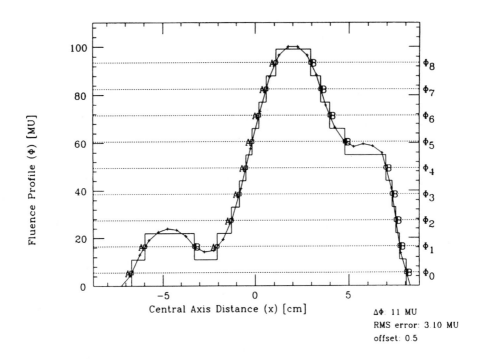

Figure 23-3b.

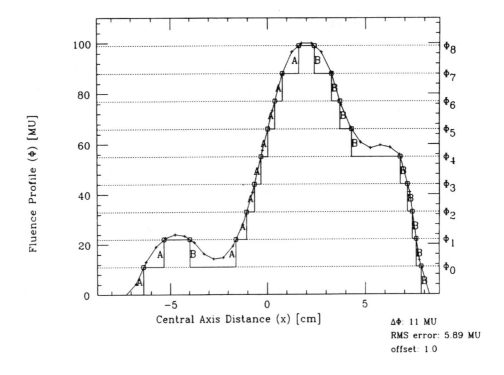

Figure 23-3c.

Figure 23-3.   *A- and B-leaf settings for offset = 0 (a), offset = 0.5 (b), and offset = 1 (c). The solid vertical lines indicate the positions of the leaf ends.*

The total number of intersection points, M, required to represent the whole fluence profile is given by

$$M = \sum_i M_i$$

Thus, besides the obvious proportional dependence of M on the resolution $\Delta\Phi$ and on the maximum number of MUs in the required fluence profile, there is a further dependence on the number of intersections for each level i. The representation of a profile that is oscillating around a mean value will require many more points, M, than a profile that has a broad plateau.

Leaf Positions

Next the positions of the leaves must be determined. An efficient leaf-setting algorithm should not require more steps than are necessary for the representation of the profile at any exposure delivery resolution $\Delta\Phi$. In particular, since at every step two leaves are set, the number of steps required, N, should be equal to M / 2.

The left leaf is labeled as the "A leaf" and the right leaf the "B leaf." We will make the assumption that the beam is totally blocked below the leaves, and we will disregard penumbra. These assumptions cause small errors in the calculated dose, but these will be corrected for later. Under these assumptions we can use a Heaviside step function,

$$H(x) = \begin{cases} 0 & \text{if} \quad x \langle\ 0 \\ 1/2 & \text{if} \quad x = 0 \\ 1 & \text{if} \quad x \rangle\ 0, \end{cases}$$

to describe the fluence profile delivered by a single leaf, A or B. Let Φ_a be the profile resulting from positioning the edge of leaf A at x=a with leaf B retracted completely, and Φ_b be the profile for positioning leaf B at x=b with leaf A retracted, both for the dose delivery increment represented by $\Delta\Phi$. Then Φ_a and Φ_b are given by:

$$\Phi_a = \Delta\Phi H(x - a) \qquad \text{and}$$
$$\Phi_b = \Delta\Phi H(-x + b).$$

If $M_i = 2$, the positioning of the leaves is trivial: leaf A must be set at position $a = x_1(\Phi_i)$ and leaf B at $b = x_2(\Phi_i)$, resulting in the rectangular profile

$$\Phi_{ab}(x) = \Delta\Phi H(x - a)H(-x + b).$$

In the general case ($M_i \geq 2$) the problem is similar to a familiar problem from computer graphics, namely, to fill a region within a contour (7). In our case the region to fill is the one below the profile, where fluence must be delivered. The solution to this problem is to open the beam within x intervals $[x_{m-1}(\Phi_i), x_m(\Phi_i)]$ if and only if m is even. This is achieved by setting the A leaf at positions $x_m(\Phi_i)$ where m is odd and the B leaf at positions where m is even, i.e.

$$\left. \begin{array}{ll} a_{n,i} = x_m(\Phi_i) & \ni m = 2n - 1 \\ b_{n,i} = x_m(\Phi_i) & \ni m = 2n \end{array} \right\} \quad n = 1,...,N_i$$

Here $a_{n,i}$ and $b_{n,i}$ denote the positions of leaf A and B, respectively, and $N_i = M_i/2$. Note, incidentally, that leaf A is always positioned at segments of $\Phi(x)$ for which $\partial\Phi/\partial x$ is positive, and leaf B at segments for which the slope is negative. Note also that the number of steps required to produce the fluence profile beneath the leaf pair is $N = \sum_i N_i = M/2$.

The discrete approximation, $\Phi_\Delta(x)$, of the desired fluence profile is now obtained by summing the rectangular fluence increments $\Phi_{a_{n,i}b_{n,i}}$;

$$\Phi_\Delta(x) = \sum_i \sum_{n-1}^{N_i} \Delta\Phi H(x - a_{n,i}) H(-x + b_{n,i}).$$

Since the maximum deviation between $\Phi(x)$ and $\Phi_\Delta(x)$ is always smaller than $\Delta\Phi$, it is clear that

$$\lim_{\Delta\Phi \to 0} \Phi_\Delta(x) = \Phi(x)$$

Determination of the Leaf-setting trajectories

From the known leaf positions $a_{n,i}$ and $b_{n,i}$, we must now find the leaf trajectories a_j and b_j, i.e. the positions of the leaves as functions of the step number, j, in the sequence of delivery:

$$\left.\begin{array}{c} a_{n,i} \to a_j \\ b_{n,i} \to b_j \end{array}\right\} \quad j = 1, ..., N.$$

Any combination of the known A and B leaf positions (i.e. any transformation F_A: $n,i \to j$ for leaf A and any other transformation F_B: $n,i \to j$ for leaf B) that does not lead to leaf collisions can be used to deliver the required fluence profile. In particular, the "sweep" (8) and "close-in" (12) techniques can be generated. The first is obtained by simply sorting separately the a's and b's by magnitude. Consequently, this technique requires the smallest amount of overall leaf travel.

The "close in" technique is implemented by positioning opposing A and B leaves on opposite sides of a local maximum of the fluence distribution at the same fluence level Φ_i, in other words by forming $a_{n,i} b_{n,i}$ pairs. *These pairs* are then simply sorted so that the a_j's in the resulting a_j b_j sequence are ordered by magnitude. Figure 23-4a and Figure 23-4b show the leaf trajectories for the sweep and close-in methods. In most cases we believe the sweep technique to be the most efficient.

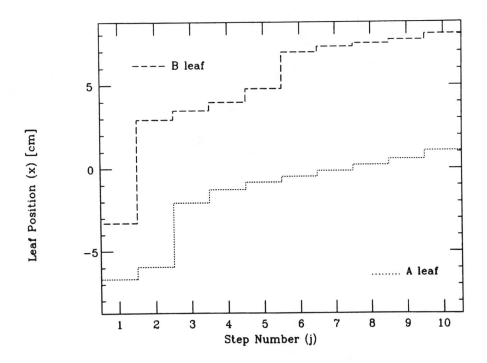

Figure 23-4a.

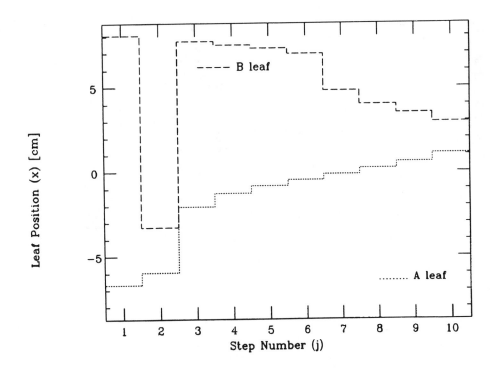

Figure 23-4b.

Figure 23-4.   *Leaf trajectories generated using the sweep technique (a) and the close-in technique (b).*

Error Estimation

These concepts have been implemented in a computer program that allows the calculation of the root-mean-square (RMS) error of the (theoretically) realized fluence with respect to the desired profile. The maximum tolerable RMS error can be entered into the program as a parameter. The algorithm then iterates through the four steps described above, decrementing $\Delta\Phi$ and calculating the error until it falls below the upper limit. For an offset of 0.5 there is a simple approximate relationship between the RMS error and $\Delta\Phi$, namely:

$$\text{RMS error} \approx \frac{\Delta\Phi}{2\sqrt{3}}$$

Figure 23-5a and Figure 23-5b show fluence profiles, $\Phi_\Delta(x)$, with RMS errors of 2 MUs and 5 MUs for two examples.

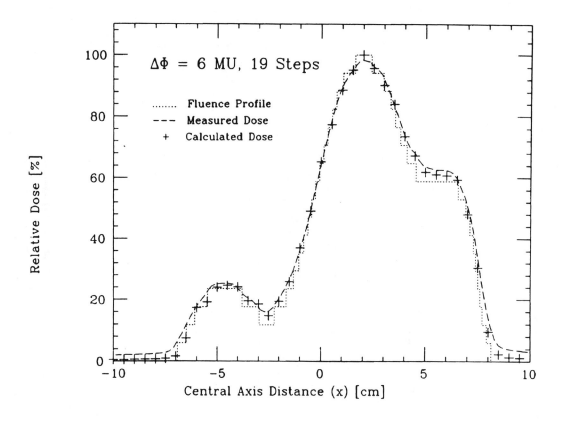

Figure 23-5a.

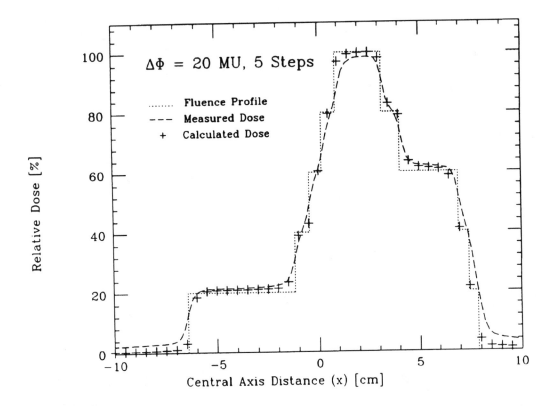

Fig 3-5b.

Figure 23-5.   *Comparison of fluence, measured dose, and calculated dose for the profile from Figure 23-2-through 23-4. The calculated RMS errors were 2 MUs (a) and 5 MUs (b).*

Conversion From Fluence to Dose

The x-ray fluence distributions were converted to dose distributions using an x-ray convolution computer code (22). The MLC-modulated fluence distribution was modeled by five discrete energy components and appropriately attenuated to model a water-equivalent phantom with a planar incident surface. The five energy components were convolved in three dimensions with dose deposition kernels to account for radiation transport effects.

Verification of MLC Leaf Sequence

Film was used to verify the leaf-setting algorithm. We have tested the algorithm both on one-dimensional profiles and on a two-dimensional distribution. Leaf-setting sequences were calculated at two resolutions for the one-dimensional distribution. The dose delivery, however, was simulated using the asymmetric jaws of a medical linear accelerator (Varian Assoc., Clinac 600C, Palo Alto, CA).

The accelerator gantry and collimator were positioned to direct a 6-MV x-ray beam vertically downward on a horizontally oriented film sandwiched at a 1.5-cm depth in a 7.5-cm x 30-cm x 30-cm "solid water" phantom (RMI, Inc., Middleton, WI). A 100-cm source-to-surface distance (SSD) was used in irradiating the film that was protected by a light-tight paper film pack (Eastman Kodak XV-II, Rochester, NY). The asymmetric jaws were set to the positions calculated by the algorithm. The non-asymmetric collimators produced a 20-cm-wide field throughout the experiment.

Irradiations were performed in the accelerator's service mode, and the machine's internal dosimetry system was used to control the MU levels delivered. Five films (four irradiated films and one unirradiated base-fog film) were processed together and analyzed using a PTW/Macbeth (Newburgh, NY) scanning densitometer with a 1-mm-diameter aperture. A base-fog was established by averaging four point density measurements of the unexposed film. Each film was scanned along the axis centered on the irradiated area in 2-mm steps. The resulting density data were converted to values of dose using a density-to-dose conversion calibration based on exposure of calibration films to known doses.

Implementation of a Combined Dose Distribution

The fluence profiles for each of the nine fields calculated by the inverse planning algorithm, described in (3) and above, were implemented using a multileaf collimator (Varian Associates, Mark 0, Palo Alto, CA), that was attached to a medical linear accelerator (Varian Associates, Clinac 2100C, Palo Alto, CA). For each of nine fields, the leaves were moved through a sequence of 20 to 30 different settings.

Phantom Measurement of the Dose Distribution

Dose was measured in a homogeneous polystyrene phantom consisting of 9 slices of 1-cm thickness. The slices were cut to match the contour of the patient for whom the dose was optimized. Three holes of 2mm diameter were drilled into each slice in order to register the slices. The slices were hold together by two lucite rods.

The phantom was assembled with seven films interspersed between polystyrene slices, to measure the dose distribution throughout the entire target volume. Each of the films was protected by a light-tight paper film pack (Eastman Kodak XV-II, Rochester, NY). After the films were assembled in the phantom, three pins were punched through the holes of the polystyrene slices and through the films in order to be able to position the films relative to the phantom later. The pins were then removed and replaced by thin (0.8 mm diameter) steel wires in order to hold the films in their position. The positioning of the phantom was done with the help of the lasers installed in the treatment room.

The phantom was irradiated with the collimator set at an angle such that each slice was covered by one leaf pair. The collimator jaws were set individually for each of the nine fields. The average collimator opening was approximately 8 x 8 cm^2. For each field, i.e. for each gantry angle, dose was delivered in 20 - 30 steps, with one monitor unit delivered at each step.

After irradiation and subsequent film development, the optical density distribution was determined using the densitometer and film scanner described above. The spatial resolution was 3 mm. The film background was determined from an unirradiated film and subtracted from the distribution. The dose distribution was then calculated from the optical density distribution with a precalculated density to dose conversion curve.

Results

The one-dimensional profiles were generated for two different degrees of accuracy: one at a calculated error of 2% RMS, the other at 5% RMS. The first profile tested was taken from a series of profiles used in the optimization of horseshoe-shaped dose distributions (1). A bin width $\Delta\Phi$ of 6 MU and 19 steps had to be used to keep the RMS error below 2%, whereas $\Delta\Phi$ of 20 MU and five steps sufficed for the 5% accuracy. The results are shown in Figure 23-5. In this figure the relative calculated and measured doses, as well as the relative incident fluence, are plotted against the distance from the central axis of the beam.

The relative fluence (plotted as a dotted line) exhibits the original stair-step characteristic created by the discrete MLC leaf positions. The calculated dose, plotted as plus signs, reflects the smoothing out of the fluence as a result of radiation transport and scatter. The fil/m-based measurement of dose, plotted as a dashed line, can be compared with the calculated dose. Agreement between the measurements and the calculations was generally within 1%, with differences as great as 3% appearing mainly at the field margin or just outside the field.

The two-dimensional case was a saddle-shaped profile. It was realized in 34 steps using a $\Delta\Phi$ of 5 MU. The calculated fluence and dose are compared with the measured dose in Figure 23-6. The agreement between the measured and calculated doses is generally better than 2%. Most significant, the effects of the finite steps as well as the finite leaf widths are for the most part smoothed away by radiation transport. The peaks at the edges of the saddles are not as great for the measured dose as for the calculated dose. The reason for this discrepency is not yet clear but may be caused by the failure of the leaf-setting algorithm to take into account details of the output factor that become important for small, narrow fields.

The full three-dimensional capability was tested by the experiment employing the multiple films exposed edge-on in the quasi-anatomical polystyrene phantom. Figure 23-7 shows the copy of a film exposed near the plane containing the central axes of the coplanar beams. Figure 23-8 displays the copies of the six off-axis films, arranged consecutively, from inferior (a,b,c) to superior (d,e,f). The isocenter plane lies at the superior margin of the slice in Figure 23-7 (at the interface with slice d in Figure 23-8), with isocenter positioned at the geometric center of the prostate target volume. Moving through the progression of slices, it can be seen that the high dose region at the center of the prostate moves posterially. In each case, the dose distribution displays the desired region of concavity that conforms to the contour of the anatomy between the rectum and the prostate.

Figure 23-9 shows the isodose curves resulting from the film scans and conversion of optical density to dose superimposed on the anatomical structures. The dashed lines outline the contours of the bladder, the rectum, the left and right pelvis, and the femoral heads. The shading indicates the prostate target volume and the crosses indicate the axis of rotation of the gantry. The isodose values range from 10% to 100% in increments of 10%. The 95% line is also shown. The 100% isodose line occurs only in slice number five, and corresponds to the maximum measured value of 91.1 cGy. The calculated maximum dose is 90.0 cGy. The maximum isodose value occuring in slice d is 70% since this slice lies in the penumbral region of the treatment field.

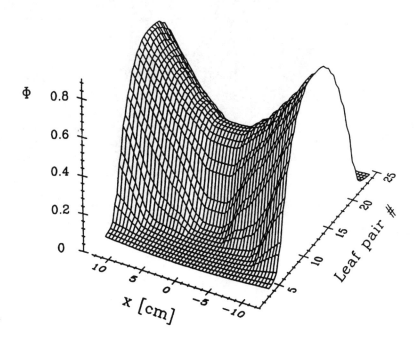

Figure 23-6a.

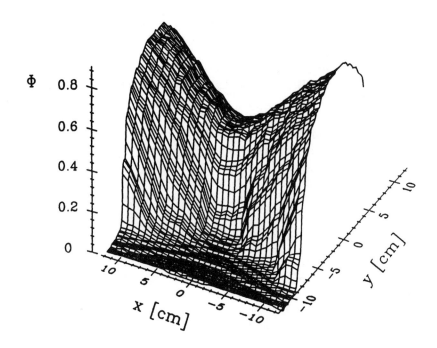

Figure 23-6b.

Figure 23-6. *Comparison of calculated fluence (a) and measured dose (b) for a two-dimensional saddle-shaped profile.*

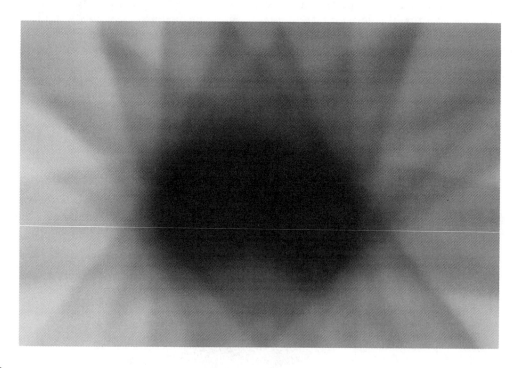

Figure 23-7a.

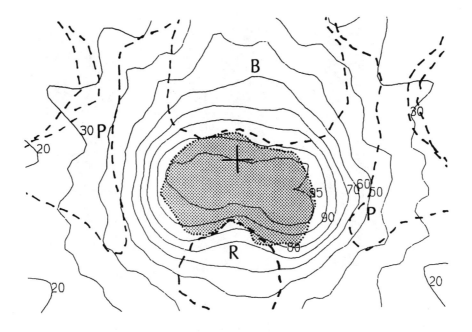

Figure 23-7b.

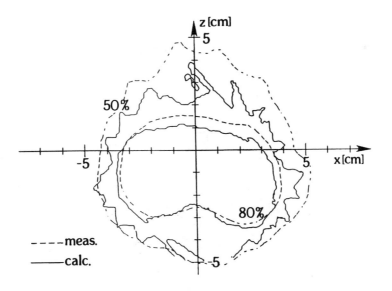

Figure 23-7c.

Figure 23-7. *Results of the full three-dimensional experiment using seven film sheets in a quasi-anatomical polystyrene phantom. Representations of the dose distribution measured by the film in the transverse slice containing isocenter. (a) Copy of the exposed and developed film (negative display). (b) Superposition of the measured isodose distribution onto the anatomy; R, rectum; B, bladder; P, pelvis. Isodose values are in % of the global maximum dose. The dotted area is the target. The cross indicates the isocenter. (c) Comparison of measured and calculated isodose lines (50% and 80%).*

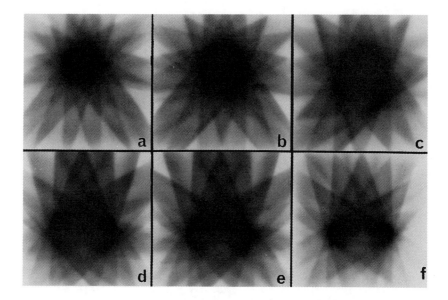

Figure 23-8. *Films exposed superior to and inferior to isocenter (negative display), Top: Inferior at distances -3 cm (a), -2 cm (b), and -1 cm (c) from the isocenter slice. Bottom: Superior at distances 1 cm (d), 2 cm (e), and 3 cm (f) from the isocenter slice.*

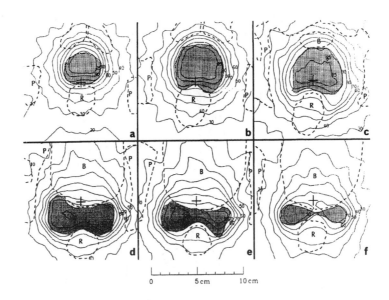

Figure 23-9. *Evaluation of the film scans. Isodose lines superimposed on the anatomy for slices at distances of -3 cm (a), -2 cm (b), -1 cm (c), 1 cm (e), 2 cm (f), and 3 cm (g) from the central slice. Isodose values are plotted in 10% increments from 10% to 100% relative to the largest dose measured globally on all seven films. This maximum dose was found, as prediced, in the slice 1cm superior to the isocenter slice. The 95% isodose line is also shown. The 100% isodose line appears only in slice (d), which contains the dose maximum. Anatomical structures are: R, rectum; B, bladder; and P, pelvis. The target is displayed by the shaded areas. The crosses mark the axis of rotation.*

The highest dose gradient is present within the area between the prostate and rectum corresponding to the concave region appearing in the films. The shape of the high dose region conforms well to the shape of the target volume for all of the slices. However, in some of the slices, there is an apparent shift of up to 4 mm of the isodose lines with respect to the anatomy contours. The observed shift may be due to a combination of five factors: the positioning of the film in the phantom; the positioning of the phantom on the treatment table; the positioning of the film on the film scanner; the coincidence of the lasers with the machine isocenter; and any error in the MLC calibration. However, it is estimated that the error resulting from these factors should be no more than ±2 mm. The reason for the larger discrepancy is not yet quite clear.

Discussion

This work has demonstrated that it is possible to arbitrarily modulate x-ray beams with a MLC using a sequence of discrete leaf settings to deliver a sequence of small dose increments. The effects of the discrete dose delivery can be reduced to arbitrarily small levels by using many leaf steps. However, we have demonstrated that relatively small numbers of steps (on the order of 10 to 30 for fields with widths up to 20 cm) can be used to deliver distributions that exhibit an accuracy of 2-5%.

The advantage of using discrete steps is that the control systems required to deliver doses in this fashion may be much simplier than those required to deliver dose at a controlled and varying rate. Controlling and verifying instantaneous dose rate and leaf motion velocity simultaneously is difficult; controlling the delivery of a sequence of small doses and discrete leaf settings in rapid sucession is a simple extension of existing linear accelerator control.

In Figure 23-5 the dose is reduced to nearly zero in one valley of the beam profile. With this algorithm, it is possible to create points or regions of no dose. As a consequence, it is possible to generate the leaf-setting sequence required to produce internal blocks within a field. The generality of the methodology allows its application to both internal partial blocks and compensators as well as to total protection of portions of the treatment field.

We have demonstrated that modulated beam conformal radiotherapy can be realized in a phantom experiment. The equipment utilized for this purpose was a conventional linear accelerator and a prototype comercial MLC. The actual irradiation time in the experiment was only 34 seconds. For a fractionated treament with 3 Gy delivered at the dose maximum in each fraction, the irradiation time will increase to a little less than 2 minutes. However, the whole process of dose delivery with the method described took several hours, and at the present stage it is consequently not possible to perform patient treatments. The reasons for this extensive delivery time are manifold.

The Varian mark 0 MLC that was used for the intensity modulation is a prototype and it was not designed for this type of treatment. Every step in the leaf setting sequence had to be selected manually, and the dose delivery had to be initialized manually at every step, as well.

A considerable speed-up and reduction of the idle time could be achieved with relatively little effort. It is necessary to use a faster MLC control computer, to increase the velocity of the leaves (which is already realized in newer versions of the MLC), to add a piece of software that allows automatic cycling through a given sequence of leaf settings, and to leave the bending magnet current, electron gun, and microwave production on throughout the entire procedure. It is estimated that with all these improvements, the average leaf setting time for each step in the delivery sequence could easily be reduced to 1 - 4 seconds, resulting in an overall machine setting time for the 225 steps of less than 15 minutes, and an overall treatment time of less than 20 minutes. This is in the order of magnitude of conventional multiple blocked field techniques, where most of the time is required for the personnel to enter the room, change the blocks, and leave the room.

It was demonstrated that the approach proposed here allows for a very precise conformation of the shape of the high dose region to the target volume. In particular, concave regions in the target volume can be matched accurately. The superposition of the measured dose distribution and the patient's anatomy shows an apparent shift of 3 mm - 4 mm within some of the transverse slices. The reason for this discrepency is not quite clear yet. The statistical positioning error was estimated to be only about ±2 mm. One problem that partially causes such a shift lies in the fact that the thickness of the leaves (1 cm) was two times as large as the thickness of the CT-slices. In other words, each leaf pair covered two CT slices. Now, since the shape of the target varies from one CT slice to the other, the optimization algorithm has to find a compromise that satisfies the objectives and the constraints in both of the slices covered. Obviously, this compromise is not in general optimal for either of the slices, and that is one possible explanation for the lateral shifts. It is interesting to note that these are real 3-D problems; they don't occur, if the problem is simplified to a 2-D slice-by slice geometry, as it is done in many other investigations.

It is anticipated that, with the development of appropriate control software by accelerator vendors, this technique could be applied to conventional compensators as well as to field modulation for conformal therapy. The methodology can be applied to create effective missing-tissue compensators or compensators for internal heterogeneities for single fields. Nevertheless, its potential to provide a practical means of delivering optimized conformal therapy is the technique most interesting for future application.

Acknowledgments

This investigation was supported in part by PHS grant number CA43840 awarded by the National Cancer Institute, DHHS and grant 15-091 awarded by the Advanced Technology Program for the Texas Higher Education Coordinating Board.

References

1. Bortfeld, T.; Bürkelbach, J; Boesecke, R.; Schlegel, W. Methods of image reconstruction from projections applied to conformation radiotherapy. Phys. Med. Biol. 35:1423-1434;1990.

2. Bortfeld, T.; Bürkelbach, J; Schlegel, W. Three-dimensional solution of the inverse problem in conformation radiotherapy. In: Advanced Radiation Therapy Tumor Response Monitoring and Treatment Planning, Breit (ed.). Berlin Heidelberg: Springer-Verlag, 0000-0000;1992.

3. Bortfeld, T.R.; Kahler, D.L.; Waldron, T.J., Boyer, A.L. X-ray field compensation with multileaf collimators. Int. J. Radiat. Oncol. Biol. Phys. (in press);1994.

4. Boyer, A.L.; Desobry, G.E.; Wells, N.H. Potential and limitations of invariant kernel conformal therapy. Med. Phys. 18(4):703-712;1991.

5. Brace, J.A.; Davy, J.G.; Skeggs, D.B.L. Computer-controlled cobalt unit for radiotherapy. Med. & Biol. Eng. & Comput. 19:612-616;1981.

6. Brace, J.A.; Davy, J.G.; Skeggs, D.B.L.; Williams, H.S. Conformation therapy at the royal free hospital. A progress report on the tracking cobalt project. Br. J. Radiol. 54:1068-1074;1981.

7. Brahme, A. Optimization of stationary and moving beam radiation therapy techniques. Radiother. Oncol. 12:129-140;1988.

8. Convery, D.J.; Rosenbloom, M.E. The generation of intensity-modulated fields for conformal radiotherapy by dynamic collimation. Phys. Med. Biol. 37(6):1359-1374; 1992.

9. Foley, J.D.; Van Dam, A. Fundamentals of interactive computer graphics. Reading, MA: Addison-Wesley; 1982.

10. Green, A. Tracking cobalt project. Nature 207:1311;1946.

11. Jennings, W.A. The tracking cobalt project: from moving-beam therapy to three-dimensional programmed irradiation. In:Orton, C.G., ed. Progress in medical radiation physics, Vol. 2. New York:Plenum Press;1985;1-44.

12. Källman, P.; Lind, B.; Eklöf, A.; Brahme, A. Shaping of arbitrary dose distributions by dynamic multileaf collimation. Phys. Med. Biol. 33(11):1291-1300;1988.

13. Kijewski, P.K.; Chin L.M.; Bjarngard B.E. Wedge-shaped dose distributions by computer-controlled collimator motion. Med Phys 5:5;1978.

14. Lane, R.G.; Loyd, M.D.; Chow, C.H.; Ekwelundu, E.; Rosen, I.I. Improved dose homogeneity in the head and neck using computer controlled radiation therapy. Int. J. Radiat. Oncol. Biol. Phys. 19:1531-1538;1990.

15. Lane, R.G.; Loyd, M.D.; Chow, C.H.; Ekwelundu, E.; Rosen, I.I. Custom beam profiles in computer-controlled radiation therapy. Int. J. Radiat. Oncol. Biol. Phys. 22:167-174;1992.

16. Leavitt, D.D.; Martin, M.; Moeller, J.H.; Lee, W.L. Dynamic wedge field techniques through computer-controlled collimator motion and dose delivery. Med. Phys. 17 (1):87-91;1990.

17. Levene, M.B.; Kijewski, P.K.; Chin, L.M.; Bengt, S.M.; Bjärngard, B.; Hellman, S. Computer-controlled radiation therapy. Radiology 129:769-775;1978.

18. Morita, K.; Takahashi, S. Rotatory conformation radiotherapy of cancer of larynx. Studies on telecobalt therapy II. Report. Studies on rotatory conformation radiotherapy. III. Report. Nippon Acta Radiol. 21:13;1961.

19. Siddon, R.L. Solution to treatment planning problems using coordinate transformations. Med. Phys. 8(6):766-774;1991.

20. Sofia, J.W. Computer-controlled multileaf collimator for rotational radiation therapy. AJR 133:956-957;1979.

21. Starkschall, G.; Bujnowski, S.W.; Wang, L.L.; Shiu, A.S.; Boyer, A.L.; Desobry, G.E.; Wells, N.H.; Baker, W.L.; Hogstrom, K.R. A full three-dimensional radiotherapy treatment planning system (abstr.). Med. Phys. 18:647;1991.

22. Takahashi, S. Conformation radiotherapy-rotation techniques as applied to radiography and radiotherapy of cancer. Acta Radiol. (Suppl. 242): 1965.

23. Trump, J.G.; Wright, K.A.; Smedal, M.I.; Salzman, F.A. Synchronous field shaping and protection in 2-million-volt rotational therapy. Radiology 76:275-;1961.

24. Webb, S. Optimization by simulated annealing of three-dimensional conformal treatment planning for radiation fields defined by a multileaf collimator. Phys. Med. Biol. 36(9):1201-1226;1991.

25. Wright, K.A.; Proimos, B.S.; Trump, J.G.; Smedal, M.I.; Johns, D.O.; Salzman, F.A. Field shaping and selective protection in megavolt radiation therapy. Radiology 72:101- ;1959.

26. Zhu, Y.; Boyer, A.L. X-ray dose computations in heterogeneous media using 3-dimensional FFT convolution. Phys. Med. Biol. 35: 351-368;1990.

Chapter 24

3-D Electron Beam Dose Algorithms

Kenneth R. Hogstrom, Ph.D.

Dept of Radiation Physics, The University of Texas, M. D. Anderson Cancer Center, Houston, Texas

Electron beam therapy is inherently three dimensional (3-D) in that treatment planning requires not only designing the lateral extent of the treatment field but also determining the energy appropriate to provide the desired penetration of the dose distribution. Therefore, a 3-D treatment planning system that utilizes a 3-D electron beam dose algorithm is clinically desirable.

The purpose of the present paper is to review the present status of 3-D electron beam dose algorithms and their utilization in a 3-D treatment planning system. This is accomplished by first discussing what we expect of a 3-D electron algorithm so as to provide a basis to compare different algorithms. Second, 3-D implementation of the Fermi-Eyges-based Hogstrom algorithm is critically discussed. Third, the other 3-D dose algorithms developed as a result of known inaccuracies in this method are categorized. Fourth, the significance of algorithm verification is emphasized. Finally, clinical applications of 3-D electron beam dose algorithms are presented that demonstrate the utility of this technology.

Expectations of 3-D Algorithms

Electron beam dose algorithms used in 3-D treatment planning systems should be capable of modeling clinical electron beams in 3-D. If the algorithm cannot model the clinical electron beam, then the treatment planning system cannot adequately simulate electron beam therapy. Albeit an obvious requirement, this is often the most serious deficiency in treatment planning computer systems. To comply with the requirement, the dose algorithm should model all beam parameters: (1) treatment machine and beam energy, (2) machine geometry (gantry angle, collimator angle, couch and patient position), (3) arc angle (rotational therapy only), (4) field shape (applicator or trimmer selection, secondary collimator insert, skin collimation), (5) bolus, and (6) monitor units.

Second, 3-D electron dose algorithms should calculate dose to each point considering the entire 3-D anatomy. Dose algorithms can be classified as making a 1-D, 2-D, or 3-D heterogeneity correction, as illustrated in Figure 24-1. In calculating dose to a specific point, the 3-D, heterogeneity-corrected dose algorithm considers the anatomy in three dimensions. In calculating the dose to a specific point within a plane of interest, the 2-D, heterogeneity-corrected dose algorithm considers only the anatomy within the plane. In calculating the dose to a specific point, the 1-D heterogeneity-corrected dose algorithm considers only the anatomy between it and the virtual source.

Third, the accuracy of a 3-D electron dose algorithm, evaluated for 3-D clinical geometries, should be within 5% of the given dose at any dose point lying outside of regions of high dose gradient (e.g. penumbra)[1]. The accuracy refers to 5% of the given dose not 5% of the dose at a point. For example, at a point where the dose is 80% of given dose, the calculated dose should be in the range of 75-85%. Evaluation of the accuracy of the algorithm should be the responsibility of the researchers who develop or study an algorithm, and an algorithm should not be used clinically or marketed until it has been evaluated. On the other hand, it is the medical physicist's responsibility to clinically assess the inaccuracies of dose calculations and to advise the radiation oncologists on their use.

---

[1] Given dose is the maximum central-axis dose in a water phantom positioned at the patient's SSD for the rectangular field that circumscribes the irregular field defined by the insert placed into the electron applicator.

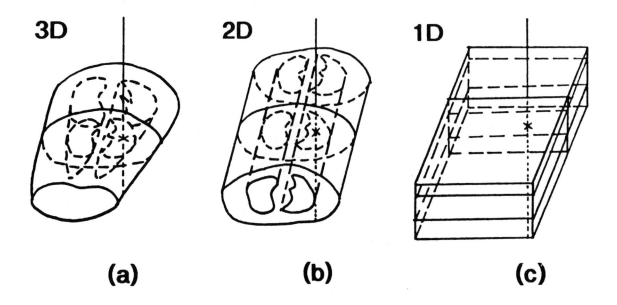

Figure 24-1. *In calculation of dose to an arbitrary point in the dose calculation volume, the anatomy used is (a) the full 3-D anatomy, (b) only anatomy in a 2-D plane, and (c) only the anatomy along a line between the source and the point of calculation, referred to as a 1-D, 2-D, and 3-D heterogeneity-corrected calculation respectively.*

3-D Pencil Beam Dose Algorithm

The 3-D electron pencil-beam dose algorithms whose accuracies have been adequtely evaluated are based on the Eyges pencil-beam theory of Hogstrom et al. (1981). Primarily due to lack of low cost computing power, its original clinical implementation was 2-D (planar dose calculation with a 2-D heterogeneity-correction), as described by Hogstrom et al. (1984) and Hogstrom (1987). As computing power increased in the late 1980's, the algorithm was implemented in 3-D by many investigators (Hogstrom, 1991), being best described by Starkschall et al. (1991).

The concept of the Hogstrom pencil-beam model is illustrated in Figure 24-2. In Figure 24-2a, an arbitrary irregularly shaped field is modeled by a set of pixels, typically 2 mm square at 100 cm SSD. A pencil beam is defined as all electrons passing through a pixel; hence, all pencil beams approximate the irregular field. Figure 24-2b shows a side view of a single pencil beam incident on the patient. The teardrop-shaped dose distribution from a pencil beam is symmetrical about the central axis because of the assumption that the electron fluence can be calculated assuming a slab phantom geometry that is unique for each pencil beam. The dose distribution for every pencil beam is summed to give the broad beam dose distribution in the patient. The strength of the Hogstrom pencil-beam algorithm is its accurate calculation of dose for irregular fields, varying air gaps, and irregular patient surfaces (Hogstrom et al. 1984), the latter two being illustrated in Figures 24-3a and b, respectively. The algorithm's accuracy has been the subject of studies too numerous to discuss or list in this work.

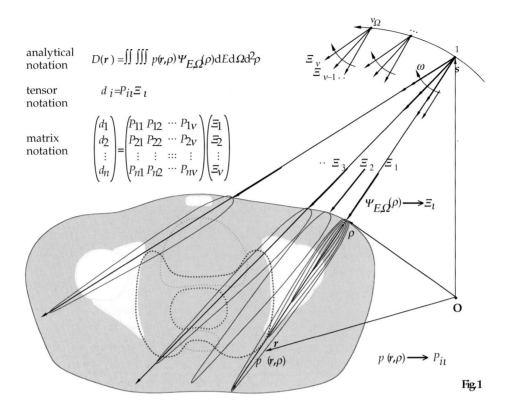

analytical notation

$$D(r) = \iint \iiint p(r,\rho)\Psi_{E,\Omega}(\rho)\,dE\,d\Omega\,d^2\rho$$

tensor notation

$$d_i = P_{il}\Xi_l$$

matrix notation

$$\begin{pmatrix} d_1 \\ d_2 \\ \vdots \\ d_n \end{pmatrix} = \begin{pmatrix} P_{11} & P_{12} & \cdots & P_{1v} \\ P_{21} & P_{22} & \cdots & P_{2v} \\ \vdots & \vdots & \cdots & \vdots \\ P_{n1} & P_{n2} & \cdots & P_{nv} \end{pmatrix} \begin{pmatrix} \Xi_1 \\ \Xi_2 \\ \vdots \\ \Xi_v \end{pmatrix}$$

$$\Psi_{E,\Omega}(\rho) \longrightarrow \Xi_l$$

$$p(r,\rho) \longrightarrow P_{il}$$

Fig.1

Plate 1. The mapping of Ψ through P on D(r) and the basic structure of Eq. (6).

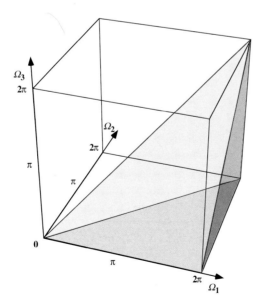

Plate 2. The shaded tetrahedral volume is the actually calculated data set of the cubical volume making up the of the three-dimensional P+ phase space (one sixth of the whole cube).

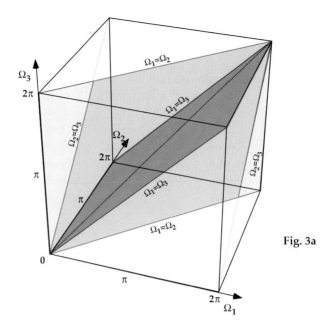

Fig. 3a

Plate 3. The three planes in the three-dimensional P+ phase space representing a reduction of the number of used beam portals from three to two. The line representing a reduction of the number of used beam portals from three to one is located on the spatial diagonal where the three above mentioned planes cross each other.

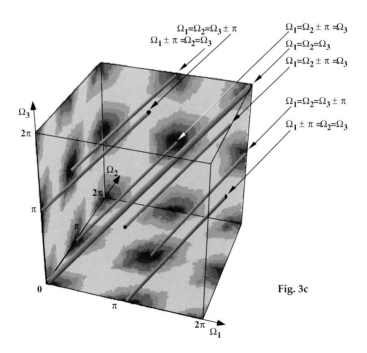

Fig. 3c

Plate 4. The lines in the three-dimensional P+ phase space representing intrinsic low P+ levels. The central thicker line represents a reduction of the number of used beam portals from three to one as previously shown in figure 1 and plate 3. The thinner six lines in the three-dimensional P+ phase space are located where planes representing a reduction of the number of used beam portals from three to two and planes representing parallel opposed beams. Along these lines two parallel opposed beams are used.

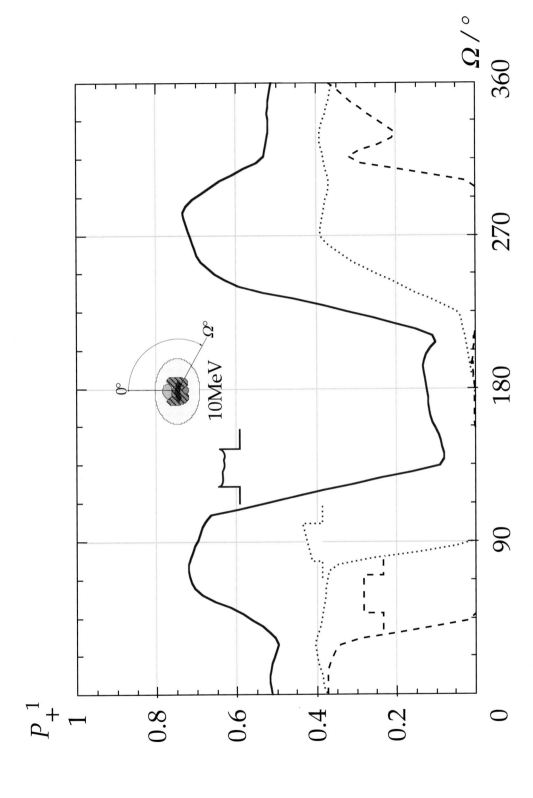

Plate 5. The one-dimensional P+ phase space, $P_{+,\psi}(\Omega)$, for treatment of an advanced cervix cancer with 10MeV monoenergetic photons using different degrees of freedom in the optimized beam profiles. The dashed line shows the result when the dose level of the homogeneous beam is the only free variable. The dotted line shows the result if there are two free variables for each optimized beam profile, the beam weight and the wedge angle. The solid line shows the result if the beam has 64 free variables corresponding to fully non-homogeneous beams.

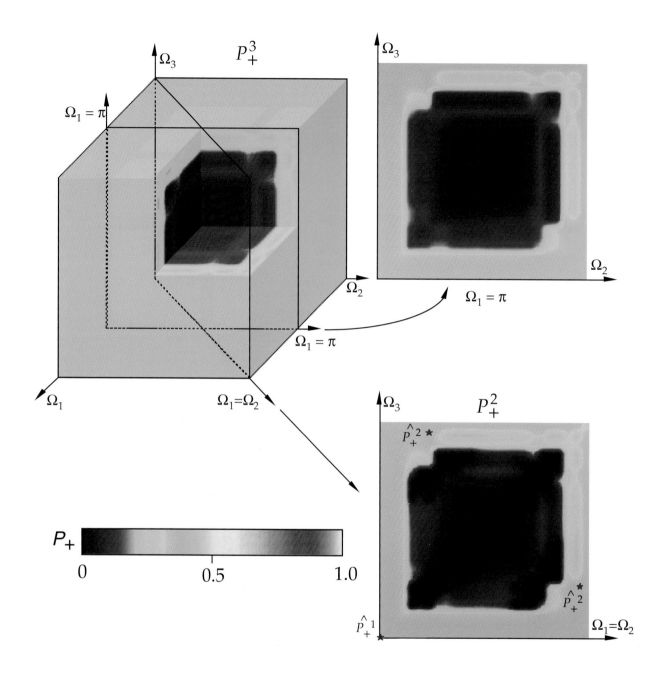

Plate 6. The three-dimensional P3+ phase space for the cervix target using only homogeneous beams. The cubical data set is shown with one corner cut out to show the interior structures. One slice of the cube is also extracted to better show interior structure. To illustrate the properties of the two-dimensional P+ phase space the diagonal plane where W1=W2 have also be extracted from the cube.

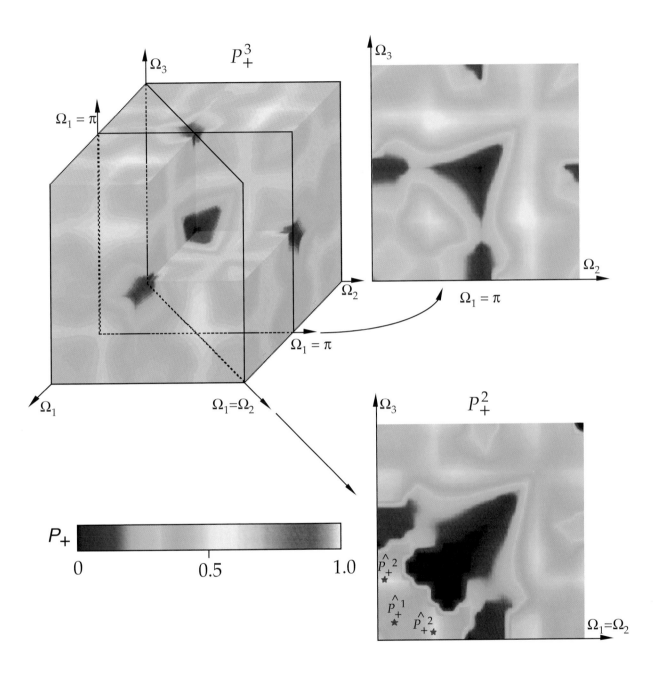

Plate 7. The same three-dimensional P3+ phase space as in plate 6 but for optimized wedged beams.

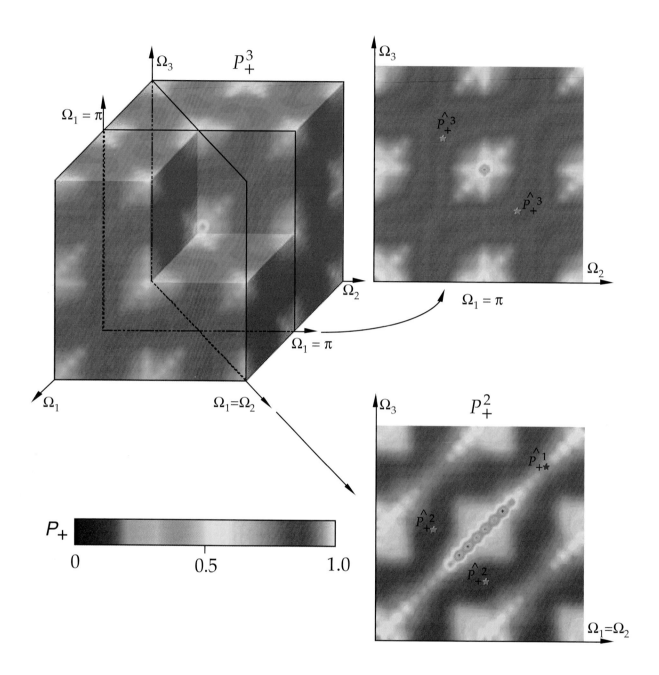

Plate 8. The same three-dimensional P3+ phase space as in plate 6 but for optimized non-homogeneous beams.

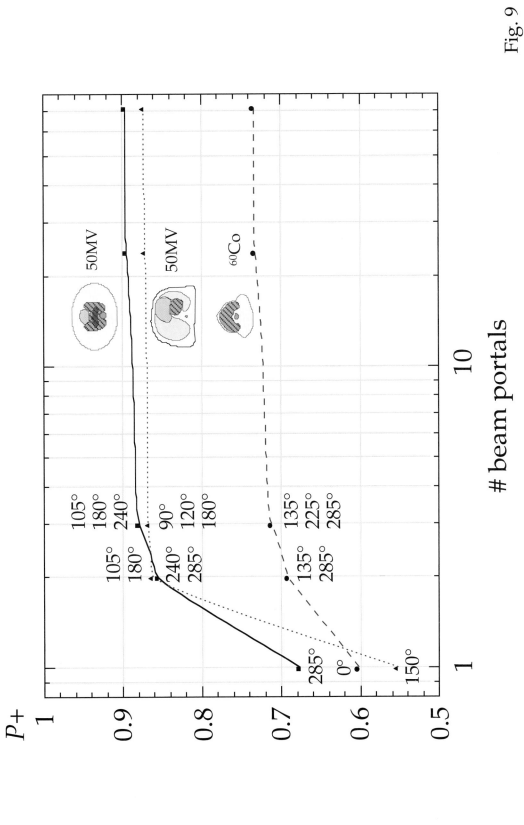

Plate 9. The probability to achieve tumor control without severe complications using increasing number of beams for the treatment of the three different target. The treatments with one, two, and three beam portals are performed using optimal beam entry directions. The 24 and 72 beam treatments are performed using beams equidistant in angle. Solid squares show the results obtained with the cervix target using 50 MV photons. Solid triangles show the result for the thorax target also using 50MV photons. Solid circles show the results for the head and neck target using a 60Co beam.

Fig. 9

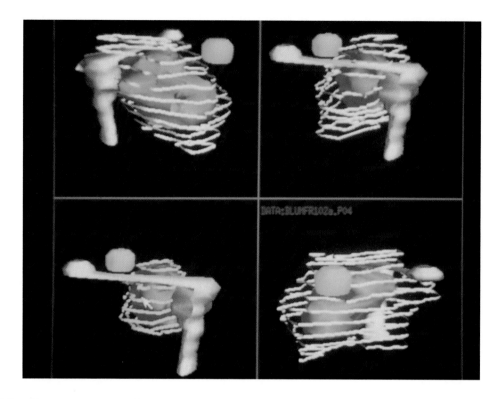

Plate 10. 3D computer visualization of a base of skull target, the organs at risk eyes, optic nerves, brain stem, and the 80, 90, and 50% isodose ribbon surrounding the target.

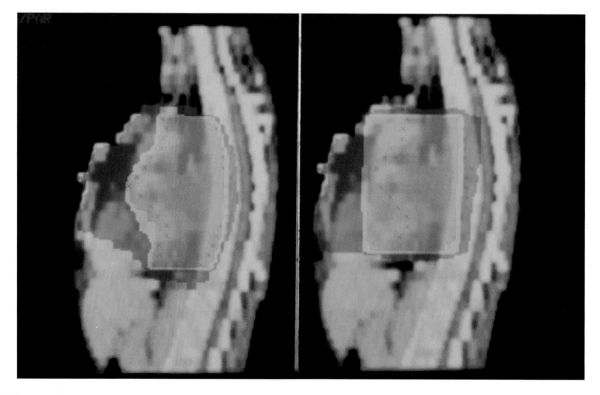

Plate 11. 2D versus 3D planning comparison in a larger mediastinal mass. The paraxial and irregularly formed beams result in an improved protection of the myocard, the lung and the spinal cord.

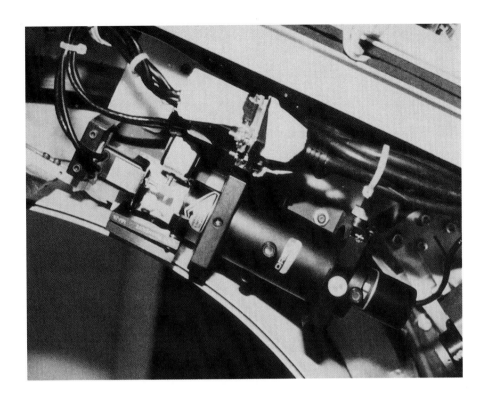

Plate 12. Laser beam portal outline transfer device mounted on the Siemens CT gantry.

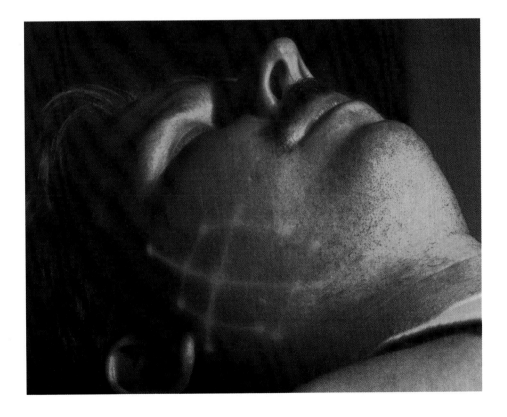

Plate 13. Lateral portal projected on the patient's skin prior to marking.

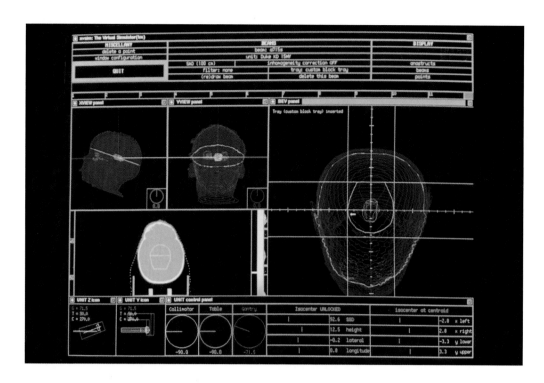

Plate 14. A typical display of the Virtual SimulatorTM. The control panel at the bottom provides the same controls as the hand control of a conventional simulator. The BEV panel serves the same purpose as a physical fluoroscopy display. The two small windows in the lower left show the current machine position. The XVIEW and YVIEW allow visualization of the depth of isocenter.

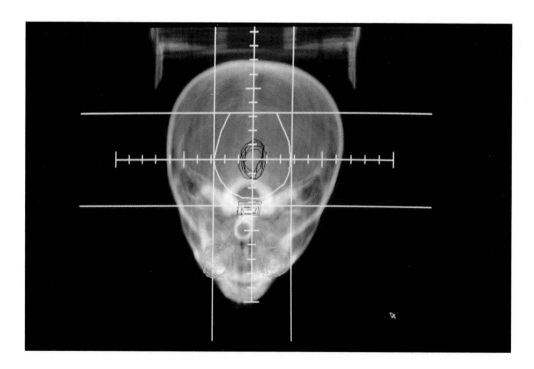

Plate 15. A DRR. This image is computed directly from the beam geometry and the planning CT dataset. It is overlayed with contours drawn on the CT scans, the port outline, the collimator position and axes, and centimeter tick marks. These are printed to film and stored in the patient's film jacket.

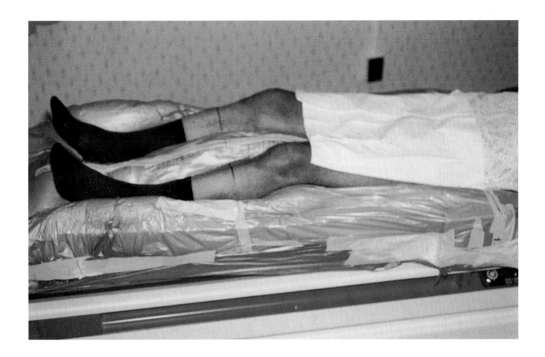

Plate 16. An immobilization cast for a prostate patient. Note the elevation of the knees, discussed in the text. Also of interest are reference marks on the patient's legs just below the knee and corresponding marks on the cast. These registration marks are used as an additional aid in reproducing the patient's position in the cast.

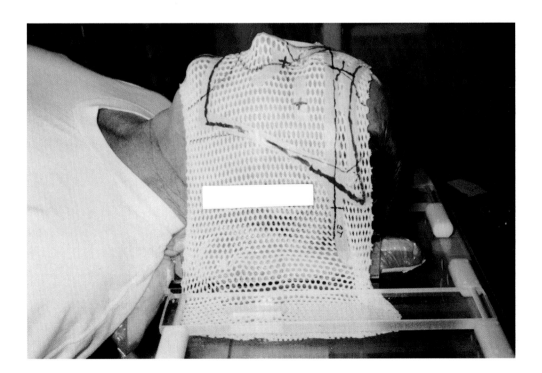

Plate 17. An immobilization cast for a head and neck patient. The custom polyurethane head sponge and thermal plastic mask form a nearly zero-tolerance encasement of the patient's head.

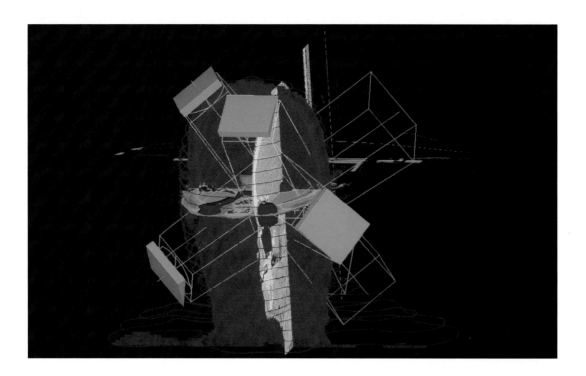

Plate 18. A non-coplanar four field treatment for a tumor of the ear. This kind of unorthodox treatment plan geometry can be planned and delivered with high confidence using the methods described here.

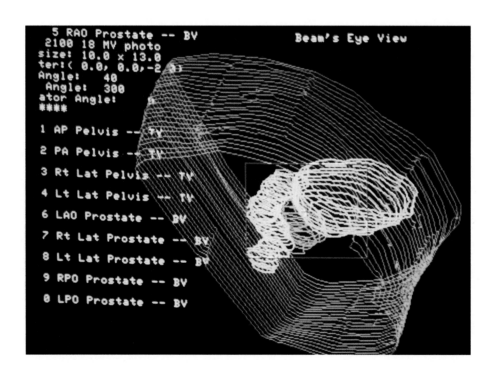

Plate 19. Wire frame display of the target and the organs at risk. The outer skin, prostate, rectum and bladder have been contoured.

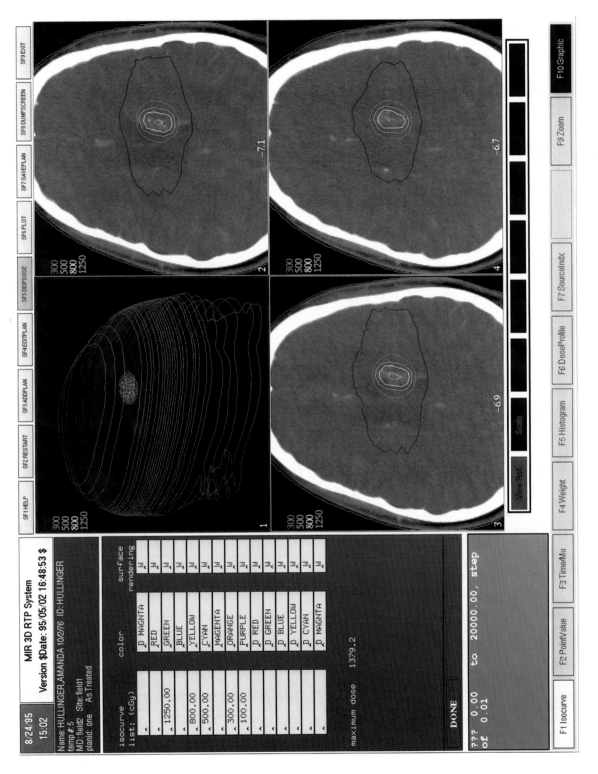

Plate 20. A multiformat window can depict a combination of 2-D and 3-D representations simultaneously.

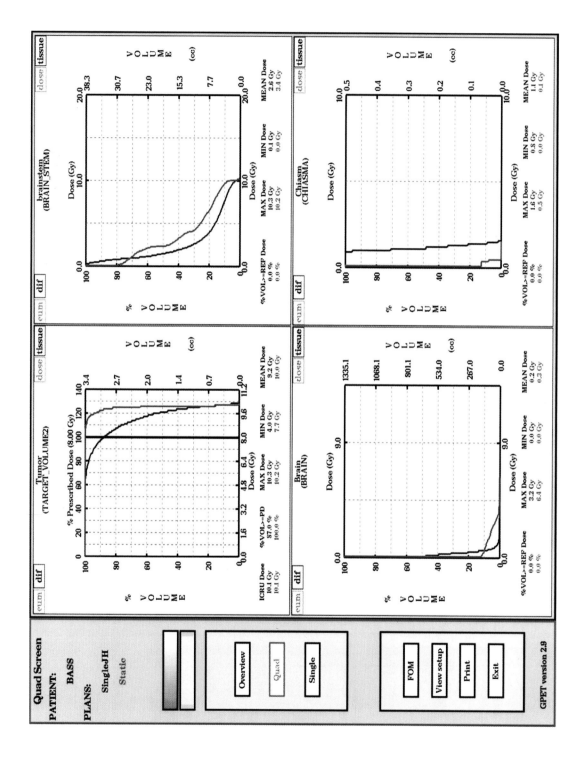

Plate 21. The Graphical Plan Evaluation Tool that was developed for the Radiotherapy Tools contract can simultaneously show dose volume histograms for multiple organs and up to three rival treatment plans.

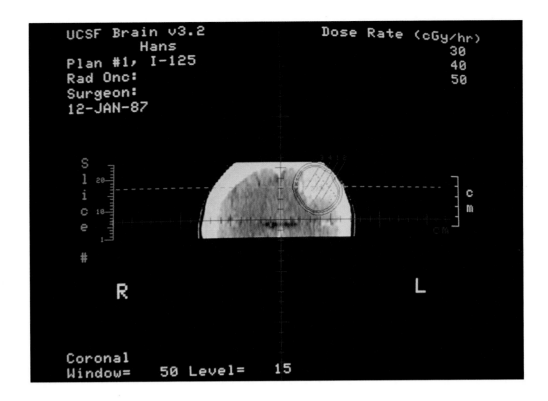

Plate 22. Coronal view of a four-catheter implant of a brain lesion. Isodose-rate contours of 30, 40, and 50 cGy/hr in this plane are displayed.

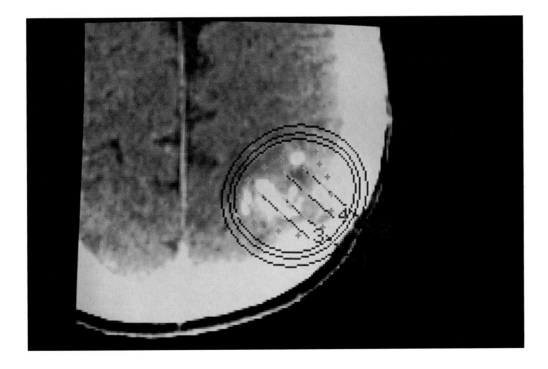

Plate 23. Close-up of a mid-transverse slice, again showing the projected catheter images and iso-dose-rate contours.

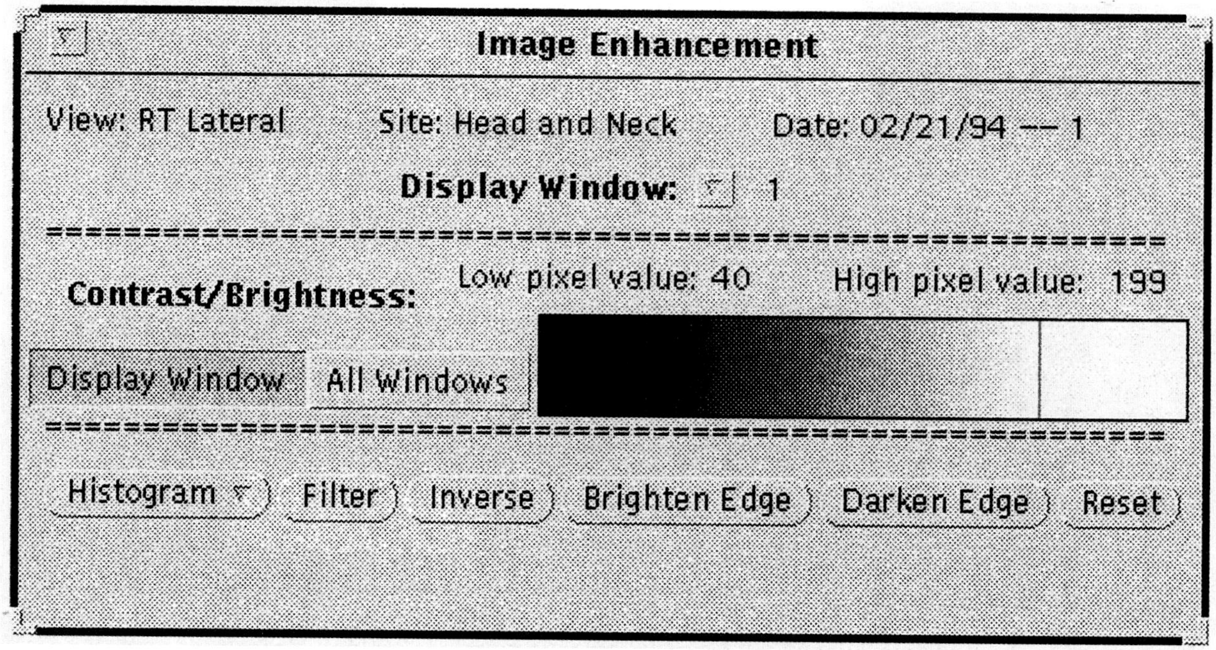

Plate 24. Image-enhancement window.

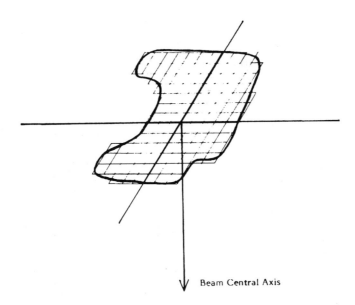

Figure 24-2a.

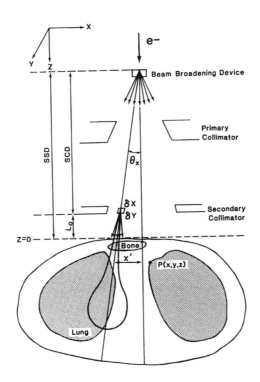

Figure 24-2b.

Figure 24-2   *Schematic representation of the electron pencil-beam dose calculation. (a) An irregular field is approximated by many pixels. (b) Each pencil beam has a size (Δx, Δy), a mean direction $\left(\overline{\theta}_x, \overline{\theta}_y\right)$, an RMS angular spread about the mean direction (σ_{θ_x}), an energy $(E_{p,o})$, and a planar fluence (electrons cm^{-2}). Only the anatomy along the central axis of the pencil beam is used to calculate the dose contribution to the patient from that pencil beam, as illustrated by the teardrop-shaped dose distribution.*

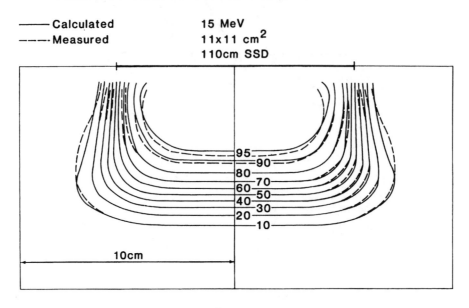

Figure 24-3a.

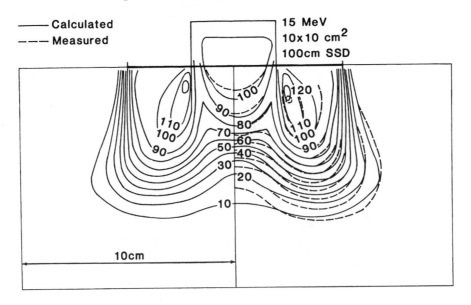

Figure 24-3b.

Figure 24-3 Comparison of pencil-beam calculated ionization distributions with those measured by a 0.1 cm³ ionization chamber: (a) extended treatment distance and (b) irregular surface (from Hogstrom et al. 1984).

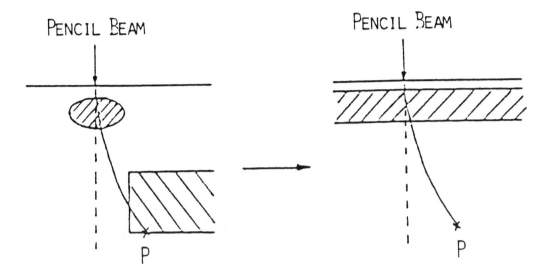

CENTRAL-AXIS APPROXIMATION

Figure 24-4a.

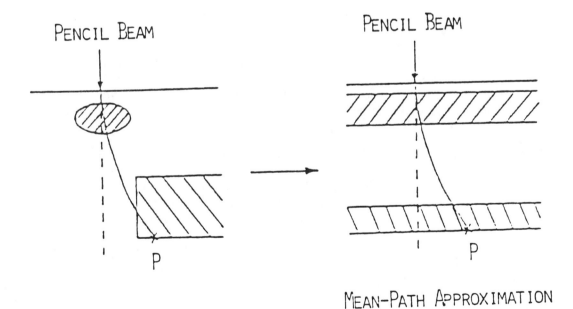

MEAN-PATH APPROXIMATION

Figure 24-4b.

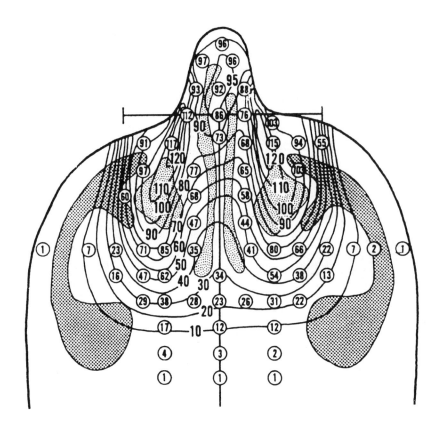

Figure 24-4c.

Figure 24-4. *(a) The anatomy along the central axis of the pencil beam (dashed line) defines the slab anatomy used to calculate dose to the point P. This results in the deep inhomogeneity being ignored. (b) The anatomy along the mean path (solid line) of electrons from the pencil beam that reach the point P defines the slab anatomy used to calculate dose to point P. This would result in the most accurate dose calculation. (c) Comparison of TLD measured with pencil-beam calculated dose in a 2-D anthropomorphic phantom irradiated by 13-MeV electrons, simulating the geometry for treatment of carcinoma of the nose (from Hogstrom et al. 1984).*

Inaccuracies that exceed 5% exist in the algorithm and can be primarily attributed to four physical properties of the algorithm: (1) the slab geometry assumption, (2) its being a planar fluence-based dose model, (3) the Eyges, Gaussian scatter distribution function, and (4) its inability to model secondary electrons. Each of these is discussed in more detail in the review article by Hogstrom et al. (1991), and in this work, only the most significant, the slab geometry assumption, will be reviewed.

As illustrated in Figure 24-4a, b, the anatomy along the central axis of a pencil beam can be significantly different from that along the mean path of the electrons from the surface to the point of dose calculation. This is most significant for patient inhomogeneities that are deep below the surface or ones with an edge long and parallel to the beam. The effect of the latter is illustrated in Figure 24-4c, where we can compare TLD-measured doses at specific points with those calculated for a 2-D nose phantom (Hogstrom et al. 1984). Agreement at most points is within our 5% goal; however, dose points in the septum (location of tumor) show the algorithm underestimating the reduction in dose by as much as 13% due to the long nasal air cavities. Inaccuracies like these have motivated additional research into electron beam dose algorithms.

Other 3-D Dose Algorithms

A variety of algorithms designed to overcome the major weaknesses of the Hogstrom pencil-beam algorithm have been studied. Here we will discuss those few that we believe are representative of the algorithms with the most potential for sufficient accuracy and applicability to clinical use.

The natural extension of the pencil-beam algorithm was to solve the Fermi-Eyges transport equation by adding higher order terms and by allowing the linear scattering power to be a function of .position, T = T (x, y, z) (Jette and Walker, 1992). A major concern with this model is its assumption that T can be determined for an effective electron energy at (x, y, z) while ignoring the presence of an energy distribution in patients, particularly in the vicinity of patient inhomogeneities, as illustrated in Figure 24-5. Also, the nonexplicit modeling of the energy distribution requires corrections for range straggling. Nonetheless, the early results of Jette and Walker (1992) are promising as illustrated in Figure 24-6. For the simple half-slab air inhomogeneity, the accuracy of the Jette algorithm is clearly a significant improvement over that of the Hogstrom algorithm.

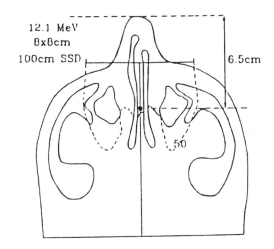

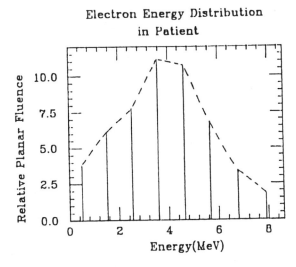

Figure 24-5.   *Energy distribution at a point in the nasal septum for the phantom of Figure 24-4c is calculated by the redefinition pencil beam algorithm. This illustrates the need to model the energy spectrum in patient electron beam dose calculations (from Shiu, 1988).*

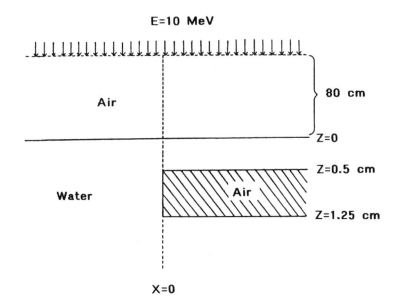

Figure 24-6a.

Calculated Dose Profile Comparison

(Water–Air Interface)

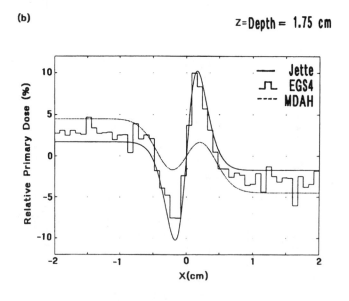

Figure 24-6b.

Figure 24-6.   *(a) Calculation geometry consisting of a broad, parallel 10-MeV electron beam normally incident on a water phantom containing a semi-infinite slab of air. (b) Comparison of dose calculations generated by EGS4 Monte Carlo, Hogstrom pencil-beam algorithm (MDAH), and Jette's pencil-beam algorithm (from Jette and Walker, 1992).*

The second category of algorithms will be referred to as phase-space algorithms, and their objective is to calculate the entire phase space of the beam at each dose point, i.e. the electron distribution differential in energy and angle at each position. The first of this type of algorithms to be discussed is the redefinition pencil beam (RPB) algorithm. It was originally reported in 2-D without modeling the energy distribution, by Storchi and Huizenga (1985), and subsequently in 3-D with modeling of the energy distribution by Shiu and Hogstrom (1991). The RPB algorithm is a natural extension of the original Hogstrom algorithm (Hogstrom et al. 1981), in which dose calculations beneath an irregular surface were made more accurate by redefining the pencil beams at the patient's surface. Shiu and Hogstrom (1991) concluded that the pencil beam algorithm's accuracy could be improved by continually redefining the pencil beams with depth. This algorithm is illustrated in Figure 24-7, which schematically shows the pencil beams at Z and how they contribute to pencil beams at Z + ΔZ. The Fermi-Eyges theory is still used in propagating the electrons from Z to Z + ΔZ with the exception that energy loss is calculated based on the path length of the pencil beam from the point of origin to destination, resulting in each pencil beam having an energy distribution associated with it. The improvement in accuracy of the algorithm is demonstrated in Figure 24-8, which calculates the dose profile 1 cm beneath a 1-cm thick air cavity that lies 2 cm below the surface. A similar concept is the phase-space time evoluation (PTSE) model of Huizenga and Storchi (1989) and Morawska-Kaczynska and Huizenga (1992). To date the PSTE model has emphasized the physics development, whereas the RPB model has emphasized its clinical implementation with 3-D inhomogeneities.

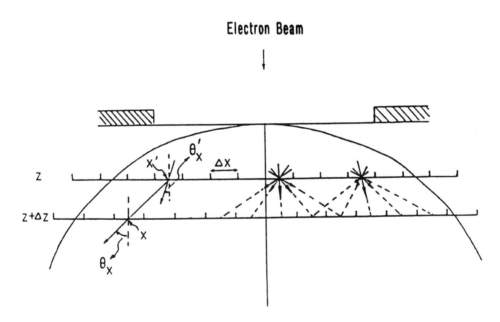

Figure 24-7. *Schematic representation of pencil beams at Z being transported to Z + ΔZ, where new pencil beams are defined (from Shiu and Hogstrom, 1991).*

The third category of 3-D dose algorithms under investigation are those based on the Monte Carlo (MC) technique. Such techniques offer the potential of the greatest accuracy, as more physical interactions can be modeled. The price paid for increased accuracy is reduced precision in that computational time to achieve suitable precision is longer. Recent efforts by Al-Beteri and Raeside (1992) have demonstrated the utility of MC calculations for the use of small-field electron beams in treating retinoblastoma. Another important consideration for MC-based dose algorithms is that they require a detailed specification of the initial particle distribution resulting from the beam design; at present this requires a separate MC calculation (Udale-Smith, 1992). The EGS4 MC code (Nelson et al. 1985) is publicly available and can be used for patient dose calculations. Methods of correlated sampling have been studied by Holmes et al. (1993) for reducing its time of calculation.

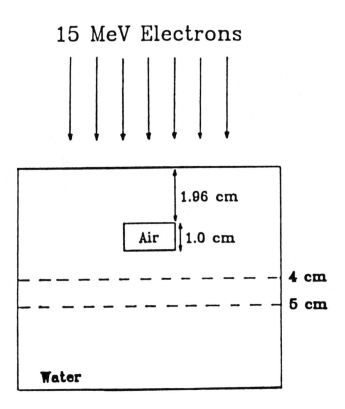

Figure 24-8a.

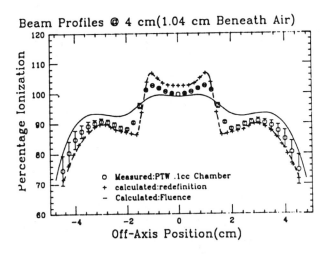

Figure 24-8b.

Figure 24-8   *Comparison of measured with calculated dosimetry to demonstrate improved accuracy of redefinition pencil beam model. (a) Measurement geometry shows a long air cavity with a 1 cm x 2 cm cross-section, 2 cm beneath the surface in a 15-MeV electron beam. (b) Comparison of measured dose with that calculated by the redefinition pencil beam algorithm (dashed line), showing improvement over a fluence-based conventional pencil beam algorithm (solid line) (from Shiu 1988).*

An interesting technique, first discussed by Mackie and Battista (1984), is the macro Monte Carlo (MMC) algorithm. This has been implemented by Neuenschwander and Born (1992) and is schematized in Figure 24-9. In this method, the exit position and momentum are randomly selected for an electron with a known momentum incident on the axis of a sphere (c.f. Figure 24-9a). Random selections are made from tables of pre-Monte Carlo computed transport of different electron energies through spheres of differing materials (density and composition). The track can then be randomly constructed by connecting spheres that intersect the previous sphere at the exit point of the electron and whose axis coincides with the exit electron's momentum vector (c.f. Figure 24-10b). Energy deposited in each sphere can be converted to dose. Results of the MMC algorithm are demonstrated for a 1-cm thick semi-infinite air slab in a 10-MeV electron beam (Neuenschwander and Born, 1992). From the isodose contours in Figure 24-10a, the calculated profile 1 cm beneath the interface is compared with measurement in Figure 24-10b, showing excellent agreement.

Macro Monte Carlo Method

EGS4 Precalculation Geometry

One Particle History

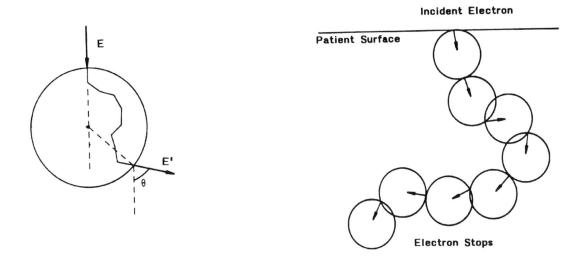

Figure 24-9a. *Figure 24-9b.*

Figure 24-9. (a) *Schematic representation of a single history for an electron perpendicularly incident on a sphere of a specific material type that exits with spherical angles* (θ, ϕ) *and a new energy* (E'). *Precalculated histories as a function on incident electron energy, E, and material type provide distribution functions for random selection of exit momentum vector (from Neuenschwander and Born, 1992). (b) Schematic representation of the MMC algorithm shows the methodology for tracking the history of one electron. The arrow indicates the direction of motion of the electron exiting the previous sphere. Note that the arrow points to the center of the next sphere (from Neuenschwander and Born, 1992).*

MMC Calculated Isodose Contours

10 MeV, 6 x 6-cm Broad Beam

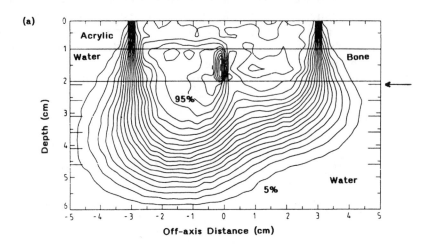

Figure 24-10a.

Dose Profile Comparison

Depth = 2.1 cm

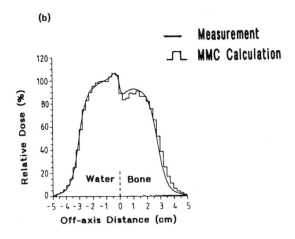

Figure 24-10b.

Figure 24-10a & b.   (a) Planar isodose contours (every 5%) for a MMC calculated dose distribution of a 10-MeV, 6 x 6-cm electron beam incident on a water phantom with a water-bone interface located 1cm beneath a 1cm thick acrylic slab. (b) Comparison of measured with calculated off-axis relative dose profiles from the data of (a) at a depth of 2.1 cm (see arrow) (from Neuenschwander and Born, 1992).

Algorithm Verification

Algorithm verification implies that the accuracy of an algorithm has been evaluated for clinically applicable test cases and that the algorithm's input data have been verified for a particular therapy machine. The former is the responsibility of research medical physicists, and with these results, clinical medical physicists can interpret clinical dose distributions calculated by the algorithm. The latter is the responsibility of the clinical medical physicist and is not the subject of this discussion.

Evaluation of an algorithm's accuracy should be done for irradiation conditions that simulate patient ones. Recently a comprehensive study was undertaken by a National Cancer Institute (NCI) Collaborative Working Group. In this study 14 experiments were performed that resulted in 78 2-D dose distributions measured for 28 unique irradiation conditions (Shiu et al. 1992). Those measurements studied the influence of energy, field shaping, air gap, irregular patient surface, and internal inhomogeneities on dose. Figure 24-11a illustrates the irradiation conditions for one of the experiments, that simulated irradiation through the ramus of the mandible. Figure 24-11b shows a comparison of the measured and calculated dose distribution in a plane parallel to the central axis of the beam and 1 cm superior to the edge simulating the lower mandible. The dose distribution was calculated using the Hogstrom 3-D pencil beam algorithm (Starkschall et al. 1991). The set of data serves as an excellent benchmark for comparing the accuracy of dose algorithms and is publicly available (Shiu et al. 1992).

The above data, although an excellent benchmark data set, must be interpreted for clinical use. Comparison data for clinical use could be improved by measuring dose distribution in more site-specific, anthropomorphic phantoms. At The University of Texas M. D. Anderson Cancer Center, measurements in 3-D anthropomorphic phantoms have been made in the eye (Kirsner et al. 1987), the spinal cord (Dominiak, 1991), and the nose (Hogstrom and Almond, 1983). Figure 24-12a shows a sagittal CT scan slice of the eye phantom, and Figure 24-12b shows the dose distribution measured in the globe using film dosimetry.

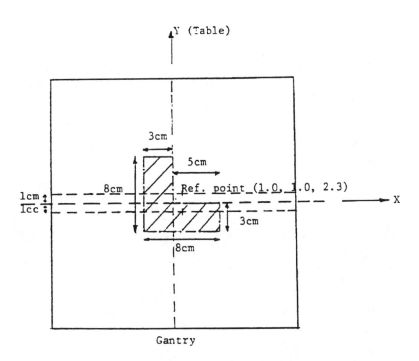

Figure 24-11a.

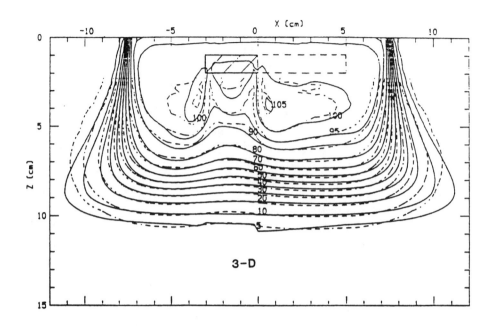

Figure 24-11b.

Figure 24-11. (a) Beam's-eye view of irradiation geometry simulating the ramus of the mandible. The L-shaped hard bone substitute was 1-cm thick and its upstream surface was 1 cm below the surface of a water phantom. (b) Comparison of measured dose (dashed contours) with dose calculated by Hogstrom pencil-beam algorithm as implemented by Starkschall et al. (1991). The dose plane is in water 1 cm from the bone substitute in the lower portion of the "L" (y = +1 cm) (from Shiu et al. 1992).

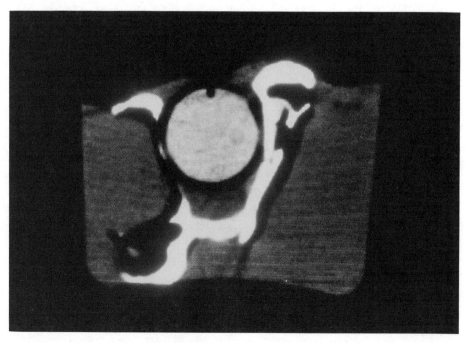

Figure 24-12a.

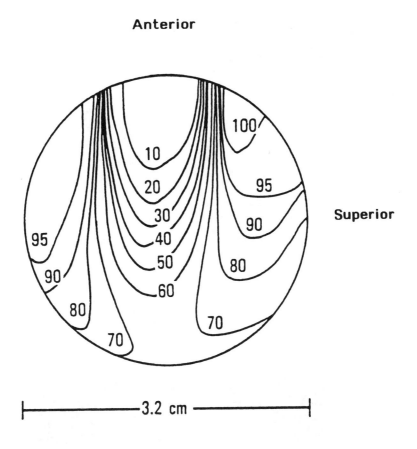

Anterior

Superior

3.2 cm

Figure 24-12b.

Figure 24-12. (a) Sagittal plane CT scan of eye phantom. Rehydrated bones are imbedded in beeswax to simulate normal tissues. A 28-mm diameter polystyrene sphere simulates the globe. Machined in two halves, it allows planar film dosimetry in sagittal and transverse planes. The niche in the anterior portion of the sphere holds a 1-cm diameter copper lens block. (b) Dose distribution measured for a 10-MeV, 5-cm diameter electron field with a 1-cm diameter lens block. This is a field configuration that can be used for anterior electron irradiation of retinoblastoma. Isodose contours are expressed as a percent of central-axis dose maximum in a water phantom without lens block (from Kirsner et al. 1987).

Utilization of 3-D Electron Beam Algorithms

We have found the 3-D electron beam dose algorithm's implementation into our 3-D treatment planning system (Starkschall et al. 1991) to be an integral part of 3-D electron beam treatment planning. Its utilization has been key in three areas: (1) dosimetric evaluation of new treatment techniques, (2) design of bolus for electron conformal therapy, and (3) dosimetric evaluation of the effects of tissue inhomogeneities.

One example of development of a new treatment technique is total scalp treatment in which lateral electron fields are abutted to parallel-opposed x-ray fields used to treat a rind of the scalp (Tung et al. 1993). As illustrated in Figure 24-13a, field overlap of 3 mm is required to optimize uniformity. The resulting dose distribution in a coronal plane is shown in Figure 24-13b.

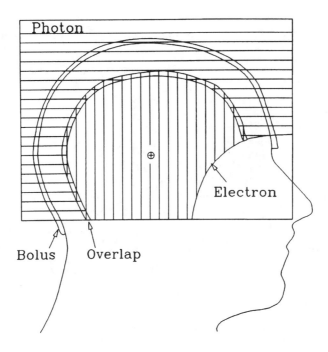

Figure 24-13a.

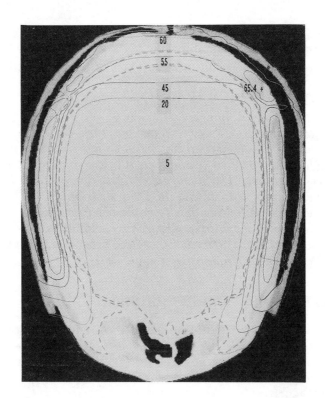

Figure 24-13b.

Figure 24-13. (a) *Schematics of electron-photon total scalp irradiation. The right and left lateral scalp are treated with electron fields. The rind of the scalp (superior and posterior) is treated with parallel-opposed 6 MV x-ray fields slightly overlapping the electron fields. The patients wears a 6 mm thick wax bolus cap. (b) Resulting dose distribution in mid-coronal plane of resulting 3-D dose distribution.*

An example of the use of Low et al. (1992) algorithm for bolus design has been discussed elsewhere in the proceedings. In one example, a posterior surgical bed of the right paraspinal muscles was treated using 17-MeV electrons and a custom wax bolus. This technique limits dose to the spinal cord and lung, while treating the paraspinal muscles.

Another use of the algorithm is to study the effect of tissue inhomogeneities on the dose distribution, which can be done by comparing the dose calculation with one calculated assuming the patient to be water. We have found this particularly interesting in the head and neck where air cavities can have a major impact on the homogeneity of the dose distribution.

Summary

We have presented a number of points that have a significant effect on the present use and future development of electron algorithms for 3-D treatment planning. The keys to a successful 3-D dose algorithm for electrons are (1) that it model all beam components necessary to treat the patient, (2) that the physics knowledge and beam data input required to clinically implement the algorithm and to verify its operation be within the grasp of the clinical medical physicist, and (3) that the algorithm's accuracy, assessed for clinical treatment geometries, be within 5%. The existing pencil beam algorithms based on the Hogstrom et al. model (1981) come closest to meeting the above keys for success. These have been demonstrated to be generally useful in 3-D treatment planning and more specifically for evaluation of the effects of inhomogeneities, development of new treatment techniques, and design of electron bolus. These algorithms can have clinically significant inaccuracies; however, a variety of new dose algorithms are being investigated that have the potential to improve accuracy of dose calculations to less than 5%. When such algorithms meet the criteria summarized here, we will have completed the next major step in 3-D electron beam treatment planning.

Acknowledgements

I would like to acknowledge members of the electron beam research team at the M.D. Anderson Cancer Center, whose contributions over the past 13 years have contributed to a better understanding of clinical electron beam dose algorithms for treatment planning, particularly Almon Shiu, George Starkschall, and the many graduate students and postdoctoral trainees.

References

1. Al-Beteri, A.A.; Raeside, D.E. Optimal electron-beam treatment planning for retinoblastoma using a new three-dimensional Monte Carlo-based treatment planning system. Med. Phys. 19:125-135, 1992.

2. Dominiak, G. S. Dose in spinal cord following electron irradiation. M.S. Thesis, The University of Texas Graduate School of Biomedical Sciences, Houston, TX, 1991.

3. Hogstrom, K.R. Evaluation of electron pencil beam dose calculations. In: Elson, H., Born, C., eds. Radiation Oncology Physics - 1986: Proceedings of the 1986 Summer School of the AAPM. New York: American Institute of Physics; 1987:532-557.

4. Hogstrom, K.R.; Almond, P.R. Comparison of experimental and calculated dose distributions: a review of electron beam dose planning at the M.D. Anderson Hospital. Acta Radiol. Suppl., No. 364:89-99, 1983.

5. Hogstrom, K.R.; Mills, M.D.; Almond, P.R. Electron beam dose calculations. Phys. Med. Biol., 26:445-459, 1981.

6. Hogstrom, K.R.; Mills, M.D.; Meyer, J.A.; Palta, J.R.; Mellenberg, D.E.; Meoz, R.T.; Fields, R.S. Dosimetric evaluation of a pencil-beam algorithm for electrons employing a two-dimensional heterogeneity correction. Int. J. Rad. Oncol., Biol., Phys., 10:561-569, 1984.

7. Hogstrom, K.R.; Starkschall, G.; Shiu, A.S. Dose calculation algorithms for electron beams. In: Purdy, J. ed. Advances in Radiation Oncology Physics - 1990 Proceedings of the Summer School of the AAPM. New York: American Institute of Physics; 1991:900-924.

8. Holmes, M.A.; Mackie, T. R.; Sohn, W.; Reckwerdt, P.J.; Kinsella, T.J.; Bielajew, A.F.; Rogers, D.W. The application of correlated sampling to the computation of electron beam dose distributions in heterogeneous phantoms using the Monte Carlo method. Phys. Med. Biol., 38:675-688, 1993.

9. Huizenga, H.; Storchi, P.R.M. Numerical calculation of energy deposition by broad high-energy electron beams. Phys. Med. Biol., 34:1371-1396, 1989.

10. Jette, D.; Walker, S. Electron dose calculation using multiple-scattering theory: Evaluation of a new model for inhomogeneities. Med. Phys. 19:1241-1254, 1992.

11. Kirsner, S.M.; Hogstrom, K.R.; Kurup, R.G.; Moyers, M.F. Dosimetric evaluation in heterogeneous tissue of anterior electron beam irradiation for treating retinoblastoma. Med. Phys. 14:772-779, 1987.

12. Low, D.A.; Starkschall, G.; Hogstrom, K.R. Electron bolus design for radiotherapy treatment planning: Bolus design algorithms. Med. Phys. 19:115-124, 1992.

13. Mackie, T.R.; Battista, J.J. A macroscopic Monte Carlo method for electron beam dose calculations: A proposal. In: Proceedings of the Eight International Conference on the Use of Computers in Radiation Therapy. Toronto, Canada: IEE Computer Society Press; 1984:123-131.

14. Morawska-Kaczynska, M.; Huizenga, H. Numerical calculation of energy deposition by broad high-energy electron beams: II. Multi-layered geometry. Phys. Med. Biol., 37(11):2103-2116, 1992.

15. Nelson, W.R.; Hirayama, H,.; and Rogers, D.W.O. The EGS4 code system SLAC-265, Stanford University, Stanford, CA, 1985.

16. Neuenschwander, H.; Born, E.J. A macro Monte Carlo method for electron beam dose calculations. Phys. Med. Biol., 37:107-125, 1992.

17. Shiu, A.S. Three dimensional electron beam dose calculations. Ph.D. Dissertation, The University of Texas Graduate School of Biomedical Sciences, Houston, TX, 1988.

18. Shiu, A.S.; Hogstrom, K.R. Pencil-beam redefinition algorithm for electron dose distributions. Med. Phys. 18:7-18, 1991.

19. Shiu, A.S.; Tung, S.; Hogstrom, K.R.; Wong, J.W.; Gerber, R.L.; Harms, W.B.; Purdy, J.A.; Ten Haken, R.K.; McShan, D.L.; Fraass, B.A. Verification data for electron beam dose algorithms. Med. Phys. 19:623-636, 1992.

20. Starkschall, G.; Bujnowski, S.W.; Wang, L.L.; Shiu, A.S.; Boyer, A.L.; Desobry, G.E.; Wells, N.H.; Baker, W.L.; Hogstrom, K.R. A full three-dimensional radiotherapy treatment planning system. Med. Phys. 18:647 (abstract), 1991.

21. Starkschall, G.; Shiu, A.S.; Bujnowski, S.W.; Wang, L.L.; Low, D.A.; Hogstrom, K.R. Effect of dimensionality of heterogeneity corrections on the implementation of a three-dimensional electron pencil-beam algorithm. Phy. Med. Biol., 36, 207-222, 1991.

22. Storchi, P.R.M.; Huizenga, H. On a numerical approach of the pencil-beam model. Phys. Med. Biol., 30:467-473, 1985.

23. Tung, S.S.; Shiu, A.S.; Starkschall, G.; Morrison, W.H.; and Hogstrom, K.R. Dosimetric evaluation of total scalp irradiation using a lateral electron-photon technique. Int. J. Rad. Oncol. Biol., Phys., 27:153-160, 1993.

24. Udale-Smith, M. Monte Carlo calculations of the electron beam parameters for three Phillips linear accelerators. Phys. Med. Biol., 37:85-106, 1992.

Chapter 25

Electron Beam Bolus for 3-D Conformal Radiation Therapy[1]

George Starkschall, Ph.D., John A. Antolak, Ph.D., and Kenneth R. Hogstrom, Ph.D.

Dept of Radiation Physics, The University of Texas, M. D. Anderson Cancer Center, Houston, Texas

This paper describes a method for delivering electron conformal radiation therapy with the aid of electron bolus. In this work, electron bolus is defined as tissue-equivalent material that is placed at or near the patient skin surface; the bolus shapes the dose distribution to conform to the target volume and to provide a more uniform dose inside the target volume (Hogstrom 1992). While electron conformal therapy can also be achieved with moving electron beams (Hogstrom 1992), this paper will be limited to fixed-beam electron conformal therapy. In addition, fixed-beam electron bolus can be used to modify the proximal patient surface so that it presents a flat surface perpendicular to the beam central axis, for example, in the treatment of the nasal cavity, but this approach to bolus design will not be discussed in this paper.

This paper comprises five sections: The first section defines electron conformal radiation therapy and identifies the differences between photon conformal radiation therapy and electron conformal radiation therapy. The second section describes electron bolus and the methodology for its design, and the third describes how the design methodology is incorporated into a three-dimensional radiotherapy treatment planning system. The fourth section describes the transfer of bolus information from the treatment planning system to a computer-driven milling machine and the fabrication of bolus using the milling machine. Finally, the fifth section describes an example of the clinical implementation of electron bolus at The University of Texas M. D. Anderson Cancer Center.

Definition of Electron Conformal Radiation Therapy

Electron conformal radiation can be defined by comparing it with photon conformal radiation therapy. The aim of conformal therapy, whether it be photon or electron, is to deliver the radiation dose so that the dose to the target volume is limited only by the tolerance of the uninvolved tissue within the target volume. Generally, this aim is achieved by configuring the beam parameters so that the region of high dose encloses the target volume while closely conforming to its boundaries. This configuration can be achieved (at least in principle) when irradiating with photons by means of customized blocking and compensation for multiple treatment portals (Boyer et al. 1993). The use of customized blocking ensures that uninvolved tissue lateral to the target volume is spared, while the use of compensation and multiple treatment portals ensures sparing of uninvolved tissue external to the target volume.

Photon conformal therapy can be used for tumors located throughout the body; however, it may be possible to treat superficial tumor volumes with electron conformal therapy, often using a single field. To generate a beam configuration for electron conformal therapy, customized blocking is also used to spare uninvolved tissue lateral to the target volume, but uninvolved tissue distal to the target volume is spared by taking advantage of the finite penetration of the electrons through the use of bolus. Once a target volume has been defined, an electron energy is selected so that the target volume is encompassed within 90% (or any other appropriate minimum dose) of the given

1 Work supported in part by Texas Higher Education Coordinating Board grant ATP050.

dose (AAPM 1991). If the distal surface of the target volume were situated at a nearly uniform depth beneath the external patient surface, an electron beam of a suitable energy with a treatment portal defined by secondary (end-of-cone) or tertiary (skin) collimation could provide electron conformal therapy. The distal surface of a real target volume, however, does not lie at a constant depth from the surface. Moreover, a critical structure may lie at a depth shallower than the deepest part of the target volume in another region of the treatment field. Thus, an electron beam with a spatially uniform energy would not be appropriate.

The following example illustrates this situation: Figure 25-1a depicts a hypothetical phantom with target volume whose distal surface varies between 1.0 cm depth and 3.0 cm depth. We wish to deliver a minimum dose of 54 Gy to the entire target volume, but we want to limit the dose to a critical structure lateral to the target volume to 45 Gy. While a 12-MeV electron beam with a given dose of 60 Gy delivers a suitable dose to the target volume, a significant and unacceptable portion of the critical structure will receive a dose in excess of the maximum allowed dose of 45 Gy. The unacceptability of the treatment plan can be easily recognized by examining the dose-volume histograms (DVH) for the target volume and critical structure in Figures 25-1b and 1c.

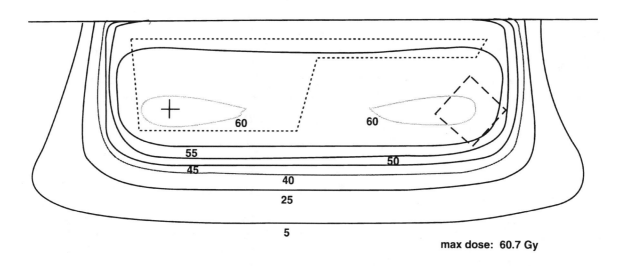

Figure 25-1a.

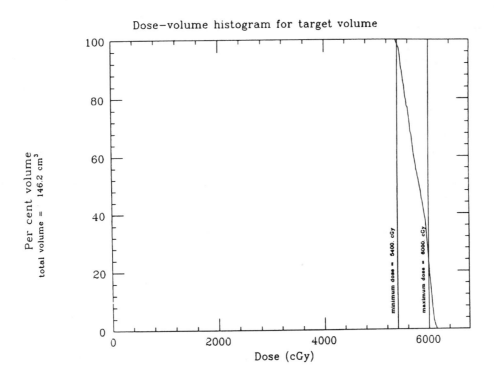

Figure 25-1b.

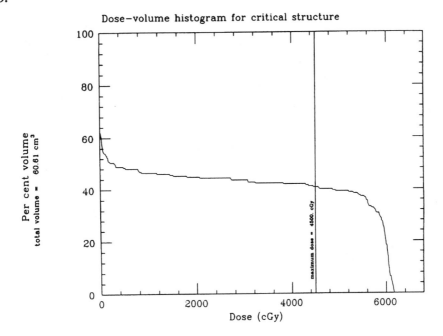

Figure 25-1c.

Figure 25-1.   *A hypothetical example of the use of electron bolus. A dose of 54 Gy is prescribed to a target volume with a distal surface that varies in depth between 1.0 cm and 3.0 cm. In addition, the critical structure adjacent to the target volume may not receive a dose in excess of 45 Gy. (b) The DVH for the target volume. (c) The DVH for the critical structure.*

The solution to the problem of over-irradiating a shallow critical structure is to use an electron beam whose energy depends on location in the treatment field. This beam would have a higher energy where more penetration is necessary, and a lower energy where less penetration is necessary. Electron bolus is used to provide this spatial modulation of the electron-beam energy and achieve electron conformal therapy.

Design of Electron Bolus

In the context of electron conformal therapy as described above, electron bolus is defined to be tissue-equivalent material placed in the path of an electron beam to modulate the energy of the beam. Although electron bolus and photon compensators are both placed in the radiation beam for the purpose of spatial modulation, the use of electron bolus is clearly different from that of photon compensating filters. A photon compensating filter is placed in the path of the photon beam to spatially vary the beam intensity, whereas an electron bolus is placed in the path of the electron beam to spatially vary the beam energy. Photon compensators are placed far from the patient surface to maximize skin sparing, while electron bolus is normally placed in contact with the patient surface. Although electron bolus is generally placed on or near the patient's skin surface, it is better considered as part of the electron beam, with coordinates described in a coordinate system that moves with the beam.

By spatially modulating the energy of the electron beam, the electron bolus shapes the electron-beam dose distribution so that the prescription isodose can track the distal surface of the target volume. The solution to the design of electron bolus would be quite simple if the magnitude of multiple Coulomb scattering were small, as in the case for protons (Urie et al. 1983); however, this is not the case. The effects of scatter can result in increased dose inhomogeneity in the target volume. Therefore, the design of electron bolus is always a tradeoff between conforming the prescription isodose to the target volume and ensuring reasonable dose homogeneity.

The first step in bolus design is bolus creation (Low et al. 1992). In this step, bolus thickness is determined so that the distal surface of the target volume is placed at a constant specified depth. To create a bolus using this method, one first generates a two-dimensional grid of fan lines emanating from the (virtual) source of electrons. Along each fan line, denoted by the indices i and j, the depth of the distal surface of the target volume, d_{ij}, is determined. The bolus thickness at the ij fan line, b_{ij}, is then given by

$$b_{ij} = (1/\rho b)[(R_{prescr})_{ij} - d_{ij}\},$$

(1)

where ρ_b is the effective density of the bolus material (ratio of bolus linear collision stopping power to that of water), and $(R_{prescr})_{ij}$ is the depth of the prescription isodose at the ij fan line. This method provides a simple algorithm for designing an electron bolus, ignoring internal patient inhomogeneity. It is possible to account for these internal inhomogeneities by replacing the physical depth along each fan line by the density-weighted radiological depth, but we have found this to be less desirable (Low et al. 1992).

Figures 25-2a, 2b, and 2c illustrate the results from designing a bolus to place the distal surface of the target volume at a specified depth. The example used is the same as that in Figure 25-1. The bolus is designed to place the distal surface of the target volume at a depth of 3.2 cm, corresponding to the depth of the 90% isodose for 12-MeV electrons. Figure 25-2a illustrates the dose distribution along the transverse plane containing the central axis of the beam, while figures 25-2b and 2c illustrate the DVH for the target volume and critical structure, respectively.

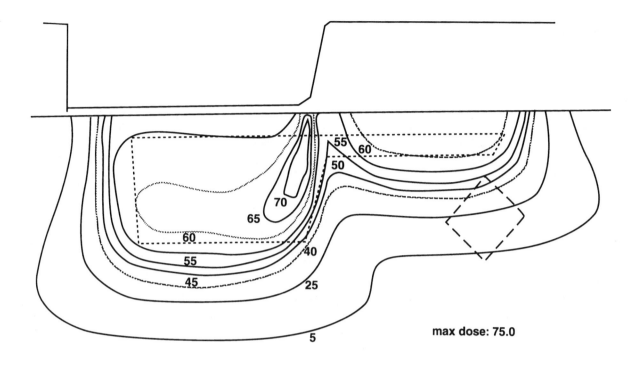

Figure 25-2a.

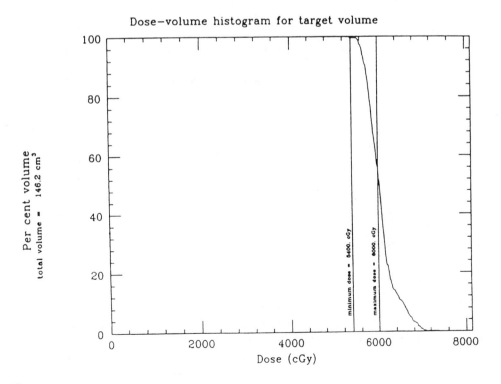

Figure 25-2b.

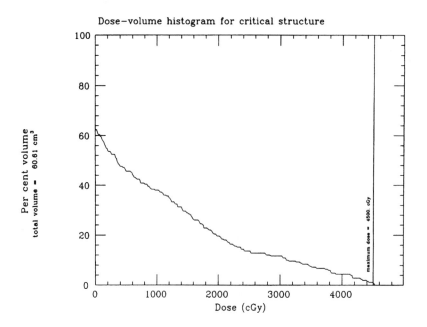

Dose–volume histogram for critical structure

Figure 25-2c.

Figure 25-2. *The previous case with a bolus designed to place the distal surface of the target volume at a constant depth of 3.2 cm. (a) The dose distribution in the transverse plane containing the central axis of a 12-MeV electron bean. The given dose is 60 Gy. (b) The DVH for the target volume. (c) The DVH for the critical structure.*

In treatment planning with electron bolus, we have observed that, at the lateral boundaries of the target volume, the distal surface tends to be rounded towards the skin surface. Designing a bolus so that the entire distal surface of the target volume were to lie at a specified constant depth would result in unnecessarily thick bolus at the edges of the treatment portal. This problem is overcome by defining a bolus margin, Δ, inside the beam's eye view projection of the target volume. For points between this margin boundary and the edge of the treatment portal, bolus thicknesses are not calculated. Bolus thicknesses are calculated everywhere else inside this region and then extended to outside the region of design. This normally suffices to resolve this problem, as the normal curvature Of the 90% isodose near the edge of the treatment field will approximately track the distal surface of the target volume in the region near the lateral boundaries. In the example illustrated in Figure 25-2, a bolus margin of 0.5 cm was used.

A second problem encountered when using a simple bolus design is more difficult to overcome. Because of the multiple Coulomb scattering of electrons, regions of bolus with steep gradients in the proximal surface will cause hot and cold spots to appear in the dose distribution. The hot and cold spots are well known and are evident in the dose distribution in Figure 25-2a, as well as in the DVH for the target volume in Figure 25-2b. The increased scatter into the hot spot results in a significant area of the target volume irradiated in excess of 70 Gy, while the decreased scatter away from the cold spot results in a significant area of target volume irradiated to less than 54 Gy. Low et al. (1992) have indicated how modification operators can act on the designed bolus to overcome this problem.

Bolus modification operators are of two types, those that modify the bolus to overcome the effects of multiple Coulomb scatter of electrons, and those that modify the bolus to facilitate the fabrication process. The latter class of bolus modification operators will be discussed later in this paper. The bolus modification operators that mitigate the effects of electron scatter may compromise the isodose tracking of the distal surface or the target volume by smoothing the proximal surface of the bolus. One such operator limits the bolus slope to a maximum gradient. We have found a useful maximum bolus gradient to be either 30° for electron energies less than or equal to 6 MeV, or 45° for energies greater than 6 MeV. Figure 25-3 illustrates application of this modification operator. In this case a slope limitation operator limiting the bolus slope to 45° was added to the bolus parameters in Figure 25-2. Figure 25-3a illustrates the dose distribution in the transverse plane containing the beam central axis, Figure 25-3b the DVH for the target volume, and Figure 25-3c the DVH for the critical structure with this slope limitation operator implemented. The maximum dose to the target volume is decreased from 75.0 Gy to 69.9 Gy, while the entire target volume is irradiated to a dose above the desired minimum of 54 Gy. The maximum dose to the critical structure remains below 45 Gy.

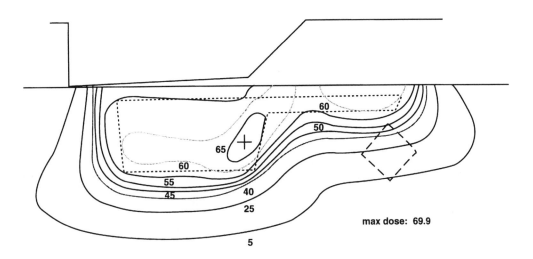

Figure 25-3a.

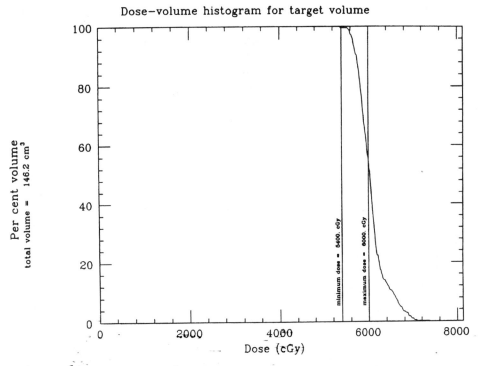

Figure 25-3b.

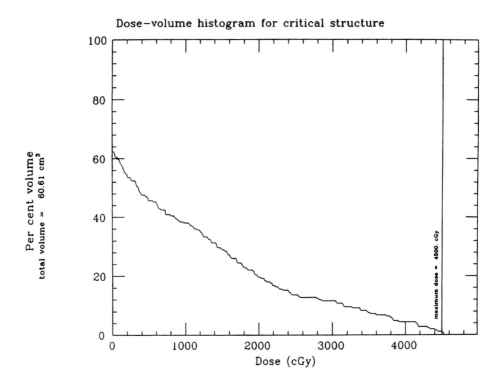

Figure 25-3c.

Figure 25-3. *The previous case with a slope limitation operator invoked to limit the slope of the proximal surface of the bolus to 45°. (a) The dose distribution in the transverse plane containing the central axis of a 12-MeV electron beam. The given dose is 60 Gy. (b) The DVH for the target volume. (c) The DVH for the critical structure.*

Several other operators can be used to modify the bolus. One of these bolus modification operators compares the depth of the calculated 90% isodose with the desired depth of the isodose and adds or removes bolus to bring the isodose line closer to the desired depth. Another modification operator adds bolus to points overlying a critical structure to decrease the dose to the critical structure, while another operator smoothes the proximal surface of the bolus by calculating a weighted average of coordinates of neighborhood surface points for each point on the proximal surface of the bolus. Bolus modification operators can be combined, but it should be noted that these operators are not commutative; hence, the order in which bolus modification operators are presented is significant A more thorough discussion of these operators is given by Low et al. (1992).

Interface With 3-D Treatment Planning System

The code for designing electron bolus has been incorporated into a three-dimensional radiotherapy treatment planning system (Starkschall 1991a). In the present version, because of the length of time required for some of the calculations, bolus design is a non-interactive process. Parameters for the bolus design are entered via a menu at the same time that other beam parameters are entered. Figure 25-4a illustrates the menu displayed on the treatment planning system for selection of bolus modification operators. The treatment planner can select one or more bolus operators. For many bolus operators, additional parameters must be selected. Figure 25-4b illustrates an example of the display of the bolus operators and parameters after all have been entered. The bolus design operators and parameters are stored in a file along with other parameters relating to the electron beam. A module in the treatment planning system then calculates the bolus geometry based on these design parameters.

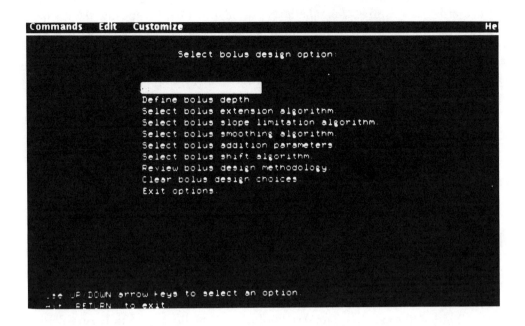

Figure 25-4a.

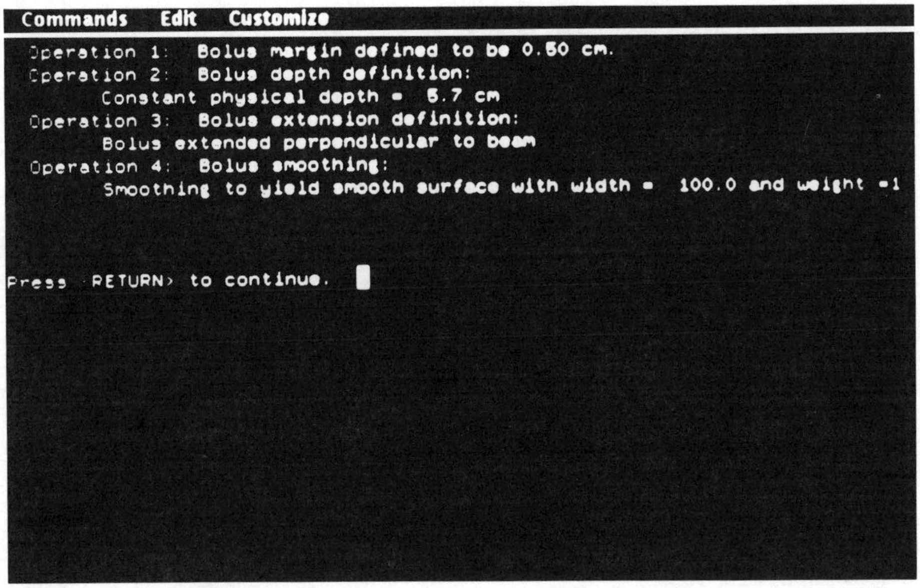

Figure 25-4b.

Figure 25-4. Menus displayed on the treatment planning system for bolus design operations. (a) The menu for selection of bolus modification operators. (b) Display of bolus parameters.

After the bolus geometry has been calculated, dose distributions incorporating the bolus are computed using the three-dimensional implementation of the pencil-beam algorithm (Starkschall 1991b). The presence of bolus modifies the calculation of effective depth and a2. These quantities are calculated by ray-tracing through a three-dimensional matrix of CT numbers. The algorithm identifies the point along each ray where the ray intersects the bolus proximal surface. From that point until the ray intersects the bolus distal surface, the effective depth and a2 are calculated using the linear collision stopping power and linear angular scattering power of the bolus material. Beyond the bolus distal surface, the effective depth and a2 are calculated using a table that relates CT number to stopping power and angular scattering power (Hogstrom et al. 1981). Figure 25-5 illustrates the regions encountered during the ray-tracing process.

Fabrication of Electron Bolus

In addition to the bolus design operators used to produce a suitable dose distribution (Low et al. 1992) and reviewed above, additional bolus design operators are needed to facilitate the fabrication. One of these fabrication operators modifies the proximal surface of the electron bolus so that a 0.5-cm border is created around the machined proximal surface. This "rim" serves as a base for machining the distal surface of the bolus. To ensure that the rim does not perturb the dose distribution, one must place the rim at least 0.8 cm outside the projection of the treatment portal. This 0.8-cm margin allows for both beam divergence and scattering in the air space between the secondary collimator (cone) and the bolus. The design of the rim is illustrated in Figure 25-6.

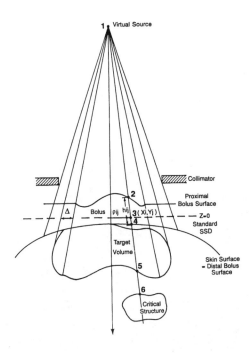

Figure 25-5. *Ray-tracing involved in the dose calculation accounting for the presence of bolus. Rays emanate from the virtual source (1). From the ray intersection with the proximal bolus surface (2) to the intersection with the distal bolus surface (4), the effective depth and a2 are calculated using the linear collision stopping power and linear angular scattering power of the bolus material. Beyond the intersection of the ray with the distal bolus surface, executive depth and a2 are calculated based on the CT numbers of voxels through which the ray passes (from Low et al. 1992).*

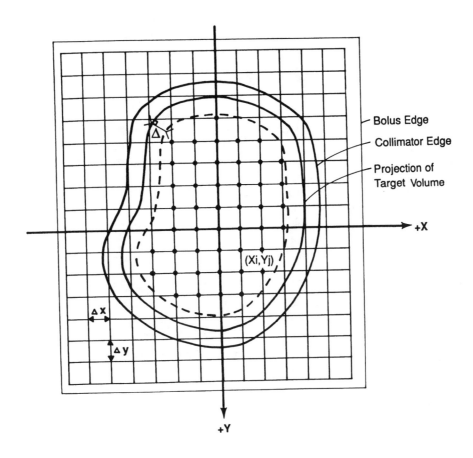

Figure 25-6. *A rim is placed around the fabricated bolus a distance of 1.5 cm from the collimator edge (from Low et al. 1992).*

A second fabrication operator determines the minimum amount of bolus wax material required to fabricate the bolus and modifies the design of the distal surface outside the projection of the treatment field. If there are any skin surfaces that slope dramatically away from the source outside the treatment portal, it is neither necessary nor desirable for the bolus to match the skin surfaces. In such a case, the distal surface of the bolus is set to the distal surface of the wax blank so that no milling in that region is required. The bolus wax is manufactured in thicknesses of 5.08 cm (2 in) or 7.62 cm (3 in), so that using one or two thicknesses of wax to fabricate the bolus allows for blanks of thicknesses of from 2 in to 6 in, at 1-in intervals. The minimum required bolus wax thickness is equal to the maximum source-to-skin distance within the treatment portal, minus the minimum source-to-bolus-surface distance within the treatment portal, rounded up to the nearest inch. Along fan lines outside the treatment portal, the distal surface of the bolus is set to the minimum of the source-to-skin distance and the minimum source-to-bolus distance plus the thickness of the minimum amount of bolus wax material required. The determination of minimum amount of bolus wax material and its application to a steeply sloping surface is illustrated in Figure 25-7.

Bolus based on the final design is then fabricated using a computer-driven milling machine[2] (Figure 25-8). The bolus is machined from modeling wax, which is very close to unit density. A computer program has been written to calculate the tool path required to mill each surface. Running on a 486 personal computer,

---

[2] Roland CAMM-3 Milling Machine.

the computer calculates the entire tool path in a few seconds, and text files containing machining instructions are created for each surface. These text files are then downloaded to the milling machine to mill the surface.

In some cases, the size of the desired electron bolus may exceed the capabilities of the small milling machine. If the lateral extent of the bolus exceeds the maximum milling area of 15 cm x 18 cm, the bolus can be machined in two or four multiple sectors. If the bolus thickness exceeds the maximum wax thickness of 2 in or 3 in, then the software designs the bolus to be milled in two thicknesses of wax.

To simplify the fabrication process, a single 0.3-cm radius ball mill is used. The proximal and distal surfaces are machined in several passes, each of which removes approximately 0.6 cm of wax material. Final smoothing passes may be necessary, depending on the original grid spacing of the designed bolus and the desired smoothness. A typical bolus for 10 x 10-cm field that is 7.62 cm thick requires approximately 1.5 hr to fabricate, with almost all of the time being used to machine the surfaces.

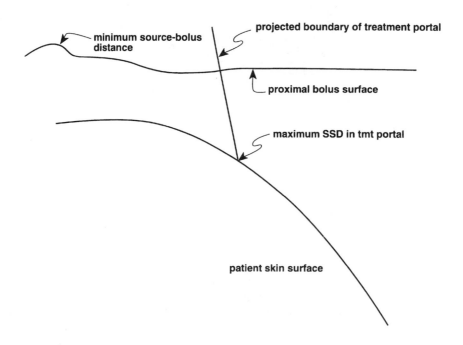

Figure 25-7.   *Distances used in the calculation of maximum bolus thickness outside the treatment portal. The maximum bolus thickness is equal to the maximum SSD in the treatment portal minus the minimum source to bolus distance in the treatment portal rounded up to the nearest inch. Outside the treatment portal, the distal surface is set so that the bolus thickness does not exceed this maximum value.*

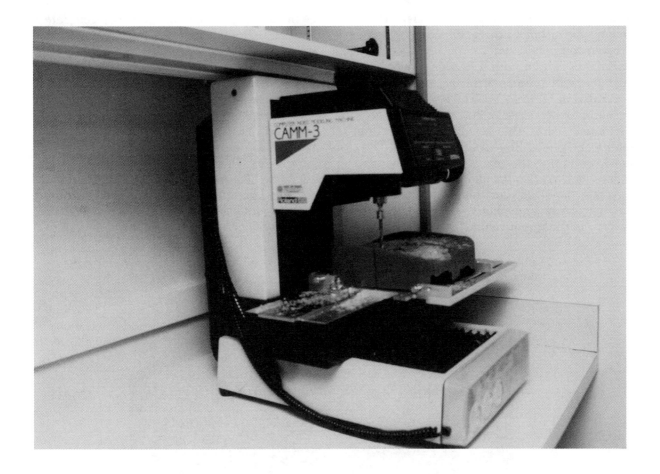

Figure 25-8. The milling machine used for bolus fabrication

Clinical Implementation of Electron Bolus

The following case describes an example of the clinical implementation of electron bolus as designed and fabricated using the methods presented in this paper (Low et al. 1991). In this case, a 17-year-old female presented with mesenchymal chondrosarcoma of the right paraspinal muscles. The patient was to undergo external-beam radiotherapy prior to surgical excision of the tumor. The target volume, as delineated by the physician, overlay parts of both lungs, kidneys, and the spinal cord. Because of a favorable prognosis combined with the patient's age, care was taken to spare as much of the lungs and spinal cord as possible. A course of 44.4 Gy given dose delivered via 17-MeV electrons with bolus combined with 11.1 Gy given dose via 6-MV photons at 2.22 Gy per fraction was prescribed.

Treatment planning CT scans were obtained at 1.0 cm spacing encompassing a volume from 5 cm superior to 5 cm inferior to the target volume. The additional CT slices at least 3 cm outside the intended field were necessary to determine the patient surface beneath portions of bolus designed outside the treatment field to allow for electron scatter and provide structural integrity. The physician outlined the target volume on the CT images and delineated a treatment field that allowed for approximately 1 cm margin around the target volume.

Bolus was designed so that the physical depth of the distal surface of the target volume was uniform 5.4 cm, which was the maximum depth of the distal surface of the target volume. This design ensured that the entire target volume lay within the 90% depth of 5.5 cm for the 17-MeV electron beam. So that the steep gradients near the periphery of the target volume would not generate a steeply sloped bolus, the bolus margin was designed to be 0.7 cm. The bolus was extended in a direction perpendicular to the beam central axis beyond the designed volume. The bolus slope limitation operator with a maximum slope of 45° was invoked as was the bolus smoothing operator with a weight parameter of 0.8 and a width parameter of 100.0. The bolus that was designed is illustrated in Figure 25-9. The electron-beam dose distribution was calculated using the pencil-beam algorithm with these bolus design parameters, while the photon-beam dose distribution was calculated using the convolution algorithm of Boyer et al. (1989) with modifications for heterogeneities by Zhu and Boyer (1990). The resulting electron dose distributions in the transverse plane containing the central axis is illustrated in Figure 25-10. The Figure indicates how the 90% isodose line tracks the distal surface of the target volume. Figures 25-11a, 11b, 11c, and 11d illustrate the DVH's for the target volume, spinal cord, right lung, and right kidney for the total plan (electrons and photons). The dose-volume histograms indicate a clinically acceptable dose delivery to the target volume coupled with sparing of the spinal cord, lung, and kidney.

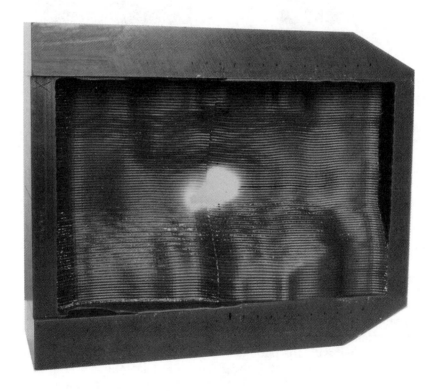

Figure 25-9. The bolus used to treat a sarcoma of the paraspinal muscles

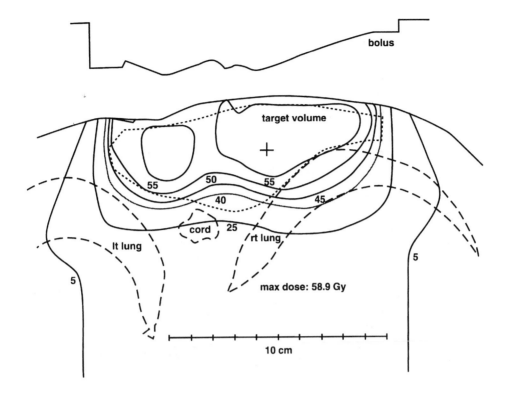

Figure 25-10. Dose distribution for electron-beam treatment of a sarcoma of the paraspinal muscles using electron bolus to reduce dose to the lungs and right kidney.

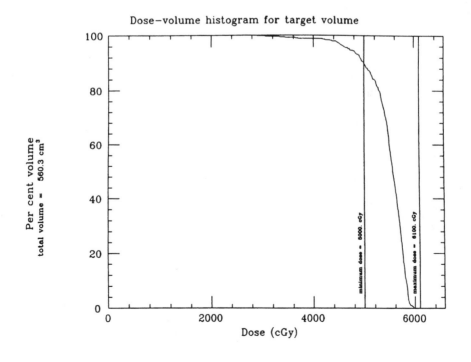

Figure 25-11a.

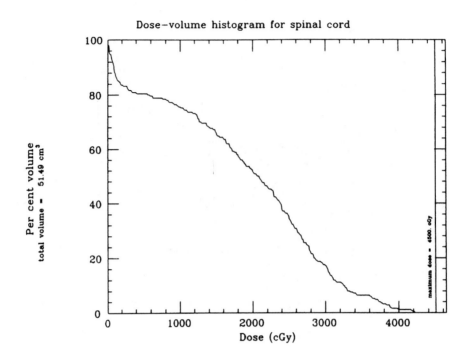

Figure 25-11b.

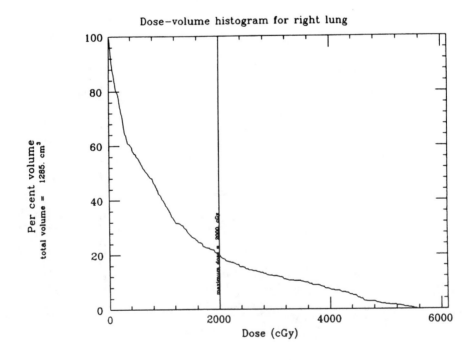

Figure 25-11c.

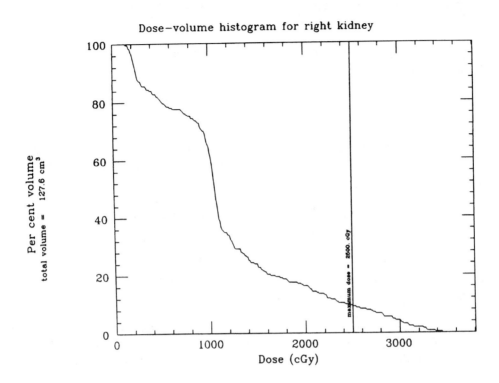

Figure 25-11d.

Figure 25-11. *Dose-volume histograms for delivery of given dose of 44.4 Gy with 17-MeV electrons with electron bolus and 11.1 Gy with 6-MV photons. (a) DVH for target volume. (b) DVH for spinal cord. (c) DVH for right lung. (d) DVH for right kidney.*

Summary

A series of operators have been developed to design electron bolus to achieve electron conformal radiotherapy. These operators are based on the work of Low et al.(1992), with practical modifications necessary for optimal machining of the electron bolus. The bolus design system has been implemented in a three-dimensional radiotherapy treatment planning system. A process has been developed for automatic milling of the wax bolus using a small computer-driven bench-top milling machine. Clinical use of the bolus design and fabrication system is currently under evaluation. In addition to the paraspinal sarcoma test case shown, we expect electron conformal therapy to be useful for treating other sites including, but not limited to, chest wall, scalp, and base of tongue.

References

1. AAPM Radiation Therapy Committee Task Group No. 25, "Clinical electron-beam dosimetry," Med. Phys. 18:73-109 (1991).

2. Boyer, A.L., Zhu, Y., Wang, L., and Francois, P., "Fast Fourier transform convolution calculations of x-ray isodose distributions in homogeneous media," Med. Phys. 16:248-253 (1989).

3. Boyer, A.L., Bortfeld, T., Kahler, D., Starkschall, G., Waldron, T., "Multileaf collimation for 3-D conformal therapy," in J.A. Purdy and B. Emami, 3-D *Radiation Treatment Planning* (Medical Physics Publishing Co, Madison, WI, 1993).

4. Hogstrom, K.R., Mills, M.D., and Almond, P.R., "Electron beam dose calculations," Phys. Med. Biol. 26:445-459 (1981).

5. Hogstrom, K.R., "Conformal therapy with electron beams," in *Proceedings of the Varian 14th Users Meeting*, Waikoloa Hawaii, May 3-5, 1992.

6. Low, D.A., Starkschall, G., Sherman, N.E., Bujnowski, S.W., Ewton, J.E., and Hogstrom, K.R., "Design and construction of a 3-D electron bolus for treatment of the paraspinal muscles," Med. Phys. 18:606 (1991).

7. Low, D.A., Starkschall, G., Bujnowski, S.W., Wang, L.L., and Hogstrom, K.R., "Electron bolus design for radiotherapy treatment planning: Bolus design algorithms," Med. Phys. 19:115-124 (1992).

8. Starkschall, G., Bujnowski, S.W., Wang, L.L., Shiu, A.S., Boyer, A.L., Desobray, G.E., Wells, N.H., Baker, W.L., and Hogstrom, K.R., "A full three-dimensional radiotherapy treatment planning system," Med. Phys. 18:647 (1991a).

9. Starkschall, G., Bujnowski, S.W., Wang, L.L., Low, D.A., and Hogstrom, K.R., "Effect of dimensionality of heterogeneity corrections on the implementation of a three-dimensional electron pencil-beam algorithm," Phys. Med. Biol. 36:207-227 (1991b).

10. Urie, M.M., Goitein, M., and Wagner, M., "Compensating for heterogeneities in proton radiation therapy," Phys. Med. Biol. 29:553-566 (1983).

11. Zhu Y., and Boyer, A.L, "X-ray dose computations in heterogeneous media using 3-dimensional FFT convolution," Phys. Med. Biol. 35:351-368 (1990).

Chapter 26

Stereotactic Radiosurgery: Physical Principles

Robert E. Drzymala, Ph.D.

Washington University School of Medicine, Mallinckrodt Institute of Radiology, St. Louis, Missouri

Stereotactic radiosurgery (7, 12, 26, 28, 30, 31, 37, 43) is a highly accurate radiation treatment technique that involves a multidisciplanary team effort from neurosurgeons, radiation oncologists, radiation physics and radiation oncology staff. Since the appearance of this method around 1950 (28), it has been used to irradiate a wide variety of relatively small brain abnormalities with a single or a limited few treatments of ionizing radiation. The aberrations that are treated can be functional or vascular lesions, as well as tumors (27).

Stereotactic radiosurgery involves procedures and accessories that are not usually employed in conventional radiation therapy. An example is the use of a stereotactic frame that can provide superior patient immobilization and millimeter targeting accuracy for the lesion. Likewise, the technique also requires strict tolerances (< 1mm) for the positioning accuracy of radiations beams. Determining the target volume location and shape is almost exclusively guided by computed tomography (CT), magnetic resonance (MR) or angiography. This contrasts with conventional radiotherapy, in which the target volume is typically obtained using a radiotherapy simulator and radiographs. Furthermore, multiple, small, isocentric beams are used, usually configured as four or more rotational arcs, which can enter the patient through an angular extent of 2π radians.

Taken in their entirety, the methodologies and capabilities of radiosurgery allow one to give a dose distribution that has tight margins around the target volume, thereby conforming to its shape with great accuracy.

Targeting and Imaging

A critical requirement of stereotactic radiosurgery is accurate localization of the target volume and the surrounding tissues. A localizer accessory to stereotactic frame provides the means for defining anatomy of the patient's head within the accurate stereotactic coordinate system (40, 45). The localizer typically appears as fiducial marks in images obtained either by CT, MR or angiography. In some instances, positron emission tomography (PET) has been used to loosely corroborate the location of the lesion and to follow the patient's response after irradiation (39). PET's poor resolution precludes its use as an accurate localization modality, however, and requires spatial correlation of these images with with other imaging modalities, such as CT and MR (34).

Locating the fiducials in an image allows computation of a mathematical relationship that associates the location of any point in the image set to stereotactic frame coordinates. Accuracy at this stage in treatment plan development impacts significantly on the confidence with which one positions treatment beams and designs their shape and extent. Localization accuracy is limited by the geometric accuracy and resolution of the imaging modality employed as well as by the precision and stability of the stereotactic frame. Particular care must be exercised when using MR to locate the patient anatomy. Although MR offers superior contrast for the brain, it has been shown that these images can harbor local geometric distortions (22, 35) which may not be detectable by cursory visual inspection. The overall accuracy and precision of the targeting procedure must be verified prior to clinical implementation of the technique and continually monitored thereafter.

Depending on the type of stereotactic frame can be fitted to the patient either invasively or non-invasively. An invasive frame mounts rigidly by pins fixed into the patient's skull and is attached to the patient throughout imaging and treatment. The Brown-Roberts-Wells[1] (21), the Leksell[2] (29), Fischer[3],Komai[4] and Sugita[5] frames are examples of this type. In contrast, non-invasive stereotactic frames do not pierce the patient's skin, but conform to specific "stable" anatomical features of the head, such as the maxilla, the bridge of the nose and/or the ear canal (8, 16, 18, 19, 25, 32).

The high level of patient immobilization required by stereotactic radiosurgery can be facilitated by the use of the appropriate stereotactic frame. Usually, only the invasive variety provides a direct means to immobilize the patient's head during treatment. Relocatable frames generally require an auxiliary device for immobilization. The relocatable frames are useful, however, in that they are relatively comfortable for the patient to wear. Of various design, they also provide a convenient means to subsequently repositioning the patient for fractionated stereotactic radiotherapy, although fractionation has been performed with an invasive frame as well (42). Relocatable frames are very useful to help monitor and correlate patient response with the volume irradiated during follow up scans.

Methods are currently being developed that involve the use of a 3-D digitizer in order to eliminate the need for a stereotactic frame to define a coordinate system that rely on optical[6], mechanical (47), or acoustical feedback (1) to locate the patient. They offer a flexible approach to monitoring the relative locations of the patient and treatment devices (e.g. linac, surgical probes) in a 3-D coordinate system. The precision of these methods is on the order of 1-2 mm, so these techniques can offer a novel ways to reposition the patient for fractionated treatments in radiation therapy as well as to monitor treatment effectiveness.

Variations of Technique

An assortment of radiation modalities have been used for stereotactic radiosurgery. These include charged particle beams, gamma rays and x-rays. Since the use of charged particles for radiosurgery is confined to only at the few institutions, we will not discuss the use of particle beams further. The reader is referred elsewhere (12, 23) to review the use of this modality in radiosurgery. We will restrict our discussion, henceforth, to photon treatment techniques.

A commercial treatment machine that is dedicated to radiosurgery and is available to the modern clinic is the Leksell Gamma Unit (3, 30). It employs up to 201 cobalt sources arranged in an almost 2π radian arrangement about the vertex of patient's head. Interposed between the patient and cobalt sources, is a large hemispherical helmet that contains a circular collimator for each cobalt source to sharply define beam edges and to center each beam to within 0.1 mm of a fixed point in space. In order to bring the focus of radiation to the correct anatomical location, the patient's head is mechanically translated within the helmet by means of a stereotactic frame.

The Gamma Unit is a relatively simple device, offers exceptional geometrical accuracy, but it's utility is limited to head lesions and it is expensive to install. The dose distribution can be effectively shaped to match the target volume by selectively blocking collimator helmet apertures (13, 48). However, the beam apertures of the Gamma Unit are only circular and limited to 18 mm, so that dose distributions covering larger, irregulaly-shaped targets can be achieved solely by using multiple isocenters. Packing the spherical-shaped dose distributions associated with each isocenter

---

[1] Radionics, Inc., Burlington, MA, BRW stereotaxis system.
[2] Elekta Instuments, AB, Stockholm Sweden, Leksell stereotaxic system.
[3] F.L. Fisher, Ltd., Freiburg, Germany, Convergent Beam Irradiation System.
[4] Mizuho Medical Industry, Inc., Tokyo, Japan, Komai stereotactic system.
[5] Tokai Rika-denki Seisakusho, Inc., Tokyo, Japan, Sugita stereotactic system.
[6] Pixsys, Inc., Pixsys System, Boulder, CO.

when they lie within the target volume and, conversely, high doses in regions where beams overlap in the normal brain parenchyma adjacent to the target or circumscribed by an arterial venous malformation are also undesirable.

Adaptation of a linear accelerator (linac) to radiosurgery can achieve similar dose distributions to the Gamma Unit but permits more flexibility in the treatment technique which may be of greater interest to the radiotherapy community at large. This can be a relatively cost effective approach as well, since the linac may otherwise be used for conventional radiotherapy. With the inherent greater complexity of the linac over the Gamma Unit, however, comes the need for more quality assurance checks in order to maintain the appropriate accuracy and precision of the technique (9, 31, 44, 46). The precision of the final treatment is a direct result of the summation of all targeting, patient alignment and treatment planning errors. Mechanical specifications of the linear accelerator, therefore, must be more stringent than with conventional radiotherapy to minimize isocenter wobble. Irradiation positioning errors typically range from 0.2 mm (14) to 0.5 mm (31), which is slightly greater than that with the Gamma Unit.

There exists a variety of treatment approaches to linac-based stereotactic radiosurgery which range from the use of multiple converging arcs to dynamic therapy. The particular approach taken for radiosurgery was dependent upon goals of treatment and the facilities at each site. The beam configurations for the major techniques employed on the linac fall into five general categories (Figure 26-1). These include single plane rotation, converging arc rotation, dynamic rotation, rotating chair and fixed conformal beam. The orientation of beams is optimized either to avoid critical normal structures and/or to spread the superficial doses over a larger volume. The ultimate goal in planning the configuration of beams is to achieve the greatest therapeutic ratio, that is, to increase dose in the lesion relative to that of the surrounding normal tissue. By varying a beam's trajectory and weight relative to others, one can modify the figure of the isodoses around the lesion. Additionally, the dose distributions can be altered by varying the size and shape of the beam aperture.

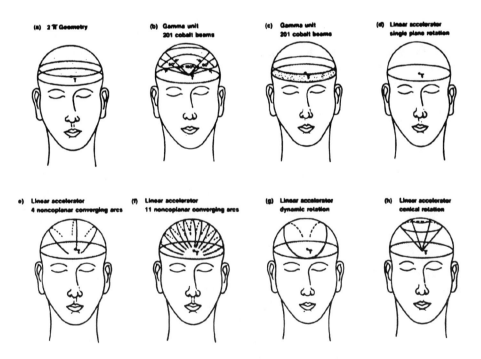

Figure 26-1. *Depicted are the various beam arrangements used for stereotactic radiosurgery. Reprinted with permission: First appeared in Neurosurgery Clinics of North America 3(1): 9-33, 1992.*

Converging Arcs

One of the earliest radiosurgical techniques that employed the megavoltage linac was developed by a group at City Hospital, Vicenza, Italy (6, 7). This approach used 9 to 16 converging arcs. The large number of arcs was necessary since only primary collimator jaws were used to define the rectangular beam apertures employed. By integrating the use of the BRW frame to localize with CT or angiography and to immobilize and position the patient on the linac directly in stereotactic coordinates, a group at the Joint Center, Harvard Medical Schools in Boston, (31) advanced the technique in the U.S.A. Their approach uses 4 converging arcs with secondary circular collimation that is closer to the patient to reduce geometric penumbra. Schell et al. (41) found by analyzing a limited number of cases with dose volume histograms that little improvement is made by using greater than 5-6 arcs.

Improvements in the accuracy of the convergent arc technique continued at the University of Florida (14) by decoupling the stereotactic collimation system from the linac gantry by means of a flexible connection. Moving the collimation to a separate uniquely designed collimator gantry, positioned close to the patient, reduced penumbra and kept the central axis of the beam aperture directed at the isocenter of couch and gantry rotation as the trajectory of a beam is changed. This resulted in less deviation of the beam from the target point in the patient than is typically found for conventional linacs.

Rotating Chair

A somewhat different approach was taken at the Emory Clinic (33) in which a rotating chair was incorporated into the technique. The chair aligns and immobilizes the patient's head in a stationary radiation beam. As the chair is rotated during treatment, the radiation beam delineates a conical rind of dose with its apex at the selected patient target coordinates. The aperture of the radiation beam determines the thickness of the rind. By fixing the gantry at different angles, but directed to the same point in the patient, the higher surface doses are distributed over a larger volume.

Dynamic Rotation

Dynamic radiosurgery was developed at McGill University (37). As the patient rests horizontally, the linac's treatment couch and the gantry are simultaneously rotated during irradiation. The beam traces one continuous path shaped like the seam of a baseball. An advantage to this approach is that the exit of the beam at any one combination of couch and gantry angles is not collinear with another. The result is rapid dosimetric fall-off at the edges of the beam aperture.

Articulated Arm Linac

The Neurotron 5000[7] takes a unique approach to radiosurgery. It employs a 6 MV linac on an articulated arm (Figure 26-2). It employs a unique method of precomputing radiographs that represent views of the patient resulting from small movements and misalignments during treatment. The arm of the linac tries to compensate for these movements to give the programmed isodose shape to the lesion. In a well shielded room, this device has few limitations for beam trajectory as compared with a conventional linac, since gantry motion is not confined to a plane or even to a point of rotation. An advantage to using this linac is that arm motion can be programmed to have different dwell times and movement speeds to shape the dose distributions. Having unconstrained motion, it has the potential to very accurately "paint" the radiation within an irregularly shaped treatment volume without using multiple centers of rotation. Limited to field sizes less than about 10 cm square, this linac can be used for conformal boosts in sites other than the head, thereby preserving cost-savings and utility for the radiotherapy clinic.

---

[7] Accuray, Inc., Neurotron 5000, Santa Clara, CA.

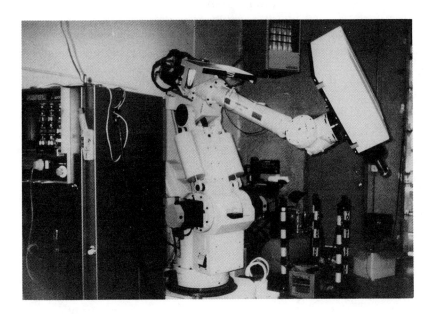

Figure 26-2. *The Neurotron 5000 is a specialized linear accelerator that is available for small field irradiation. It has the unique ability to give a treatment from any angle without moving the patient.*

Shaping Doses on a Linac

Historically, the apertures of stereotactic beams have generally been circular which will give an approximately spherical dose distributions when using multiple converging arcs if the each is weighted to the same dose per degree at a single isocenter. Brain lesions are usually not shaped like spheres, however, and some degree of dose shaping is desirable. Classically, isodose distributions are manipulated by combining the beam trajectories, weights and aperture shapes in various ways (17).

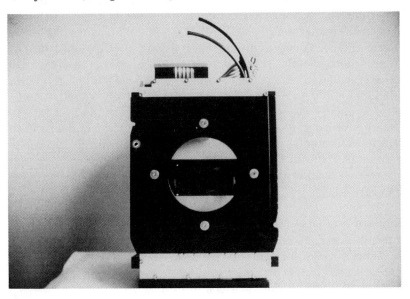

Figure 26-3. *The Peacock System, as shown from looking from the beam-exit side, is a multileaf collimator attachment for the linear accelerator. Although it is general purpose for typical field sizes, it can provide shaping of small radiation fields.*

In an attempt to approach truly 3-D conformal radiosurgery treatments, there has been interest recently in using irregularly shaped apertures to match the boundaries of the target volume. A limited number of static beams, shaped, angled and weighted appropriately, can produce a prescription isodose surface that matches the target shape very closely. Using just a few static beams results in increased dose in tissues, superficial to deep lesions. One solution to the problem rests in determining the minimal number of static beams that must be used to maintain acceptable superficial doses. Another solution is to use shaped beams with rotational arcs. Serago et al. (43) developed a convergent arc technique at the Miami Stereotactic Radiosurgery Center, Baptist Hospital of Miami, in which the shape of the beam aperture is an ellipse fit to the composite shape of the lesion, as seen by the beam. The authors claim better optimized dose distributions using this method compared to that attainable with circular collimators. Attempting to better conform the beam aperture to the shape of the lesion, Leavitt et al. (26) engineered a mechanical collimator that dynamically shapes the beam in accordance with beam's-eye-view of the lesion and linac rotation. The most complex specialized collimator available for radiosurgery to date is the Peacock System[8] Figure 26-3 shows this specialized multileaf collimator which "optimizes" doses within transverse sections of the patient. The ability to manipulate dose distributions within the patient volume using the Peacock System is quite impressive. For a detailed description of this device and its capabilities, the reader is referred to another paper in this series.

Dosimetric Parameters

The beam apertures used in radiosurgery can be very small with sizes ranging from 0.4 mm to 40 mm. As mentioned previously, the use of additional collimation is commonly used to sharpen beam penumbra. Dose gradients at beam edges are typically 7-20% per millimeter (20, 36-38, 48) for a stereotactic treatment. Under these conditions and depending on the energy of the beam, electronic equilibrium may not be achieved for the smaller apertures. One could measure the output of a radiosurgery beam at depths where the beam aperture is large enough to provide electronic equilibrium and relate the ionization at shallower depths relative to this. These problems provides a challenge to measure and quantify the dosimetric characteristics of these beams.

Any dosimeter that is employed to measure these beams must also be small with dimensions significantly less than the beam. Thermoluminescent dosimeters (TLDs), diodes and ionization chambers have been used successfully (2, 5, 36, 38, 46) to measure the necessary beam data: the percent depth dose (PDD), tissue phantom ratio (TPR), profiles, and output factor. Ideally, one wishes to use an appropriately small waterproof ionization chamber because of its energy independence. The typical ionization chamber has dimensions too large, however, while reducing its size is constrained by limited sensitivity. Diodes have relatively sensitive and small active volumes, but their response is energy dependent. Film dosimetry offers the highest resolution and is useful for measuring beam profiles at fixed depth, but again energy dependence limits its convenience for PDD and TPR measurements. Film dosimetry has been used successfully for 3-D relative measurements in small volumes (9). TLDs are available in 1 mm x 1 mm rods and can be use for absolute measurements. A calibration factor for each rod must be determined, however, for accuracy better than a few percent.

Water is the standard tissue-equivalent medium in which one can measure the irradiated volume of the beam. The use of other media, such as solid water or polystyrene, can have advantages when determining a beam's constancy on a periodic basis. Determining the correct dosimetric characteristics of the small beams and maintaining their constancy impacts greatly on the quality of computerized treatment planning and dose computation.

---

[8] Nomos, Corp., Peacock™ System, South Miami, FL.

Computerized Treatment Planning:

Only one FDA approved treatment planning system is currently available for stereotactic radiosurgery, the RSA System.[9] Many other planning systems have been developed in-house, however, (11, 15, 24, 35). Computerized planning can serve to conveniently integrate several aspects of the radiosurgery procedure. These include image retrieval, target localization, setting up the appropriate beam configurations, computing the doses and discriminating between competing treatment plans. In order to be useful, planning software must utilize the functionality of the stereotactic frame and permit an accuracy greater than that usually found in the conventional planning systems.

Stereotaxis

As mentioned earlier, one must be able to compute the mathematical transformations from the patient image(s) to the stereotactic coordinate system. This usually requires digitization of fiducial markers in the images. Selected target points and contoured boundaries of the lesion and normal anatomical structures can then be specified in stereotactic coordinates. The fidelity with which the planning system must represent these points and contours is on the order of a few tenths of a millimeter in order to not degrade the accuracy afforded by the stereotactic frame.

Beam Setup

Beam configuration required for a treatment may be complex with static beams, arcs and/or isocenters, depending on the technique, lesion shape or size and the proximity of adjacent normal structures. A particularly useful feature in a planning system is the ability to define beam aperture and position of a group of beams with one command. For example, using convergent arc technique, multiple arcs are tied together with a common isocenter. It would be convenient if the rotational-arc-beams could be repositioned collectively by moving their isocenter to a new location. Similarly, specifying, in one step, the beam aperture for all arcs associated with an isocenter may be desirable. To carry this idea a bit further, the availability of "standard" beam setup files is useful if they define beam arrangements corresponding to a standard treatment approach or specific treatment protocols.

Dose Computation

Only a simple dose computation need be employed for radiosurgery. Circular beam apertures, having radial symmetry, require only a central axis depth dose and profile measurements in a radial plane at an appropriate number of depths to describe the beam. Furthermore, the relatively homogeneous electron density of the head precludes the need to account for tissue heterogeneity's. Under these conditions an algorithm computing dose employing ratio TAR with an off-axis ratio (RTAR/OAR) correction seems adequate.

Radiosurgery treatments require a significant number of dose point calculations in order to be simulated on the computer with a high degree of spatial accuracy, since one wishes to compute doses on the same order of spatial accuracy ($\sim$ 0.5 mm) as the treatment or better. Rotational arcs are typically approximated by a series of stationary beams that are spaced every 5 or 10 degrees and summed, which depends on the distance of critical structures from the isocenter and the size of the beam aperture. As an example of the number of calculations required, let us do some simple math. For a treatment totaling 560 degrees divided over 4 arcs converging on a single isocenter, such as in the Joint Center technique (31), 60 beams would be used every 10 degrees. Each beam would require about 250,000 dose points to be computed in order to handle the penumbra correctly. The treatment plan would require 15 million dose points for all beams and about 18,000 tri-linear interpolations to fill the dose matrix. It soon becomes obvious that in order for the isodoses to be

---

[9] Radiosurgical and Stereotactic Applications, Inc., Xknife™ Radiosurgery System, Winchester, MA.

computed quickly, one must use either a fast computer, a simple dose computation algorithm or both. The former requirement is satisfied by today's RISC-based UNIX workstations and the latter is satisfied by the use of the RTAR/OAR algorithm without heterogeneity correction. Since "optimization" of the beam configuration for a specific patient with an irregularly shaped lesion is an iterative process, computation times accumulate and can be a significant part to the time-critical planning process. We have employed a RTAR/OAR algorithm on a Silicon Graphics workstation that will compute the 3-D dose distribution for a 4 converging arc treatment in less than 5 minutes.

Displaying Doses

Isodose distributions and patient anatomy can be depicted in many ways. A format that is familiar to the neurosurgeon and the radiation oncologist is the superposition of isodose lines on 2-D images. It allows one to limit attention to a particular image plane without the potential confusion of information overload. MR seems to be preferred by neurosurgeon, because of its superiority of contrast for brain structures and its ability to provide images at high resolution in arbitrary planar views. CT images can be reconstructed into arbitrary planes, but with reduced resolution. The merits of MR versus CT images with respect to spatial fidelity has been discussed earlier.

Depicting 3-D wireframe anatomy with beam trajectories and target points in a room view of the patient can orient the physician for a global overview of the treatment. Visualizing anatomy as 3-D solid surfaces combined with solid, transparent or wire contour dose surfaces, one can determine the location of overdosed or underdosed regions in the target volume and the beams producing them. Interactive treatment planning is important these representations to get a true appreciation for the 3-D spatial relationships.

Combining the different formats on one screen is a most useful approach to understand the dose distribution in the patient. Color Plate 20 shows a multiformat window in which a combination of 2-D and 3-D representations can appear simultaneously.

Comparing Rival Plans

By inspection of 2-D and 3-D isodose distributions, one might arrive at two or more treatment plans that appear, at first glance, to be equivalent. Discerning the differences, merits and shortcomings of one plan relative to the others can be extremely difficult for the non-coplanar 3-D beam configurations that are common to radiosurgery. The amount of dose information that needs to be analyzed is immense. One tool that has been found to be extremely useful is the dose volume histogram (DVH) (4, 10). Without looking at isodose distributions it can show the presence of overdosed and underdosed regions in the irradiated volume by quick inspection of the plot. A major drawback of the DVH is that it contains no spatial information in the plot about the location of the doses. It must be used in combination with 3-D dose distributions in an attempt to understand the full impact of a plan on patient outcome and complications. A DVH screen obtained using the Graphical Plan Evaluation Tool that was developed for the NCI-sponsored Radiotherapy Treatment Planning (RTP) Tools contract[10] appears in color Plate 21. The DVHs show comparisons for two treatment plans. One plan results from using converging arc rotation, the other is from an arrangement of six static conformal beams. Inspection of the DVHs shows the larger volume of brain tissue irradiated to low doses as would be expected for the rotational technique compared to that from the static conformal beams.

---

[10] NCI Contract N01-CM-97564.

Summary

The overall accuracy and precision of state-of-the-art stereotactic radiosurgery depends on each step of computerized planning and its execution in the clinic. This technique differs from conventional radiotherapy in that the treatment is given in one or just a few treatment sessions and that highly accurate targeting apparatus and unusual patient positioning devices are used. An attempt is made to reduce geometrical treatment errors to less than 1 mm which tightens the tolerances for the performance of the linear acelerator, treatment planning and imaging systems. Atypically small beams are used to treat small volumes, usually less than 30 cm^3, with beam edges that are sharply defined by additional collimation close to the patient. The techniques that have been developed are quite varied in their beam configurations and irradiators. Considerable effort has been made in order to shape dose distributions to the treatment volumes and reduce dose to surrounding tissues. Rotational arcs as well as static non-coplanar conformal beams are employed, which require truly 3-D, but rapid computerized treatment planning.

References

1. Barnett, G.H.; Kormos, D.W.; Steiner, C.P.; Weisenberger, J. Intraoperative localization using an armless, frameless stereotactic wand. J. Neurosurg. 78:510-514; 1993.

2. Bjarngard, B.E.; Tsai, J.-S.; Rice, R.K. Doses on the central axes of narrow 6 MV x-ray beams. Med. Phys. 17:794-806; 1990.

3. Bradshaw, J.D. Special report. The stereotactic radiosurgery unit in Sheffield. Clinical Radiol. 37:277-279; 1986.

4. Chen, G.T.Y.; Austin-Seymour, M.; Castro, J.R.; Collier, J.M.; Lyman, J.T.; Pitluck, S.; Saunders, W.M.; Zink, S.R. Dose volume histograms in treatment planning evaluation of carcinoma of the pancreas. In: Eighth International Conference on the Use of Computer in Radiation Therapy. IEEE Computer Society Press; 1984:264-268.

5. Chierego, G.; Marchetti, C.; Avanzo, R.C.; Pozza, F.; Colombo, F. Dosimetric considerations on multiple arc stereotaxic radiotherapy. Radioth. Oncol. 12:141-152; 1988.

6. Colombo, F.; Bendetti, A.; Pozza, F.; Avanzo, R.C.; Chierego, G.; Marchetti, C.; Zanardo, A. Stereotactic external irradiation by linear accelerator. Neurosurg 16:154-160; 1985.

7. Columbo, F.; Benedetti, A.; Pozza, F.; Zanardo, A.; Avanzo, R.C.; Chierego, G.; Marchetti, C. Stereotactic radiosurgery utilizing a linear accelerator. Appl. Neurophysiol. 48:133-145; 1985.

8. Delannes, M.; Daly, N.J.; Bonnet, J.; Sabatier, J.; Tremoulet, M. Fractionated radiotherapy of small inoperable lesions of the brain using a non-invasive stereotactic frame. Int. J. Radiat. Oncol. Biol, Phys. 21:749-755; 1991.

9. Drzymala, R.E. Quality Assurance for linac-based stereotactic radiosurgery. In: Starkschall, G.; Horton, J., Quality Assurance in Radiotherapy Physics. Proceedings of an American College of Medical Physics Symposium. Galveston, TX: Medical Physics Publishing, Madison WI; 1991:121-138.

10. Drzymala, R.E.; Mohan, R.; Brewster, L.; Chu, J.; Goitein, M.; Harms, W.; Urie, M. Dose volume histograms. Int. J. Radiat. Oncol. Biol. Phys. 21:71-78; 1991.

11. Drzymala, R.E.; Narayan, P.; Simpson, J.R.; Rich, K.M.; Klein, E.E.; Wasserman, T.H. A computerized three-dimensional planning system for stereotactic radiosurgery. In: Lunsford, L.D., Stereotactic Radiosurgery Update. Pittsburgh, PA: Elsevier, New York; 1991:251-256.

12. Fabrikant, J.I.; Lyman, J.T.; Hosobuchi, Y. Stereotactic heavy-ion Bragg peak radiosurgery for intra-cranial vascular disorders: Method for treatment of deep arteriovenous malformations. Br. J. Radiol. 57:479-490; 1984.

13. Flickinger, J.C.; Maitz, A.; Kalend, A.; Lundsford, L.D.; Wu, A. Treatment volume shaping with selective beam blocking using the Leksell Gamma Unit. Int. J. Radiat. Oncol. Biol. Phys. 19:783-789; 1990.

14. Friedman, W.A.; Bova, F.J. The University of Florida radiosurgery system. Surg Neurol 32:334-342; 1989.

15. Gehring, M.A.; Mackie, T.R.; Kubsad, S.S.; Paliwal, B.R.; Mehta, M.P.; Kinsella, T.J. A three-dimensional volume visualization package aplied to stereotactic radiosurgery treatment planning. Int. J. Radiat. Oncol. Biol. Phys. 21:491-500; 1991.

16. Gill, S.S.; Thomas, D.G.T.; Warrington, A.P.; Brada, M. Relocatable frame for stereotactic external beam radiotherapy. Int. J. Rad. Oncol. Biol. Phys. 20:599-603; 1991.

17. Goitein, M.; Laughlin, J.; Purdy, J.A.; Sontag, M.; al., e. State-of-the-art of external photon beam radiation treatment planning. Int. J. Radiat. Oncol. Biol. Phys. 21:9-23; 1991.

18. Graham, J.D.; Warrington, A.P.; Gill, S.S.; Brada, M. A non-invasive, relocatable stereotactic frame for fractionated radiotherapy and multiple imaging. Radiotherapy and Oncology 21:60-62; 1991.

19. Hariz, M.I.; Henriksson, R.; Lofroth, P.; Laitinen, L.V.; Saterborg, N. A non-invasive method for fractionated stereotactic irradiation of brain tumors with linear accelerator. Radiother. Oncol. 17:57-72; 1990.

20. Hartmann, G.H.; Schlegel, W.; Sturm, V.; Kober, B.; Pastyr, O.; Lorenz, W.J. Cerebral radiation surgery using moving field irradiation at a linear accelerator facility. Int. J. Radiat. Oncol. Biol. Phys. 11:1185-1192; 1985.

21. Heilbrun, M.P.; Roberts, T.S.; Apuzza, M.L.J.; Wells, T.H.; Sabsin, J.K. Preliminary experience with Brown-Roberts-Wells computerized tomograph stereotaxic guidance system. J. Neurosurg 59:217-220; 1983.

22. Henkelman, R.M.; Poon, P.Y.; Bronskill, M.J. Is magnetic resonance imaging useful for radiation therapy planning? In: I. Proceedings of Eighth International Conference on the Use of Computers in Radiation Therapy. Toronto, Canada: IEEE Computer Society; 1984:181-185.

23. Kjellberg, R.N. Stereotactic Bragg peak photon beam radiosurgery for cerebral arteriovenous malformations. Ann. Clin. Res. 18:17-19; 1986.

24. Kooy, H.M.; Nedzi, L.A.; Loeffler, J.S.; Alexander III, E.; Cheng, C.-W.; Mannarino, E.G.; Holupka, E.J.; Siddon, R.L. Treatment planning for stereotactic radiosurgery of intra-cranial lesions. Int J. Radiat. Oncol. Biol. Phys. 21:683-693; 1991.

25. Laitinen, L.V. Non-invasive multipurpose stereoadapter. Neurol. Res. 9:137-141; 1987.

26. Leavitt, D.D.; Gibbs, F.A.; Heilbrun, M.P.; Moeller, J.H.; Takach, G.A. Dynamic field shaping to optimize stereotactic radiosurgery. Int. J. Radiat. Oncol. Biol. Phys. 21:1247-1255; 1991.

27. Leksell, D.G. Stereotactic radiosurgery. Present status and future trends. Neruological Research 9:60-68; 1987.

28. Leksell, L. The stereotaxic method and radiosurgery of the brain. Acta. Chir. Scand. 102:316-319; 1951.

29. Leksell, L.; Jernberg, B. Stereotaxis and tomography. Acta Neurochurg. 52:1-7; 1980.

30. Lunsford, L.D.; Flickinger, J.; Lindner, G.; Maitz, A. Stereotactic radiosurgery of the brain using the first United States 201 cobalt-60 source Gamma Knife. Neurosurgery 24:151-159; 1989.

31. Lutz, W.; Winston, K.R.; Maleki, N. A system for stereotactic radiosurgery with a linear accelerator. Int. J. Radiat. Oncol. Biol. Phys. 14:373-381; 1988.

32. Lyman, J.T.; Phillips, M.H.; Frankel, K.A.; Fabrikant, J.I. Stereotactic frame for neuroradiology and charged particle Bragg peak radiosurgery of intracrantial disorders. Int. J. Radiat. Oncol. Biol. Phys. 16:1615-1621; 1989.

33. McGinley, P.H.; Butker, E.K.; Crocker, I.R.; Landry, J.C. A patient rotator for stereotactic radiosurgery. Phys. Med. Biol. 35:649-657; 1990.

34. Pelizzari, C.A.; Chen, G.T.; Halpern, H.; Chen, C.T.C., M.D. Three-correlation of PET, CT and MRI images. J. Nucl. Med 28:528; 1987.

35. Peters, T.M.; Clark, J.A.; Pike, G.B.; Collins, H.L.; Leksell, D.; Jeppsson, O. Stereotactic neurosurgery planning on a personalcomputer-based workstation. J. Digit Imaging 2:75-81; 1989.

36. Pike, G.B.; Pdogorsak, E.B.; Peters, T.M.; Pla, C.; Olivier, A.; Souhami, L. Dose distributions in radiosurgery. Med. Phys. 17:296-309; 1990.

37. Podgorsak, E.B.; Olivier, A.; Pla, M.; Lefebvre, P.-Y.; Hazel, J. Dynamic stereotactic radiosurgery. Int. J. Radiat. Oncol. Biol. Phys. 14:115-126; 1988.

38. Rice, R.K.; Hansen, J.L.; Svensson, G.K.; Siddon, R.L. Measurement of dose distributions in small beams of 6 MV x-rays. Phys. Med. Biol. 32:1087-1099; 1987.

39. Rich, K.M.; Griffeth, L.K.; Dehdashti, F.; Drzymala, R.E.; Klein, E.E.; Feigenbutz, J.E.; Simpson, J.R.; Wasserman, T.H. The role of FDG-PET scan in the imaging of malignant CNS tumors after stereotactic radiosurgery. In: Lunsford, L.D., Stereotactic Radiosurgery Update. Pittsburgh, PA: Elsevier, New York; 1991:411-413.

40. Saw, W.M.; Winston, K.R.; Siddon, R.L.; et, a. Coordinate transformations and calculation of the angular and depth parameters for a stereotactic system. Med. Phys. 14:1042-1044; 1987.

41. Schell, M.C.; Smith, V.; Larson, D.A.; Wu, A.; Flickinger, J.C. Evaluation of radiosurgery techniques with cumulative dose volume histograms in LINAC-based stereotactic external beam irradiation. Int. J. Radiat. Oncol. Biol. Phys. 20:1325-1330; 1991.

42. Schwade, J.G.; Houdek, P.V.; Landy, H.J.; Bujnoski, J.L.; Lewin, A.A.; Abitol, A.A.; Serago, C.F.; Fisciotta, V.J. Small-field stereotactic external-beam radiation therapy of intracranial lesions: Fractionated treatment with a fixed-halo imobilization device. Radiology 176:563-565; 1990.

43. Serago, C.F.; Lewin, A.A.; Houdek, P.V.; Gonzales-Arias, S.; Abitbol, A.A.; Marcial-Vega, V.A.; Pisciotti, V.; Schwade, J.G. Improved linac dose distributions for radiosurgery with elliptically shaped fields. Int. J. Radiat. Oncol, Biol. Phys. 21:1321-1325; 1991.

44. Serago, C.F.; Lewin, A.A.; Houdek, P.V.; Gonzalez-Arias, S.; Hartmann, G.H.; Abitbol, A.A.; Schwade, J.G. Stereotactic target point verification of an x ray CT localizer. Int. J. Radiat. Oncol. Biol. Phys. 20:517-523; 1991.

45. Siddon, R.L.; Barth, N.H. Stereotaxic location of intracranial targets. Int. J. Radiat. Oncol. Biol. Phys. 13:1241-1246; 1987.

46. Tsai, J.S.; Buck, B.A.; Svensson, G.K.; Alexander, E.; Cheng, C.W.; Mannarino, E.G.; Loeffler, J.S. Quality assurance in stereotaxic radiosurgery using a standard linear accelerator. Int. J. Radiat. Oncol. Biol. Phys. 21:737-748; 1991.

47. Watanabe, E.; Mayanagi, Y.; Kosugi, Y.; Manaka, S.; Takakura, K. Open surgery assisted by the Neuronavigator, a stereotactic articulated sensiive arm. Neurosurgery 28:792-800; 1991.

48. Wu, A.; Lindner, G.; Maitz, A.H.; Kalend, A.M.; Lunsford, L.D.; Flickinger, J.C.; Bloomer, W.D. Physics of Gamma Knife approach on convergent beams in stereotactic radiosurgery. Int J. Radiat. Oncol. Biol. Phys. 18:941-949; 1990.

Chapter 27

Stereotactic External Beam Irradiation (SEBI) with a Linear Accelerator: The Washington University Experience[1]

Joseph R. Simpson, M.D, Keith M. Rich, M.D., Robert E. Drzymala, Ph.D., Todd H. Wasserman, M.D., Eric A. Klein, M.S., Martha L. Michaletz, R.T.T., C.M.D., and Janet Maurath, R.T.T.

Radiation Oncology Center and Neurosurgery Department, Washington University School of Medicine, Jewish Hospital of St. Louis, St. Louis, Missouri

In February 1989, a method of treating small intracranial lesions with a modified Varian 6 MV linear accelerator and special treatment collimators was initiated. It was modeled on the technique published from the Joint Center for Radiation Therapy in Boston.[13] The fundamental requirement of stereotactic external beam irradiation is the ability to plan and deliver doses to a precisely identified target. This requires identification of the target within a well-defined stereotactic space which can be reproduced in the treatment targeting and dose delivery process. The problem has been resolved by the use of a stereotactic headframe, e.g., the Brown-Roberts-Wells (BRW) stereotactic frame, which can be used with both CT and angiography. An angiography localizing box is added for treatment of arteriovenous malformations. A separate BRW frame, compatible with MR (non-ferromagnetic), is used for this imaging modality. The frames are each able to define the target points precisely to within 1 mm accuracy compared with their actual locations. The linear accelerator used for treatment should have an isocenter that similarly remains within 1 mm as it traverses its required arcs for dose delivery. The base ring assembly must also precisely set up the target points in the treatment room as obtained from the CT, MR, or angiogram images. The verification of each of these steps was carried out in extensive physics testing of our system prior to its first use. This paper summarizes the development of our 3-D treatment planning system and initial clinical experience with 103 patients with a variety of CNS lesions.

Materials and Methods

Patients were referred for evaluation for SEBI with recurrent tumors, primary or metastatic, which were ≤4.5 cm in maximum diameter and where additional surgical therapy was not advisable in the opinion of the referring and consulting neurosurgeons and radiation oncologists. Patients with AVM's ≤4.5 cm, located in inoperable locations, who refused surgery, or following partial occlusion with embolization(s), were also offered SEBI. There were 99 adult patients and 4 children (under 16 years of age) treated. Four adult patients (two male and two female) were treated on two occasions. There were thus 64 male and 43 female patients. Up to three lesions at a given session could be treated although most patients had a single lesion irradiated. The beam arrangement usually consisted of four to eight non-coplanar arcs intersecting at the isocenter of the linear accelerator. The isocenter was always within 1 mm on verification filming prior to patient treatment. Figure 27-1 shows a photograph of a patient in the treatment position. A quality assurance protocol was performed on each treatment day to verify the continued accuracy of the isocenter localization from the 3-dimensional imaging space to the treatment location at the isocenter of the linac and the constancy of the accelerator isocenter targeting throughout the required arcs. This protocol has been previously described.[1]

---

[1] Key Words: Radiosurgery, 3D treatment planning.

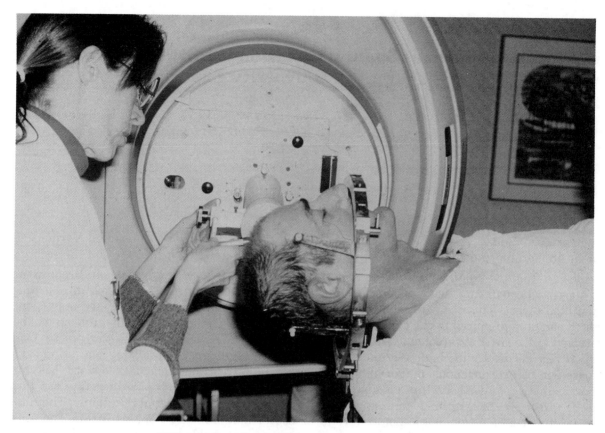

Figure 27-1. Patient in treatment position

Our first treatments were performed based on prior experimental verification of targeting, but without the ability to prospectively visualize the treatment isodoses in all three dimensions. These initial treatments, delivered to patients with recurrent brain metastases or malignant gliomas, helped to clinically verify the accuracy of our system. Subsequently, our 3-D treatment planning capability has evolved from initially using a combination of a commercially available 2-D treatment planning computer modified for 3-D planning (Modulex, Computer Medical Systems, St. Louis, MO) along with a Microvax II (Digital Equipment Corp.), and a real time display computer system (MMSX, developed by the Washington University Computer System Laboratory).[2] We next adapted the system utilizing Macintosh compatible software made available from the University of Arizona treatment planning group, which allowed calculation of isodose on all three orthogonal axes, which could then be overlaid on the images from the CT or MR scans. Finally, computer enhancements were developed in-house allowing transfer of images directly to a Silicon Graphics Iris work station, where contouring of targets on successive MR images, and computation of dose and its display in real time was possible, such that alternative isocenters and beam weightings could be evaluated prior to patient treatment. The analysis of treatment plans is further enhanced by the ability to produce dose volume histograms for both target tissues and normal surrounding tissues of interest. We are currently in the process of developing a Figure of merit scoring system which will hopefully facilitate systematic evaluation of alternative beam arrangements and geometries.

All patients underwent imaging studies either with angiography, CT, MR, or both angiography and MR, while wearing a BRW stereotactic frame and treatment was delivered on the same day. Treatment was carried out following completion of the quality assurance protocol and treatment planning. The stereotactic frame was removed immediately after delivery of the planned dose and patients were observed overnight prior to discharge. Treatment cone sizes ranged from 10 mm to 35 mm. The doses of irradiation were chosen to reflect the projected 1-3% risk of necrosis, which depends on field size.[3,4,6] The range of doses used in this series varied from 1200 to 3000 cGy in a single fraction calculated at the 50 to 90% isodose line. This resulted in maximum doses within the treated volumes of 1500 to 4500 cGy. The categories and number of patients treated in each category are shown in Table 27-1.

Table 27-1. Patient Type

Diagnosis	Number	Sex	
		M	F
Anaplastic Astrocytoma	7	4	3
Acoustic Neuroma/Schwannoma	9	6	3
Arteriovenous Malformation	16	9	7
Glioblastoma Multiforme	14	9	5
Juvenile Pilocytic Astrocytoma	4	3	1
Meningioma	3	1	2
Metastatic	41	23	18
Miscellaneous	11	8	3
Pituitary	2	1	1
Total	107	64	43

Results

The end point for assessing treatment outcome differed depending on lesion type. For AVM's, it was obliteration of the nidus on follow-up angiography. This study has been performed in 14 of 22 patients to date. Figure 27-2 shows an example of a before and after arteriogram for a patient with a 3.2 cm AVM of the posterior frontal lobe treated to 1800 cGy at the 80% isodose line using a 35 mm collimator. At one year follow-up, there is no residual AVM visualized. Tumor endpoints were either the disappearance of a lesion on follow-up MR or CT, or lack of growth on serial studies. Patients with malignant disease also showed significant responses to stereotactic external beam therapy. Figure 27-3 shows a before and after CT scan for a patient with several brain metastases treated with whole brain irradiation plus a stereotactic boost to two of the larger lesions. The scan remained normal for over one year following treatment. Figure 27-4 shows a CT scan of a patient with an acoustic schwannoma before and 7 months following SEBI with 1500 cGy at 90% using a 25 mm cone. Our longest survivor with a recurrent malignant glioma is a man who had a glioblastoma multiforme and was treated for relapse three months after initial therapy with surgery and irradiation plus BCNU. He is now 24 months following stereotactic irradiation and continuing to work and function normally. Therapy was generally quite well tolerated. Four patients with seizure history experienced transient increases in seizure frequency within 24 hours of treatment. One patient with a recurrent acoustic neuroma developed a persistent facial nerve palsy several months after treatment. One patient with a large recurrent glioblastoma multiforme developed an increasing mass on follow-up CT scanning and was reoperated with a finding of radiation necrosis and no viable tumor.

With MR based treatment planning, targets very close to critical locations could be evaluated and treatment selected with clearer recognition of potential side effects. Figure 27-5 shows an example of isodoses displayed on MR images. We have been gratified that patients treated to lesions close to the optic chiasm or in the brain stem have tolerated treatment without side effects.

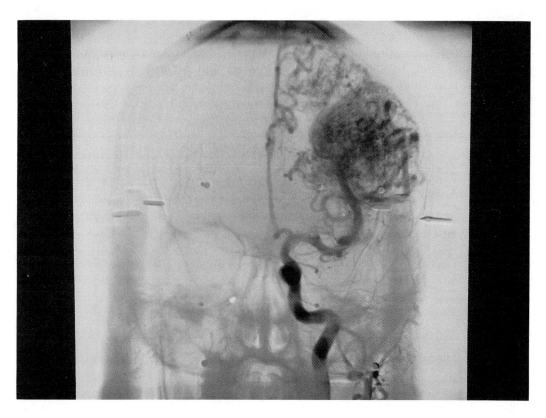

Figure 27-2a.

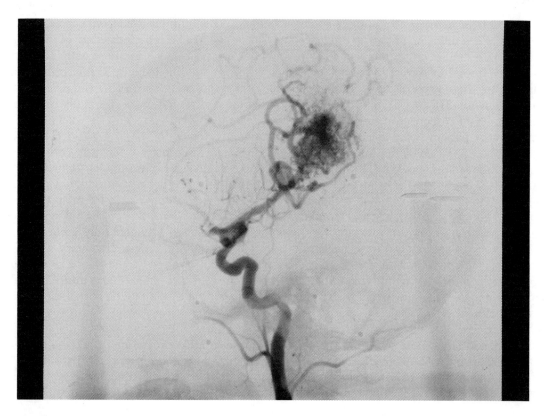

Figure 27-2b.

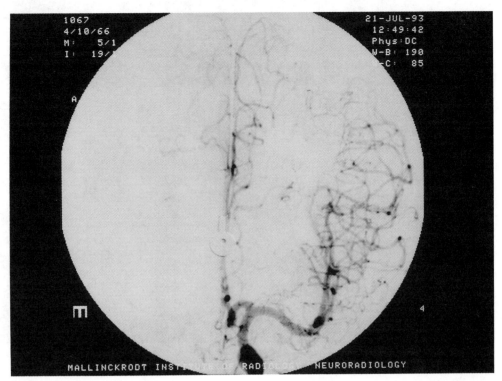

Figure 27-2c.

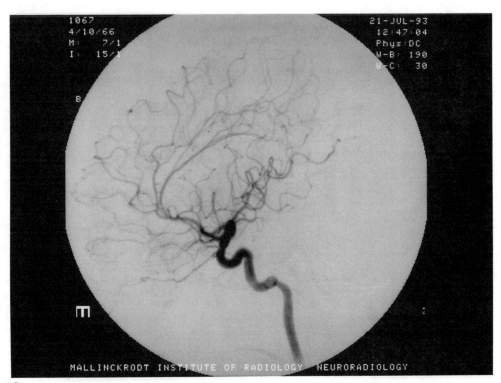

Figure 27-2d.

Figure 27-2.   *Arteriograms: (a,b) before and (c,d) after treatment with 1800 cGy at 80% isodose line using 3.5 cm cone.*

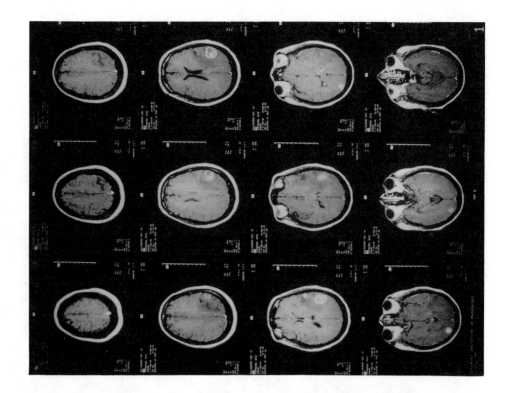

Figure 27-3a.

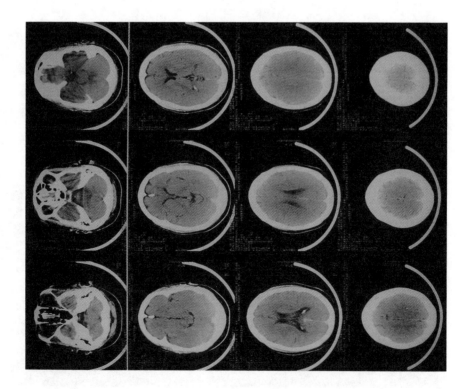

Figure 27-3b.

Figure 27-3. *MR scan (a) before and CT scan (b) after treatment of brain metastases with 2500 cGy at 80% isodose line using 3 cm cone and 3500 cGy whole brain.*

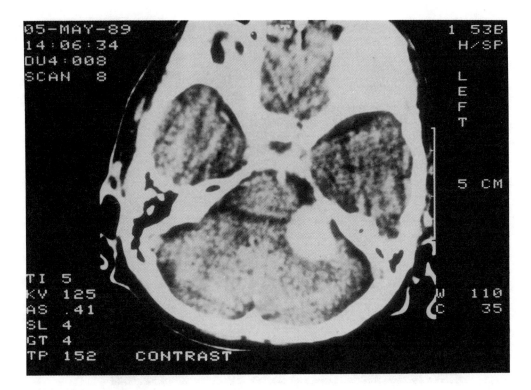

Figure 27-4a.

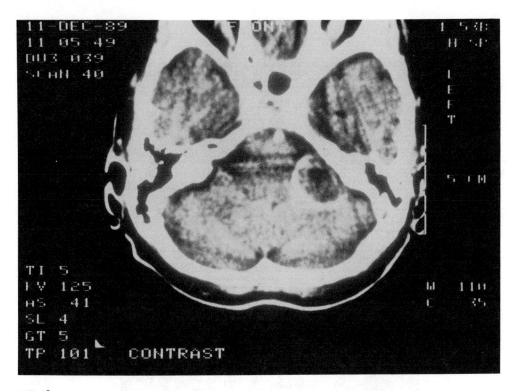

Figure 27-4b.

Figure 27-4.   *CT scans of acoustic schwannoma (a) before and 7 months (b) following treatment with 1500 cGy at 90% isodose line using 2.5 cm cone.*

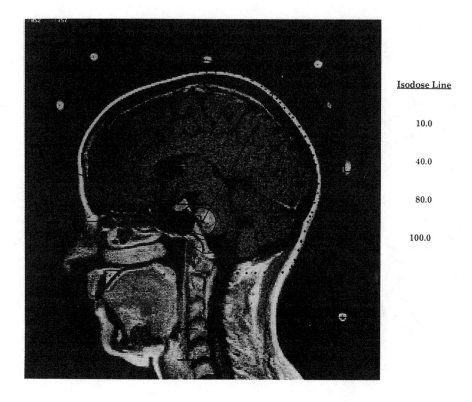

Isodose Line

10.0

40.0

80.0

100.0

Figure 27-5a.

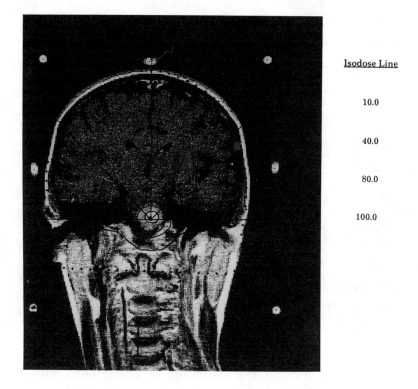

Isodose Line

10.0

40.0

80.0

100.0

Figure 27-5b.

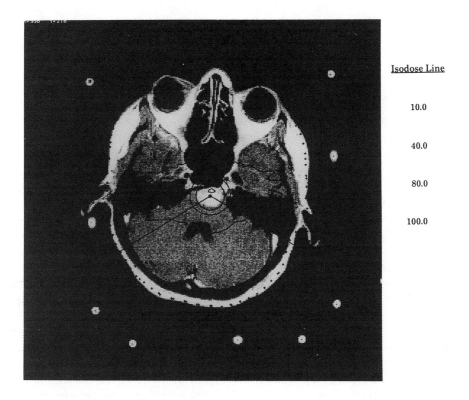

Isodose Line

10.0

40.0

80.0

100.0

Figure 27-5c.

Figure 27-5.   *Isodose curves shown on magnetic resonance images (a) sagittal, (b) coronal and (c) axial.*

Discussion

While the efficacy of SEBI in treating AVM's has been well established,[6,9,10,11] the concept of managing tumors,[12] both primary and metastatic, initially and at recurrence, is of more recent vintage in the United States.[7] Benign tumors such as meningiomas and acoustic neuromas, which displace rather than infiltrate normal brain tissue, may be particularly suitable for treatment with SEBI.[8] There have, however, been reports from both here[10,11,12] and abroad,[9] suggesting that SEBI might provide significant advantages over other therapies in both primary and metastatic malignant tumors as well. A dose-seeking trial is currently being carried out nationally by the Radiation Therapy Oncology Group (RTOG 90-05) in an effort to determine maximum tolerated dose of SEBI therapy in a multi-institutional group-wide setting, using either a gamma unit or linear accelerator. Encouraging pilot studies of this treatment in primary brain tumor management have also been reported.[12] Our experience has confirmed other reports of SEBI efficacy for metastases and AVM's as well as some recurrent malignant gliomas. Our experience with positron emission tomography suggests that this modality may help predict outcome of SEBI treatment in certain patients with metastatic disease.[5] The successive enhancements of our 3-D treatment planning system have allowed delivery of treatment to proceed with confidence and efficiency. Suitable lesions would be ≤4.5 cm. in greatest diameter and located in areas where excessive dose to critical normal structures could be avoided. We conclude that this treatment offers potential for improving treatment results for several groups of patients with circumscribed brain tumors and vascular malformations. In addition, the experience in three dimensional treatment planning and dose delivery, as well as more precise patient set up, may well yield improvement in techniques and strategies used in conventional radiation therapy.

Acknowledgements

The authors gratefully acknowledge the computer programming efforts of Prithvi Narayan, M.S.

References

1. Drzymala, RE. Quality assurance for linac-based stereotactic radiosurgery Proceedings of an American College of Medical Physics Symposium. Galveston, TX: Medical Physics Publishing, Madison, WI; 1991:121-138.

2. Drzymala, RE; Narayan, PI; Simpson, J.R.; Rich, K.M.; Klein E.E.; Wasserman, T.H. A computerized three-dimensional planning system for stereotactic radiosurgery. Lunsford, L.D. (ed.)., In. Stereotactic Radiosurgery Update., Proceedings of the International Stereotactic Radiosurgery Symposium, Pittsburgh, PA, 1991. Elsevier Science Publishing Co. Inc.; New York.

3. Flickinger, J.C.; Lunsford, L.D.; Kondziolka, D.; Maitz, A.H.; Epstein, A.H.; Simons, S.R.; Wu, A. Radiosurgery and brain tolerance: An analysis of neurodiagnostic imaging changes after gamma knife radiosurgery for arteriovenous malformations. Int. J. Radiat. Oncol. Biol. Phys. 25:19-25;1993.

4. Flickinger, J.C. An integrated logistic formula for prediction of complications from radiosurgery. Int. J. Radiat. Oncol. Biol. Phys. 17:879-885; 1989.

5. Griffeth, L.K.; Rich, K.M.; Dehdashti, F.; Simpson, J.R.: Fusselman, M.J.; McGuire, A.H.; Siegel, B.A. Brain metastases from non-central nervous system tumors: Evaluation with PET. Radiology 186:37-44, 1993.

6. Kjellberg, R.N. Stereotactic bragg peak proton beam radiosurgery for cerebral arteriovenous malformations. Ann. Clin. Res. Suppl. 47:17-19; 1986.

7. Larson, D.A.;Wasserman, T.H.; Drzymala, R.E.;Simpson, J.R. Stereotactic External-Beam Irradiation. In: Principles and Practice of Radiation Oncology, 2nd Edition, Perez, C.A. and Brady, L.W. , eds., Philadelphia, PA: Lippincott Co.; 1992:553-563.

8. Larson, D.A.; Flickinger, J.C.; Loeffler, J.S. The radiobiology of radiosurgery. Int. J. Radiat. Oncol. Biol. Phys. 25:557-561, 1993.

9. Leksell, D.G. Stereotactic radiosurgery: Present status and future trends. Neurological Research 9:60-68, 1987.

10. Loeffler , J.S.; Alexander, E.; Alexander, E., III; Siddon, R.L.; Saunders, W.M.; Winston , K.R.; Coleman, C.N.; Black, P.M. Stereotactic radiosurgery for intracranial arteriovenous malformations using a standard linear accelerator. Int. J. Radiat. Oncol. Biol. Phys. 17:673-677, 1989.

11. Loeffler, J.S.; Siddon, R.L.; Wen, P.Y.; Nedzi, L.A.; Alexander, E. Stereotactic radiosurgery of the brain using a standard linear accelerator: A study of early and late effects. Radiother. & Oncol. 17:311-321, 1990.

12. Loeffler, J.S.; Alexander, E.; Shea, M.; Wen, P.Y.; Fine, H.A.; Kooy, H.M.; Black, P. McL. Radiosurgery as part of the initial management of patients with malignant gliomas. J. Clin. Oncol. 10:1379-1385; 1992.

13. Lutz, W.; Winston, K.R.; Maleki, N. A system for stereotactic radiosurgery with a linear accelerator. Int. J. Radiat. Oncol. Biol. Phys. 14:373-381, 1988.

Chapter 28

Three-Dimensional Dose Calculation in Brachytherapy

Jeffrey F. Williamson, Ph.D.

Mallinckrodt Institute of Radiology, Washington University School of Medicine, St. Louis, Missouri

Three-dimensional (3-D) dose calculation, as defined in this chapter, is an emerging area of research in brachytherapy dosimetry. A dose-calculation algorithm is 3-D if it accounts for dependence of the scattered photon dose-distribution on the 3-D geometric structure of the source, any applicator or local shielding heterogeneities, and heterogeneities in tissue composition. The widely-used Sievert integral model is a one-dimensional (1-D) rather than a 3-D algorithm. In this model, both the scattered- and primary-photon dose components contributed by each volume element (See Figure 28-1) are functions only of the thicknesses of active source, capsule and other non-water media intersected by the primary photon flight path connecting the source element and the point of interest. In a 3-D calculation, the scatter dose contribution depends on the cross-sectional area and location of any nontissue-like object in proximity of the source.

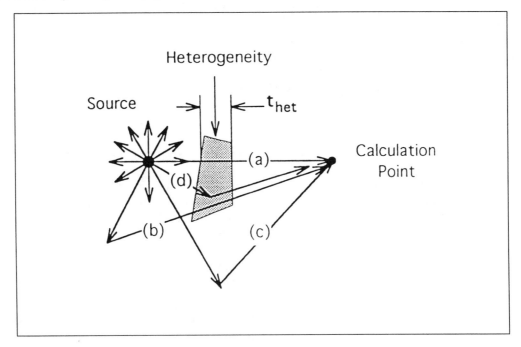

Figure 28-1. *Schematic illustration of 1- and 3-D treatment of an irregular bounded heterogeneity by the underlying dose-calculation algorithm. In a 1-D algorithm, the perturbing effect of the heterogeneity is a function only of the thickness of heterogeneous algorithm, t_{het}, traversed by primary photon flight paths between the source and the point of interest. The fraction of scattering volume screened by the scattered-photon dose contributed by the heterogeneity (trajectories c and d) and its effect on the multiple-scattered photon dose component (trajectory d) are ignored. These effects, which depend on heterogeneity size, shape and location as well as thickness, are treated by 3-D algorithms.*

Interest in 3-D dose calculation is being driven by several current developments in clinical brachytherapy including:

(1) A growing emphasis on physical optimization of the dose distribution a means of improving clinical efficacy of brachytherapy. In high dose-rate (HDR) brachytherapy, the loss of therapeutic ratio characteristic of low dose-rate brachytherapy must be balanced by additional dose sparing of critical normal tissues. Image-based 3-D treatment planning (Ling et al. 1987, Schoeppel et al. 1993) bases dose specification on a 3-D quantitative geometric model of the target volume and any dose-limiting normal tissues. Both of these treatment modalities allow for varying physical parameters, such as source locations and strengths, in order to optimize the tradeoff between target volume coverage and irradiation of dose-limiting normal tissues.

(2) Intensive investigation of the dose perturbations arising from applicator shielding, inter-source and -applicator attenuation, and variations in tissue density and composition. These investigations demonstrate that the resultant dose distributions often have a complex dependence on the size, shape and relative locations of the heterogeneity, source and calculation point which cannot be accurately modelled by 1-D heterogeneity corrections.

(3) Development of new low-energy isotopes for brachytherapy, including ^{103}Pd, ^{241}Am, ^{143}Sm, and ^{169}Yb, with photon energies in the range of 23-100 keV (Williamson 1995). Conventional 1-D dose calculation models breakdown in this energy range. A major rationale for investigating many of these sources is the ease with which sensitive tissues can be shielded from low-energy photons.

(4) Validation of brachytherapy dose measurement and Monte Carlo photon-transport simulation as accurate and reliable tools for characterizing brachytherapy dose distributions. These dosimetry tools have made possible investigation dosimetric characterization of low-energy brachytherapy sources as well as tissue and applicator heterogeneities. These experiences have made clear the limitations of the universally-used 1-D Sievert models.

Collectively, these developments constitute a significant departure from the conventional approach to brachytherapy dosimetry. Historically, brachytherapy treatment techniques, dose prescriptions, and knowledge of normal-tissue and tumor dose-response relationships have evolved empirically, guided by observed control and complication rates in large groups of patients treated in a uniform fashion over many years. This evolutionary dynamic placed relatively little emphasis on physically-accurate dose computation and 'physics-based' optimization, especially in gynecological brachytherapy. Prior to 1980, treatment planning and dosimetric evaluation of brachytherapy had changed relatively little since the introduction of afterloading techniques and new reactor-produced radium substitutes such as ^{137}Cs and ^{192}Ir in the 1950's and early 1960's. With the exception of ^{125}I interstitial sources, the armamentarium of brachytherapy sources and techniques was relatively stable. Dose distributions were calculated by superposition, which approximates dose at a point by the sum of contributions from each source. Each source contribution was estimated from a single-source dose matrix, usually derived from simple semi-empirical models such as the Sievert integral (Sievert 1921, Young and Batho, 1964). These models assumed unbounded water medium and accounted only for oblique filtration of primary photons by the source capsule. Heterogeneities were ignored, including tissue-composition and density variations, applicator attenuation and shielding effects, air-tissue interfaces and inter-source and -applicator shielding effects. Direct measurement of absorbed dose near brachytherapy sources, using thermoluminescent dosimeters, radiographic film, solid-state detectors or small ion chambers was relatively rare even in the research laboratory and had little impact on clinical practice.

In contrast to the traditional 'minimalist' philosophy of brachytherapy physics, interest in the current developments, listed above, is motivated by the premise that physical and radiobiological optimization of implant therapy can improve clinical outcome. Accurate, prospective and reasonably rapid estimation of dose-rate distributions, often in the presence of tissue and applicator heterogeneities, is essential to each of these developments.

The goal of this paper is to review the current state of brachytherapy dose-calculation algorithms. We begin by reviewing what is known of the dosimetric effects of shielding and tissue heterogeneities on single-source dose distributions. The next section reviews the current status of empirical and theoretical brachytherapy dosimetry techniques. Finally, emerging trends in brachytherapy dose-calculation algorithm development are reviewed.

Dosimetry of Tissue and Shielding Heterogeneities

In contrast to external beam, comparatively little work has been done either to empirically characterize dose in heterogeneous brachytherapy geometries or to develop clinically-useful heterogeneity-correction algorithms. Commercially-available treatment planning programs almost universally ignore heterogeneities such as air-tissue interfaces, local tungsten shielding in vaginal applicators, and tissue-composition variations in ^{125}I seed implants despite the fact that such heterogeneities may perturb dose by as much as 50% (Dale 1983, Williamson 1990). Fortunately, this topic has received increasing attention over the last 10 years. In this section, the published literature dealing with brachytherapy heterogeneity effects will be briefly reviewed and number of new approaches to dose-calculation in heterogeneous geometries discussed.

The most extensively-studied heterogeneity effect is the influence of shielded gynecological colpostats on ^{137}Cs dose distributions. Both experimental studies (Ling 1984, Meertens 1985, Mohan 1985, Saylor 1976 and Weeks 1990) and Monte Carlo calculations (Williamson 1990) show that applicator shielding reduces doses by as much as 50% for a single applicator (Figure 28-2). For typical clinical combinations of applicators, dose computation by superposition, which accounts only for source filtration, overestimates doses at bladder and rectal reference points by 12-25% (Williamson 1990, Ling 1984).[1] One-dimensional algorithms (Van der Laarse 1984 and Weeks 1990) have been developed which apply effective path-length attenuation corrections to those primary photons passing through the high-density applicators or shields. These approaches, reviewed in detail below, ignore shield size and location which significantly influence the dose distribution, especially for low- and medium-energy sources. An alternative approach, described by Mohan et al. (1985) uses a 3-D relative dose matrix measured about a single applicator, using a silicon diode detector, directly in treatment planning. However, all of these methods have serious limitations. Purely empirical approaches can not be used to optimize shielding or applicator design without constructing a prototype at each iteration of the design cycle. The 1-D computational approaches require extensive comparison with Monte Carlo or measured data before they can yield accurate dose estimates for a given source-heterogeneity combination.

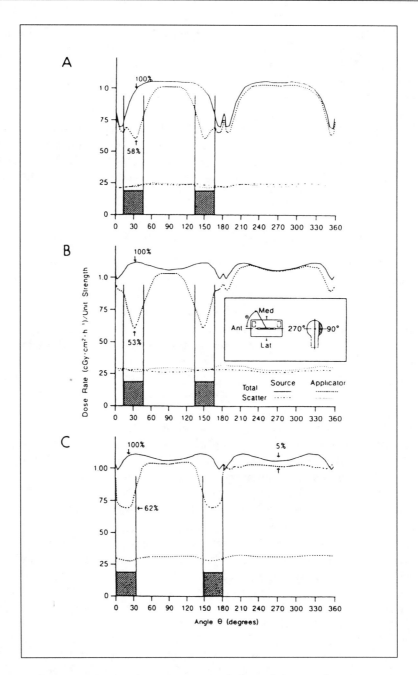

Figure 28-2   *Angular dose profiles in the transverse planes of three colpostat-source combinations containing sources of air-kerma strength 1 $\mu Gy \cdot m^2 \cdot h^{-1}$.*

A = Fletcher-Suit rectangular-handled colpostat loaded with a 226 Ra tube (1 mm Pt)

B = Fletcher-Suit rectangular-handled colpostat loaded with a ^{137}Cs tube

C = 3M Fletcher-Suit-Delclos colp[ostat loaded with a ^{137}Cs tube

The total and scattered dose rates (multiplied by a distance squared) are plotted as a function angle from the anterior ovoid axis at a constant distance of 3 cm from the active source center. Profiles for the source alone in water (solid lines) and the source-applicator combination (broken lines) are shown. Shaded regions denote the angular regions shadowed by the shields. From Williamson (1990) with permission.

In interstitial implant dosimetry, few publications treat heterogeneity phenomena. Meisberger (1968) has shown that implantation of ^{192}Ir seeds near an air-water interface results in dose underestimates of 7%. For ^{137}Cs sources in the presence of 2 cm thick aluminum, air, and bone slabs, Prasad (1983) has reported dose correction factors, based upon film dosimetry, ranging from 3% to 8%, suggesting that tissue heterogeneities are probably not significant for higher-energy brachytherapy sources. Both shielded [241]Am intracavitary applicators (Muench 1992) and shielded ^{125}I episcleral plaques, giving rise to a 8% dose reduction (Weaver 1986) in the unshielded region, have been described. For [241]Am, Nath (1987a) has shown that lead shielding correction factors are highly dependent upon lateral shielding dimensions (See Figure 28-3), indicating that heterogeneity corrections in this energy range depend significantly on geometric boundary conditions.

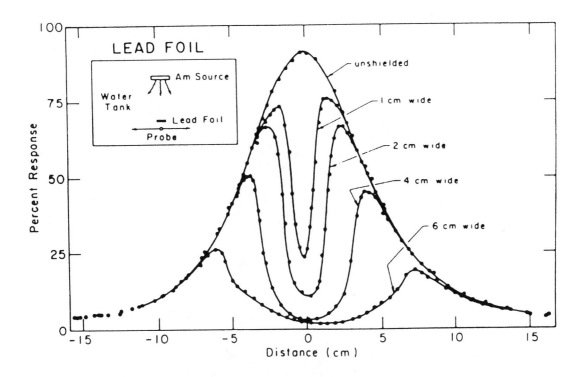

Figure 28-3. *Dose profiles, measured by a scintillation probe, perpendicular to the axis of a disk-shaped* [241]*Am source downstream of 1 mm thick lead shields of various widths. From Nath (1987a) with permission.*

Low-energy (≤ 40 keV) sources pose an additional challenge since absorbed dose is highly dependent on the atomic composition of the tissue. Dale (1983), using 1-D Monte Carlo calculations, demonstrated that the specific dose rate constant for ^{125}I in adipose tissue is 40% smaller than in water. Experimentally, Huang (1990) has demonstrated that the ^{125}I dose-rate constant for breast phantom material is only 76% that of liquid water (See Figure 28-4). For ^{125}I breast implants, such sparing of normal adipose tissue has been hypothesized to confer therapeutic benefit (Ling 1989). In the first published study of bounded tissue heterogeneities near low-energy sources. Meigooni, et al. (1992c) showed that a 2.1 cm cylindrical annulus of polystyrene perturbed doses by as much as 125%, 53% and 10% for [103]Pd, ^{125}I and [241]Am sources respectively (See Figure 28-5).

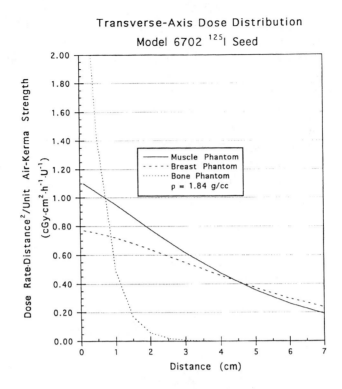

Figure 28-4. *Transverse axis dose-rate distributions (Huang 1990) for a Model 6702 ^{125}I seed in muscle phantom, breast phantom and bone phantom. Dose is expressed as dose to the surrounding medium.*

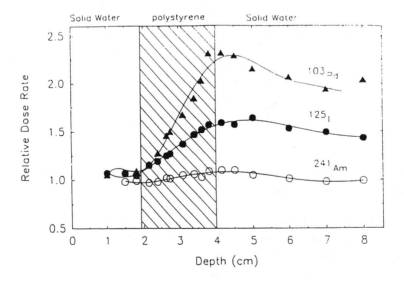

Figure 28-5. *Heterogeneity correction fractors, defined as dose to water with a 2.1 cylindrical annulus of polystyrene positioned in solid-water phantom relative to dose at the same point in a uniform solid-water phantom. Correction factors are plotted as a function of transverse-axis distance for ^{241}Am, ^{125}I and ^{103}Pd sources placed at the center of the polystyrene annulus. From Meigooni (1992) with permission.*

Measured and Calculated Single-source Heterogeneity Correction Factors

The complexity of single-source heterogeneity corrections (HCF's), and the potential role Monte-Carlo Photon-Transport (MCPT) calculations can play in characterizing these phenomena, is illustrated by the measurements and calculations recently published by author's group (Williamson 1993b and Perera 1994). Their goals were (a) to systematically study HCF's as a function of thickness, lateral dimensions, composition and location relative to the point of measurement and (b) to obtain a set of precision benchmarks for assessing the accuracy of MCPT in predicting dose distributions in the presence of bounded heterogeneities. Using a Scanditronix silicon diode detector (electron field type), HCF's in water were measured downstream of cylindrical heterogeneities of lead, steel, titanium, silver, aluminum and air positioned on the transverse axes of ^{125}I, ^{137}Cs ^{169}Yb and ^{192}Ir sources as illustrated by Figure 28-6. Cylindrical heterogeneities were positioned with their axes aligned with the transverse source bisector and their centers positioned 15 mm from the source center. Manual diode readings were obtained at 5-15 points along the transverse source axis spanning the source center-to-detector face distances of 1.8 to 16 cm. Generally, for each source-material combination, measurements were made for 4 different geometries: small- and large-diameter (6.3 mm and 19 mm) cylinders of two thicknesses (15-25% or 35-60% transmission) each. To quantify the effects of heterogeneities, the measured heterogeneity correction factor (HCF) was defined as:

$$\text{HCF}_{\text{det}}^{\text{meas}} = \frac{\text{Diode Reading with Heterogeneity}}{\text{Diode Reading without Heterogeneity}} \quad \text{at Same Point in Space} \qquad (1)$$

Each of the measurements was simulated using Monte Carlo photon-transport (MCPT) calculations, which took into account the 3-D geometric structure of the source, measurement phantom, heterogeneity, and detector. For each measured HCF, the corresponding theoretical ratio, $\text{HCF}_{\text{det}}^{\text{mcpt}}$, defined as the ratio of simulated detector readings, was calculated. The corresponding $\text{HCF}_{\text{wat}}^{\text{mcpt}}$, defined as the ratio of MCPT dose rates in water, was also calculated. The directly measured heterogeneity correction was corrected for diode energy response artifacts by MCPT simulation giving rise to a measured ratio of dose rates in water, $\text{HCF}_{\text{wat}}^{\text{meas}}$

$$\text{HCF}_{\text{wat}}^{\text{meas}} = \text{HCF}_{\text{det}}^{\text{meas}} \cdot \frac{\text{HCF}_{\text{wat}}^{\text{mcpt}}}{\text{HCF}_{\text{det}}^{\text{mcpt}}} \qquad (2)$$

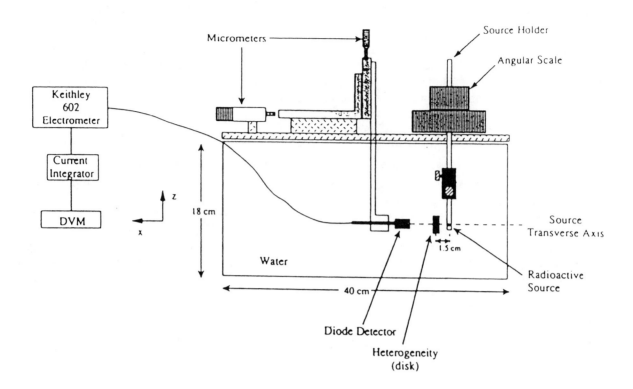

Figure 28-6. *Illustration of the micrometer-driven source positioning jig and associated water phantom used to measure silicon diode response as a function of distance along the transverse axis of a brachytherapy source. The source holder is mounted on a micrometer-driven turn-table allowing angular dose profiles to be measured. Micrometers allow positioning of the detector holder along the axis parallel to the source bisector and along its axis of symmetry. In addition, the source holder has fine adjustment screws allowing the source to be moved in the X-Y plane to ensure that the longitudinal source axis intersects and is bisected by the axis of turntable rotation. Source alignment is observed through a magnifying periscope to reduce personnel exposure. Not illustrated is the lead-brick vault surrounding the apparatus. From Williamson (1993b) with permission.*

Figures 28-7 to 28-9 compare $\mathrm{HCF}_{wat}^{meas}$ to its MCPT counterpart, $\mathrm{HCF}_{wat}^{mcpt}$, for a sample of the nearly 1,800 manually-measured diode readings. Agreement was excellent, rarely exceeding 5% and generally was in the 1-3% range. Several conclusions can be drawn:

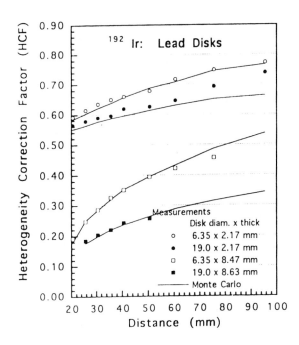
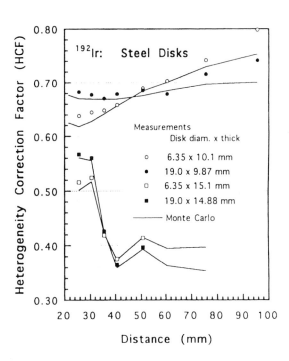

Figure 28-7. *Comparison of heterogeneity correction factors, as measured with a Scanditronix silicon diode detector to Monte Carlo calculations for a steel-clad Ir-192 interstitial seed in the presence of disk-shaped lead (left panel) and steel (right panel) heterogeneities. The measurements are represented. The solid and open symbols denote large- and small-diameter heterogeneities while circles and squares denote thin and thick heterogeneities respectively. From Williamson (1993b) with permission.*

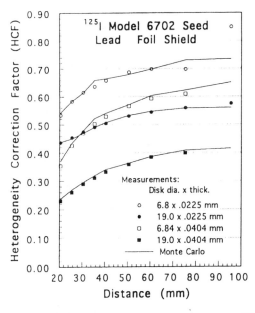
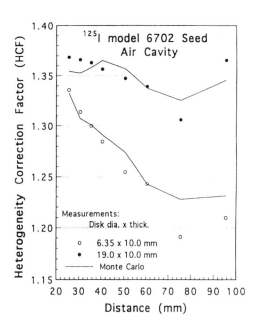

Figure 28-8. *Same as in Figure 28-7 for an ^{125}I Model 6702 seed in the presence of lead-foil shields (left panel) and cylindrical air cavities (right panel). From Williamson (1993b) with permission.*

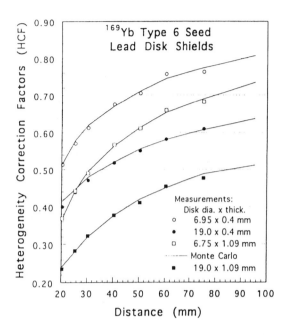
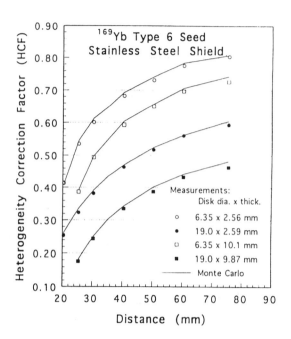

Figure 28-9. *Same as in Figure 28-7 for a type 6 ^{169}Yb seed Model 6702 seed in the presence of lead shields (left panel) and steel shields (right panel). From Perera (1994) with permission.*

(a) Heterogeneity effects can be quite large. A 1 cm-thick air void near an ^{125}I seed increases dose downstream by 21-37%. The magnitude of HCF is often significantly smaller (by 50-90%) than predicted by attenuation of the primary photons, emphasizing the importance of scattered radiation to these phenomena.

(b) Even for relatively high-energy sources such as ^{192}Ir, measured HCF's vary significantly with heterogeneity diameter (up to 50% variation) and measurement distance (up to factor-of-three). For ^{125}I, HCF variations with distance and heterogeneity diameter exceed the importance of thickness as a variable, with the larger thin disk sometimes conferring more protection than the small thick disk. In general, HCF behavior is complex, involving an interplay between primary photons transmitted by the barrier, scattered photons diffusing around the barrier, and scattered photons originating in the barrier. For clinical source arrangements that approximate a single-source geometry, dose calculation in the presence of bounded high-density heterogeneities is intrinsically a three-dimensional problem that can not be successfully attacked by simple 1-D algorithms.

(c) Comparison of measured HCF's with those calculated by MCPT, reveals excellent agreement, on the order of 1-3% for distances up to 7.5 cm, at which point the precision of the experimental readings begins to deteriorate. The mean of percentage deviations of theory from measurement is +1.1%, -0.6% and -1.1% for ^{125}I, ^{137}Cs and ^{192}Ir sources respectively. Our experience suggests that Monte Carlo simulation is powerful, convenient and accurate tool for investigating this long-neglected area.

Many important questions remain to be studied, including (a) the effects of bounded tissue-composition heterogeneities on low-energy seed dosimetry and (b) the conditions under which the complex behavior of single-source heterogeneities is ameliorated by the presence of multiple sources in clinical implants.

Quantitative Brachytherapy Dosimetry in Complex Geometries

Meaningful dose-calculation algorithm development is possible only if reliable and accurate benchmark dose distributions exist against which such algorithms can be validated. Until about 1980, direct measurement of dose around brachytherapy sources and applicators in support of clinical treatment planning and quality assurance was relatively uncommon even within the research setting, let alone the clinical environment. Historically, this arose not only because of the difficulties and labor-intensity of such measurements, but to a consensus view that objective and reproducible dose measurement was impossible and that even simplistic theoretical models were more reliable. Simple Sievert and point-source models continue to be treated as primary sources of brachytherapy dose distributions for ^{137}Cs, ^{192}Ir and other radium-substitute radionuclides. A major accomplishment of the last decade is validation and acceptance of TLD dosimetry as an accurate and comprehensive source of directly-measured single-source dose distributions for clinical treatment planning. The availability of measured brachytherapy dose distributions has made possible another major development in basic brachytherapy dosimetry: the validation of Monte Carlo photon-transport (MCPT) simulation, a fundamental theoretical computational method, as a clinical dosimetry tool in this area. Both of these developments will be briefly reviewed.

Experimental Brachytherapy Dosimetry

Brachytherapy dosimetry places severe demands on dose detectors: its dose distributions are characterized by steep dose gradients, a large range of dose rates, and relatively low photon energies. A suitable detector must have a wide dynamic range, flat energy response, small size, and high sensitivity. All detectors, including organic detectors such as radiochromic film and plastic scintillator, are subject to artifacts: volume-averaging, self-attenuation, directional anisotropy and energy-response. The most severe artifact of all is the exquisite sensitivity detector response to positioning errors: measurement of dose near a point source with 2% accuracy requires that the source-to-detector distance be specified with an accuracy of 20 μm, 50 μm, 100 μm, and 200 μm, respectively, at distances of 2, 5, 10 and 20 mm. Small ion chambers (Saylor et al. 1976, Meertens et al. 1985) are unsuitable because of their large size and poor sensitivity while silver-halide radiographic film fails because of excessive energy response although it has excellent spatial resolution and sensitivity. Energy response artifacts, which arise whenever the atomic composition of the active detector differs from that of the measurement medium, result in a detector response per unit dose in medium that varies with position in the phantom. This is due to softening of the photon spectrum with increasing distance from the source secondary to buildup of lower-energy scattered photons and attenuation of primary photons. Emerging detector technologies such as GAF-radiochromic film (McLaughlin 1991 and Muench 1992) and plastic scintillator (Perera 1992), utilize organic detector elements to avoid this problem. Diode detectors (Mohan 1985, Metcalfe 1988, Ling 1983), have excellent sensitivity and small size. However, their response with respect to photon energy is so poorly matched to tissue that they are unsuitable for absolute dose-rate measurements and, for most brachytherapy radionuclides, are not suitable for even relative measurements. Diode response per unit dose to water has been shown to vary by 15% to 75% with distance from ^{137}Cs, ^{192}Ir and ^{169}Yb sources (Williamson 1993b, Perera 1994). Only for ultra-low energy sources such as ^{125}I and ^{103}Pd, is diode response/unit dose independent of measurement distance in the phantom (Li 1993).

Thermolumiscent dosimetry (TLD), using TLD-100 LiF chips or extruded ribbons, has emerged as the detector offering the best compromise between small size, sensitivity, good energy response and ease of accurate positioning: it is currently accepted as the experimental "gold standard" for measurement of absolute dose rates in brachytherapy. Even though TLD-100 has very poor intrinsic sensitivity, its practical response per unit volume approaches that of ion chamber, largely because TLD is solid. By irradiating TLD's long enough (30 minutes to 120 hours), integrated signals with good signal-to-noise ratio characteristics have been obtained over the distance range of 1-7.5 cm low dose-rate (LDR) sources. Meigooni (1995) has recently shown that 5% accuracy can achieved for doses as small as 0.2 cGy. In contrast to ion chamber, long irradiations are practical since many TLD detectors can be simultaneously irradiated in a single experiment. The distance-dependence of TLD response/unit dose is moderate; 10% for [192]Ir (Meigooni 1988a), 3-4% for [169]Yb (MacPherson 1995 and Piermattei 1992) and is negligible for [125]I (Perera 1992).

Validation of TLD-based brachytherapy dosimetry is largely, but not exclusively, due to the efforts of the recently-completed Interstitial Brachytherapy Dosimetry Contract supported by the National Cancer Institute (Anderson et al. 1990). The associated collaborative working group (ICWG) consisted of independent teams of researchers based at three institutions (Yale University, Memorial Sloan-Kettering Institute, and the University of California at San Francisco). The ICWG made available three independently-measured sets (Weaver 1989, Nath 1990b, and Chiu-Tsao 1990) of dose distributions for ^{125}I and ^{192}Ir interstitial sources for comparison to validate their TLD measurement methodology. Other groups deserve credit as well, most notably the TLD measurements of Luxton, et al. (1990) and Piermatti (1988) and the relative diode measurements of Ling (1983,1985) and Schell (1987). The TLD methodology developed by these investigators has been extended to provide complete 2-D dose distributions about ^{125}I, ^{192}Ir and [103]Pd brachytherapy sources (Nath 1993, Chiu-Tsao 1990). Positioning artifacts are controlled by using solid water plastic phantoms (Meigooni 1988b) with precisely-machined detector slots whose location relative to the source can be accurately measured. The precision of source-to-detector positioning is on the order of 100 cm, making this technique suitable for measurement at distances of 1 cm or more.

Although instrumentation and TLD annealing practices vary from investigator to investigator, potential experimental artifacts such as volume averaging, angular anisotropy, energy response, positioning inaccuracies, background corrections and inter-chip attenuation and scattering effects must be carefully controlled and correction factors derived from ancillary experiments or Monte Carlo simulations (Meigooni 1988a). To extract estimates of dose rate (cGy/h) per unit strength near a brachytherapy source, rather than dose relative to a reference point, an accurate TLD reading (TL)/unit absorbed dose calibration must be established. This is achieved by exposing TLD's to a known dose in free space in an x-ray beam which has a spectrum that matches that of the brachytherapy source of interest.

The ICWG investigators claim an accuracy of 3-6% for transverse-axis TLD dosimetry for LDR ^{125}I and ^{192}Ir seeds. Review of the data published by the three participating institutions (Figure 28-10) reveals agreement in absolute dose rate (not relative) ranging from 2-5% over the 1-5 cm distance range supporting this claim. However, at shorter and longer distances, discrepancies of 10-30% appear, indicating that signal-to-noise ratio problems limit TLD precision at large distances while positioning or volume-averaging artifacts limit measurement accuracy at distances of less than 10 mm. Comparison of measured and Monte Carlo-based brachytherapy dose distributions is discussed below.

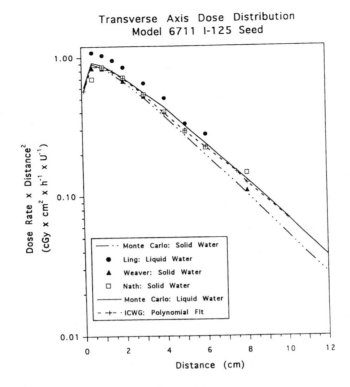

Figure 28-10. *Comparison of measured and calculated (Monte Carlo) absolute dose rates per unit air kerma strength for the Model 6711 seed. Monte Carlo estimates (from Williamson, 1991b) of dose rate to water are plotted for both liquid- and solid-water measurement medium. The measured data are taken from the following references: Ling (1983), Weaver (1989), Nath (1990b) and Anderson (1990). From Williamson (1991b) with permission. Agreement between the TLD measurements and the Monte Carlo calculations (assuming solid-water measurement medium) average 1-3% while the conventional used data of Ling (1983) overestimates true absorbed dose by 18%.*

Monte Carlo Simulation: A New Clinical Dosimetry Tool

Another important development in brachytherapy dosimetry is the emergence of Monte Carlo photon-transport (MCPT) simulation as a reliable and accurate source of brachytherapy dosimetry data. This approach is made feasible by the availability of more accurate photon cross-section libraries and 3-D geometric modeling techniques allowing the effects of internal source structure, dose measurement geometry, and source calibration geometry to be modeled (Williamson 1989). Under certain conditions, Monte Carlo simulation can be used to calculate actual dose rates in medium per unit source strength, as well as relative dose distributions.

Monte Carlo simulation is a specific numerical solution to a general problem, namely the Boltzmann transport equation. The solution to this equation, given the distribution of ionizing radiation sources and absorbing media along with a description of the collisional dynamics underlying the transport, scattering and absorption of ionizing radiation in matter, completely characterizes the resultant dose distribution. Unfortunately, this integro-differential equation is too complex to be solved accurately by analytic or even deterministic numerical methods in any but the simplest of 1- and 2-D geometries. Thus, Monte Carlo simulation, which solves the transport equation by random sampling, is currently the only practical theoretical method of calculating absorbed dose in the presence of geometrically complex boundary conditions (Miller and Lewis, 1984 and Jenkins et al. 1988). Using probability distributions derived from total and differential cross sections, a small (10^5-10^7) subset of photon or electron histories is randomly constructed by following each photon from birth through successive scattering events and, eventually, to absorption or escape from the system, using random sampling to decide its fate at each decision point. The result is equivalent to randomly selecting a small number of photon histories from the set of all those possible. A statistical estimate of absorbed dose rate at a point is obtained by calculating the dose contribution from each simulated collision (a process known as "estimation") and taking the average over all contributions (Williamson 1987). Because particle histories can be accurately and efficiently constructed even in the presence of complex, 3-D boundary conditions, "exact" but statistically uncertain solutions, derived from first principles with little reliance on approximations, are possible for a wide range of clinically-relevant brachytherapy problems.

In principle, it is straightforward to include transport of secondary electrons in the simulation, which is clearly necessary to solve problems of clinical interest in megavoltage photon domain. Although the influence of secondary electron transport has not been studied in brachytherapy, significant CPE-failure artifacts are expected only near media interfaces and very close to (< 5 mm) higher-energy sources since brachytherapy photon energies are relatively low (Roesch 1958). By approximating absorbed dose in medium as collision kerma, highly complex MCPT problems can be readily solved on small mini-computers or workstations. Realistic modeling of brachytherapy source, applicator and detector geometries has proven to be essential for accurate results. The development and technical aspects of Monte Carlo-based brachytherapy dosimetry have recently been reviewed by Williamson (1995).

Accurate and reliable MCPT-based dosimetry requires painstaking attention to many technical details including: choice of physical model of photon scattering, choice of cross-section library, accuracy and reliability of the underlying geometric model and appropriate choice of estimators and other variance-reduction techniques (Williamson 1995). In particular, a flexible and general system of geometric modeling and realistic modelling of source and detector internal structure are required. Brachytherapy sources and applicators have complex internal designs often leading to highly anisotropic dose distributions. In addition, dose distributions around sources emitting photons with energies greater than 40 keV are sensitive to the shape and size of the surrounding scattering medium. Calculation of absolute dose rates may require simulation of the experimental geometry used to standardize air-kerma strength for the source (Williamson 1988b). Finally, comparison of MCPT predictions with measured results may require simulation of detector response. Under these conditions excellent agreement (1-5%) has been found between TLD dose-rate measurements and MCPT calculations has been observed. Figure 28-10 shows the agreement between the ICWG TLD measurements and the author's MCPT calculations for a model 6711 ^{125}I interstitial seed.

Summary: Empirical and Theoretical Dosimetry Methods

Monte Carlo simulation overcomes many of the limitations of purely empirical dosimetry approaches. Errors due detector displacement and volume-averaging artifacts near sources and signal-to-noise ratio problems far from sources can be limited to a few percent through selection of appropriate estimators and variance-reduction techniques. Monte Carlo simulations are not subject to positioning or energy-response artifacts. However, in contrast to experimental methodologies, meaningful simulation requires precise knowledge of the geometric configuration of sources and applicators. In addition, the influence of relatively small uncertainties ($\pm$2-3%) in low-energy photon cross sections is amplified at large distances. To calculate absolute dose rates knowing only the source strength, the method of source-strength standardization must be well understood. Any deviation of stated air-kerma strength from its formal definition will introduce errors into the calculated dose rates. The available evidence indicates that when all of these conditions are met, Monte Carlo dose-rate estimates have an accuracy on the order of a few percent.

The optimal approach to brachytherapy dosimetry is probably a combination of empirical and Monte Carlo dose-estimation techniques. Because its accuracy depends on many types of input data, Monte Carlo simulation should not be used as the sole source of clinical dosimetry data. Among the documented 'surprises' that a purely theoretical method may fail to anticipate are the contamination of the NIST ^{125}I calibration standard by low-energy photons (Williamson 1988b) and contamination of a prototype ^{103}Pd seed by high-energy photons due to neutron activation of trace elements (Meigooni 1990). Monte Carlo (or any other theoretical) dose calculations about any source or applicator involving previously unverified geometry, photon spectrum or calibration standards should be experimentally verified. At minimum, the measured benchmark data should include transverse-axis measurements and at least one angular dose profile. A calibrated detector, which allows measurement of absolute dose rates (not just relative doses), is necessary. As work from the author's group shows, the detector need not respond linearly to dose in medium: for the purpose of verification, it is sufficient to compare measured and simulated detector responses per unit air-kerma strength. Having verified accuracy of MCPT for the given source type, the 2-D dose-rate distribution in water may be calculated.

Experimentally-verified MCPT simulation is a powerful clinical dosimetry tool. In addition to providing artifact-free single-source dose-rate distributions, MCPT calculations can be performed prospectively without construction of prototype sources. Thus Monte Carlo simulation can serve as a design tool, helping to identify the mechanical specifications of sources and applicators that give rise to desired dosimetric characteristics. Monte Carlo can also be used to calculate basic dosimetry data which, in practice or in principle, is inaccessible to measurement. Examples include scatter-to-primary ratios and dose-spread arrays needed as input data to clinical dose-computation algorithms. Characterization of poorly-understood phenomena, such as dosimetric influence of applicator shielding and tissue heterogeneities, can be greatly accelerated. Finally, an emerging application of MCPT is characterization of dosimeter artifacts and optimization of dose detector design.

Practical Dose-Calculation Algorithms for Heterogeneous Geometries

Accurate but practical dose-calculation algorithms are needed both to facilitate applicator design for low-energy isotopes and to extract meaningful normal-tissue and tumor-control dose response data from image-based evaluation of patients treated with intracavitary therapy. In addition, accurate dosimetric treatment of applicator shielding and tissue composition variations is a prerequisite to incorporating physical optimization into clinical brachytherapy. A useful dose calculation algorithm must be fast enough to allow evaluation of absorbed dose throughout large 3-D dose matrices with reasonable turnaround time, must be accurate, and must be sufficiently general to handle the range of source arrangements, applicator geometries, and tissue heterogeneities likely to be encountered in the targeted clinical applications. Ideally, such an algorithm should be applicable to both high- and low-energy radionuclides, should require only a limited base of well-defined physical data, and should be fully three dimensional. Monte Carlo simulation, although highly general and accurate, is at present too CPU-intensive to support the volume of dose calculations required by clinical treatment planning given the computing resources currently available for this task. This has stimulated a revival in brachytherapy algorithm development with the goal of striking a more practical compromise between accuracy and speed.

One-Dimensional Primary-Photon Pathlength Algorithms

One-dimensional (1-D) heterogeneity corrections depend only on the thickness, t_h, of heterogeneity traversed by primary photons. These models are fundamentally generalizations of the Sievert integral, which is widely used to calculate dose distributions about sources that can be approximated by radioactivity uniformly distributed along a line segment which is encapsulated in a cylindrical filter, usually stainless steel or platinum. In the case of an isotropic point source, the essential feature of the 1-D primary-photon pathlength approach can be expressed simply

$$\dot{D}_{het}(\bar{r}) = \dot{D}_{hom}(\bar{r}) \cdot e^{-\mu_h \cdot t_h} \tag{3}$$

where $\dot{D}_{hom}$ and $\dot{D}_{het}(\vec{r})$ denote dose rates at the point of interest in homogeneous medium and in the presence of the heterogeneity, respectively. The thickness of heterogeneous material traversed by primary photons traveling from the source to the point of interest, $\vec{r}$, is denoted by t_h and μ_h is the effective linear attenuation coefficient of the heterogeneous medium. The 1-D pathlength model assumes that heterogeneity alters both the primary and scattered-photon dose contributions by the same exponential correction factor, i.e., the scatter-to-primary ratio (SPR) is a function only of the thickness of tissue-equivalent medium traversed by the primary photons. Figure 28-11 shows that this assumption is false for a cylindrical HDR source in uniform medium: the SPR at a fixed distance of 2 cm from the active center varies by more than a factor of two with respect to polar angle. The SPR increases near the longitudinal axis due to partial 'filling in' of the oblique-filtration induced primary-dose deficit by scattered photons originating elsewhere in the medium. As shown by Figures 28-5 to 28-7, the distribution of scattered photons depends on the 3D heterogeneity geometry and is only weakly correlated with the local primary-photon dose rate. The pathlength model handles this problem by treating μ_h as an empirical parameter that can deviate significantly from either the linear attenuation or energy absorption coefficients. Inaccurate treatment of the scatter-dose distribution is compensated by primary-dose calculation errors of equal magnitude but opposite direction.

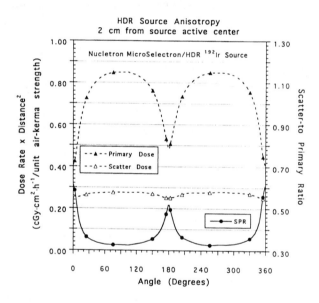

Figure 28-11. *Polar dose profile at a fixed distance of 2 cm from the active source center of a Nucletron MicroSelectron/HDR ^{192}Ir source in water. The left-hand scale shows the scattered- and primary-photon dose components as a function of polar angle with respect to the source cable while the right-hand scale shows the scatter-to-primary (SPR) dose ratio.*

The principal advantages of 1-D pathlength algorithms are speed and simplicity: ray tracing need only be applied between each active source element and each point of interest. The 1-D pathlength algorithm, along with its empirical multi-dimensional generalizations, are the only clinically-usable computational models for heterogeneous geometries currently available. The main drawback is limited applicability: acceptable accuracy results only when HCF's are modestly dependent on heterogeneity cross-sectional geometry. So far, development and validation of this approach have been limited to high-density, high-atomic number heterogeneities, such as applicator shielding, active source core, and source encapsulation.

A general form of the 1-D pathlength model (Nath 1987b and Williamson 1988a) applicable to geometrically-complex shielded source geometries, is illustrated by Figure 28-12. The problem geometry consists of a brachytherapy source, consisting of an active source core of radius, s, encapsulated in a metal filter of radial thickness, t, in the presence of a high-density metal internal shield. The active source is decomposed into N_i small elements each of volume ΔV_i and located at $\vec{r_i}$. Then, just as in the Sievert integral, inverse square-law, tissue-attenuation and -buildup corrections, and effective attenuation corrections are separately applied to each source element, ΔV_i. The N_i dose-rate contributions are then summed, giving an estimate of the dose rate at the point of interest, $\vec{r}$. The dose rate is given by

$$\dot{D}_{het}(\vec{r}) = S_K \cdot \left(\mu_{en}/\rho\right)_{air}^{wat} \cdot \frac{\displaystyle\sum_{i=1}^{N_s}\left[\Delta V_i \cdot B(\lambda_{i3}) \cdot \left(\vec{r} - \vec{r_i}'\right)^{-2} \cdot \exp\left(-\sum_{j=1}^{4}\mu_j \cdot \lambda_{ij}\right)\right]}{|\vec{r_c}|^2 \cdot \displaystyle\sum_{i=1}^{N_s}\left[\Delta V_i \cdot \left(\vec{r_c} - \vec{r_i}'\right)^{-2} \cdot \exp\left(-\mu_1 \cdot s - \mu_2 \cdot t\right)\right]} \qquad (4)$$

where the indices j = 1,...,4 denote the media composing the active source core, the source (Williamson 1988a, Nath 1987a) encapsulation, the surrounding water and the internal shielding, respectively. The variables $\lambda_{i1},...,\lambda_{i4}$ denote the distances traversed by primary photons through each of these four media as they travel from the source element ΔV_i a t$\vec{r_i}$ to the point of interest, $\vec{r}$. The other symbols in equation (4) are defined as follows:

S_K =   strength of the source in terms of air-kerma strength in units of $\mu Gy \cdot m^2 \cdot h^{-1}$ where $1\mu Gy \cdot m^2 \cdot h^{-1} = 1cGy \cdot cm^2 \cdot h^{-1} = 1\,U$. The point on the transverse source axis (usually 1m from the source) where the air-kerma rate in free space specified, is denoted by $\vec{r_c}$.

$\left(\mu_{en}/\rho\right)_{air}^{wat}$ =   the mean ratio of mass-energy absorption coefficients, averaged over the photon spectrum in free space with respect to air-kerma, for water to that of air.

$B(d)$ = $\dfrac{\text{total dose in water}}{\text{primary dose in water}}$ at distance d from an isotropic point source, i.e., the buildup factor for water

μ_j =   the effective attenuation coefficient for active source, filter and shielding material for j = 1, 2 and 4 respectively. For the special case of water (j = 3), μ_j denotes the narrow-beam attenuation coefficient, as required by the definition of buildup factor.

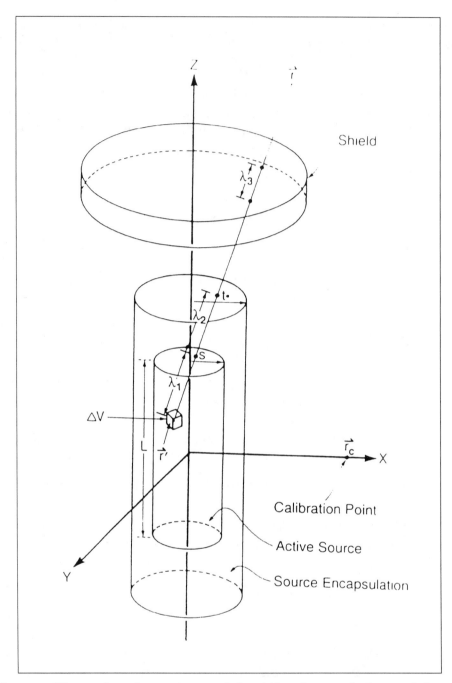

Figure 28-12. *Diagram illustrating the geometry of the 1-D primary-photon path-length dose-calculation model for calculating absorbed dose about geometrically complex sources and shielded applicators. The diagram illustrates an intracavitary source consisting of uniformly distributed radioactivity in a cylindrical region of volume V, length L and radius s which is concentrically and symmetrically placed in a larger cylinder of radius t which denotes the source capsule. Also pictured is a disk-shaped shield located above the source. dV' denotes a differential volume element located at r'. Adapted from Williamson (1988a).*

A 3-D ray-tracing subroutine library required to calculate the sequence of path-lengths, $\lambda_{i1},...,\lambda_{i4}$ for each pair of points ($\vec{r_i}$, $\vec{r}$) from a model of the source-shielding geometry. Mathematically, λ_{ij} for a given $\vec{r}$ can be represented by:

$$\lambda_{ij} = \int_0^{|\vec{r_i}-\vec{r}|} \pi_j(\vec{r_i} + \frac{\vec{r}-\vec{r_i}}{|\vec{r}-\vec{r_i}|}\cdot s)\cdot ds \quad \text{where } \pi_j(\vec{r}) = 1 \text{ if } \vec{r} \text{ lies in medium j and } \pi_j(\vec{r}) = 0 \text{ if not} \quad (5)$$

$\pi_j(\vec{r})$ is the point classification function, which simply classifies an arbitrary point, $\vec{r}$, as to whether it is inside or outside the union of regions composed of medium j. The sums in the numerator and denominator of equation (4) are proportional to the dose rate in water and air-kerma strength, respectively, <u>per unit activity contained in the source</u>. The denominator is required to renormalize the numerator (dose rate in water) to the quantity air-kerma strength, which is the output produced by the <u>filtered</u> source. Omitting this correction will result in a 'double' oblique filtration correction. It is obvious that the above model could easily be generalized to more than four media and to extended sources of arbitrary shape.

The 1-D primary path-length approach was introduced independently by Van der Laarse and Meertens (1984, 1985) and Weeks and Dennett (1990) for ^{137}Cs sources positioned in vaginal colpostats containing tungsten-alloy shielding, although not in the general form just described. Weeks used a small ion chamber to measure the dose downstream of a sample of each material in the problem (tungsten, steel, styrofoam, Lucite and nylon) with cross-sectional dimensions of 1 x 5 cm and known thicknesses. By normalizing each measurement to the reading measured in homogeneous water at the same point, he was able to calculate the effective 'water replacement' attenuation coefficient, μ_j, for each material in this representative geometry. Weeks verified his model by comparing its predictions to extensive diode measurements made around a plastic colpostat containing tungsten-alloy shields, which were converted to absolute dose rates by normalizing homogeneous-medium readings to corresponding calculated dose rates. He found excellent agreement (3%) between the measured and calculated results. The model of Meertens and Van der Laarse is very similar except that the effective attenuation coefficient, μ_h, is treated as a parameter of best fit. These investigators used a small ion chamber to map the relative dose distribution in several planes arising from a Selectron shielded colpostat containing a sequence of 4 spherical ^{137}Cs sources. Since the distance between each measurement plane and applicator center could not be specified exactly, they varied both the distance and μ_h until the optimal fit between measured and calculated isotransmission lines was achieved. They claimed an accuracy of 4% away from the shield edges and 10% or 3 mm near the boundaries of the region shadowed by the shields. Interestingly, Meertens' value of μ_h (0.10 mm^{-1}) for tungsten was reasonably close to that of Weeks and Dennett (0.12 mm^{-1}). In comparison, the linear attenuation and energy absorption coefficients take the values 0.170 and 0.091 mm^{-1}, respectively, assuming that the tungsten alloy has a density of 17 g/cm^3. Figure 28-13 shows the isotransmission lines (dose with shields/dose without shields) calculated by Meertens and Van der Laarse for a typical clinical loading consisting of two colpostats and an intrauterine tandem.

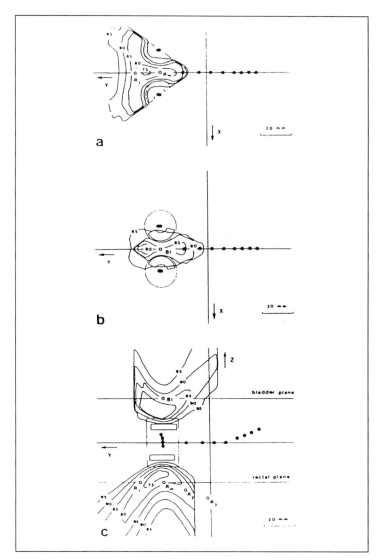

Figure 28-13. *Isotransmission curves produced by a typical clinical loading of a pair of shielded Fletcher-Suit colpostats (4 spherical ^{137}Cs sources each) and an intrauterine tandem (8 sources) manufactured by Nucletron corporation for the Selectron remote-afterloading device. The data are calculated by the 1-D path-length model developed by Meertens and Van der Laarse (1985). The internal shields consist of 3.5 mm-thick tungsten. Isotransmission curves are shown for (a) the rectal plane (coronal plane 25 mm posterior to the tandem), (b) the bladder plane (coronal plane 27 mm anterior to the tandem) and (c) a sagittal plane containing the tandem. From Meertens et al. (1985) with permission.*

Although one could argue that the dose measurement techniques used to validate the 1-D primary-photon pathlength models have an accuracy no better than 10%, the model probably has an accuracy better than 5% for multiple-applicator combinations typically used in clinical practice. Under these conditions, dose sparing due to internal shields is limited to approximately 25%. This level of accuracy is quite remarkable in view of the fact that the 1-D path-length model completely neglects the influence of shield location and cross-sectional area on the resultant HCF. For a ^{137}Cs point source, Figure 28-14 shows the effect of tungsten shield-diameter on the dose downstream of the heterogeneity. This figure shows, that up to distances of 5 cm, the variation of HCF with respect to distance is 17% and with respect to shield diameter is about 20%. Thus for points of interest less than 2 cm downstream of the shield (the region of most clinical relevance), the 3-D scattering effects neglected by the 1-D pathlength model probably introduce errors on the order of ±5%, especially when large fractions of the dose are delivered by unshielded sources. Although one should be cautious in applying this model to unidirectional applicators, e.g., segmentally-shielded vaginal cylinders, this simple and reasonably accurate approach can be recommended to those interested in more accurate dose calculation around intracavitary implants utilizing [137]Cs.

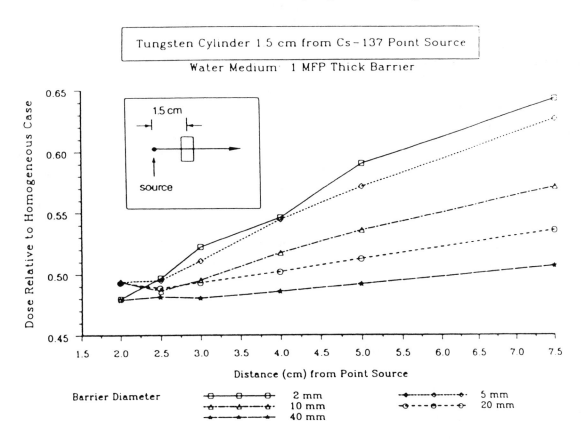

Figure 28-14. *Transmission ratios along the axis of a one mean-free path (5.4 mm) cylindrical tungsten shield located 1.5 cm from a ^{137}Cs point source in water. The data were calculated by Monte Carlo simulation for shields ranging from 2 to 40 mm in diameter. The right scale denotes dose in water with the shield in place relative to dose in water at the same point in homogeneous medium. From Williamson (1990) with permission.*

(1) Generalizations of 1-D Primary-Photon Pathlength Algorithms

Figures 28-5 to 28-7 indicate that for photon energies at and below that of ^{192}Ir, shielding correction factors become more dependent on shield dimensions and locations. For unidirectional ^{192}Ir applicators, variations as large as 45% with respect to shield diameter and distance from the shield penumbra can be expected. It is unlikely that the 1-D pathlength approach is applicable to lower energy sources such as ^{192}Ir and [169]Yb, which have larger scatter-to-primary ratios, and photon scattering interactions that more closely approximate elastic collisions. This has stimulated development of more sophisticated and accurate algorithms. In an effort both to retain the efficiency characteristic of primary-photon ray tracing and to improve upon the accuracy of the basic 1-D pathlength model, some investigators have turned to empirical modeling of the scatter-dose distribution. These approaches (a) explicitly separate the primary and scattered-photon dose components and (b) use empirical corrections to model dependence of the scatter dose component on the 3-D geometry of interest point, source, and heterogeneity. Thus, the complex 3-D behavior of the often-dominant scatter-dose distribution is partially re-introduced into the 1-D pathlength model.

The simplest example of an empirical 3-D scatter-correction model is the scatter-separation method developed by the author (Williamson 1990). This method evolved from the observation that, despite factor-of-two variations in primary dose around shielded vaginal applicators containing ^{137}Cs and ^{226}Ra sources, the scatter-dose component is approximately (within 20%) isotropically distributed. This suggested that scatter-dose can be treated as distant-dependent but angle-independent term obviating the need to calculate scatter dose at each point by Monte Carlo. Most of the residual anisotropy was eliminated by observing that the perturbation of the scatter dose by the applicator at each point was linearly related to the additional primary-photon attenuation contributed by the applicator, expressed in mean-free paths, MFP (see Figure 28-15). Basic data for the model was derived from Monte Carlo simulations: scattered-photon dose rates at 30 polar angles with respect to the longitudinal source axis at distances of 1.2, 1.5, 2.0, 3.0 and 5.0 cm in the transverse plane of each source-applicator combination. These simulations were based upon realistic geometric models of the source internal structure, colpostat body, source restraining mechanism and bladder and rectal shields, involving as many as 55 different geometric shapes and seven media. In addition, scatter dose rates per unit air-kerma strength for the filtered source alone, $\dot{D}_{s,s}(\vec{r})$, were calculated at the same at the same points. By applying curve fitting to this limited base of data, the ratio of scatter with applicator to scatter from source alone, $\alpha(r, \text{MFP}) = \dot{D}_{s,a}(\vec{r})/\dot{D}_{s,s}(\vec{r})$, was reduced to a coarse 2-D table depending only on distance from the applicator center, and applicator attenuation in MFP. Then the total dose rate, $\dot{D}_a(\vec{r})$ at any point $\vec{r}$ in the presence of a shielded applicator is given by:

$$\dot{D}_a(\vec{r}) = S_K \cdot \left[\dot{D}_{p,a}(\vec{r}) + \dot{D}_{s,s}(|\vec{r}|, \cos\theta) \cdot \alpha(|\vec{r}|, \text{MFP}) \right] \quad (6)$$

where $\dot{D}_{p,a}(\vec{r})$ and $\dot{D}_{p,s}(\vec{r})$ denote the primary dose rate per U with the shielded applicator and for the filtered source alone. The primary-photon attenuation due to the applicator, $\text{MFP}(\vec{r})$, is given by

$$\text{MFP}(\vec{r}) = -\ln\left[\frac{\dot{D}_{p,a}(\vec{r})}{\dot{D}_{p,s}(|\vec{r}|, \cos\theta)} \right] \quad (7)$$

Thus calculation of scatter dose at any point around an applicator requires exact calculation of the primary dose, three 2-D table lookups from pre-calculated arrays: scatter dose, $\dot{D}_{s,s}(r, \cos\theta)$, and primary dose, $\dot{D}_{p,s}(r, \cos\theta)$, from the source alone and the scatter perturbation correction, $\alpha(r, \text{MFP})$. For three widely-used applicator-source combinations (3M applicator with Cs-137 and rectangular-handled Fletcher-Suit applicator with Cs-137 and Ra-226), dose calculation accuracy and computational efficiency, both relative to Monte Carlo simulation, were found to be 3% and 15,000, respectively. Although computational complexity is similar to that of the simple primary ray-path correction models, scatter-separation explicitly corrects for distance-dependence of heterogeneity corrections and anisotropy of the scattered- and primary-photon dose profiles arising from the source alone. Our model ignores the variation of HCF with shield area at a fixed distance.

A different approach to empirical scatter correction has been developed by Nath et al. (1987a and 1990a) in an effort to model the dose distribution around vaginal plaques containing multiple ^{241}Am sources. Nath's basic model is very similar to the generic 1-D primary ray-tracing model described by equation (4) above, expect that his geometric model includes as many as five 1 cm-diameter cylindrical sources (see Figure 28-16). However, the buildup factor, B, for water medium is replaced by an anisotropic buildup factor, B_{anis}:

$$B_{anis} = 1 + (B_{iso} - 1) \cdot a(\theta)^n \tag{8}$$

where B_{iso} is the isotropic point-source buildup factor and θ is the angle between the longitudinal axis of the source currently being calculated and the point of interest, $\vec{r}$. The function $a(\theta)$ corrects for the anisotropic distribution of scatter around each single source and has the form $a + (1-a) \cdot \cos\theta$ for a cylindrical source where a is an empirical value varying from 0.75 to 0.85. The integer n denotes the number of sources in the plaque and corrects for global reduction of the multiply-scattered photon dose-rate component due to the presence of multiple, bulky extended sources. The generally good agreement between the model predictions and dose rates measured by thermoluminescent dosimetry is illustrated in Figure 28-17 for a 5-4-5 Ci vaginal applicator. The RMS average deviation of the model predictions from the measurements varied from 7% to 13% although relative errors at individual points as large as 35% were reported. That the average errors are somewhat larger than those of the 1-D primary-photon pathlength model is a reflection of how much more difficult algorithm design is for 60 keV photons than for ^{137}Cs γ-rays. Of interest is Nath's conclusion (1990a) that multiple-source arrays give rise to nearly factor-of-two source-to-source or 'line-of-sight' shielding corrections and additional 'indirect' dose correction factors averaging 19% due to reduction of multiply-scattered photon fluence. Use of partial- or full-transmission lead-foil shields further complicates the problem, giving rise to a dose distribution that is highly dependent on cross-sectional shield shape as well as thickness (Muench 1992). A major lesson of the Yale experience is that simple Sievert-like models, based on the universally-used dose-superposition principle, do not model dose distributions with adequate accuracy in this energy range.

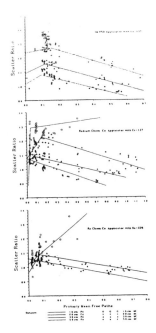

Figure 28-15. *Scatter-dose ratio, a (scatter dose with colpostat / scatter dose from encapsulated source only), plotted as a function of average primary photon attenuation expressed in units of mean-free path, contributed by the applicator. The symbols denote the Monte Carlo data for rectangular handled Fletcher-Suit colpostats or 3M Fletcher-Suit-Delclos colpostats and the lines indicated the piece-wise linear fit to the data. From Williamson (1990) with permission.*

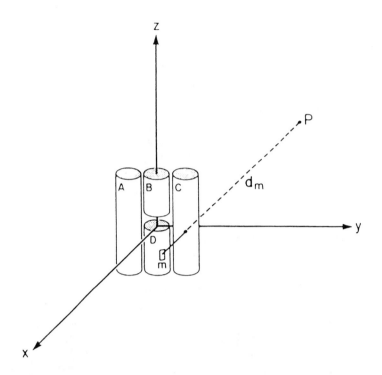

Figure 28-16. *Schematic diagram, showing the 5-4-5 Ci ^{241}Am vaginal plaque, illustrating the geometry used by Nath's generalized 1-D path-length model for calculation of dose rate near multiple, bulky source arrays. The angle, q, used to correct for anisotropic distribution of scatter dose, is that between the Z axis and the line segment PE. Integration over surface-area elements, E, is used to obtain line-of-sight primary- and scattered-photon source-to-source shielding corrections. From Nath et al. (1990a) with permission.*

Despite the advantage of computational simplicity, empirical generalizations of the 1-D path-length model have several shortcomings. First, dose-calculation accuracy for low-energy (< 400 keV) sources appears to be limited to 10% for typical multiple-source arrays characteristic of clinical practice. In addition, these models require extensive validation against measured or Monte Carlo dose rates in order to define the empirical scatter-dose corrections. This laborious process must be repeated for each applicator-source combination. For multiple source arrays of new low-energy sources such as ^{241}Am, each type of shielding geometry requires empirical validation. Clearly, to fully exploit the potential of customized shielding of low-energy source implants, a more general and accurate dose-calculation algorithm is necessary. An important potential application of the 1-D algorithms is the computational dosimetry of Ir-192 high dose-rate intracavitary therapy, for which no validated dose-calculation algorithm has been reported to date.

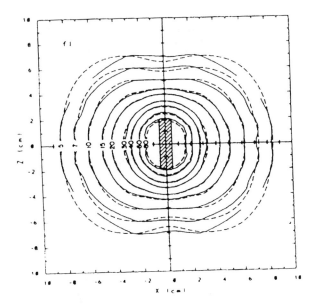

Figure 28-17. *Measured (solid lines) and calculated (broken lines) isodose-rate curves (cGy/hr) produced by a 5-4-5 Ci suit ^{241}Am vaginal applicator. The top panel shows the dose distribution in a plane through the center and perpendicular to the source axes and the bottom panel represents the dose distribution in a plane perpendicular to the plaque through the center of the central source. The dose calculations, based on Nath's model, include corrections for both line-of-sight corrections and corrections for global reduction in scatter dose. From Nath (1990a) with permission.*

Emerging Developments in Dose Calculation: Explicitly 3-D Algorithms

Our review of the brachytherapy dosimetry literature suggests that in many clinical applications of low-energy sources, inter-source shielding, local shielding and possibly tissue heterogeneities give rise to large dose perturbations that have a complex dependence upon the geometric distribution of sources and applicators, and upon the lateral dimensions and location of shielding media. An algorithm which is efficient, is fully three-dimensional, is derived from principles of radiation transport, and supports accurate prospective dose calculation over a wide range of heterogeneous geometries would significantly enhance our capability to optimize dose distributions in brachytherapy. Unfortunately, no such algorithm exists in clinically-usable form as of this writing. In fact, the only published contributions in the area of explicitly 3-D dose calculation are those of the present author. His group has developed two 3-D algorithms: 3-D scatter convolution (Williamson 1991a) and scatter subtraction (Williamson 1993a). Current implementations of these approaches are limited to point sources in the presence of geometrically-simple heterogeneities and demonstrate, at best, proof of underlying principles. However, these studies demonstrate that (a) a high level of accuracy is potentially achievable without resorting to Monte Carlo simulation, (b) the tradeoff between accuracy and numerical complexity is steep and (c) that there at least two promising pathways for future work in this area.

3-D Convolution Algorithm for Brachytherapy Dosimetry

The convolution method was first proposed for megavoltage photon-beam dose calculations (Boyer 1985, Mackie 1985, and Mohan 1986) in heterogeneous media and was successfully adapted to brachytherapy dose calculation by the author's group (Williamson 1991a). The algorithm requires a limited base of well-defined physical data, is fully three dimensional and predicts absolute dose rates as well as relative correction factors. It takes into account not only the thickness of heterogeneities, but their composition, size, and location relative to the source and point of interest as well. Our prototype brachytherapy convolution is accurate within 3% for both low- (^{125}I) and high-energy (^{137}Cs) sources in the presence of shields, air-voids and air-tissue boundaries. The basic principle of the convolution method is illustrated by Figure 28-18, which shows a point source near an irregularly-shaped heterogeneity.

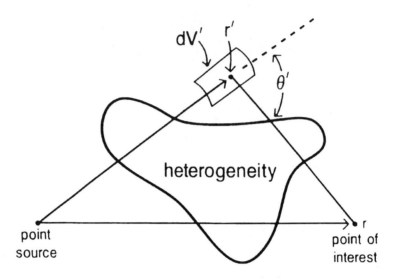

Figure 28-18. *Geometry of the dose-convolution method. dV' denotes a typical scatter-dose voxel, defined as a differential volume-centered about the primary photon collision point $\vec{r}$ in a spherical coordinate system. From Williamson et al. (1991a) with permission.*

The 3-D space surrounding the source is partitioned into small scattering voxels of volume dV'. The primary energy-fluence rate, per unit air-kerma strength, $\dot{\Psi}(\bar{r}')$, is calculated at the center $\bar{r}'$ of each voxel, including the attenuating effects of heterogeneities. The scatter-dose contribution to the point of interest, $\bar{r}$, from each voxel, $\bar{r}'$, is estimated from the scatter-dose kernel, $K(\bar{r} - \bar{r}')$. The process of adding together these differential scattered-photon dose contributions amounts to convolving energy fluence density, $\dot{\Psi}(\bar{r}')\cdot\mu$ (r') against the scatter-dose kernel, $K(\bar{r} - \bar{r}')$. Thus, the total dose rate, $\dot{D}(\bar{r})$, at point ($\bar{r}$) is

$$\dot{D}(\bar{r}) = S_K \cdot \left[\dot{D}_p(\bar{r}) + \int_V \dot{\Psi}(\vec{r}') \cdot \mu(\vec{r}') \cdot K(|\vec{r}' - \vec{r}|, \theta') \cdot dV' \right] \qquad (9)$$

The basic data required by the algorithm is the "dose-spread array" or scatter-dose kernel, $K(t,\theta)$, which gives the distribution of scatter dose arising from mono-directional primary photons going into first collision at t = 0. These data were precalculated by Monte Carlo simulation, illustrating its utility in calculating basic treatment planning data that is inaccessible to direct measurement. Isodose curves of ^{125}I and ^{137}Cs dose spread arrays are shown in Figure 28-19. Our prototype convolution code used 3-D numerical integration to evaluate the integral and required 100,000 to 200,000 integrand evaluations and careful attention to integrand singularities at r' = 0 and r' = r to obtain numerically stable and accurate results.

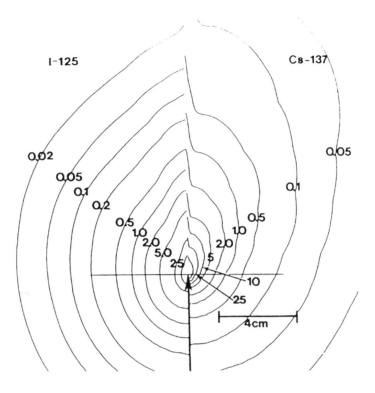

Figure 28-19. *Isodose representation of dose-spread arrays or scatter-dose kernels calculated for unbounded water medium by Monte Carlo simulation. The curves to the left and right of the bold arrow represent the dose-spread arrays for the ^{125}I and ^{137}Cs photon spectra, respectively. The bold arrow represents the primary-photon and collision site. The display in normalized to a value of 100 at a point of 1 cm downstream of the primary-photon collision site. From Williamson (1991a) with permission.*

Our results show that correcting only the primary-photon energy fluence rate for heterogeneities upstream of the scatter voxel at $\bar{r}'$ is inadequate: scaling corrections to the scattering kernel, $K(t,\theta)$, to account for the perturbing effect of heterogeneities intersecting the scattered-photon path between $\bar{r}'$ and $\bar{r}$ were necessary as well. This gave rise to the following scaling correction :

$$K_{het}(t',\theta') = K_{wat}(\rho',\theta') \cdot \left(\frac{\rho'}{t'}\right)^2 \cdot \left(1 - \frac{\mu_{en}(\vec{r}')}{\mu(\vec{r}')}\right)^{het}_{wat} \tag{10}$$

where $t = |\bar{r} - \bar{r}'|$, $\cos\theta' = (\bar{r} - \bar{r}') \cdot \bar{r}'/t$ and K_{wat} is the scattering kernel calculated for homogeneous water medium. r' represents the effective pathlength relative to water over which the scattered photons are attenuated and is given by:

$$\rho' = \frac{1}{\mu'_{wat}} \cdot \int_0^{t'} \mu'\left[\vec{r}' + \ell \cdot \frac{(\vec{r} - \vec{r}')}{|\vec{r} - \vec{r}'|}\right] \cdot d\ell \tag{11}$$

$\mu'(\bar{r})$ and μ'_{wat} denote the linear attenuation coefficients in the heterogeneous and homogeneous geometries respectively. The last bracketed term in equation (10) is the ratio of scattered photon energy emitted per primary photon collision in the heterogeneity relative to that in water. This correction, important for low-energy sources such as ^{125}I, varies from unity only when the scatter voxel at $\bar{r}'$ falls inside a heterogeneity of composition different than that of water. Figure 28-20 shows that the model accurately predicts the HCF arising from a 1 MFP-thick titanium disk near an ^{125}I point source, including the 30% variation in dose with disk diameter.

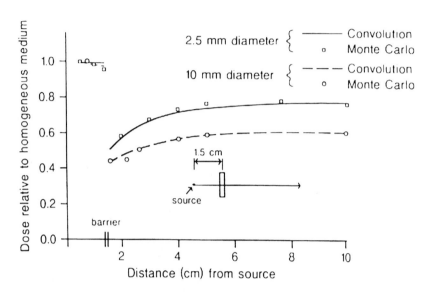

Figure 28-20. *Dose correction factors (dose in heterogeneous geometry/dose in unbounded homogeneous water) as a function of distance from a ^{125}I point source in the presence of a flat disk (0.4 mm thick by 2.5 or 10 mm diameter) of titanium aligned perpendicular to the dose-profile axis and located at 1.5 cm downstream from the source. The lines indicate the results of the convolution calculation and the symbols the corresponding Monte Carlo estimates. From Williamson (1991a) with permission.*

The form of the kernel-scaling correction, equation (10), has important implications for practical implementation of the algorithm. The corrected scattering kernel is spatially variant, i.e., K depends not only on $|\bar{r} - \bar{r}'|$ but on $\bar{r}$ and $\bar{r}'$ individually. First, evaluation of the integral, equation 9, (actually a superposition integral) requires ray tracing between every scattering voxel $\bar{r}'$ and every point of interest, $\bar{r}$. Such algorithms have been classified as "scatter ray-trace methods" by Wong and Purdy (1990). Secondly, spatial variance implies that 3-D Fast-Fourier Transform (FFT) techniques (Boyer 1986b), which require a spatially invariant kernel, can not be used to accelerate numerical evaluation of the integral. Although convolution calculations are very accurate, our implementation (not optimized for speed) was only 20-50 times faster than Monte Carlo simulation, which is clearly too slow for treatment planning. We found that the first-order Taylor expansion of K_{het}, successfully used by Boyer (1986a) in external-beam dosimetry to eliminate explicit scatter-voxel ray tracing and to make the convolution integral spatially invariant, fails in the presence of high-density brachytherapy shields. Thus methods such as adaptive multi-dimensional integration and exploitation of parallel processing, rather than FFT methods, will have to be used to accelerate the calculations. These approaches, along with adaptive recursively-defined 3-D calculation grids, e.g., octrees (Yau and Shihari 1983), offer the potential of reducing the computational burden by as much as two orders of magnitude. Common to adaptive approaches is selective concentration of grid points and integrand evaluations to those spatial regions in which dose gradients are large.

(2) The Scatter-Subtraction Method of Brachytherapy Dose Calculation

To achieve a better compromise between computational efficiency and physical accuracy, the author's group (Williamson 1993a) has developed a variant of the 3-D scatter-integration approach, called the "scatter-subtraction" method. The underlying principle, scatter subtraction, is widely utilized in external beam dosimetry to estimate the scatter dose under small blocks positioned in extended photon-beam fields: scatter dose contributed by an extended field of cross-sectional area F to a point under a small block of area B at depth d is proportional to SMR(d,F) - SMR(d,B). Lulu and Bjarngard (1982) first applied scatter subtraction to 2-D bounded heterogeneities in ^{60}Co beams, reducing these problems to simpler 1-D slab problems that could be solved with conventional heterogeneity corrections, such as the Batho method. Our prototype scatter-subtraction computer code for brachytherapy exploits this principle to reduce the problem of calculating the dose behind a 2-D bounded heterogeneity to two simpler 1-D problems. Thus scatter subtraction reduces the dimensionality of the scatter-convolution integral by one, in principle allowing 3-D heterogeneity problems to be solved using 2-D numerical integration.

The scatter-subtraction algorithm describes the perturbing effect of bounded heterogeneities on the scattered-photon dose distribution in terms of a fundamental dosimetric ratio: the collimated point source scatter-to-primary ratio or SPR(r,θ). Mathematically, SPR(r,θ) is defined (see Figure 28-21) as

$$SPR(r, \theta) = \frac{\text{scatter dose in water}}{\text{primary dose in water}} \quad \text{at distance r from a collimated point source} \qquad (12)$$

Isotropic emission of primary photons is understood to be restricted or collimated to a cone of half-angle θ relative to the line connecting the source and calculation point. These data are precalculated by Monte Carlo simulation for homogeneous liquid-water medium and stored as a 2-D look-up table for use in subsequent dose calculations. Figure 28-22 graphically illustrates SPR(r,θ) data sets for the ^{125}I photon spectrum. The collimated SPR is functionally similar to the SMR of external beam dosimetry except that the angle 2·θ serves as a measure of "brachytherapy field size."

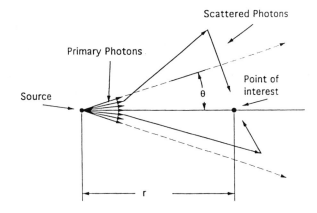

$$SPR(r, \theta) = \frac{\text{Scatter Dose in water}}{\text{Primary Dose in water}} \quad \text{at distance r from a point source collimated to angle } \theta$$

Figure 28-21. *Drawing illustrating the concept of collimated scatter-to primary ratio, SPR(r,θ). Primary photon emission from an isotropic point source, embedded in homogeneous liquid-water medium, is theoretically restricted to a cone of half-angle q, with respect to the source-to-calculation point axis by the Monte Carlo code subroutine which samples the primary-photon trajectories. Both first- and multiply-scattered photon dose contributions are then calculated. For θ = π, SPR (r, θ) is equivalent to the isotropic point-source build-up factor. From Williamson et al. (1993a) with permission.*

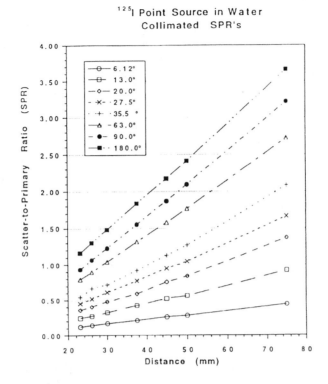

Figure 28-22. *θ) Graphical representation of SPR(r, is plotted as a function of distance along the cone axis for various angles q, for primary-photon spectra consisting of (A)^{125}I photons (B) 100 keV monoenergetic photons and (C) the ^{192}Ir photons. All data were calculated by Monte Carlo simulation. From Williamson et al. (1993a) with permission.*

Figure 28-23 illustrates the simple 2-D benchmark problem our prototype code is designed to solve: find the dose rate at distance r from a point source positioned on the axis of a cylindrical water-equivalent heterogeneity. This 2-D problem is reduced to two more tractable 1-D cylindrically-symmetric problems by partitioning the point source into two disjoint collimated sources. These conical scattering regions are bounded by the cone of half-angle q which subtends the heterogeneity at its center when the cone apex is positioned at the source point. The smaller cone defines a brachytherapy 'mini-beam' in the presence of a slab heterogeneity, while the complementary-cone primary photons interact only with homogeneous medium, contributing scatter-dose to the point of interest by diffusion of multiply-scattered photons around and through the barrier. The mini-beam problem can be solved by a 1-D correction functionally similar to those of external beam dosimetry. Applying the scatter subtraction principle, the dose rate per unit air-kerma strength, $\dot{D}_i(r)$ in the inhomogeneous geometry, can be written as

$$\dot{D}_i(r) = \dot{D}_{p,i}(r) \cdot \left[1 + SPR(r,\theta) \cdot C_1\right] + \dot{D}_{p,h}(r) \cdot \left[SPR(r,\pi) - SPR(r,\theta)\right] \cdot C_2 \qquad (13)$$

where $\dot{D}_{p,i}(r)$ and $\dot{D}_{p,h}(r)$ denote the primary dose rates for the inhomogeneous and homogeneous geometries respectively. The first term represents the primary and scatter dose arising at r from primary photons initially confined to the mini-beam. The second term represents scatter dose that diffuses around and through the heterogeneity due to primary photons colliding in the homogeneous medium outside of the mini-beam. C_1 is the heterogeneity correction factor for the mini-beam slab problem and C_2 is a barrier attenuation correction to the scatter contribution originating outside the mini-beam.

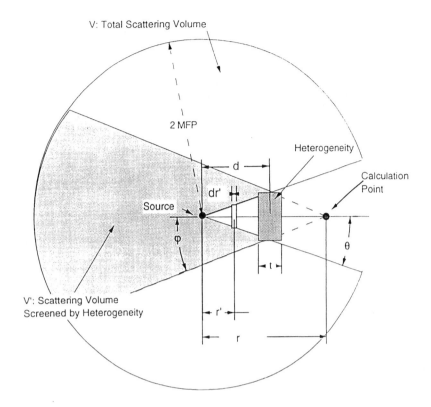

Figure 28-23. *Geometry of the scatter-subtraction model, as applied to a two-dimensional cylindrically-symmetric heterogeneous geometry. The mini-beam boundaries are formed by the cone with its apex located at the photon source, its axis passing through the calculation point and solid angle which subtends the disk-shaped heterogeneity at its center. From Williamson et al. (1993a) with permission.*

The factor C_1 corrects the homogeneous mini-beam SPR for the presence of the slab heterogeneity accounting for (a) attenuation of primary photons by the barrier which influences the magnitude of scattered-photon dose accumulated downstream of the barrier (b) perturbation of scatter radiation accumulating downstream of the barrier due to changes in scatter production within the barrier and (c) perturbation of the scattered radiation component generated upstream of the barrier due to traversing the barrier. Evaluation of this parameter is more complex in brachytherapy than in external beam because the mini-beam can not be approximated by a non-divergent beam. The scatter-subtraction method uses a relatively simple SPR-rescaling approximation that we call "1-D scatter integration." Despite its simplicity, the approach is sufficiently accurate because both numerator and denominator of C_1 use the same simplistic assumptions resulting in significant cancellation of errors.

$$C_1 = \frac{\left[\int_0^\infty \overline{\mu}(r') \cdot \exp(-\int_0^{r'} \mu(\ell) \cdot d\ell) \cdot G(r' \cdot \tan\theta, |r - r'|) \cdot T(\int_{r'}^{r} \mu(\ell) \cdot d\ell) \cdot dr' \right] / \dot{D}_{p,i}(r)}{\left[\int_0^\infty \overline{\mu}(r') \cdot e^{-\overline{\mu} \cdot r'} \cdot G(r' \cdot \tan\theta, |r - r'|) \cdot T(|r' - r|) \cdot dr' \right] / \dot{D}_{p,h}(r)} \tag{14}$$

The numerator and denominator of equation (14) are proportional, respectively, to the heterogeneous and homogeneous SPR's in the mini-beam geometry, both evaluated in the 1-D scatter-integration approximation. Each integral term is approximately proportional to scatter dose which is approximated by the sum of infinitesimal disk-source contributions. This approximation is derived by partitioning the mini-beam into thin disk-shaped scattering sources (see Figure 28-23), and correcting each scattering element for (a) number of once-scattered photons liberated due to primary collisions (b) correcting the first-order scatter fluence for inverse square law and (c) correcting for attenuation of once-scattered photons and subsequent buildup of multiply-scattered photons. The function G(B,r) corrects the once-scattered photon fluence at r for the fact that each disk is a geometrically extended source of scattered photons:

$$G(B,r) = \frac{1}{4\pi B^2} \cdot \ln\left[\frac{B^2 + r^2}{r^2}\right] \qquad (15)$$

where r is distance from a disk-source of radius B to the point of interest. The function T(r) accounts for the attenuation of once-scattered photons emitted by the disk and the consequent buildup of multiply-scattered photons over the distance r-r':

$$T(r) = e^{-\overline{\mu} \cdot r} \cdot [1 + SPR(r,\pi)] = \frac{\text{Total dose in water}}{\text{Dose in free space}} \text{ at distance r from a point source} \qquad (16)$$

and is approximated by the primary-photon SPR data. The terms of the form $\int_{r'}^{r} \mu(\ell) \cdot d\ell$ described 1-D ray-tracing along the mini-beam central ray and account for the attenuating effect of the heterogeneity on the primary- and scattered-photon dose components.

Since the non-unit density of the heterogeneity modifies the transmission of first- and multiply-scattered leakage photons that traverse the heterogeneity, simple subtraction of SPR's does not adequately characterize this scatter-dose component. This phenomenon gives rise to the scatter-subtraction correction, C_2, in equation (13). A simple geometric correction factor was found to model this phenomenon with an adequate degree of accuracy. This correction assumes that the fraction of leakage scatter which is screened by the heterogeneity (volume V' in Figure 28-23) is equal to that fraction of the total scattering volume (volume V) that is shadowed by the barrier with respect to the calculation point. Photons originating in the unscreened region are assumed to be unperturbed while those shadowed by the barrier are assumed to be exponentially attenuated so that C_2 becomes:

$$C_2 = \left(1 - \frac{V'}{V}\right) + \left(\frac{V'}{V}\right) \cdot e^{-\overline{\mu} \cdot (\rho_{het} - 1) \cdot t} \qquad (17)$$

where ρ_{het} and t denote the mass density and axial thickness of the heterogeneous region respectively. The volumes V and V' are given by simple analytic formulae.

Scatter-subtraction predictions were compared to extensive Monte Carlo calculations for ^{125}I, ^{192}Ir and 100 keV point sources near disk-shaped water-equivalent barriers ranging in diameter from 3.6 mm to 24 mm, and in primary-photon transmission from +36% to -70%. Figure 28-24 illustrates these comparisons for ^{125}I and ^{192}Ir sources near 36% transmission disks. For all problems evaluated, the RMS error in our absolute dose-rate predictions ranges from 0.6% to 6.6% with a maximum error of 7% in the worst case. Relative to Monte Carlo simulation, scatter subtraction was 500-1000 times faster. Extension of this promising approach to 3-D geometries, high-atomic-number shields of irregular shape, and to tissue composition heterogeneities is underway.

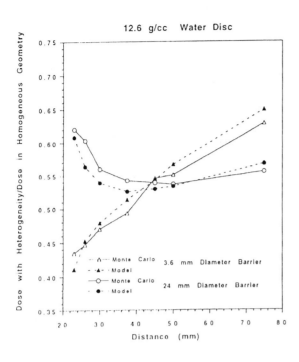
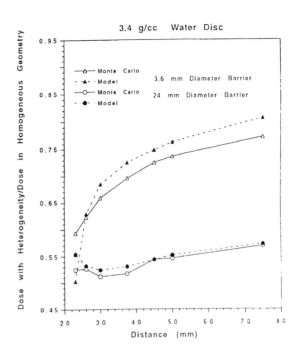

Figure 28-24. *Comparison of 1-D scatter-subtraction predictions (closed symbols) with corresponding Monte Carlo calculations (open symbols) for water- equivalent disk-shaped density heterogeneities located 15 mm from isotropic point sources. The left panel shows a 12.6 g/cc water disk near ^{192}Ir point source. The right panel shows a 3.4 gm/cm cube disk shaped water heterogeneity in the presence of a suit ^{125}I point source. Both graphs compare the model predictions to Monte Carlo calculations for a small 3.6 mm-diameter as well as large 24 mm-diameter barriers. From Williamson et al. (1993a) with permission.*

Conclusions

The status of 3-D dose calculations in brachytherapy have been reviewed. The central problem to solved by such algorithms is accurate prospective calculation of absorbed dose. We have reviewed a number of new and promising developments in basic brachytherapy dosimetry that have emerged during the last decade. These include development of new low-energy sources that offer greatly enhanced potential for radiobiological and physical optimization of implant therapy, and new uses for conventional sources, such as ^{192}Ir in high dose-rate brachytherapy. These opportunities for physical optimization of brachytherapy have reawakened interest in basic experimental and theoretical brachytherapy dosimetry. Through the efforts of a relatively small number of investigators, both dose measurement and Monte Carlo simulation techniques have been perfected and validated, resulting in accurate and reliable clinical treatment planning data for low-energy sources such as ^{125}I and ^{103}Pd and basic single-source dosimetry data for developmental brachytherapy sources. An area of current investigation is development of algorithms capable of supporting accurate, fast and prospective calculation of absorbed dose in the presence of tissue-heterogeneities, applicator shielding, and inter-applicator and source shielding effects. Success of these efforts is essential to large-scale clinical exploitation of the opportunities offered by new isotopes, high dose-rate remote afterloading and image-based treatment planning for improving clinical outcome. While much has been achieved and a number of promising new directions identified, this practical problem remains unsolved.

References

1. Anderson LL, Nath R, Weaver, KA, Nori D, Phillips TL, Son YH, Chiu-Tsao ST, Meigooni AS, Meli JA, Smith V (Interstitial Collaborative Working Group) (1990) Interstitial Brachytherapy, Physical, Biological, and Clinical Considerations, Raven Press, New York.

2. Boyer AL, Mok EC (1985) A photon dose distribution model employing convolution calculations. Med Phys 12:169-177.

3. Boyer AL and Mok EC (1986a) Calculation of photon dose distribution in an inhomogeneous medium using convolutions. Med Phys 13: 503-509.

4. Boyer AL and Mok EC (1986b) Brachytherapy seed dose distribution calculation employing the fast Fourier transform. Med Phys 13: 525-529.

5. Chiu-Tsao S-T, Anderson LL, O'Brien K, Sanna R (1990) Dose Rate Determination for ^{125}I Seeds. Med Phys 17: 815-825.

6. Dale RG (1983) Some theoretical derivations relating to the tissue dosimetry of brachytherapy nuclides with particular reference to iodine-125. Med Phys 10: 176-183.

7. Huang DYC, Schell MC, Weaver KA, Ling CC (1990) Dose distribution of ^{125}I sources in different tissues. Med Phys 17:826-832.

8. Jenkins TM, Nelson WR, Rindi A (1988) Monte Carlo Transport of Electrons and Photons, Plenum Press, New York.

9. Li Z, Williamson JF, Perera H (1993) Monte Carlo calculation of kerma to a point in the vicinity of media interfaces. Phys Med Biol 38:1825-1840.

10. Ling CC, Yorke ED, Spiro IJ, Kubiatowicz D, Bennett D (1983) Physical dosimetry of ^{125}I seeds of a new design for interstitial implant. Int J Radiat Oncol Biol Phys 9:1747-1752.

11. Ling CC, Spiro IJ (1984) Measurement of dose distribution around Fletcher-Suit-Delcos colpostats using a Therados radiation field analyzer (RFA-3). Med Phys 11:326-330.

12. Ling CC, Schell MC, Yorke ED (1985) Two-dimensional dose distribution of ^{125}I seeds. Med Phys 12:652-655.

13. Ling CC, Schell MC, Working KR, Jentzsch K, Harisiadis L, Carabell S, Rogers CC (1987) CT-Assisted Assessment of Bladder and Rectum Dose in Gynecological Implants. Int J Radiat Onc Biol Phys 13:1577-1582.

14. Ling CC, Yorke ED (1989) Interface dosimetry for ^{125}I seeds. Med Phys 16:376-381.

15. Lulu BA, Bjarngard BE (1982) Batho's correction factor combined with scatter summation. Med Phys 9:372-377.

16. Luxton G, Astrahan MA, Findley DO, Petrovich Z (1990) Measurement of dose rate from exposure-calibrated ^{125}I seeds. Int J Radiat Oncol Phys 18:1199-1207.

17. Mackie TR, Scrimger JW, Battista JJ (1985) A convolution method for calculating dose for 15-MV x rays. Med Phys 12:188-196.

18. MacPherson MS, Battista JJ (1995) Dose Distributions and Dose Rate Constants for New Ytterbium-169 Brachytherapy Seeds. Med Phys 22(1):89-96.

19. McLaughlin WL, Yun-Dong C, Soares CG, Miller A, Van Dyk G, Lewis DF (1991) Sensitometry of the response of a new radiochromic film dosimeter to gamma radiation and electron beams. Nuclear Instruments and Methods in Physics Research A302:165-176.

20. Meertens H, van der Laarse R (1985) Screens in ovoids of a Selectron cervix applicator. Radiotherapy and Oncology 3:69-80

21. Meigooni AS, Meli JA, Nath R (1988a) Influence of the variation of energy spectra with depth in the dosimetry of ^{192}Ir using LiF TLD. Phys Med Biol 33:1159-1170.

22. Meigooni AS, Meli JA, Nath R (1988b) A comparison of solid phantoms with water for dosimetry of ^{125}I brachytherapy sources. Med Phys 15:695-701.

23. Meigooni AS, Sabnis S, Nath R (1990) Dosimetry of Palladium-103 Brachytherapy Sources for Permanent Implants. Endocurie Hypertherm Oncol 6:107-117.

24. Meigooni AS, Nath R (1992) Tissue inhomogeneity correction for brachytherapy sources in a heterogeneous phantom with cylindrical symmetry. Med Phys 19:401-407.

25. Meigooni AS, Mishra V., Panth H., Mishra V, Williamson J.F. "Instrumentation and Dosimeter-Size Artifacts in Thermoluminescent Dosimetry of Low-Dose Fields. Med Phys 22:555-561, 1995.

26. Meisberger LL, Keller RJ, Shalek RJ (1968) The Effective Attenuation in Water of the Gamma Rays of Gold 198, Iridium 192, Cesium 137, Radium 226, and cobalt 60. Radiology 90: 953-957.

27. Metcalfe PE (1988) Experimental verification of cesium brachytherapy line source emission using a semiconductor detector. Med Phys 15:702-706.

28. Miller WF, Lewis EE (1984) Computational Methods of Neutron Transport, John Wiley & Sons, New York.

29. Mohan R, Ding IY, Martel MK, Anderson LL, Nori D (1985) Measurements of Radiation Dose Distributions for Shielded Cervical Applicators. Int J Radiat Oncol Biol Phys 11:861-868.

30. Mohan R, Chui C, Lidofsky L (1986) Differential pencil beam dose computation model for photons. Med Phys 13:64-73.

31. Muench PJ, Nath R (1992) Dose distributions produced by shielded applicators using ^{241}Am for intracavitary irradiation of tumors in the vagina. Med Phys 19(5):1299-1306.

32. Nath R, Gray L (1987a) Dosimetry Studies on Prototype ^{241}Am Sources for Brachytherapy. Int J Radiat Oncol Biol Phys 13:897-905.

33. Nath R, Gray L, Park CH (1987b) Dose distributions around cylindrical ^{241}Am sources for a clinical intracavitary applicator. Med Phys 14:809-817.

34. Nath R, Park CH, King CR, Muench P (1990a) A dose computation model for ^{241}Am vaginal applicators including the source-to-source shielding effects. Med Phys 17: 833-842.

35. Nath R, Meigooni AS, Meli JA (1990b) Dosimetry on the transverse axes of ^{125}I and ^{192}Ir interstitial brachytherapy sources. Med Phys 17:1032-1040.

36. Nath R, Meigooni AS, Muench P, Melillo A (1993) Anisotropy Functions for ^{103}Pd, ^{125}I, and ^{192}Ir Interstitial Brachytherapy Sources. Med Phys 20(5):1465-1473.

37. Perera H, Williamson JF, Monthofer SP, Binns WR, Klammen JC, Fuller GA, Wong JW (1992) Rapid Two-dimensional Dose Measurement in Brachytherapy using Plastic Scintillator Sheet: Linearity, Signal-to-Noise Ratio and Energy Response Characteristics. Int J Radiat Oncol Biol Phys 23:1059-1069.

38. Perera H, Williamson JF, Li Z, Mishra V, Meigooni AS (1994) Dosimetric characteristics, air-kerma strength calibration and verification of Monte Carlo simulation for a new ytterbium-169 brachytherapy source. Int J Radiat Oncol Biol Phys 28(4):953-970.

39. Piermattei A, Arcovito G, Bassi FA (1988) Experimental dosimetry of ^{125}I new seeds (Model 6711) for brachytherapy treatments. Physica Medica 1:59-70.

40. Piermattei A, Arcovito G, Azario, L, Rossi, G, Soriani, A and Montemaggi, P. (1992) Experimental dosimetry of ^{169}Yb seeds prototype 6 for brachytherapy treatment. Physica Medica 8: 163-169.

41. Prasad SC, Bassano DA, Kubsada SS (1983) Buildup factors and dose around a ^{137}Cs source in the presence of inhomogeneities. Med Phys 10:705-708.

42. Roesch WC (1958) Dose for Nonelectronic Equilibrium Conditions. Radiation Research 9:399-410.

43. Saylor WL, Dillard M (1976) Dosimetry of ^{137}Cs sources with the Fletcher-Suit gynecological applicator. Med Phys 3:117-119.

44. Schell MC, Ling CC, Gromadzki ZC, Working KR (1987) Dose distributions of model 6702 ^{125}I seeds in water. Int J Radiat Oncol Biol Phys 13:795-799.

45. Schoeppel SL, LaVigne ML, Martel MK, McShan DL, Fraass BA, Roberts JA (1993) Three-Dimensional Treatment Planning of Intracavitary Gynecologic Implants: Analysis of Ten Cases and Implications for Dose Specification. Int J Radiat Onc Biol Phys 28:277-283.

46. Sievert RM (1921) Die Intensitätsverteilung der primaren -Strählung in der Nähe medizinischer Radiumpräparate. Acta Radiologica 1:89-128.

47. Van der Laarse R, Meertens H (1984) An algorithm for ovoid shielding of a cervix applicator. The Proceedings 8th International Conference on the Use of Computers in Radiation Therapy, Toronto, Canada, edited by Cunningham JR, Ragan D, Van Dyk D, Los Angeles, CA, IEEE Computer Society, 365-369.

48. Weaver KA, (1986) The dosimetry of ^{125}I seed eye plaques. Med Phys 13:78-83.

49. Weaver KA, Smith V, Huang D, Barnett C, Schell MC, Ling C (1989) Dose parameters of ^{125}I and ^{192}Ir seed sources. Med Phys 16:636-643.

50. Weeks KJ, Dennett JC (1990) Dose Calculation and Measurements for a CT-Compatible Version of the Fletcher Applicator. Int J Radiat Oncol Biol Phys 18:1191-1198.

51. Williamson JF (1987) Monte Carlo evaluation of kerma at a point for photon transport problems. Med Phys 14:567-576.

52. Williamson JF (1988a) Monte Carlo and Analytic Calculation of Absorbed Dose near ^{137}Cs Intracavitary Sources. Int J Radiat Oncol Biol Phys 15:227-237.

53. Williamson JF (1988b) Monte Carlo evaluation of specific dose constants in water for ^{125}I seeds. Med Phys 15:686-694.

54. Williamson JF (1989) Radiation Transport Calculations in Treatment Planning. Computerized Medical Imaging and Graphics 13:251-268.

55. Williamson JF (1990) Dose Calculations About Shielded Gynecological Colpostats. Int J Radiat Onc Biol Phys 19:167-178.

56. Williamson JF, Baker R, Li Z, (1991a) A convolution algorithm for brachytherapy dose computations in heterogeneous geometries. Med Phys 18:1256-1265.

57. Williamson JF (1991b) Comparison of measured and calculated dose rates in water near I-125 and Ir-192 seeds. Med Phys 18(4):776-786.

58. Williamson JF, Li Z, Wong JW (1993a) One-Dimensional Scatter-Subtraction Method for Brachytherapy Dose Calculation near Bounded Heterogeneities. Med Phys 20:233-244.

59. Williamson JF, Perera H, Li Z and Lutz WR (1993b) Comparison of Calculated and Measured Heterogeneity Correction Factors for ^{125}I, ^{137}Cs and ^{192}Ir Brachytherapy Sources near Localized Heterogeneities. Med Phys 20:209-222.

60. Williamson J.F. (1995) Recent Advances in Brachytherapy Dosimetry. In: Smith AR (ed) Radiation Therapy Physics. Berlin; Springer-Verlag pp. 247-302 .

61. Wong JW, Purdy JA (1990) On methods of Inhomogeneity Corrections for Photon Transport. Med Phys 17:807-814.

62. Yau MM and Shirhari SN (1983) A Hierarchical Data Structure for Multidimensional Digital Images. Communications of the ACM Journal 26: 504-515.

63. Young MEJ, Batho HF (1964) Dose tables for linear radium sources calculated by an electronic computer. Brit J Radiol 37:38-44.

Chapter 29

3-D Brachytherapy: Clinical Experience

Theodore L. Phillips, M.D. and Keith Weaver, Ph.D.

Dept of Radiation Oncology, University of California San Francisco, San Francisco, California

The introduction of image-based tumor localization, normal tissue localization, and treatment planning has made significant strides in megavoltage teletherapy. It remains, however, in its infancy in terms of application to brachytherapy. There are a number of reasons for the delay in implementation which will be discussed below, but a number of solutions are also available that will see application in the next few years. We have had experience at UCSF in several body areas using three dimensional (3-D) planning and are developing systems to apply this generally.

Reasons for Difficulty in Introduction of 3-D Planning to Brachytherapy

In order to fully apply the advantages of image-based dose localization, it is necessary to locate in three dimensional space the position of anatomical structures and tumor tissue, as well as the radiation dose distribution. In the case of brachytherapy, radiation is emitted by interstitial sources which may either be permanent, hand afterloaded or placed by remote afterloading machines. It is relatively simple to locate the anatomic structures based on CT (computed tomography) with fiducial marks. It is often much more difficult to delineate the tumor. In general, this is done best with MRI (magnetic resonance imaging) which must then be integrated into the planning system with CT as the gold standard for exact dimensions. Finally, the most difficult task is locating the position of the sources relative to the anatomic structures. This is usually done with orthogonal or stereo-radiographs which can obtain high precision. Recently several efficient programs have been developed that calculate dose distributions in 3-D.(1) Unfortunately, these do not display the anatomic structures, with the exception of the bones, in any detail. The use of stereotactic frames solves this problem, and they have been widely applied for CNS implants. Transferring this technology to other body sites is in process, but not yet a satisfactory clinical tool. The use of multiple bony landmarks in conjunction with catheter, source or seed locations is an interim solution which appears to have reasonable accuracy.

A number of attempts have been made to localize sources using the actual CT or MRI images. The spatial resolution available makes it often difficult to precisely localize each source. Many of the needles and applicators are not suitable for use with MRI and cause, in addition, artifacts in CT.

Solutions to the Problem

The initial and obvious solution is the use of CT and MRI with stereotactic frames or other immobilization devices. These are well known for CNS implants, and a fair amount of work has been done in developing a generally applicable body stereotactic device. Significant progress in this direction has been made by Bruce Lulu at the University of Arizona, and by others. Various persons have proposed the insertion of mounting screws in bony structures such as the pelvis to which a removable stereotactic frame could be attached for accurate localization. CT and MRI compatible applicators are under development and have been tested in a limited fashion at UCSF for pelvic MRI.

For maximum accuracy in placing the dose distribution within and about the tumor, it will be necessary to guide the applicators, needles or sources directly into the tumor, using fluoroscopic imaging techniques or either stereotaxis or remote arms which are linked in 3-D space to the imaging program. Several methods for doing this have been developed, using either direct linkage with sensors or laser localization techniques. These techniques will allow not only the accurate recording of where the actual dose is deposited but with preplanning, the accurate placement of the carriers and sources into an ideal distribution within the tumor.

The flexibility allowed with remote afterloaders, either high-dose rate or pulsed low-dose rate, allows for correction of some of the maldistribution of needles or catheters through weighting of source dwell time. This is only a partial correction, however, and the patient would be better served by more accurate placement of these needles and catheters.

UCSF Experience to Date

The largest experience with 3-D planned and executed interstitial radiotherapy is in the central nervous system. The placement of a frame for localization prior to CT and MRI imaging allows exact fiducial marking and 3-D space identification of the location of tumor and normal structures. Needle insertion guides and templates attached to the stereotactic frame allow for accurate positioning of source carriers (catheters) in the tumor volume with accuracy to within a few millimeters. The UCSF computer program BRAIN for planning and evaluating stereotactic implants has been described in detail by Weaver, et al. (9,10) color Plates 22 and 23 shows how BRAIN allows catheters, sources, and isodoses to be superposed over the CT images. More than 600 patients have had successful stereotactic implants for malignant gliomas using this planning system. The results have been quite encouraging with improvement in survival to 88 weeks in glioblastoma multiforme.(5) Results in anaplastic astrocytoma have not been superior to conventional management, and the technique is reserved for failure of initial therapy. The experience with gliomas has proven the efficacy of 3-D planning for brachytherapy.

Until now, 3-D imaging has only been used as a planning aid for sites other than the brain. We have had limited experience with gynecologic malignancies. CT and MRI are used to plan template implants, using either the Martinez or the Syed templates, and either conventional iridium with flexiguides or pulsed low-dose rate iridium using the Selectron Martinez template. Planning processes have been remarkably improved by the use of 3-D data, and delivery is relatively close to the plan because the template is placed on the perineum and the obturator in the vagina at the time of preimplant scanning. In a number of patients, scans have also been obtained with the needles in place, using the flexiguides. We are currently in the process of evaluating CT and MR compatible needles for use with the pulsed Selectron.

Applications in the head and neck and other sites have so far been limited to exercises in preplanning. However, currently undergoing testing is a generalized version of BRAIN called CTBRACHY. This program incorporates CT imaging into a general-purpose brachytherapy planning software package. No stereotactic frame is used - source positions are obtained with conventional orthogonal or stereo-shift radiographs. The program uses images of three non-collinear points that are visible both on the films and on CT reconstructions to transform seed positions to CT space. In addition to iodine seeds, allowed source types include low and high activity iridium and cesium pellets. Figure 29-1 and 2 illustrate the output of this program for a permanent iodine implant of the falx for a meningioma. We expect to add MRI to the program in the near future. This program should largely solve the problem of localizing sources accurately with respect to the tumor and other anatomic structures.

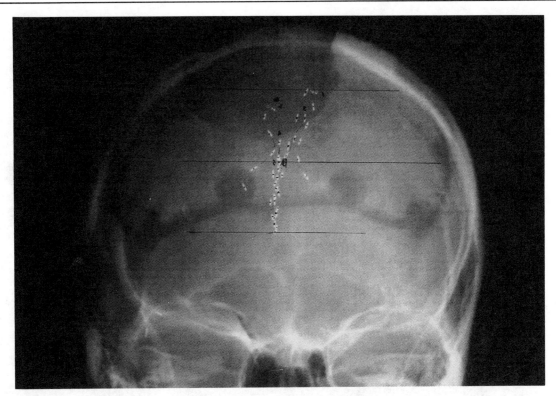

Figure 29-1a.

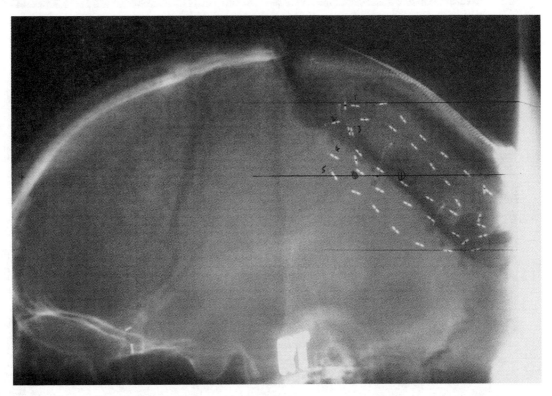

Figure 29-1b.

Figure 29-1. *Orthogonal radiographs of the skull of a patient with meningioma of the Falx cerebri.and a permanent iodine 125 implant. Panel A is an AP view and panel B a lateral view.*

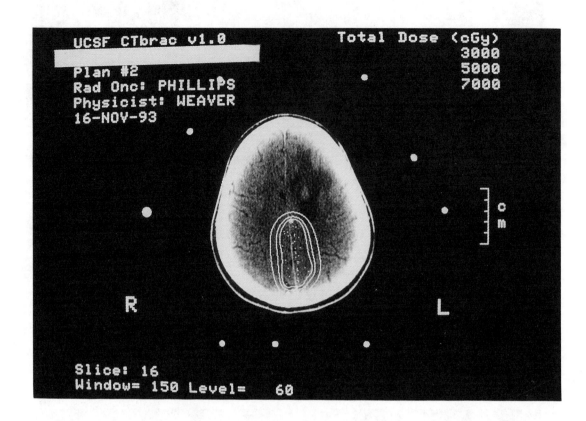

Figure 29-2a.

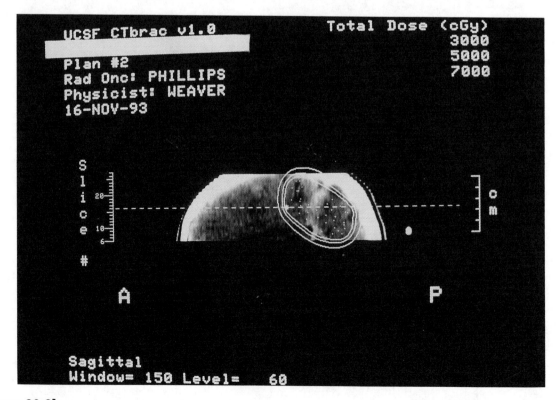

Figure 29-2b.

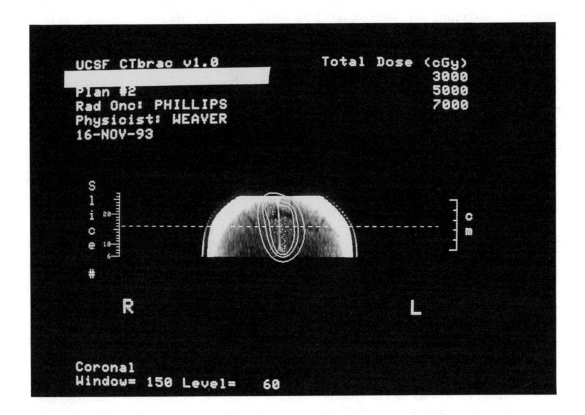

Figure 29-2c.

Figure 29-2. *Output form the new CTBRACHY program showing the distribution of dose for a permanent iodine 125 implant in the same patient as FIgure 29-2. Panel A: Axial view. Panel B: Sagittal view. Panel C: Coronal view.*

Discussion

A number of groups are working on the use of axial scans with CT and MRI. Much of the work has used axial images in planning but not in dose calculation and in selection of prescription dose. Stereotactic implants of the CNS required not only displays of dose on CT images but three dimensional images and 3-D dose calculations, allowing displays of dose in any arbitrary plane, thus allowing dose optimization and conformation of the dose to the tumor target. In addition to UCSF several research groups and more recently commercial companies have produced such software.

Applying these principles to other brachytherapy sites is more difficult as outlined above. Indexing of the CT space to the images of sources or applicators was a nominal problem in the 'CNS with stereotactic frames. Little distortion of the anatomy occurs due to the implant. At other sites, although the sources can be placed accurately relative to the bony anatomy, distortion of the soft tissue due to edema and hemorrhage as well as mechanical pressure from the applicators or needles will be a problem. The amount of this problem as determined by clinical experience will determine if a post-implant CT is required or whether the pre-implant planning CT will suffice, as it has for brain implants.

Roy and co-authors have described a method for planning permanent implants of the prostate using CT. (4) The prostate is outlined on each 5 mm slice and related to a template placed against the perineum during the planning CT. Trajectories are them calculated to limit needle tracks outside the prostate and achieve coverage of the prostate with at least 90% of the prescribed dose. They found that this method more accurately depicted the actual dose as compared to nomogram methods and often required twice the radioactivity to achieve the nominal dose to 90% or more of the gland. This suggests that actual calculations on CT are far superior to nomograms in permanent implants.

In a study of orthogonal films, CT and TLD measurements, Kapp and coworkers found that single point calculations of bladder and rectal dose seriously underestimate the maximum dose by 140% in 13.8% of patients.(2) They suggest that multiple points be calculated. This study indicates that CT planning and verification of dose could reduce toxicity through calculations of dose at many points in critical structures. Indeed, dose volume histograms may be of even more value.

Warszawski explored the use of isodose curves from brachytherapy determined from radiographs superimposed on CT images.(8) They found their technique superior for displaying doses to target and critical organs for flexible catheter implants. This technique is similar to the one we propose.

The University of Michigan group has developed CT and MRI compatible gynecologic applicators and template techniques and evaluated dose distributions on both CT and MRI. (3,6,7) They found that interstitial implants could be optimized and that MRI gave superior information on tumor location and dose. Their approach uses MRI or CT with compatible applicators in place. It remains to be seen if orthogonal radiographs can produce source position data that is accurate enough to avoid the need for a scan with applicators in place.

Plans for the Future

Programs are under development for accurate alignment of the localization points for needles, catheters and sources with CT, and MRI in 3-D. These programs are using identifiable bony anatomic landmarks, and will also be capable of using implanted fiducial seeds. A stereotactic device is also under investigation for use in the pelvis.

A system which uses multiple laser beams and CCD cameras to determine the position of the handle of a wand in 3-D space is also being considered. This will allow the accurate implantation of needles in 3-D space. A similar apparatus using LED's and CCD cameras is already under application in conjunction with the Peacock system for 3-D conformal therapy using modulated beams and multileaf collimation. We plan to work on developing a stereotactic remote wand system for brachytherapy insertions.

References

1. Elbern, A.W. Computation of dose distribution for linear radioactive sources in brachytherapy. *Computers in Biology and Medicine* 22(4):263268, 1992.

2. Kapp, K.S., Stuecklschweiger, G.F., Kapp, D.S., and Hackl, A.G. Dosimetry of intracavitary placements for uterine and cervical carcinoma: results of orthogonal film, TLD and CT-assisted techniques. *Radiotherapy and Oncology* 24:137-146. 1992.

3. LaVigne, M.L,Schoeppel, S.L, and .,McShan, D. L. The use of CT based 3-D anatomical modeling. in the design of customized perineal templates for interstitial gynecologic implants. *Medical Dosimetry* 16:187-192 1991.

4. Roy, J.N, Wallner, K.E., Harrington, P.J., Ling, C.C., Anderson, L.L. A CT-based evaluation method for permanent implants: application to the prostate. *International Journal of Radiation Oncology Biology Physics* 26:163-169, 1993.

5. Scharfen, C.S.; Sneed, P.K.; Wara, W.M.; Larson, D.A; Phillips, T.L.; Prados, M.D.; Weaver, K.A.; Malec, M.; Lamborn K.R.; Lamb, S.A.; Ham, B.; Gutin, P.H. High activity Iodine-125 interstitial implant for gliomas. *International Journal of Radiation Oncology Biology Physics* 24:583-591, 1992.

6. Schoeppel, S.L., Ellis, J.H., LaVigne M.L., Schea, R.A., Roberts, J.A. Magnetic resonance imaging during intracavitary gynecologic brachytherapy. *International Journal of Radiation Oncology Biology Physics* 23:169-174. 1992.

7. Schoeppel, S.L., Fraass, B.A., Hopkins, M.P., LaVigne M.L., Lichter, A.S., McShan, D.L., Noffsinger, S, Perez-Tomayo, C., and Roberts, J.A. A CT compatible version of the Fletcher system intracavitary applicator: clinical application and 3-dimensional treatment planning. *International Journal of Radiation Oncology Biology Physics* 17:1103-1109, 1989.

8. Warszawski, N.; Bleher, M.; Bratengeier, K.; Bohndorf, W. The use of isodose curves on radiographs and on CT scans in interstitial brachytherapy. *Clinical Oncology (Royal College of Radiologists)* 4(4):228-231, 1992.

9. Weaver, K.A.; Smith, V.; Lewis, J.; Lulu, B.; Barnett, C.; Leibel, S.; Gutin, P.; Phillips, T.L. A CT-based computerized treatment planning system for I-125 stereotactic brain implants. *International Journal of Radiation Oncology Biology Physics* 18:445, 1990.

10. Weaver, K.A. "Stereotactic Brachytherapy Physics" in Radiation Therapy Physics, Alfred Smith ed., Springer-Verlag GmbH, in press.

Chapter 30

Radiation Therapy Electronic Portal Imaging Devices

Daniel A. Low, Ph. D.

Mallinckrodt Institute of Radiology, Washington University School of Medicine, St. Louis, Missouri

There has been a surge of interest in the development of on-line portal imaging for radiotherapy driven by the development of electronic portal imaging devices (EPIDs). Two outstanding reviews have appeared recently that cover the state of the art in the design and use of EPIDs (11, 44). Most of the clinical and scientific investigation of on-line portal imaging has taken place with developmental units. This has confined the studies and utilization of this technology to research-driven radiotherapy departments. However, the recent development and sale of commercial systems [1,2,3,4] will result in the spread of on-line imaging to smaller clinics.

The introduction of EPIDs into the clinic demands an improved understanding by physicists of their characteristics, capabilities and limitations. The physicist will be involved in the evaluation of competing commercial devices and must be able to develop specifications for the acquisition of the imager. An understanding of the types of available imagers, imaging techniques and concepts will be important for the generation of acceptance tests and commissioning procedures. Image analysis software will likely be included with the EPID, and the physicist should have an understanding of how the software affects the presented image. Image alignment and registration software may also be included and will have to be evaluated.

This paper starts with a discussion of the imaging concepts borrowed from diagnostic radiology and modified for use in radiation therapy. It then considers currently available imaging techniques along with one promising technology. Finally, image enhancement, evaluation and alignment software are discussed.

Imaging Parameters

Developers have utilized concepts based on those found in diagnostic radiology and digital imaging to describe the imaging characteristics of EPIDs. While in most cases the parameters can be applied directly, there are characteristics of radiation therapy imaging that make it unique. For example, the pixel sizes required in digital radiography range from 0.05 cm in cardiac and gastro-intestinal imaging to 0.01 cm in mammography and chest imaging (43). This is smaller than the pixel sizes currently offered with commercial EPID products (typically 0.05 cm to 0.1 cm at isocenter). Physical processes also alter the environment in which the image is acquired. Figure 30-1 shows the subject contrasts (defined below) of a 1-cm thick air cavity and a 1-cm thick bony structure imbedded in a 20-cm thick water phantom as a function of incident monoenergetic photon energy (11). The subject contrast is 10-20 times lo wer for radiation therapy energies than diagnostic energies due to the increase in the fraction of scattered photons and the decrease in the difference in relative photon attenuation of the object to water.

---

[1] Varian Associates, Palo Alto, CA.
[2] Siemens Medical Systems, Concord, CA.
[3] Philips Medical Systems, Shelton, CO.
[4] InfiMed Inc, Liverpool, NY

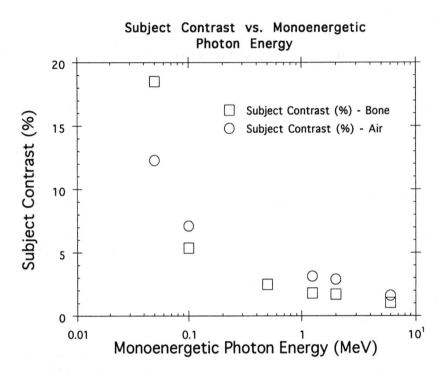

Figure 30-1. *The subject contrast of a 1-cm thick bony structure imbedded in a 20-cm thick water phantom as a function of incident monoenergetic photon energy. The subject contrast drops dramatically with increasing photon energy due to the reduction of the photoelectric cross section relative to the Compton cross section as well as the increased scatter fraction at higher energies.*

The ability to distinguish an object, such as a bone, from background tissues requires that the number of photons passing through the object differs from the number of photons passing through the neighboring tissues. The quantity that describes the presentation of the object at the image plane is the subject contrast. Motz and Danos (11, 41) defined the subject contrast as the ratio of the difference in the signal beneath the object (n) to

that of the background (n') normalized to the mean signal.

$$S = \frac{n - n'}{(n + n')/2}$$

(1)

For an object of thickness L_x and linear attenuation coefficient μ_x imbedded in a homogeneous medium of thickness L and linear attenuation coefficient μ, the subject contrast can be written as:

$$S = \frac{2\left(1 - e^{-L_x(\mu_x - \mu)}\right)}{1 + e^{-L_x(\mu_x - \mu)} + (2F)/(1 - F)}$$

(2)

where F is the scatter fraction, equal to the fraction of photons incident on the detector stemming from scatter. Equation 2 shows that the subject contrast improves with increasing object thickness and decreasing scatter fraction (from, for example, a thinner medium or increased object-to-detector distance). As the scatter fraction approaches 1, the subject contrast goes to zero, as expected. In addition, the subject contrast improves as the difference in the between the linear attenuation of the subject and the background increases.

While equation 2 gives an indication of the effects of the difference between the photon flux, it does not reveal if the object will be visible in the image. This is because there is uncertainty in the value of any pixel or pixels due to noise. Noise can arise from statistical fluctuations in the number of photons available to construct the image or from electronics used to acquire the image. Therefore, while the subject contrast is an important imaging concept, it does not necessarily indicate if an object will be detected in the image. One quantity that indicates the relationship between the ability to distinguish an object and the noise is called the signal-to-noise ratio (SNR). When the noise is associated only with the statistical fluctuation in the photons used to create the image, the SNR can be written as:

$$SNR = \frac{n - n'}{\sqrt{n + n'}}$$

(3)

The SNR can be described using the same variables as equation 2 to yield

$$SNR = \left[A\Phi \eta e^{-\mu L}\left(1 + e^{-L_x(\mu_x - \mu)} + \frac{2F}{1 - F}\right)\right]^{1/2} \frac{S}{2}$$

(4)

where A is the area of the object to be imaged, Φ is the photon flux impinging on the patient integrated over the image acquisition time, and η is the photon detection efficiency of the detector (indicating the number of "counts" collected per incident photon). The SNR improves with decreasing phantom thickness (through increased photon flux and decreased scatter fraction), increased object area, detection efficiency and subject contrast.

While the subject contrast decreases markedly from diagnostic procedures to radiation therapy procedures, the photon penetration and flux increase greatly. In the example presented earlier, the SNR remains constant up to Cobalt energies and then decreases by only a factor of two at an energy roughly equivalent to that of an 18 MV beam (see Figure 30-2) (11). This simple analysis indicates that images with contrast detail comparable to that found in diagnostic procedures are possible in radiation therapy.

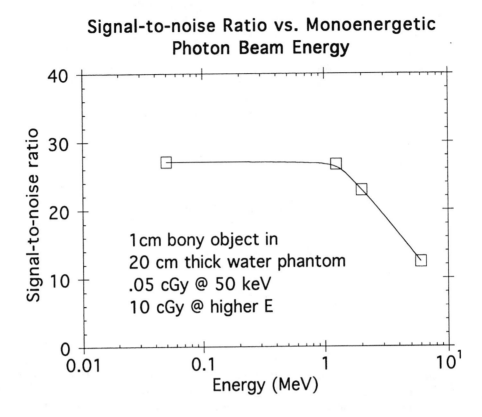

Figure 30-2. *The signal-to-noise ratio (SNR) of the same system as in Figure 30-1 plotted as a function of incident monoenergetic photon energy. The beam intensities have been established for typical diagnostic and therapy procedures, as appropriate for the incident beam energy. The SNR is roughly constant from diagnostic energies to Cobalt. The reduction in subject contrast has been compensated by the increased photon flux.*

The SNR can be used to gauge whether an image will be detectable from the background. Studies have shown that for the object to be visible, the signal-to-noise ratio must satisfy the condition (41),

$$SNR \geq 5 \tag{5}$$

The number of incident photons is not measured using clinical imagers whose output pixel values may not be linear with respect to incident photon flux. Therefore, the concept of signal-to-noise ratio must be generalized to the resulting image to be useful for clinical applications. Equation 3 can be rewritten to consider a collection of pixels by substituting the average pixel value for the number of collected photons. The imager will behave linearly over a sufficiently small range of pixel values so the SNR can be evaluated in this limit. The noise is replaced by the uncertainty in the pixel average as measured by the distribution of pixel values beneath the object of interest (28).

$$SNR = \frac{|\bar{n} - \bar{n}'|}{\left(d\bar{n}^2 + d\bar{n}'^2\right)^{1/2}} \tag{6}$$

where $\bar{n}$ and $\bar{n}'$ are the average pixel values in the image of the test object and the background, respectively, and $\delta\bar{n}$ and $\delta\bar{n}'$ are the uncertainties in the test object and background average readings, respectively.

The noise introduced by the acquisition system can be characterized by the noise-power spectrum (NPS) which is the frequency-space representation of the variance of the output signal to the input signal. While the NPS expresses the modification of the signal by the imager, the effect on the SNR caused by the imager yields a more direct indication of the influence of the imaging hardware on the quality of the image. The ratio of output SNR to input SNR yields this information. If the SNR is presented as a function of spatial frequency, the square of the ratio of output SNR to input SNR yields what is termed the Detective Quantum Efficiency (DQE) (11):

$$DQE(f) = \left[\frac{SNR_{out}(f)}{SNR_{in}(f)} \right]^2$$

(7)

The DQE is also a measure of the image receptor dose efficiency(8).

The spatial resolution of an imager is best described by its modulation transfer function (MTF), which is defined as the Fourier transform of the line-spread function (LSF). The LSF is obtained by irradiating the imaging device with a thin beam and observing the resulting image values. In general, the image will be resemble a Gaussian, with a poorer imager exhibiting a broader peak or higher tail. The Fourier transform of the peak yields the MTF.

In electronic systems, the MTF indicates the fraction of a signal with a particular frequency that is transmitted through the system. The MTF(0) is related to the DC gain of the system. Since images are inherently different than the source distributions, the MTF(0) value has no meaning, and can be arbitrarily set to 1.0 for comparison with higher frequency components (equivalent to the ability to arbitrarily normalize the resulting image). The ideal MTF has a value of 1.0 for all frequencies indicating a faithful representation of the subject. A realistic imaging device has an MTF that begins at 1.0 for zero frequency and decreases for higher frequencies. Better imaging systems retain a greater MTF at higher frequencies than poorer imagers.

The effect of non-unity MTF on an image can be illustrated by examining the region near the edge of an object. A perfect edge (indicated by the sudden change in flux over a small distance) contains very high-frequency components that must be transmitted through the imaging device to display the edge in the image. The reduction of the MTF at high frequencies indicates that this edge cannot be faithfully reproduced. The result is a blurred edge in the image. Therefore, for imaging sharp-edged or small features, the MTF must be large at wavelengths comparable to the size of the featured image.

In practice, however, the MTF of therapy imagers is difficult to measure due to scattered radiation. The measurement of the line-spread function at radiation therapy energies has been described by Droege et al. (13) and Monro et al. (37). The presence of scattered radiation complicates the derivation of the MTF from the LSF data.

The DQE can be related to the MTF by(11):

$$DQE(f) = K^2 \frac{MTF^2(f)}{\Phi NPS(f)}$$

(8)

where K is a constant that indicates the gain of the system, which for a linear digital system can be taken to be unity. The DQE indicates the relative efficiency of transfer of information (SNR) as a function of incident frequency and therefore depends upon the MTF. Since the SNR is affected by system noise, the DQE is also sensitive to noise, as indicated by the presence of the NPS in equation 8.

EPID Technology

There are two types of commercially available EPIDs. One uses a metal plate to convert photons to scattered electrons which strike a fluorescent screen producing an image(6, 23, 35, 36, 48). The image is viewed via a front-surface mirror using a television camera. The light collection is very inefficient with these systems, as only 0.01% of the light generated in the phosphor is gathered by the camera(35, 36). The size of the fluorescent screen ranges from 40 x 40 cm to 35 x 44 cm with a projected size at isocenter of from 19 x 24 cm to 26 x 33 cm. The acquisition rate of these detectors is quite rapid, with an image acquired every 1/30 of a second (the video frame rate). However, rarely is a frame rate of 1/30 of a second required for therapy imaging, and groups of images can be averaged to reduce the noise level and improve the SNR. The images are digitized using frame-grabber circuits with an analog-to-digital conversion dynamic range of 8 bits (with in one case averaging to 16 bits) and from 256 x 512 to 512 x 512 pixels.

The cameras supply a great deal of the image noise, and one method of improving these images is to improve the quality of the video camera. Wong is investigating the effects of replacing the standard video camera with a cooled CCD camera(52). The CCD chip is cooled to reduce background thermal noise resulting in the reduction of the final image noise. One difficulty with CCD cameras is their sensitivity to ionizing radiation, so the camera must be adequately shielded from scattered x-ray radiation.

The optical systems have the disadvantage that the 45 degree mirror makes them large. They cannot then be used with a beam stopper machine. However, most commercial designers have made the mounts retractable so the imager does not intrude on patient setup or on patient treatments when the patient is not being imaged.

The second commercial system utilizes a liquid ionization chamber to acquire the image (shown in Figure 30-3). It is based on a chamber developed at The Netherlands Kanker Instituut (32, 33, 46, 47). The chamber operates through the ionization of a 0.08 cm thick layer of isooctane liquid (similar to gasoline) placed between two circuit boards. A 1 mm thick steel converter plate is used to enhance the chamber photon. The active area is 32.5 x 32.5 cm (for a projected field of view of 23 x 23 cm at a target-chamber distance of 140 cm) with 256 x 256 pixels (0.127 cm on a side per pixel). One circuit board (the high-voltage board) is charged to 250 V, and the positive ions are collected on the other circuit board (the collection board). The boards are etched such that one of 256 parallel conducting strips on the high-voltage board is energized at one time and the ions are simultaneously collected from 256 parallel conducting strips on the collection board. Each strip on the collection board is connected to an electrometer and its output is multiplexed to a digital-to-analog converter and stored as a 12-bit value. The electrometers are scanned multiple times (7.5 µs per electrometer) to obtain the radiation intensity distribution at the level of the energized high-voltage line. The scans are repeated until roughly 10 or 20 milliseconds has passed, depending on the user-selected imager acquisition mode. The next high-voltage line is then energized and scanned to obtain the intensity distribution along that line. The entire scan process takes roughly 5 to 10 seconds and is synchronized with the accelerator beam pulse repetition rate to ensure that the beam intensity will remain relatively constant for the data acquisition scans. Therefore different acquisition parameters are set at the factory as a function of beam energy and pulse repetition rate. Four different acquisition modalities are provided, though only two have been found to be clinically useful. These two are the standard mode, which acquires the image with the full 256 x 256 resolution, and the fast acquisition mode, that energizes two neighboring high-voltage lines simultaneously, yielding an image with 128 x 256 pixels. The fast acquisition mode is approximately four times as fast as the standard mode and can be used when an image is required with the minimum patient dose.

The chamber signals are not directly stored. Differences in electrometer sensitivity, high voltage settings and chamber imperfections yield sensitivity differences across the chamber that would render the image clinically useless. The image is referenced to an image taken with no radiation to eliminate electrometer offsets and an image taken with an open field to eliminate sensitivity variations across the chamber. This modified image is stored in either a compressed or uncompressed format.

While not yet commercially available, hydrogenated amorphous silicon (a-Si:H) is being investigated for use in a detector for radiation therapy(2, 3, 4, 5). Crystalline silicon CCDs cannot be manufactured to sizes required for therapy imaging, unlike a-Si:H which has been manufactured to 30 x 30 cm. The size may be increased to 100 x 100 cm for display technology by 1996(1). The a-Si:H detector array is used as a light detector behind a converter plate and phosphor screen. The a-Si:H detector consists of a two-dimensional array of a-Si:H photodiodes coupled to an a-Si:H field-effect transistor (FET). The sensor converts visible light to an electrical signal which is controlled by the FET. Figure 30-4 shows a diagram of a single sensor and Figure 30-5 shows a schematic of an array. The x-rays strike the converter consisting of a metal plate/phosphor combination producing visible light which is transmitted through a transparent conducting later to the photodiode. The transparent conducting layer (indium tin oxide, ITO) allows the application of reverse bias to the photodiode while transmitting the visible light. Metal conductors are placed between adjacent pixels to distribute the reverse bias voltage which is used to deplete the intrinsic layer of the photodiode.

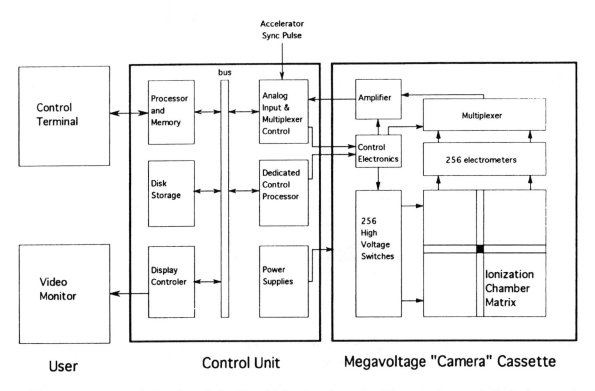

Figure 30-3. A schematic of the liquid ionization chamber and associated electronics

The signal is transferred to the source side of the FET which acts as a gate to allow the charge to be either trapped on the source side or to be transferred to the drain side, depending upon the state of the gate control bias. The gate lines are connected via FET control lines along rows of detectors while the drains are connected along data lines connected to columns of connectors. Therefore, as a particular gate row is activated, the currents collected in the row of sensors can be sampled along the columns of data lines. Each data line is connected to an external charge-sensitive preamplifier.

Data acquisition consists of the irradiation of the EPID with resulting current in the photodiode and charging of the n-layer to a value equal to the liberated electron-hole pairs in the depletion region. Readout and resetting of the bias across the photodiodes is accomplished by activating the FET control lines to allow the stored charge to flow to the preamplifiers. The FETs are then rendered nonconducting and the next column is read out. The resetting of the sensors during readout allows them to begin gathering data as soon as their readout is complete.

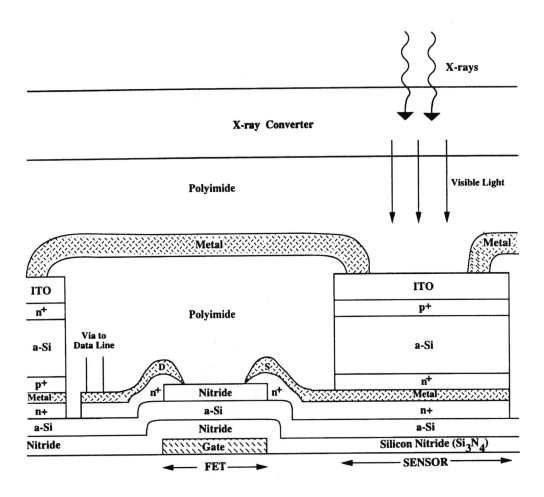

Figure 30-4. *A schematic of a single a-Si:H detector within an a-Si:H detector array. The a-Si:H field-effect transistor is shown on the left with the photodiode on the right.*

The efficiency of the charge collection as a function of incident radiation intensity is a function of the fractional area covered by the optical sensors (the fill factor). Since some of the area is taken by the FETs and other non-sensitive functions, the fill factor is not 1.00, and has ranged from 0.48 to 0.83 in test arrays. However, even with this limitation, light collection efficiency is far superior to the mirror system. In addition, the sensitivity of the sensor must match the light output characteristics of the phosphor (see Figure 30-6). The collection efficiency of the current prototype a-Si:H detector is roughly 60% to 70% from 450 nm to 650 nm and matches well the output of CsI(Tl) and Gd_2O_2S:Tb scintillators.

The advantages of a-Si:H as an imaging device are numerous. Since it has an amorphous structure, the damaging effects of radiation are minimized allowing the detector to be placed in the primary beam. Second, the devices should be relatively flat (on the order of 2 cm) allowing their use with beam-stop accelerators. In addition, their light weight may allow them to be mounted on portable cassettes to be transported to the desired site. The devices may also be used for fluoroscopy in the clinic, eliminating the bulky and cumbersome intensifier tube and eliminating the image distortion found in these systems.

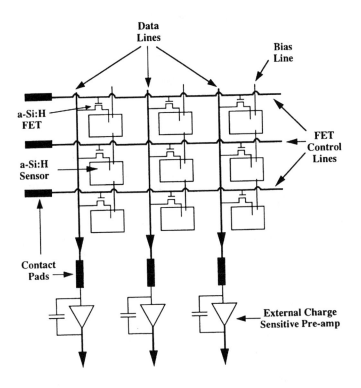

Figure 30-5. A schematic of an a-Si:H detector array

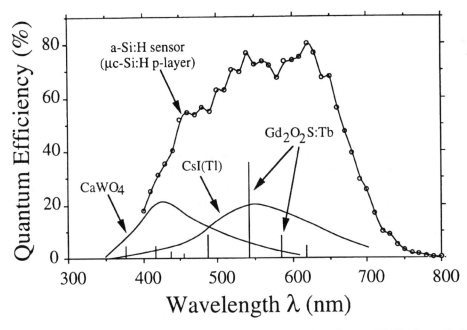

Figure 30-6. *A graph of the light-absorption characteristics of an a-Si:H photodiode and the light output characteristics of three common phosphors.*

Other detection systems that have been developed include a scintillation-based fiber optic imager, scanning ZnWO$_4$ crystal array, and a scanning diode array (18, 39, 50, 51).

Clinical Application: Quality Assurance

Commissioning procedures need to be performed before an EPID is introduced into the clinic. While the format of the commissioning procedure depends on the functions and limitations of the particular EPID, some common features can be identified.

Physical Operation and Safety

The commissioning procedure must include steps to assure the EPID is operating as specified. Motion controls, limits and interlocks must be tested. Most of the clinical systems will be equipped with collision interlocks that disable patient support assembly (PSA) motion and gantry motion. In addition, interlock bypass systems may be present in the form of buttons, switches or bypass plugs and these must also be tested. Procedures to regulate the use of interlock bypasses must also be addressed. The EPID support system may have manual and motorized motions that need to be tested. If the support system position is indexed so the positions can be transferred to the acquisition computer, the accuracy and reproducibility of that system should be checked. Any manual position indicators should also be inspected for accuracy.

It is important to assess the accuracy and reproducibility of the location of isocenter and orientation of the beam axes (radial and transverse) on the image. The beam location analysis depends upon the stability of isocenter location. The most restrictive system has the isocenter passing through a known point on the chamber regardless of gantry angle. In general, this condition is met if the imager support mount is sufficiently stable. Analysis software can therefore independently assess the locations of patient features and beam-defining apertures. If the gantry mount is not stable, the intersection of the central axis with the chamber surface may shift with gantry angle. If this shift is reproducible and is a function only of gantry angle, then the location can be measured and the information used to locate isocenter. If the isocenter location is neither fixed nor reproducible, analysis of the portal must account for the additional degree-of-freedom. For mounted blocks, the relative position of patient and block can still assessed. This may be sufficient since the clinician is concerned with the irradiated portion of the patient. However, fields are often small when using conformal therapy and images of these portals may not contain sufficient internal information to assess the location of the treated volume. In these cases, the patient can be irradiated with a fiducial tray using larger orthogonal anterior-posterior (AP) and lateral fields to locate isocenter. This technique may utilize diagnostic quality images if such a source is available on the accelerator. The location of isocenter may not determine if the treatment blocks are in the correct positions. If the beam-defining aperture is a multileaf collimator, however, the location of isocenter in the direction perpendicular to the leaf motion axis can be readily determined by locating the collimator edges. These edges are positioned at fixed increments from isocenter. For the direction parallel to leaf motion, the planned leaf positions must be known. The QA procedures for the collimator must assure that the leafs are moving to the desired positions. If so, the location of the leaf edges can be correlated with the planned leaf positions to locate the isocenter position.

The target-to-imager distance (TID) coupled with the target-to-object distance (TOD, usually located at the intersection of the plane perpendicular to the beam central axis and the prescription point) determines the magnification M factor for the image

$$M = \frac{TID}{TOD}$$

If the acquisition hardware does not record the TID with the image, this information may be lost for later analysis. When the TOD coincides with the standard treatment distance, the beam-defining edge may be used to calculate the TID and therefore the magnification factor. This is especially convenient for multileaf fields, where the leaf width is known.

Image Acquisition, Noise and Spatial Resolution

The introduction of an EPID into a clinical setting requires a detailed understanding of the limitations and benefits of on-line portal imaging, as well as those of the EPID itself. Imaging properties can be summarized in terms of contrast and spatial resolution. Contrast resolution describes the ability of an EPID to resolve a low-contrast object from a background region. Since both the image and the background signal levels have uncertainties characterized by noise, the image must differ from the background by a sufficient amount to be detected. Spatial resolution describes the imager's ability to detect small features. However, the measurement of these parameters must take into account the fact that a direct measurement of contrast is not possible since the pixel-value to photon flux conversion is not necessarily known. A number of methods have been presented to provide a straightforward measurement of contrast and spatial resolutions. A cylindrical test phantom has been described for portal film evaluation and is commercially available(29). A contrast-detail phantom has also been described(44). It is similar to one used for quality assurance in our clinic (shown in Figure 30-7). The phantom consists of a 2.5 cm thick, 14 cm wide, 14 cm long sheet of aluminum with an array of holes drilled into the surface. The holes have diameters that range from 0.1 to 1.5 cm with depths that range from 0.025 to 0.3 cm.

Contrast-detail phantoms are useful for the qualitative evaluation of EPID performance. They can be used to provide a baseline performance status. Images taken at later times can be compared to assure that the imager is operating at the same level as when it was commissioned. Contrast-detail phantom images do not indicate the contrast resolution the imager will exhibit in clinical situations. A method for determining the minimum resolvable thickness (MRT) of heterogeneity (e.g. bone) within a homogeneous phantom was developed by Low, et al. (28). Figure 30-8 shows the average pixel values when multiple thicknesses of Lucite material are placed atop a homogeneous water-equivalent phantom. The readings are linear over the range of pixels encountered in the test. The technique to measure the MRT assumes that the response of the chamber is linear when a low-contrast object is being imaged. A piece of plastic is imaged atop a water-equivalent phantom. The plastic should be roughly 1-2 cm thick and 2.5 x 2.5 cm wide. The measurement is only applicable for the employed field size, the incident photon beam energy, and the thickness of the phantom. The region beneath the plastic is selected and the average and standard deviation of the pixels is noted. The average of the pixel value in the region bordering the plastic is also noted as a background. The MRT of bone is calculated by:

$$MRT = 5 \frac{\delta n_{PMMA} t_{PMMA}}{\left| \overline{n}_{PMMA} - \overline{n}_{H_2O} \right|} \left(\frac{\mu_{PMMA}}{\mu - \mu_{H_2O}} \right) \sqrt{2 \frac{lw}{A} \frac{TOD}{TID}}$$

(9)

where for equation 9, the plastic is polymethylmethacrylate (PMMA). TOD is the distance from the target to the object (in this case, the bone), TID is the distance from the target to the imager, l and w are the length and width of the chamber pixels, respectively, A is the area of the object of interest, μ is the linear attenuation coefficient of the bone, t is the thickness of the test plastic, δn is the standard deviation of the pixel values beneath the plastic and $\overline{n}_{PMMA}$ and $\overline{n}_{H_2O}$ are the average pixel values beneath the plastic and phantom, respectively. The MRT can also be used to check performance of the imager and can be used to compare imagers from different manufacturers.

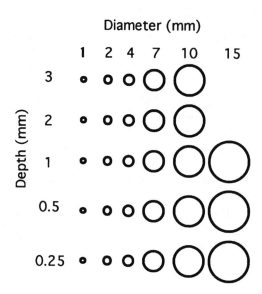

Figure 30-7. *A modified Las Vegas contrast-detail phantom that provides a simple method for the evaluation of a clinical EPID image quality during routine QA procedures. The phantom consists of an aluminum sheet 2.5 cm thick, 14 cm wide and 14 cm long. The face has a series of circular holes drilled to specified depths diameters. The diameters and depths of the holes are listed in the figure.*

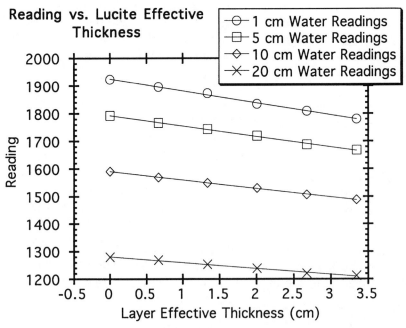

Figure 30-8. *Measured pixel values using a Varian PortalVision ionization chamber EPID measured by irradiating a series of 2.5 x 2.5 cm Lucite pieces placed atop a water-equivalent phantom by a 6 MV photon beam. The pixel values are plotted against the Lucite thickness for a number of phantom thicknesses. A linear least-squares fit is shown for each curve.*

The ability to resolve small features within an image depends on the spatial resolution of the chamber system. As previously mentioned, standard measurement techniques of spatial resolution require that the response of the chamber be known. However, the fact that the chamber response is linear over a narrow range can be used to measure the spatial resolution of the chamber when scatter from a phantom is included. This is clinically desirable, as imaged objects within a patient are always surrounded by a scattering medium. A method for obtaining the imager resolution by measuring a modified line-spread function (LSF) was developed by Low, et al. (28). A 0.9 cm thick sheet of PMMA was imaged atop a 5 cm thick PMMA phantom (Figure 30-9). The edge of the PMMA was placed along the central axis so that the front face was tangent to the incident photon beam and was aligned with the imager pixels. The transmitted photon flux had a sharp change beneath the edge of the added PMMA. The edge was broadened due to secondary photon scatter at the phantom and the geometric broadening of the PMMA edge due to finite source size. In addition, the resulting image included the effects of the inherent resolution of the imager. Figure 30-10 shows a profile across the edge for four acquisition modes averaged over 11.3 cm (125 pixels) to reduce the effects of noise in the determination of the edge width. The derivative of this function is proportional to the line-spread function (LSF) of the imager/phantom combination and is shown in Figure 30-11 for one of the acquisition modes. The noise in the low-contrast image precludes the calculation of the MTF from these data. However, for clinical purposes, the width of the LSF is sufficient to characterize the spatial resolution of the system. A parameter, termed the line-spread width (LSW), was developed to characterize the LSF of the system and is defined as twice the standard deviation of a Gaussian function fit to the measured LSF:

$$LSW = 2\sigma_{LSF} \tag{10}$$

Because the scattered edge may be as little as 1 or 2 pixels wide, the measured LSW may depend on the alignment between the plastic edge and the pixel boundaries. Multiple images taken with slight offsets may be used to determine a best and worst-case LSW.

Finally, some systems may not present a geometrically accurate representation of the image due to optical distortions. The distortions should be measured prior to clinical use of the EPID. The graticule can be imaged to provide features with known spacing. The image analysis software can be used to locate the pixels corresponding to the graticule points. A second image taken with the collimator rotated 45 degrees relative to the first image will provide a determination of distortions off-axis.

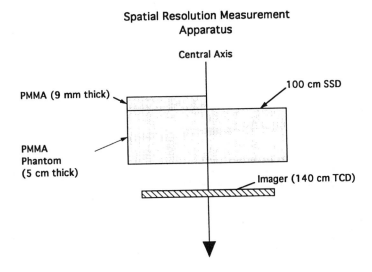

Figure 30-9. *The jig used to measure the line-spread function (LSF) of the phantom-imager combination.*

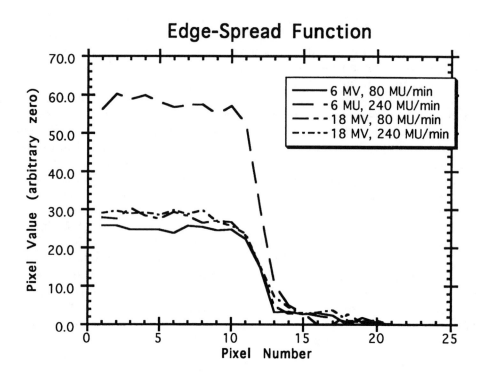

Figure 30-10. *Profiles measured using a Varian PortalVision ionization chamber EPID by irradiating the jig shown in Figure 30-9 with a 6 MV photon beam. Each curve represents one acquisition mode (accelerator repetition rate and imager acquisition technique).*

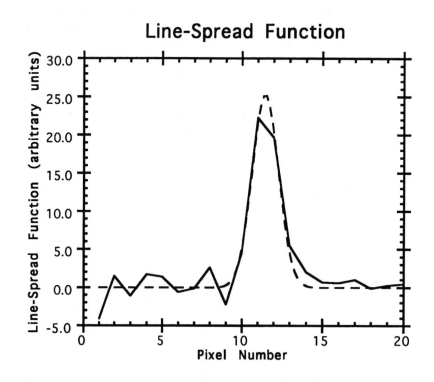

Figure 30-11. *The line-spread function (LSF) of the 240 MU/min high resolution acquisition mode. the LSF is the derivative of the appropriate profile shown in Figure 30-10.*

Image Storage, Analysis, and Handling

Commercial EPID systems will have software routines for storing and retrieving images, often using compression algorithms to conserve disk space. The accuracy of image storage can be tested by selecting a set of pixels and noting their pixel value. After image storage and retrieval, the pixel values must be identically equal to the values prior to storage. Image manipulation software must also be checked for accuracy and reproducibility. It is desirable that the software store either only the initial unaltered image or both the unaltered image and the manipulated image to assure that the original data is available for future analysis.

Image analysis software may also be present on the acquisition system and must be checked prior to clinical use. The simplest measures the average and standard deviation of a set of pixels within a user-specified rectangular region of interest. This type of software can be checked by setting the region-of-interest to one pixel and noting the pixel values of a set of pixels within a rectangular region (e.g. 5 x 5 pixel square). The same region can then be specified and the mean and standard deviation compared with a manual calculation using the known pixel values. More complex analysis schemes, such as histogramming, can be checked by preparing a test image with a known pixel-value distribution. The histogram can be calculated independently of the acquisition software and compared with the software's output.

Image enhancement software is utilized to assist in the identification of features that would otherwise be difficult to locate with simple level and window software. The utility of the software is evident if it provides the intended result, rather than to provide a specific operation to the image pixel values. Therefore, evaluation of this type of software requires the visual inspection of the resulting images, rather than a quantitative analysis . Image alignment software must be similarly treated.

Reference Image Acquisition

The acquisition software of an EPID will commonly allow the presentation of a reference image which is placed aside the acquired image for comparison. In general, the reference image is either a simulation image or a digitally reconstructed radiograph (DRR) with an indication of the desired portal outline. In some cases, the reference image may be the initial portal image. The EPID operator either visually examines the two images or utilizes software to determine if the patient was irradiated to the appropriate location to within some user-specified specification. The acquisition of the reference image may use hardware and software that is completely different than the therapy image. For example, one system utilizes a CCD camera to digitize the simulation film. The optical system for the digitization system should be checked to assure that the scale on the digitized film is correct and that there are minimal distortions. A translucent sheet of graph paper can be digitized for this determination.

Support Software

There has been a great deal of effort invested in image analysis techniques. The first part of this section will discuss algorithms that enhance the ability to visualize or detect objects in the image. The second part discusses software that locates image features and compares the on-line image with a reference image. These tools are essential to the utility of an EPID and highlight the flexibility in image analysis provided by use of a digital system for the acquisition of portal images.

The human eye is capable of resolving a finite number of gray levels on a monochrome monitor. An image may have different regions that simultaneously exhibit a large dynamic range of pixel values and subtle details. If the gray scale is set to encompass the entire dynamic range within the image, the gray-level differences corresponding to the subtle detail will not provide sufficient differentiation in gray levels to be visible. The details can be presented in the image by manipulation of the map that provides the correspondence between pixel value and gray level. The simplest image enhancement technique involves windowing and leveling of the output gray level as a function of the pixel value. The user can adjust the pixel values corresponding to the darkest and lightest gray levels. One of the difficulties with simple level and window adjustment is that only one range of pixel values can be displayed with the ideal gray levels. There are many clinical cases where the simultaneous presentation of two or more regions with differing pixel values is very useful.

There is no a priori reason that the pixel-value-to-gray scale map must be monotonic. When attempting to locate an anatomical landmark, the user does not utilize the absolute gray scale value in that region of the image. The gray scale can be adjusted on a region-by-region basis to reveal the anatomical features.

The averaging of sequentially-acquired images to reduce noise is carried out by all EPID manufacturers. Leszczynski et al. (25) modeled noise as multiplicative and additive. The value z of pixel (i,j) is equal to

$$z(i,j) = x(i,j)v(i,j) + w(i,j)$$

(11)

where $x(i,j)$ is the noise-free image, $v(i,j)$ is the multiplicative noise due to random photon counting statistics and $w(i,j)$ is due to electronic noise added to the signal. The variance in the average of a group of images decreases with increasing numbers of images used to generate the average. Figure 30-12 shows the variance of pixel intensities measured over a homogeneous region as a function of the inverse of the number of images used to calculate the average. It is clear from Figure 30-12 that the variance can be improved with increasing averaging. However, some imaging studies such as rotational or dynamic therapies demand rapid imaging. The number of images available for averaging may not be sufficient to minimize the variance. For these cases, image noise reduction would be useful.

Noise-reduction filters can be described as either linear or non-linear (49). Linear filters include local neighborhood pixel averaging and averaging using a truncated Gaussian weighting function. Linear filters tend to degrade the spatial resolution of the image. Adaptive non-linear filters can reduce noise in nearly homogeneous regions with little loss in spatial resolution. Leszczynski investigated and modified the Lee filter (19, 20, 21) for analyzing portal images. Lee assumed that the variance in a group of pixels in one image is the same as the variance in a single pixel over a sequence of images. The value of z that minimizes the mean square error is

$$\hat{z}(i,j) = \bar{z}(i,j) + k(i,j)\left[z(i,j) - \bar{z}(i,j)\right]$$

(12)

where $\bar{z}(i,j)$ is the average pixel value over a region centered about (i,j) and $k(i,j)$ is given as

$$k(i,j) = \frac{\mathrm{var}[z(i,j)] - \overline{x^2}(i,j)\sigma_v^2(i,j) - \sigma_w^2(i,j)}{\mathrm{var}[z(i,j)]}$$

(13)

where $\sigma_v^2(i,j)$ and $\sigma_w^2(i,j)$ are the local variances of the multiplicative and additive noise components, respectively. $k(i,j)$ has a value between 0 and 1, depending on whether the noise is random (k near 0) or systematic (k near 1). When the noise is random, the pixel value is set to the mean over the region ($\bar{z}$) and when the noise variance is small, the pixel value is set to the original pixel value. Leszczynski noted that the noise variance is difficult to determine and developed a method for the determination of the value of k by comparing two images that were generated by averaging a different number of individual images.

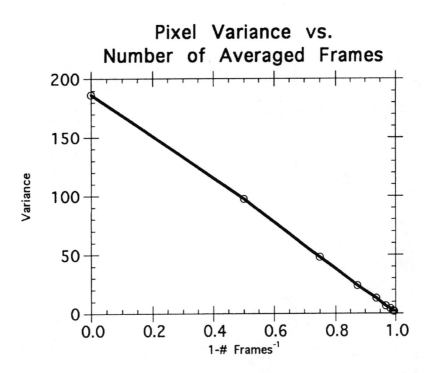

Figure 30-12. *The variance of the average of group of pixels from a set of images taken of a homogeneous physical system as a function of the number of images used to measure the average. The only difference between pixel values was due to photon statistics and random electronic noise. The graph shows that the averaging of images can reduce the effects of random noise on the resulting image.*

A number of methods for modifying the pixel-density map has been developed that utilizes the number of pixels with a particular value (image histogram) (12, 22, 26, 30, 45). One method, termed global histogram equalization (HE) sets the derivative of the gray-scale map at a particular pixel value to be proportional to the number of pixels exhibiting that pixel value. However, the region outside the radiation field consists of large areas of nearly equal pixel value, and may demand a significant portion of the available gray scale. Pizer, et al. (41) developed the algorithm by applying the HE algorithm to only local regions within the image. This algorithm, termed adaptive histogram equalization (AHE, also known as local histogram modification) (16, 27) eliminates the loss of gray-scale due to the blocked field region, but still suffers with the loss of field-edge definition (45). Leszczynski et al. (24) applied an algorithm to locate the portal edge and then applied the AHE algorithm only to the region within the field boundary. The technique is termed selective adaptive histogram equalization (SAHE) and preserves the field edge and the gray-scale range available for clinically relevant portions of the image. Figure 30-13 (provided by Leszczynski) shows an example of a portal taken with 4 MV x rays in the head and neck region. Figure 30-13a shows the image with only window and level control applied. Figure 30-13b shows the same field with global histogram equalization applied. Figure 30-13c shows the same field with adaptive histogram equalization and Figure 30-13d shows the same portal image with the SAHE algorithm applied. There is an obvious difference between the quality of the four images, with the SAHE algorithm retaining the field edge definition.

A novel technique being exploited for mammography may prove useful in radiation therapy imaging (17). Images are reconstructed from transform coefficients modified at one or more levels of transform space. While this technique is being developed for diagnostic radiology, modification for radiation therapy may be possible.

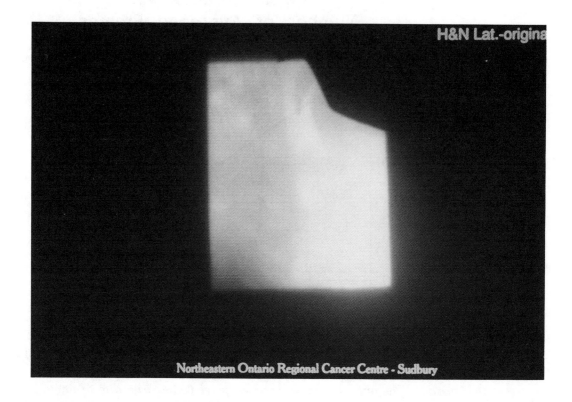

Figure 30-13a.

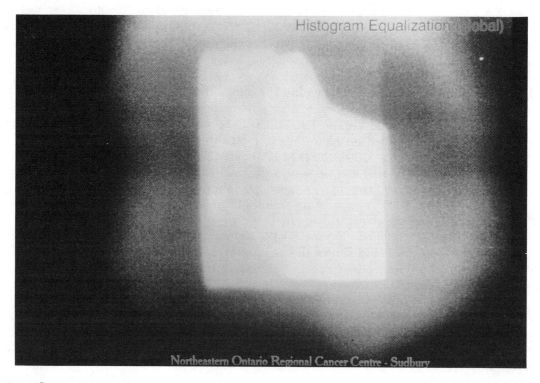

Figure 30-13b.

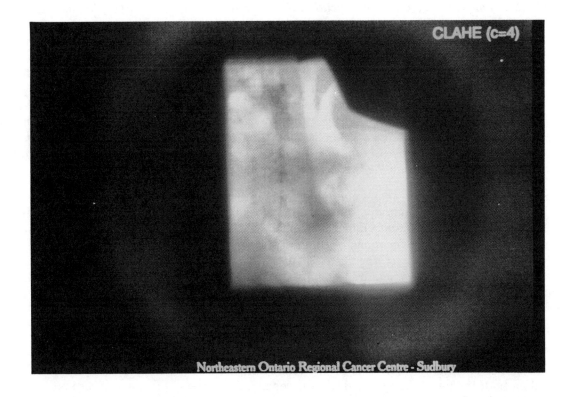

Figure 30-13c.

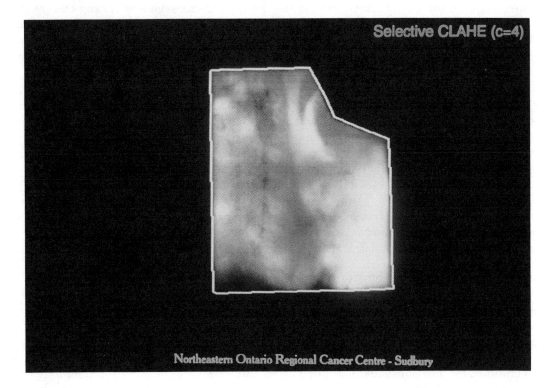

Figure 30-13d.

Figure 30-13. *A portal image taken of a head-and-neck irradiation with 4 MV photons. a) shows the image with only window and level adjustments. b) shows the same image with global histogram equalization applied. Features that were otherwise indistinct in Figure 30-13a are slightly easier to see with the applied equalization. The field edge distinction has been reduced. c) the same image as shown in Figure 30-13a with the adaptive histogram equalization applied. Features are now much clearer, although the region outside the image shows features generated by periodic noise. The field edge more difficult to see than in figures 13a and 13b. d) the same image as shown in Figure 30-13a with the selective adaptive histogram equalization algorithm applied. The features within the field edge are as distinct as with the adaptive histogram equalization, but the distinction of the field edge is retained.*

The acquisition of portal images allows clinicians to quantitatively assess the location of treatment beams with respect to patient anatomy. The portal image is inspected to locate anatomical features that can be identified on the reference image. The portal outline is also located in both the reference and portal images. The relative locations of the portal boundary and anatomical features are then used to determine the location of the treated field with respect to the reference image. This technique can be applied to each acquired portal image to yield a distribution of the treated fields. This information can be used to calculate the dose distribution delivered to the patient or to examine the quality of treatment localization procedures (e.g. immobilization techniques).

The analysis of portal images can be defined as the location of treated portal field edges on anatomy described on a reference image. To accomplish this with portal images taken in the treatment position, a number of tasks must first be completed. First, anatomical landmarks must be selected and located on both the portal images and the reference image. The description of patient anatomy can be accomplished by use of either discrete points, or curved line segments called contours. Second, the portal field outline must be located in the portal images. Alignment can then be accomplished by matching anatomical structures (equivalent to calculating a transformation matrix for the portal image) in the portal image to those in the reference image and noting the position of the portal field outline, or by matching field outlines in both the portal image and the reference image and noting the shift in the internal anatomy (31). The second method presupposes that the block outline does not change, an assumption that may not prove to be correct if, for example, the collimator is used to define one edge and is set by eye in the treatment room.

The description of anatomical landmarks by points provides some advantages with respect to image correlation (34). The advantage of describing anatomical features by points is that a transformation between locations of the points in the portal image relative to those defined in the reference field is readily available. This is similar to techniques used to correlate medical images taken with different modalities (15). The alignment of anatomical points has been utilized in automated and semi-automated techniques (31, 34, 38). The user must locate the anatomical fiducial points on the reference and the portal image and the images are aligned by calculating the image transformation (rotation, translation and scale) that minimize the sum-squared distance between corresponding anatomical points. The largest drawback of this system is that many anatomical landmarks do not have regions where points can be accurately placed.

Most landmarks visible on portal images are caused by the projections of curved bony structures. The projected thickness combined with the increased physical density generates a curved feature that is easily detected in the image. Further, many features, such as the sella tursica, present unique patterns that are easily recognizable to the trained eye. Interfaces with lower-density regions can also provide good contours for image localization, the apex of the lung being an example. The description of anatomical landmarks by continuous curved line segments is therefore a logical technique for the subsequent alignment of these features. Many alignment algorithms have utilized digitized structures to manually align images. For example, Graham, et al. (14) has developed a method for image alignment where the anatomical landmarks are contoured in the reference image. In addition to the anatomical landmarks, the portal outlines are also contoured for both the portal and reference images. The graticule tray is utilized for the initial portal image to provide scale, collimator orientation and central axis location for both the reference and portal images. Once the image coordinate systems are known, the anatomical landmarks of the reference images are superimposed on the portal image. The user can manipulate the contours as a group to best fit the corresponding features on the portal image. Once the user has determined the appropriate alignment, a coordinate transformation can be derived to describe the transformation from the portal image patient position to that in the simulation film. The digitized portal field edge location on the simulation field can then be determined. This process can be repeated for all acquired portal images to generate a map of the field overlap frequency on the simulation image.

While contours supply more natural descriptions of anatomical features than points, they provide a more difficult challenge for automated techniques. Balter, et al. (5) have developed techniques for the characterization and overlap of curve segments from different images. Their technique involves two steps and assumes that the magnification of the two images are known; 1) the determination of the overlapping segments and 2) the calculation of the coordinate transformation that best describes the overlap of the two curves. The curves are described by their local curvature, which is independent of the coordinate system (aside from the magnification factor). The local curvature is examined as a function of the distance along the contour. The two curves are shifted until there is a maximum correlation. The portions of the curves that are contained in both images are located and can be used to calculate the coordinate transformation from one image to the other. The algorithm that was developed modifies the digitized curve by interpolation to yield a smoother curve for curvature calculations. This technique yields a list of possible shifts that must be rectified. The selection of the appropriate transformation is made using the coordinates of the points within each curve. The list of possible shifts is used to locate corresponding points on each curve. The transformation that yields the minimum root-mean-squared distance between points is the chosen transformation.

One of the goals of on-line imaging is the ability for software to automatically correlate images and determine the accuracy of a treatment. Unfortunately, the complete automation of this process has not yet been developed, although there have been significant advancements towards that goal.

Automatic field edge detection is one area that has seen progression in recent years. Meertens et al. (31) utilized an edge-detection algorithm to locate the field edge once the corners of the field have been located. They utilized an edge-detection matrix which was convolved with the image. The matrix detects only gradients along a particular axis. The two matrices that correspond to "horizontal" and "vertical" gradients are:

horizontal

$$\begin{vmatrix} 1 & 0 & -1 \\ 2 & 0 & -2 \\ 1 & 0 & -1 \end{vmatrix}$$

vertical

$$\begin{vmatrix} 1 & 2 & 1 \\ 0 & 0 & 0 \\ -1 & -2 & -1 \end{vmatrix}$$

These matrices are convolved with the image to produce an array that is proportional to the horizontal gradient or the vertical gradient, as appropriate. The points that provide a maximum in the gradient are identified as edge points and a line that indicates the field edge is fit to the points. Bijhold, et al. (9) developed a two-step method for portal field edge detection. First, an approximate field edge detection scheme was developed that defined the field edge pixels as those containing a threshhold pixel value. The pixel value was obtained by investigating the histogram of pixel values. The boundary pixels appear near a minimum in the histogram. Further analysis of relative peaks heights in the histogram are used to eliminate incorrect histogram minima from consideration. The second phase utilizes gradient-locating matricies to locate the regions of maximum gradients near the defined edge positions.

The previous matricies are used in addition to two matricies that are sensitive to the gradient 45° from the horizontal or the vertical axes:

Diagonal matricies:

$$\begin{vmatrix} 2 & 1 & 0 \\ 1 & 0 & -1 \\ 0 & -1 & -2 \end{vmatrix}$$

$$\begin{vmatrix} 0 & 1 & 2 \\ -1 & 0 & 1 \\ -2 & 1 & 0 \end{vmatrix}$$

The group of Bijhold, et al. (10) describe the field edge by a set of moments m_{ab} defined by;

$$m_{ab} = \oint x^a(s)y^b(s)ds, \quad a,b \in \{0,1,2,...\}$$

(14)

where the order of moment is given by the sum of a and b. The procedures for calculating and normalizing moments is given in the paper. It is assumed that when two shapes have the same moments, their shape must be the same. Therefore, the criterion for matching images is to minimize the sum of the differences (FD) between their moments:

$$FD = \sum_{a=0}^{M} \sum_{b=0}^{M-a} \left(m_{ab_i} - m_{ab_p} \right)^2$$

(15)

where the subscript i refers to the intended shape and p to the potal outline. M is the maximum order of the moments used for the analysis. The reference contour is perturbed by rotation and translation to locate a minimum in the FD parameter. The located minimum may be only a local minimum that yields an incorrect alignment. Portal contours that are near the intended portal are aligned with improved results relative to those that differ greatly from the intended portal, especially by rotation angle.

The authors also provide a second alignment scheme, in which pixels within corresponding structures of the two images are aligned by using an analogue to attractive forces and pressures. The translation T, rotation angle ϕ and magnification M are derived from weighted sums of the distances between pixels A_i and B_j of images A and B, respectively.

$$T_A = \sum_{i=1}^{N_B} \sum_{j=1}^{N_A} W_{ij}\left(B_i - A_j\right) \tag{16}$$

$$\phi_A = \arcsin\left(\sum_{i=1}^{N_B} \sum_{j=1}^{N_A} W_{ij} \frac{B_i \times A_j}{|B_i||A_j|}\right) \tag{17}$$

$$M_A = \sum_{i=1}^{N_B} \sum_{j=1}^{N_A} W_{ij} \frac{B_i \bullet A_j}{|B_j|^2} \tag{18}$$

The W-parameters are weighting functions that determine the "strength" of the force working between the pixels. The authors chose an exponential force law due to its finite range and finite value at zero distance.

$$W_{ij} = e^{-|B_i - A_j|^2 / D^2} \bigg/ \sum_{k=1}^{N_B} \sum_{l=1}^{N_A} e^{-|B_k - A_l|^2 / D^2} \tag{19}$$

The range of the force is determined by the parameter D. The points are moved according to the force exerted on them. The range of the force is decreased slightly with each perturbation. One weakness of this algorithm is that it cannot determine the image alignment when there is a perturbation of the image shape, such as after a trim or fill. In addition, local force minima can fool the algorithm into selecting an inappropriate field shift.

Another scheme was proposed by Leszczynski, et al. (24) beginning by convolving the image with a symmetric Gaussian and then the vertical and horizontal gradient operators shown above. The Gaussian convolution reduces the effect of random noise on the field edge search. The local edge strength is the root-mean square sum of the two components. This algorithm was thoroughly tested with head-and-neck, thorax, breast, abdomen, pelvis and extremities. In all cases, the algorithm correctly located the field outline. An analysis of the displacement of the field edge with the true field edge (defined by the 50% intensity) was conducted. The algorithm was found to locate the field edge to within 0.05 cm of the true field edge for 85% of the cases.

Acknowledgments

The authors would like to acknowledge Dr. Arthur Boyer, Dr. Larry Antonuk, Dr. Konrad Leszczynski, and Varian for providing figures used in this paper.

Reference

1.   Adam, J. A. Industries transcend national boundaries, IEEE Spectrum, 27:26-31;1990.

2.   Antonuk, L. E.; Boudry J.; Yorkston, J.; Wild, C. F.; Longo, M. J.; Street, R. A. Radiation damage studies of amorphous silicon photodiode sensors for applications in radiotherapy x-r imaging, Nucl. Instr. Meth. A299:143-146;1990.

3.   Antonuk, L. E.; Boudry, J.; Huang, W.; McShan, D. L.; Morton, E. J.; Yorkston, J.; Longo, M. J.; Street, R. A. Demonstration of megavoltage and diagnostic x-ray imaging with hydrogenated amorphous silicon arrays, Med. Phys. 19:1455-1466;1992.

4.   Antonuk, L. E.; Yorkston, J.; Boudry, J.; Longo, M. J.; Street, R. A.; Large area amorphous silicon photodiode arrays for radiotherapy and diagnostic imaging, Nucl. Instr. Meth. A 310:460-464;1991.

5.   Antonuk, L. E.; Yorkston, J.; Boudry, J.; Longo, M. L.; Jimenez, J.; Street, R. A. Development of hydrogenated amorphous silicon sensors for high-energy photon radiotherapy imaging, IEEE Trans. Nucl. Sci. NS-37(2):165-170;1990.

6.   Baily, N. A.; Horn, R. A.; Kampp, T. D. Fluoroscopic visualization of megavoltage therapeutic x ray beams, Int. J Radiat. Oncol. Biol. Phys. 6:935-939;1980.

7.   Balter, J. M.; Pelizzari, C. A.; Chen, G. T. Y. Correlation of projection radiographs in radiation therapy using open curve segments and points, Med. Phys. 19:329-334;1992.

8.   Barnes, G. T. Digital x-ray image capture with image intensifier and storage phosphor plates: imaging principles, performances and limitations, Digital Imaging, proc. of the 1993 AAPM summer school, ed. by W.R. Hendee and J.H. Trueblood, 1993.

9.   Bijhold, J.; Gilhuijs, K. G. A.; van Herk, M.; Meertens, H. Radiation field edge detection in portal images, Phys. Med. Biol. 36:1705-1710;1991.

10. Bijhold, K. G.; Gilhuijs, K. G. A.; van Herk, M. Automatic verification of radiation field shape using digital portal images, Med. Phys. 19:1007-1014;1992.

11. Boyer, A. L.; Antonuk, L.; Fenster, A.; van Herk, M.; Meertens, H.; Monro, P.; Reinstein, L. E.; Wong, J. A review of electronic portal imaging devices (EPIDs), Med. Phys. 19:1-16;1992.

12. Cumberlin, R.; Rodgers, J.; Fahey, F. Digital image processing of radiation therapy portal films, Comp. Med. Imag. Graph. 13:227-233;1989.

13. Droege, R.T. A megavoltage MTF measurement technique for metal screen-film detectors, Med. Phys. 6:272-279;1979.

14. Graham, M. L.; Cheng, A. Y.; Geer, L. Y.; Binns, W. R.; Vannier, M. W.; Wong, J. W. A method to analyze 2-dimensional daily radiotherapy portal images, Int. J. Radiation Onc. Biol. Phys. 20:613-619;1991.

15. Holupka, E. J.; Kooy, H. M. A geometric algorithm for medical image correlations, Med. Phys. 19:433-438;1992.

16. Hummel, R. Image enhancement by histogram transformation, Comput. Graph. Image Process. 6:184-195;1977.

17. Laine, A.; Huda, W.; Honeyman, J. C.; Steinbach, B. Mammographic image processing using wavelet processing techniques, Med. Phys. 20:920;1993.

18. Lam, K. S.; Partowmah, M.; Lam, W. C. An on-line electronic portal imaging system for external beam radiotherapy, Brit. J. Radiol 59:1007-1013;1986.

19. Lee, J. S. Digital i d) the same image as shown in Figure 30-13a with the selective adaptive histogram equalization algorithm applied. The features within the field edge are as distinct as with the adaptive histogram equalization, but the distinction of the field edge is retained. mage smoothing and the sigma filter, Comput. Vision Graphics Image Process. 24:255-269;1983.

20. Lee, J. S. Refined filtering of image noise using local statistics, Comput. Graphics Image Process. 15:380-389;1981.

21. Lee, J. S., Digital image enhancement and noise filtering by use of local statistics, IEEE Trans. Pattern Anal. Mach. Intell., PAMI-2:165-168;1980.

22. Leong, J. A digital image processing system for high energy x-ray portal images, Phys. Med. Biol 29:1527-1535;1984.

23. Leong, J. C.; Stracher, M. A. Visualization of internal motion within a treatment portal during a radiation therapy treatment. Radiother. Oncol. 9:153-156;1987.

24. Leszczynski, K. W.; Shalev, S. The enhancement of radiotherapy verification images by an automated edge detection technique, Med. Phys. 19:611-621;1992.

25. Leszczynski, K. W.; Shalev, S.; and Cosby, N. S. An adaptive technique for digital noise suppression in on-line portal imaging, Phys. Med. Biol 35:429-439;1990.

26. Leszczynski, K.; Shalev, S. Digital contrast enhancement for on-line portal imaging, Med. Biol. Eng. Comput. 27:507-512;1989.

27. Leszczynski, K.; Shalev, S. A robust algorithm for contrast enhancement by local histogram modification, Image Vision Comput. 7:205-209;1989.

28. Low, D. A.; Klein, E. E.; Maag, D. K.; Umfleet, W. E.; Purdy, J. A. Commissioning and quality assurance of a clinical electronic portal imaging device, Submitted to Int. J. Rad Onc. Biol. Phys.

29. Lutz, W. R.; Bjarngard, B. E. A test object for evaluation of portal films, Int. J. Rad. Onc. Biol. Phys 11:631-634;1985.

30. Meertens, H. Digital processing of high-energy photon beam images, Med. Phys. 12:111-113;1985.

31. Meertens, H.; Bijhold, J.; Stackee, J. A method for the measurement of field placement errors in digital portal images, Phys. Med. Biol. 35:299-323;1990.

32. Meertens, H.; van Herk, M.; Bijhold, J.; Bartelink, H. First clinical experience with a newly developed electronic portal imaging device, Int. J Radiat. Oncol. Biol Phys 18:1173-1181;1990.

33. Meertens, H.; van Herk, M.; Weeda, J. A liquid ionization detector for digital radiography of therapeutic megavoltage photon beam, Phys. Med. Biol 30;313-321:1985.

34. Michalski, J. M.; Wong, J. W.; Bosch, W. R.; Yan, D.; Cheng, A.; Gerber, R. L.; Graham, M. V.; Halverson, K. J.; Low, D. A.; Valicenti, R. K.; Piephoff, J. V. An evaluation of two methods of anatomical alignment of radiotherapy portal images, Submitted to Int. J. Rad. Onc. Biol. Phys.

35. Monro, P.; Rawlinson, J. A.; Fenster, A. A digital fluoroscopic imaging device for radiotherapy localization. Int. J. Rad. Onc. Biol. Phys. 18:641-649;1990.

36. Monro, P.; Rawlinson, J. A.; Fenster, A. A digital fluoroscopic imaging device for radiotherapy localization. In: Proceedings of the World Congress on Medical Physics and Biomedical Engineering, Phys. Med. Biol. 33 (Suppl. 1) 45, 1988.

37. Monro, P.; Rawlinson, J. A.; Fenster, A. Therapy imaging: a signal-to-noise analysis of metal plate/film detectors, Med. Phys. 14:975-984;1987.

38. Monro, P.; Towner, J.; Jaffray, D. A.; Battista, J. J.; Fenster, A. A semi-automated method of aligning portal images Med. Phys. 18:850;1991.

39. Morton, E. J.; Swindell, W.; Lewis, D. G.; Evans, P. M. A linear scintillation-crystal photodiode detector for radiotherapy imaging, Med. Phys. 18:681-691;1991.

40. Motz, J.; Danos, M. Image information content and patient exposure. Med. Phys. 5:9-22;1978.

41. Pizer, S. M.; Amburn, E. P.; Austin, J. D.; Cromartie, R.; Geselowitz, A.; Greer, T.; Romeny, B. H.; Zimmerman, J. B.; Zuiderveld, K. Adaptive histogram equalization and its variations, Comput. Vision Graph. Image Process. 39:355-368;1987.

42. Rougeot, H. Direct x-ray photoconversion processes, Digital Imaging, proceedings of the 1993 AAPM summer school, edited by W. R. Hendee and J. H. Trueblood, 1993.

43. Shalev S, The design and clinical application of digital portal imaging systems: presented at the 34th Annual Scientific Meeting of the American Society for Therapeutic Radiology and Oncology, November 11, 1992.

44. Shalev S, The Las Vegas Phantom design developed for the AAPM spring seminar in Las Vegas, April 6, 1989.

45. Sherouse, G. W.; Rosenman, J.; McMurry, H. L.; Pizer, S. M.; Chaney, E. L. Automatic digital contrast enhancement of radiotherapy films, Int. J. Rad. Onc. Biol. Phys. 13:801-806;1987.

46. Van Herk, M.; Meertens, H. A digital system for portal verification, in Proceedings of the 9th international conference on the use of computers in radiation therapy (Elsevier North-Holland, Amsterdam, 1987), pp. 371-374.

47. Van Herk, M.; Meertens, H. A matrix ionization chamber imaging device for on-line patient setup verification during radiotherapy, Radiother. Oncol. 11:369-378;1988.

48. Visser, A. G.; Huizenga, H.; Althof, V. G. M.; Swanenburg, B. N.; Performance of a prototype fluoroscopic radiotherapy imaging system, Int. J. Radiat. Oncol. Biol. Phys. 18:43-50;1990.

49. Wang, D. C. C.; Vagnucci, A. H.; Li, C. C. Digital imaging enhancement: a survey, Comput. Vision, Graphics Image Process. 24:363-81;1983.

50. Wong, J. W.; Binns, W. R.; Cheng, A. Y.; Geer, L. Y.; Epstein, J. W.; Klarmann, J.; Purdy, J. A. On-line radiotherapy imaging with an array of fiber-optic image reducers. Int. J. Rad. Onc. Biol. Phys. 18:1477-1484;1990.

51. Wong, J. W.; Cheng, A. Y.; Binns, W. R.; Epstein, J. W.; Klarmann, J.; Perez, C. A. Development of a second-generation fiber-optic on-line image verification system. Int. J. Rad. Onc. Biol. Phys. 26:311-320;1993.

52. Wong, private communication.

Chapter 31

Patient Positioning Immobilization Devices for Conformal Therapy

Mary V. Graham, M.D. and Russell L. Gerber, M.S.

Mallinckrodt Institute of Radiology, Washington University School of Medicine, St. Louis, Missouri

The immobilization of patients to accurately reproduce fractionated radiotherapy remains a difficult technical aspect of radiation therapy. Goitein described the difference between localization error and immobilization error.[1] Localization error <u>may</u> be significantly reduced using 3-dimensional techniques provided tumors are accurately defined with the available imaging modality (e.g., CT, MRI, PET, etc.). Immobilization error, i.e. the displacement of the tumor fields relative to the intended treatment volume, <u>may</u> be decreased by improved immobilization devices. Systematic immobilization errors occur when the treatment fields fail to reproduce the simulation and/or planning situation. Random errors may occur secondary to patients being inadequately immobilized, with resultant treatment fields inaccurately aligned from treatment to treatment. Patients may also move during treatment because of either inadequate immobilization or physiologic activity. Traditional radiotherapy has allowed for variable margins to account for discrepancies in the patient setup. Provided there is good localization, margins around target volumes must account for 1) reproducibility of the daily setup and 2) physiologic or unintentional movement by the patient.

The goal of 3-dimensional technologies is to make the delivery of radiation dose conformal around the target areas. In doing this, there is the temptation to make treatment field margins tighter. The gravest danger, however, is that if margins around target areas are made too small, increased localization error will occur. Margins around target areas must take into account both the potential for systematic error and immobilization error, as well as beam penumbra characteristics. The proposed ICRU definitions for radiation therapy account for systematic and immobilization error in the planning target volume; however, beam characteristics are not included in the planning target volume as newly defined by the ICRU.[2]

Immobilization Devices

There are many types of immobilization devices available to the radiotherapist. For 3-dimensional fractionated radiotherapy, certain characteristics are desirable. Niewald analyzed several properties of immobilization materials and described an analysis with the most desirable characteristics.[3] Not only must the materials be easy to work with and adequately mold around the patients, but they must have resistance to bending and stretching and thus allow for reproducibility in the setup. The presence of the immobilization material must not significantly perturb the dose distribution in the patient. Thermoplastic masks have been studied in this regard and the increase in surface dose is insignificant. This allows one to treat through the mask without making cutouts in the material. No increase in skin reaction has been observed in our experience using this type of mask for head and neck immobilization.

All major institutions using 3-dimensional techniques for routine treatment of patients have reported increasing the amount of immobilization for treatment delivery. The majority of these institutions are using a combination of alpha cradles and thermoplastic molds. In treating head and neck areas, many have found that the accuracy of the setup can be increased by using a thermoplastic mold over the face and neck in conjunction with an alpha cradle to build up the support of the neck, shoulder, and upper thorax. Important technical aspects regarding immobilization of the head and neck area require that the mold be tightly conformal around the bridge of the nose and also the jaw so that the person cannot move within the device (Figure 31-1).

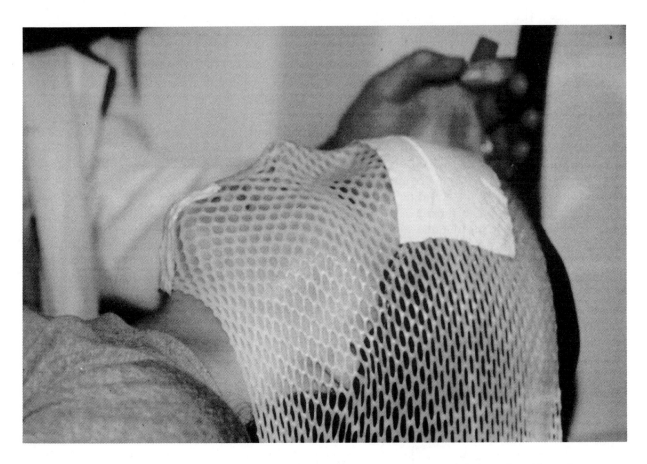

Figure 31-1. Thermoplastic immobilization mask for patients with head and neck tumor

At Washington University, patients with tumors in the thorax have been routinely immobilized with an alpha cradle (Figure 31-2). The alpha cradles must be large enough to support and reproducibly position the patient with their arms over their heads so that a variety of oblique beams will not enter through the arms. Alpha cradles need to be very supportive of the arms above the head to avoid an unstable position. The mold should also continue down to approximately the level of the hips in order to support and reproduce the tilt of the torso. In treating the thorax we have also found that multiple laser setup points that correlate the patient with the immobilization device are required because the patient may lie down in the cradle in different ways, resulting in off axis tilting.

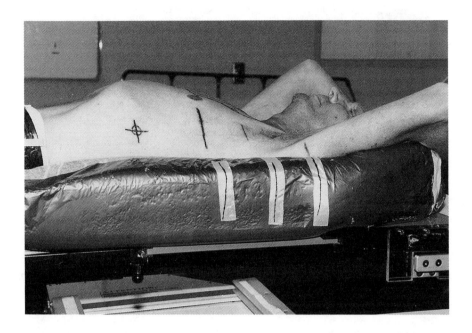

Figure 31-2. Alpha cradle immobilization and laser set up lines for patient with primary lung cancer

Several institutions have implemented 3-dimensional treatment for prostate cancer, and there appear to be at least two different types of immobilization emerging. A large number of institutions use alpha cradles with the patient lying prone. In order to give adequate support to the patient, these alpha cradles must extend from above the waist to at least the level of the knees. The cradles must have significant lateral support and also be pulled up between the legs so that the patient will have the same pelvic tilt and positioning of the legs each day (Figure 31-3). Multiple laser setup points for this type of immobilization are also desirable. The feet are immobilized either with the alpha cradle or by taping them together. A different immobilization technique used at Memorial Sloan-Kettering positions the patient in a prone position with a heavy gauge solid thermoplastic sheet mold placed over the pelvis and bolted to the table. The salient features of this type of mold are that it must be very conformal in the sacral area and in between the legs in order to reposition the patient reproducibly. Users of this immobilization device feel that the patient in the prone position has a bit more stability because the pelvic bones provide three point stabilization on the table. In addition, this type of mold is bolted directly to a custom base on the table, and thus once the patients are placed in the mold, they are essentially unable to move. With this device, patients are set up using the laser lines and again, no dose corrections are made for calculation through the base or the immobilization mold.

Once the immobilization device is chosen, it is desirable that it be indexed and mounted to the therapy couch.[4] Registration of these immobilization/repositioning devices to the treatment couch at the time of construction during the initial simulation provides a good starting point for reconciling the coordination system between the different treatment planning phases (CT data acquisition, virtual simulation, block verification).

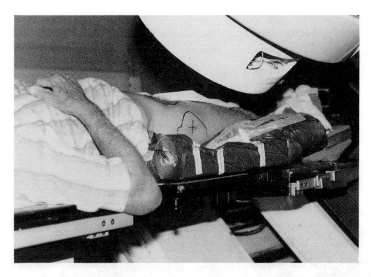

Figure 31-3. *Alpha cradle immobilization for prostate cancer treatment (Note, feet taped together.)*

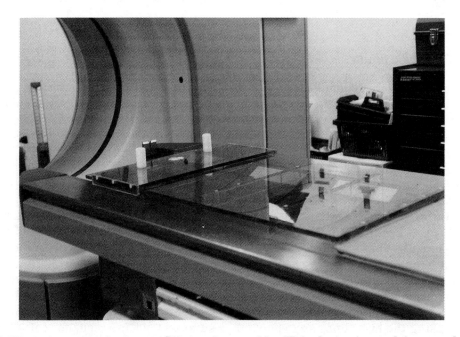

Figure 31-4. *MIR registration device on CT simulator table. This device is used for attaching and registering patient immobilization device to CT, simulator, or treatment machine.*

The registration device that is in use at MIR, shown in Figure 31-4, can be used for both thermoplastic repositioning masks as well as custom foam repositioning devices. It consists of a plastic base plate with two nylon pins, separated by 10 inches, protruding upward approximately 2 inches. The base attaches to the table providing a mounting mechanism. Since the treatment couches are different for the CT, simulators, and treatment units, a registration device was fabricated for each unit. The distance from the middle of the pins to the edge of the base and the distance between the pins was maintained for each of the devices. A reference point midway between the pins and 1.75 inches from the edge of the base was marked on each. This reference point was then set as isocenter for each of the simulators and treatment units to establish the digital table position relative to the isocenter.

The digital readouts for each unit were adjusted such that each gave the same reading relative to the isocenter.

At our institution the immobilization/repositioning devices are constructed in the simulator with the registration device attached to the table. After the physician has chosen the area of interest, the table coordinates are recorded as references for reconciling the beam coordinates established on the 3-D planning system.

The process of registering the repositioning/immobilization devices to the treatment couch provides the therapists with a set of coordinates that can be used to reproduce the patient treatment on a daily basis. Studies are being designed to evaluate the overall effect of the process on daily reproducibility of the treatments.

Another desirable characteristic of 3-D immobilization devices is that they be adaptable to multiple imaging devices including CT, MRI, and PET. In order to reference the immobilization device with the patient during image acquisition, the University of Michigan[9] has permanently glued plastic angiocatheter tubing to the laser lines of a thermoplastic mask. This angiocatheter tubing can then be filled with appropriate contrast material during imaging. For example, polyethylene 16 g tubing is placed inside the tubing for CT scans, mineral oil is instilled for MRI scans, and Fluorine-18 for PET scans. This technique allows reference points from the immobilization device to appear on the planning image and to be used as fiducial markers for the evaluation of immobilization.

Results

The effect of immobilization has been specifically reported for 3-dimensional treatment.[5,6,7,8,9] Rosenman et al. reported on the amount of systematic error occurring between virtual simulation and physical simulation for 3-dimensional patients in a variety of sites. In 78% of the evaluable patients, treatment designed with virtual simulation could be implemented on the physical simulator with a precision of ±5 mm (±3 mm for brain and head and neck sites). In his discussion of cases where setup precision was not within 5 mm, the problem was attributed to "human error." Setup errors reportedly have become progressively less frequent as the technologists have better understood the system and minor technical improvements made.

Soffen and Hanks have compared port films of 3-dimensional treatment with prostate patients casted and not casted for therapy.[8] They found significant improvement, i.e. reduction in the average daily error, in the patients who were casted. The median daily error for the casted group was 1 mm as opposed to 3 mm for the noncasted group. They also demonstrated that the 10% largest daily variations were entirely eliminated by casting and that 43% of casted patients' port films were exactly on the simulated isocenter compared to 22% with the cast.

Rosenthal and Roach have also evaluated the positioning error for 6-field conformal prostate treatments with and without alpha cradle casting.[7] Patients who were immobilized had significantly reduced errors in patient positioning. Hunt et al. evaluated systematic and random discrepancies between simulation and treatment positioning for 6 patients with nasopharyngeal carcinoma.[9] She concluded that conformal treatment may be more sensitive on a daily basis to positional uncertainty than traditional beam arrangements. Her data showed that day to day variations can potentially lead to critical structure and target doses which are different from the planned values. For this reason it is imperative that adequate margins around the target volumes (the planning target volumes as defined by ICRU 50) be studied and maintained to compensate for the uncertainties of treatment setup.[2]

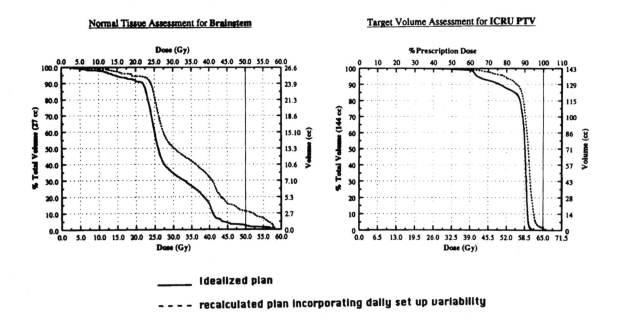

Figure 31-5. *Dose volume histograms for target volume and adjacent normal tissue (brainstem) comparing original 3-D calculations vs. recalculated doses after daily treatment error incorporated.*

Piephoff et al. evaluated the impact of daily treatment verification on 3-dimensional dose distributions for a variety of sites; incorporating daily treatment error into the 3-D calculations demonstrated differences between the original and the recalculated dose distributions by dose.[10] Dose volume histograms demonstrated a reduction in coverage of the target volumes by the prescription dose. If an adequate margin to account for daily setup error was incorporated into the planning target volume, then daily variation did not significantly reduce tumor coverage. Figure 31-5 is an example of the reduction in target volume coverage when a recalculated plan incorporated daily treatment error, as compared to an original plan without any treatment error. As target volume coverage was decreased, surrounding normal tissues or organ dose increased. This is also depicted on the dose volume histogram in Figure 31-5.

Systematic evaluation of the degree of accuracy for 3-D conformal therapy in the thorax or abdominal sites has not been reported.

Conclusions

Accurate immobilization for patients undergoing 3-dimensional treatment is imperative. Increased immobilization is required for 3-dimensional treatment as more accurate setup becomes necessary for these types of treatment delivery. Each institution must study the accuracy of its treatment setup in order to determine individual institutional margins around the site-specific target volumes. As further 3-dimensional treatment develops, we must study the effect of immobilization and patient physiologic movement in order to understand and allow for appropriate margins. As Dr. Goitein (perhaps prophetically) stated in 1975 "no amount of attention to patient positioning can [sic] compensate for failure to encompass the entire volume of disease within the planned treatment field."[1]

References

1. Goitein M and Busse J. Immobilization error: Some theoretical considerations. <u>Radiology</u> 117:407-412, 1975.

2. ICRU, Report No. 50, Prescribing, Recording, and Reporting Photon Beam Therapy (to be published). International Commission on Radiation Units and Measurements, Washington, D.C., 1993.

3. Niewald M, Lehmann W, Uhlmann, U, Schnabel K, Letz H-K,. Plastic material used to optimize radiotherapy of head and neck tumors and the mammary carcinoma. <u>Radiother. Oncol.</u> 11:55-63, 1988.

4. Thornton AF, Ten Haken RK, Weeks KJ, Gerhardsson A, Correll M, Lash RT(R)(T) and KA (R)(T). A head immobilization system for radiation simulations, CT, MRI, and PET imaging. <u>Medical Dosimetry</u> 16:51-56, 1991.

5. Thornton AF, TenHaken RK, et al. Three dimensional motion analysis of a head immobilization system for simulation, CT, MR, and PET imaging. <u>Radiotherapy and Oncology</u> 1):224-228, 1991.

6. Rosenman J, Sailer SL, Sherouse MS, Chaney EL, Tepper JE. Virtual simulation: Initial clinical results. <u>Int. J. Radiat Oncol. Biol Phys.</u> 20:843-851, 1991.

7. Rosenthal SA, Roach M III, Goldsmith BJ, Pickett B, Doggett C, Ryu JK. The accuracy of patient positioning during radiation for prostate cancer using a six field conformal technique with and without immobilization <u>Int. J. Radiat Oncol Biol Phys</u> 24 (Suppl. 1):188, 1992.

8. Soffen EM, Hanks GE, Hwang CC, Chu CH. Conformal static field therapy for low volume low grade prostate cancer with rigid immobilization. <u>Int. J. Radiat Oncol Biol Phys.</u> 20:141-146, 1991.

9. Hunt MA, Kutcher GJ, Burman C, Fass D, Harrison L, Leibel S, Fuks Z. The effect of positional uncertainties on the treatment of nasopharynx cancer. (Accepted for publication).

10. Piephoff JV, Michalski JM, Bosch WR, Graham ML, Harms WB, Purdy JA, Perez CA. A method to evaluate the impact of daily treatment variation on 3-dimensional dose distributions. Accepted for presentation at ASTRO, November 1993, New Orleans.

Chapter 32

On-Line Portal Imaging
The Mallinckrodt Institute of Radiology Experience

Jeff M. Michalski, M.D.

Mallinckrodt Institute of Radiology, Washington University School of Medicine, St. Louis, Missouri

It has been long known that uncertainty in delivery of daily radiotherapy treatments exists (4,11,12,17). The frequency and magnitude of reported field placement errors (FPE) depend on a number of factors and include anatomical site, method of immobilization, definition of what constitutes an error, and institutional treatment policy. At the Mallinckrodt Institute of Radiology we have embarked on a program to identify and reduce the clinical impact of FPE's in daily external beam radiotherapy. Integral to achieving these goals has been the development of an electronic portal imaging device (18), its clinical implementation, and the parallel development of software to analyze the images acquired with this and similar devices.

Since 1989, we have acquired daily portal images in a small population of patients treated at our radiation oncology center. These patients and their corresponding images from their treatment serve as the data base for this report.

Detection of Field Placement Errors

A field placement error is a discrepancy in the setup and orientation of a radiotherapy portal relative to its intended prescription. The identification of an error requires the registration of anatomy within a portal image relative to its beam edges and referencing that to the corresponding anatomy of a prescription image.

A number of methods have been developed to simplify the process of portal image to prescription image comparison (1,2,3,8,10,13,16). As part of an NCI contract, we have developed software tools to analyze portal images or digitized port films (14). These methods require identification of anatomical landmarks on corresponding simulation and portal images. These landmarks are then aligned and the actual position of the beam isocenters, or the block edges, are then compared to the reference film. The first method requires identification of anatomical landmarks as fiducial points, the second method requires the design of an anatomical template that is superimposed on corresponding portal images. An analysis of each method has demonstrated alignment accuracy of an anatomical phantom to within 0.8 mm. Agreement was very good between several individuals aligning the identical clinical images. These methods are soon to be introduced into clinical use for the evaluation of daily treatment setup.

Quantification and Classification of Errors

Methods have been devised to compress the large amount of on-line imaging data to succinct representations of a treatment course of external beam radiotherapy. The cumulative verification image analysis (CVIA) method reduces the variable daily block positions to a graphical representation of a percentage treatment area coverage (8,15). Block overlap isofrequency distributions (BOID) present the user with a quick overview of the treatment quality relative to the prescription (Figure 32-1).

Using alignment tools and the CVIA method we have calculated the width of BOID's for a small group of head and neck cancer patients. This may serve as a first order estimate of daily treatment variation to be inluded as margin for radiotherapy treatment planning. The range (0 to 100% block overlap) of daily variation can be as small as 6mm or as great as 14mm (8). Another study has shown that daily variation is site dependent with average 0 to 100% BIOD's widths of 7 mm in head and neck sites, 14 mm in pelvic sites, and 12 mm in thoracic sites (15).

Daily treatment variation contain both random and systematic errors (15). A random error is one which is present on any given day as a chance event. A systematic error propogates itself and will continue to be present unless an intervention to eliminate it were to take place. Distinguishing between the two types can sometime be obvious (for example, block cutting or mounting errors are systematic errors). In other situations a cumulative analysis of several days' images will reveal the presence of a systematic error. The clinical significance and solution to eliminating each of these two classes of errors is very different.

Clinical Significance of Field Placement Error

It is premature to determine if the presence of significant FPE's correlates with clinical outcome. Other factors that may relate to tumor control, such as intrinsic tumor radiosensitivity, propensity for metastatic spread, radiation dose and fractionation, and the administration of systemic therapy may prevent direct correlation of FPE's with outcome. We may be able to predict the clinical significance of FPE's by retrospectively analyzing the adequacy of target volume coverage by its prescribed radiation dose. A dose recalculation method illustrates daily FPE's impact on the adequacy of dose delivery (15). The dosimetric consequences of FPE's are small when patients are treated with generous margins and there is a predominantly random type of error. When margins are narrow, or when there is a significant systematic error present, the dose to tumor or normal tissues may be compromised. A project has been initiated to analyze the impact of daily treatment variation on dose volume relationships to tumor and normal tissue in a group of patients whose treatments were planned with the three dimensional treatment planning system.

Interactive Use of On-Line Portal Imaging Devices

A goal of many institutions using on-line portal imaging devices has been to detect and correct significant daily FPE's after a small fraction of each treatment has been delivered (5,6,7). After appropriate corrective action, if necessary, the treatment would proceed. This procedure requires rapid display of a portal image with a small radiation dose and quick comparison of the image to its reference. To date, such interventional studies have yielded mixed results. The procedure invariably increases treatment time but it is unclear as to whether clinically significant improvement in treatment delivery is achieved. At our radiation oncology center the preliminary analysis of a similar study has not demonstrated a tremendous improvement in the delivery of daily radiotherapy. Shortcomings of this study, as well as others, include (1) a lack of baseline error analysis, (2) no evaluation tools to detect clinically significant errors, and (3) no demonstrated ability to correct errors once they have been recognized.

Future interventional portal imaging studies at our radiation oncology center will include more intensive training of our technologists to identify and correct errors. Additionally, periodic off-line cumulative image analysis with the use of image alignment tools and the CVIA method to identify random versus systematic errors will be employed as a second level of error detection and correction (Figure 32-2).

The "Electronic View Box" (EVB) is a software tool that mimics the current practice of portal image or port film review with side by side comparison to a reference image. The advantage of an EVB is its ability to correct for magnification factor differences, its use of image and contrast enhancement algorithms, and the installation of image registration and alignment tools. The EVB allows for more sophisticated off-line or "backroom" analysis of portal images. Recently we have used the features of this tool to assess the quality of information derived from weekly port films relative to daily on-line portal images. Significant discrepancies may exist between the treatment record provided by daily portal images compared to periodic portal films (18).

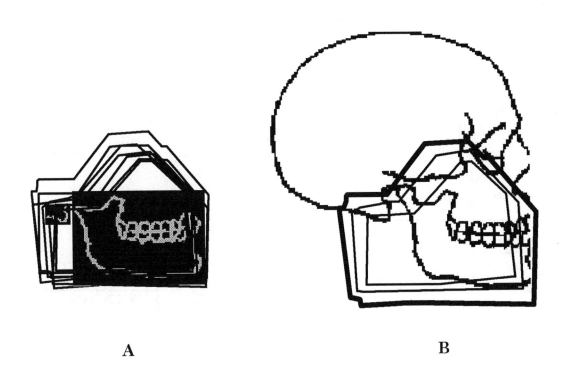

A   **B**

Figure 32-1. *The cumulative verification image analysis tool. (A) Multiple daily portal images are automatically registered to a prescription simulation image. (B) Block overlap isofrequency distributions are displayed on the simulation image and demonstrate quality of daily treatment setup.*

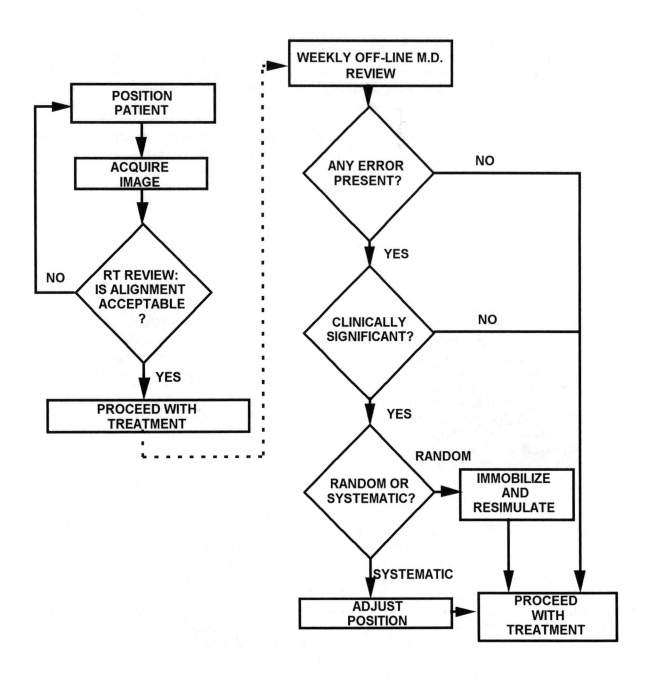

Figure 32-2. *Treatment position correction strategy with daily on line and weekly off line analysis and interventions.*

Conclusions

The use of on-line portal imaging in our clinic has allowed us to quantify and classify FPE's. These devices have spurred the development of sophisticated software tools and algorithms to facilitate the rapid identification of FPE's and to estimate their clinical significance. Studies to reduce or eliminate FPE's are currently ongoing.

As 3-dimensional treatment planning becomes more commonplace, on-line portal imaging will become necessary to: (1) quantify FPE's to determine what constitutes an appropriate planning margin in a variety of clinical circumstances and (2) to expedite the treatment verification process in these complicated multiple field radiotherapy plans.

References

1. Balter, J., Pelizzari, C., Chen, T.: Correlation of projection radiographs in radiation therapy using open curve segments and points. Med Phys 19:329-334, 1992.

2. Bijhold, J., van Herk, M., Vijlbrief, R., Lebesque, J.: Fast evaluation of patient set-up during radiotherapy by aligning features in portal and simulator images. Phys Med Biol 36:1665-1679, 1991.

3. Boyer, A., Dong, L., Starkschall, G., Hogstrom, K., A portal image correlation procedure. Med Phys 19:802, 1992.

4. Byhardt, R.W., Cox, J.D., Hornburg, A., Liermann, G.: Weekly localization films and detection of field placement errors. Int J. Radiat Oncol Biol Phys 4:881-887, 1978.

5. DeNeve, W., Van den Heuvel, F., Coghe, M., Verellen, D., De Beukeleer M., Roelstraete, A., De Roover, P., Thon, L., Storme, G.: Interactive use of on-line portal imaging in pelvic radiation. Int J. Radiat Oncol Biol Phys 25:517-524,1993.

6. DeNeve, W., Van den Heuvel, F., DeBeukeleer, M., Coghe, M., Thon, L., DeRoover, P., Van Lancker, M., Storme, G.: Routine clinical on-line portal imaging followed by immediate field adjustment using a tele-controlled patient couch. Rad Oncol 24:45-54, 1992.

7. Ezz, A., Munro, P., Porter, A., Battista, J., Jaffray, D., Fenster, A., Osborne, S.: Daily monitoring and correction of radiation field placement using a video-based portal imaging system: A pilot study. Int J. Radiat Oncol Biol Phy 22:159-165, 1992.

8. Halverson, K., Leung, T.,: Pellet, J., Gerber, R., Weinhous, M., Wong, J.: Study of treatment variation in the radiotherapy of head and neck tumors using a fiberoptic on-line radiotherapy imaging system. Int J. Radiat Oncol Biol Phys 21:1327-1336, 1991.

9. Jones, S., Boyer, A.: Investigation of an FFT-based correlation technique for verification of treatment set-up. Med Phys. 18:1116-1125, 1991.

10. Lam, W., Herman, M., Lam, K., Lee, D.: On-line portal imaging; Computer-assisted error measurements. Radiology 179:871-873, 1991.

11. Marks, J.E., Haus, A.G., Sutton, H.G., Griem, M.L.: Localization error in the radiotherapy of Hodgkin's disease and malignant lymphomas with extended mantle fields. Cancer 34:83-90, 1974.

12. Marks, J.E., Haus, A.G., Sutton, H.G., Griem, M.L.: The value of frequent treatment verification films in reducing localization error in the irradiation of complex fields. Cancer 37:2755-2761, 1976.

13. Meertens, H., Bijhold, J., Strackee, J.: A method for the measurement of field placement errors in digital portal images. Phys Med Biol 35:299-323, 1990.

14. Michalski, J.M., Wong, J.W., Yan, D., Gerber, R.L., Cheng, A., Halverson, K.J., Graham, M.V.: Comparison of two portal image alignment methods for treatment verification analysis. Int J Radiat Oncol Biol Phys 24: supplement 1 (abstract), 215, 1992.

15. Michalski, J.M., Wong, J.W., Gerber, R.L., Yan, D., Cheng, A., Graham, M.V., Renna, M.A., Sawyer, P.J., Perez, C.A.: The use of on-line image verification to estimate the variation in radiation therapy dose delivery. Accepted for publication Int J. Radiat Oncol Biol Phys, 1991.

16. Munro, P., Towner, J., Jaffray, D., Battista, J., Fenster, A.: A semi-automated method of aligning portal images. Med Phys 18:850, 1991.

17. Rabinowitz, I., Broomberg, J., Goitein, M., McCarthy, K., Leong, J.: Accuracy of radiation field alignment in clinical practice. Int J. Radiat Oncol Biol Phys 11:1857-1867, 1985.

18. Valicenti, R.K., Michalski, J.M., Bosch, W.R., Gerber, R.L., Graham, M.V., Cheng, A., Purdy, J.A.: Is weekly port filming adequate for verifying patient position in modern radiation therapy? Int. J. Radiat Oncol Biol Phys. 30(2):431-438, 1994.

19. Wong, J.W., Binns, W.R., Cheng, A., Geer, L.Y., Epstein, J.W., Klarmann, J., Purdy, J.A.: On-line radiotherapy imaging with an array of fiberoptic image reducers. Int J. Radiat Oncol Biol Phys 18:1477-1484, 1990.

Chapter 33

Automated Portal Image Correlation Techniques

Arthur L. Boyer, Ph.D., and Lei Dong, M.Eng.

Dept of Radiation Physics, University of Texas M.D. Anderson Cancer Center, Houston, Texas

Conformal radiotherapy is being considered as a means to improve the efficiency of radiation therapy for the management of cancer. The proposed techniques employ computer-controlled linear accelerators equipped with Multileaf Collimators (MLCs) that can deliver a complex treatment sequence once a patient has been positioned. Another approach to conformal radiotherapy is to use multiple non-coplaner unmodulated beams. In either case, accurate patient position verification is a fundamental requirement for high-dose conformal therapy.

Statistical studies[1-5] using either portal films or electronic portal imaging devices (EPIDs) have shown that using conventional set-up techniques 10-20% of recorded fields have setup errors of more than 10mm. One of the major reasons for this error frequency is the insensitivity of human vision to subtle differences in the images, especially for the low contrast megavoltage portal images. Computer assisted data analysis software that is fast and accurate and can give quantitative results may provide a solution to this problem.[6-13]

Here we distinguish between a localization portal image, usually taken the first time the patient is setup for treatment, and a verification portal image acquired during the subsequent course of the treatment to verify the continued alignment of the patient. The localization image is compared with a simulator image to avoid initial setup errors. Once the localization image is approved, it can be used as a reference image for comparison with subsequent daily portal verification images. In this paper we will not discuss the comparison of a simulator image with a portal localization image, which usually involves the comparison of images obtained from different modalities and requires user-assisted landmarks or anatomy registration.[6-11] This step is usually somewhat labor-intensive and time-consuming. However, it needs to be done only once for each patient.

We will describe a computer algorithm that can rapidly and accurately register two similar portal images for both translational shifts and in-plane rotations. The algorithm can be used to compare a verification portal image with a reference localization image with little user intervention.

Materials and Methods

The portal images we used were acquired from two sources: one was portal films digitized by a film digitizer (Model TZ-3X, TruvelTM Corp.), the other was an electronic portal imaging device (PortalVisionTM, Varian Oncology Systems, Palo Alto, CA). The film digitizer was equipped with a linear CCD array camera and had an 8-bit resolution in grayscale. It could scan a full size 14" x 17" x-ray film with a spatial resolution of 99 mm per pixel. The PortalVision EPID employed a square matrix of 256x256 liquid-ionization chambers to acquire a 256x256 pixel resolution and 12-bit quantization grayscale image. The EPID image cassette had a sensitive area of 32.5 cm x 32.5 cm, and the effective size of each individual ion chamber was 1.27 mm x 1.27 mm.

Moments Method to Align Radiation Field Outlines

Portal films of a head phantom (Alderson Rando™) were digitized by the film digitizer (Figure 33-1). The test image in the right panel had both translational shifts and rotational shifts in the radiation field and the anatomy (internal structure) inside the radiation field relative to the reference image in the left panel. The alignment of radiation field is particularly important for portal films because the film may slip inside the film envelope or slip inside the film cassette, and the digitizing window on the digitizer may be different each time. This is also true for an EPID equipped with rotary arm cassette holder. The position of the image cassette may change although the patient setup might be correct. However, position repeatability can be improved by a digitally controlled retractable EPID cassette holder employing pre-set positions.

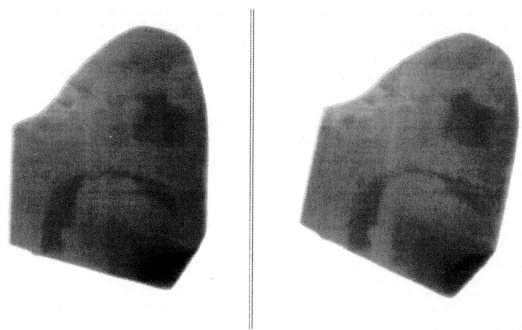

Figure 33-1. *A pair of digitized portal films of the Alderson Rando™ head phantom. The reference image is on the left, the test image is on the right. The test image has both translational shifts and rotational shifts for both radiation field and the internal structure inside the radiation field.*

Segmentation

We have found that the Moments Method worked better when images were segmented. We use a simple global thresholding method[15] to delineate the radiation field (segmentation). A typical histogram of a digitized portal film is shown in Figure 33-2. We used an empirical method to chose the threshold. We can calculate the lower grayscale limit $I1$ and the higher grayscale limit $I2$ inside the histogram. The threshold I_{th} is calculated by $I_{th}=(I_1+I_2)/2$, which is the middle of this non-zero frequency range in the histogram. A black and white segmented image can be generated by:

$$B(i,j) = \begin{cases} 1 \text{ if } I(i,j) & I_{th} \\ 0 \text{ if } I(i,j) & I_{th} \end{cases}$$

(1)

where $I(i,j)$ is the grayscale value at pixel position (i,j), and $B(i,j)$ is the black and white segmented image. This simple empirical method seems to work well for collimated or blocked radiation fields, where the histogram peak corresponding to the primary radiation area and the histogram peak corresponding to the shielded background area are separated. The same method is effective for both digitized portal films and EPID images. The segmented images in Figure 33-1 are shown in Figure 33-3.

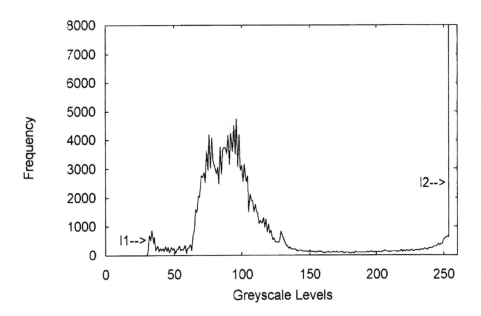

Figure 33-2. *The histogram distribution of the digitzed reference image in Figure 33-1. The digitizer had a 8-bit or 256 grayscale resolution. The peak near grayscale level 250 was from the unexposed background region of the film (brighter). Th peak near grayscale level 90 was from the region of radiation field (exposed, film is darker).*

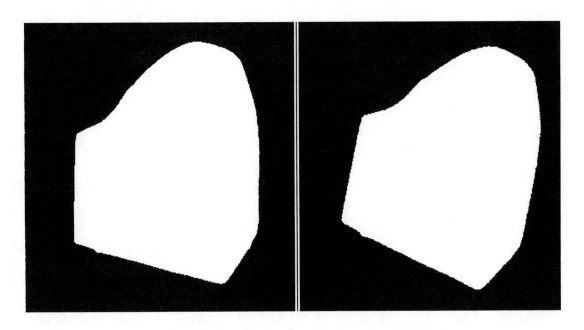

Figure 33-3. *Radiation field deliniation. The images were the segmented images in Figure 33-1 by using a global thresholding method. The reference image is on the left, the test image is on the right.*

Moments Method

One can construct the following moments:

$$M_{kl} = \sum_{ij} i^k j^l B(i, j),$$

(2)

where $B(i,j)$ is the segmented image in equation (1) at pixel position (i,j). The coordinates of the centroid are given by:

$$\bar{x} = M_{10} / M_{00}$$
$$\bar{y} = M_{01} / M_{00}$$

(3)

One can also construct the central moments by:

$$\mu_{kl} = \Sigma_{ij} (i - \bar{x})^k (j - \bar{y})^l B(i, j),$$

(4)

A moment invariant angle 14 (similar to principal axis in a rigid body) can be defined as:

$$\tan 2\theta = \frac{2\mu}{\mu_{20} - \mu_{02}}.$$

(5)

The moments method to align images includes a three-step procedure:

Step 1: Align Centroids

Calculate the centroid of both the test image and the reference image using Eqn. (3), and shift the test image to bring its centroid into alignment with the reference centroid.

Step 2: Align Rotational Angle

Calculate the difference in the moment invariant angle $\Delta\theta = \theta_{test} - \theta_{ref}$, where θ was calculated using Eqn. (5). Rotate the test image about the centroid by $\Delta\theta$ angle to align the rotation of the test image.

Step 3: Scale Image

After the images have been centered and rotationally aligned, they can be scaled about the centroid by using scaling factors in the x (i) and y (j) directions:

$$SF_x = \frac{(\mu_{20})_{test}}{(\mu_{20})_{ref}}$$
$$SF_y = \frac{(\mu_{02})_{test}}{(\mu_{02})_{ref}}$$

(6)

Note, the moments calculation uses the segmented black and white images, but the calculated shifts, rotations and scale factors are applied to the original grayscale test image to align it with the grayscale reference image. The result is shown in Figure 33-4.

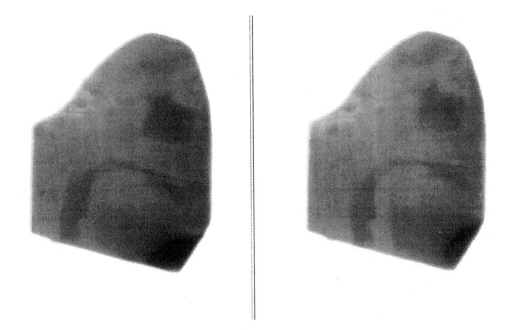

Figure 33-4. *The radiation field outline was aligned by the Moments Method. The reference image is on the left, the test image is on the right. Note, the anatomy (internal structure) inside the radiation field is still not aligned.*

We have tested the moments method in a controlled experiment in which portal films and EPID images were made by exposing an Alderson Rando™ head phantom to 6MV x-ray. The films or the EPID image cassette was shifted and rotated by measured amounts. The moments method was applied to the digitized portal films and EPID images. The results were shown in Table 33-1 and Table 33-2. In this experiment the algorithm tracked the translations to within 0.7 mm and the rotations to within 0.2° for portal films and 0.6° for EPID images. The reproducibility of the film positioning was approximately 1mm and 1°.

Table 33-1. *Test results for the Moments Method to align translational shifts of the radiation field. The test was done by moving the EPID image cassette holder towards one direction for 3 mm, 5 mm, 8 mm and 10 mm without changing other positions. These shifts were scaled to isocenter level from 127 cm SSD to 100 cm SSD. The accuracy of the EPID cassette movement is about ±1 mm. A portal film was positioned and exposed on top of the EPID cassette holder each time after the EPID image was taken. Theoretically, the portal film and the EPID image should have the same field displacement.*

	Δx (mm)	Δy (mm)	$\Delta\theta$ (°)	Δx (mm)	Δy (mm)	$\Delta\theta$ (°)	Δx (mm)	Δy (mm)	$\Delta\theta$ (°)	Δx (mm)	Δy (mm)	$\Delta\theta$ (°)
Physical Shifts	2.4	0.0	0.0	3.9	0.0	0.0	6.3	0.0	0.0	7.9	0.0	0.0
Portal Films	2.2	0.3	-0.2	4.4	0.4	-0.3	6.5	0.0	-0.2	8.5	0.3	0.3
EPID Images	2.4	0.0	0.4	4.6	0.0	0.1	6.5	0.0	0.0	8.4	0.0	-0.1

Table 33-2. *Test results for the Moments Method to align rotational shifts of the radiation field. The test was done by rotating both the couch and the collimator about the isocenter by 3°, 5°, and 8° in the same direction to simulate a net radiation field rotation. The accuracy of the couch movements is about ±1° and the accuracy of collimator rotation is less than 1°. A portal film was positioned and exposed on top of the EPID cassette holder each time after the EPID image was taken. Theoretically, the portal film and the EPID should have the same field displacement.*

	Δx (mm)	Δy (mm)	$\Delta\theta$ (°)	Δx (mm)	Δy (mm)	$\Delta\theta$ (°)	Δx (mm)	Δy (mm)	$\Delta\theta$ (°)
Physical Shifts	0.0	0.0	3.0	0.0	0.0	5.0	0.0	0.0	8.0
Portal Films	-0.3	0.7	2.8	0.2	-0.2	4.8	-0.3	-0.6	7.8
EPID Images	-0.2	-0.4	3.2	-0.2	-0.5	5.3	-0.2	-0.8	8.6

Correlation Method to Register Internal Structure

The cross-correlation (correlation in short) technique has been used to determine if an image contains a region that is similar to a region within another image. This region W is called the Region Of Interest (ROI). We use a circular ROI to avoid losing information in case there are in-plane rotations in the image. The normalized correlation function is defined as:

$$c(a,b,\theta) = \frac{\sum_{i,j}^{\Omega} I_{test}(i+a,j+b,\theta) * I_{ref}(i,j)}{\sqrt{\sum_{i,j}^{\Omega} I_{test}^2(i,j) * \sum_{i,j}^{\Omega} I_{ref}^2(i,j)}}$$

(7)

where I_{ref} (i,j) is the grayscale reference image at pixel position (i,j) inside the ROIΩ, and I_{test}(i+a,j+b,θ) is the grayscale test image after translating the center of the ROI by a vector of (a,b) and then rotating through the angle θ about this new center of the ROI. By changing a,b and θ the ROI is translated and rotated inside the test image until it matches a similar region in the reference image. The maximum correlation value in the correlation space (a,b,θ) corresponds to the best match condition between the test image and the reference image.

The calculation could be lengthy if we were to calculate for every possible position and in-plane rotation using Eqn. (7). However, clinical patient setup errors rarely exceed 20mm in translation and 10° in rotation. This gives us a chance to reduce the amount of calculation. We proposed a two-stage correlation procedure as follows:

Step 1: 2-D Global Search for Translational shifts

In this step, we first sought translational shifts ignoring any in-plane rotations of the image. In-plane rotations of patient portal images tend to be small, and we found the correlation value to be more sensitive to translations than rotations. We used a smaller circular ROI $\Omega 1$ (The region of r<R1 in Figure 33-5) to further minimize the effect of in-plane rotation in the image.

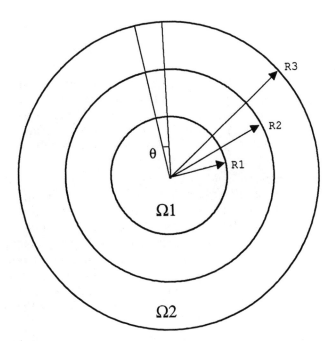

Figure 33-5. *Regions of Interest (ROIs) for the correlation technique. Smaller circular ROI (r<R1) can minimize the effect of in-plane rotations and was used in the gradient search method to located translational shifts. Larger ring-shaped ROI (R2<r<R3) can emphasize the effect of in-plane rotations and was used in the local 3-D linear search step to find the best match in the image.*

A typical 2-D normalized correlation function is shown in Figure 33-6. It can be seen that c(a,b) has many local maxima and minima. Only the global maximum position represents the best match condition. Therefore, before applying the Gradient Search Method, it was necessary to divide the search window into smaller sub-search-windows. Otherwise, the Gradient Search may climb to a local maximum position.

The idea of the gradient search is based on the fact that we can get to the peak most quickly by following the direction of maximum variation determined by,

$$\vec{\Delta}c = \frac{\partial c}{\partial x}\,\vec{i} + \frac{\partial c}{\partial y}\,\vec{j},$$

(8)

where the derivatives can be calculated approximately by:

$$\frac{\partial c}{\partial x} \cong c(i+1,j) - c(i,j)$$

$$\frac{\partial c}{\partial y} \cong c(i,j+1) - c(i,j)$$

(9)

c(i,j) is the correlation value calculated by Eqn. (7) assuming $\theta=0°$. Once the direction of the gradient was obtained, we moved our search point from position 1 to 2 as shown in Figure 33-7. The correlation value was computed at point 2 and compared with the value at point 1. If $c_1<c_2$, we had made a step toward the maximum; if $c_1>c_2$, we had overshot the maximum and needed to refine our search, e.g., reduce the step size by half, until the local maximum was reached.

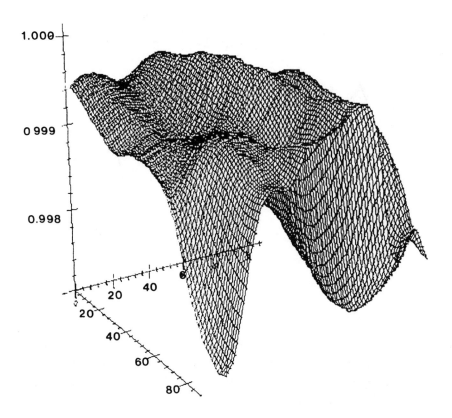

Figure 33-6. A sample distribution of the normalized correlation function of the 2-D translational shifts

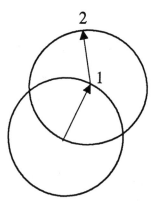

Figure 33-7. The gradient search method will pick up a direction of maximum gradient

Step 2: Local 3-D Search for Best Match

The translational shifts found in step 1 were very close to the actual shifts. Nevertheless, due to the finite in-plane rotation in the image, this position found by step 1 might be off by a few pixels. The best match was obtained by searching through a local 3-D correlation space (i, j, θ) around the translational position found in step 1. We used a linear search. The translational search window was ±3 pixels in steps of 1 pixel in each direction and the rotational search window was ±10° in step of 3°. A parabolic fitting was used at the angle of the maximum correlation value to further refine the search of maximum correlation angle without reducing the step size. In this step, we emphasized the effect of the in-plane rotation in order to get a better detection of the rotational shifts. A ring-shaped ROI $\Omega 2$ (R2<r<R3 in Figure 33-6) was used to calculate the correlation value in this step.

Results

Using the global 2-D gradient search followed by a local 3-D linear search, we obtained the best match between the test images and the reference images. The center of the ROI in the reference image was set to the position of the centroid by default, but the user could optionally change the ROI to any other positions interactively with a mouse pointer. This is the only place in the procedure that the user may need to intervene. However this step would be required if the centroid happened to be too close to a field edge or even outside of the radiation field. Another advantage of the user chosen ROI is that the user may want to know how much a particular anatomical structure was moved. Choosing a different ROI may also avoid possible artifacts in the image, since the reliability of the correlation algorithm depends on the noise inside the image.

The correlation method was carried out after the radiation field was aligned by the moments method. Hence any change obtained by the correlation method was the change of internal structure (anatomy). Table 33-3.and Table 33-4 showed the results of a controlled study using both portal films and EPID images. The phantom was moved to simulate an anatomical shift of the patient. The test results in Table 33-3 and Table 33-4 indicated that the two-step moments-correlation alignment procedure could track translational shifts to within 1mm and rotational shifts to within 1.5°. Figure 33-8 shows a test image after the moments-correlation alignment procedure. Both the radiation field and the anatomy inside the radiation field were aligned. The computing time required for the moments-correlation procedure to align a pair of EPID images (without user intervention) was about 3 seconds on Sun Sparc 10 workstation or 15 seconds on PC 486/33MHz. About 60% of computing time was spent on the 3-D linear search step.

Table 33-3. *Test results for the Correlation Method to align anatomical translational shifts. The test was done by moving the couch towards one direction for 3 mm, 5 mm, 8 mm and 10 mm without changing other parameters. The phantom was assumed to be at isocenter, and all the translational shifts were scaled to the isocenter level. The accuracy of the couch movements is about ±1 mm. A portal film was positioned and exposed on top of the EPID cassette holder each time after the EPID image was taken. Theoretically, the portal film and the EPID should be identically exposed.*

	Δx (mm)	Δy (mm)	$\Delta\theta$ (°)	Δx (mm)	Δy (mm)	$\Delta\theta$ (°)	Δx (mm)	Δy (mm)	$\Delta\theta$ (°)	Δx (mm)	Δy (mm)	$\Delta\theta$ (°)
Physical Shifts	3.0	0.0	0.0	5.0	0.0	0.0	8.0	0.0	0.0	10.0	0.0	0.0
Portal Films	3.3	0.0	0.1	5.4	0.3	0.3	8.1	0.3	0.3	10.5	0.3	0.1
EPID Images	3.0	0.0	0.1	5.0	0.0	0.1	8.0	0.0	0.0	11.0	0.0	-0.7

Table 33-4. *Test results for the Correlation Method to align rotational shifts of the anatomy inside radiation field. The test was done by rotating the couch about the isocenter by 3°, 5°, and 8° to simulate a patient in-plane rotation. The accuracy of the couch movements is about ±1°. Note, the ROI for this study was chosen at the centroid of the radiation field. If the centroid of the radiation field was not at the isocenter about which the couch was rotated, there will be a companion translational displacement for the RO1. This displacement can be significant for large rotations. A portal film was positioned and exposed on top of the EPID cassette holder each time after the EPID image was taken. Theoretically, the portal film and the EPID should be identically exposed.*

	Δx (mm)	Δy (mm)	Δθ (°)	Δx (mm)	Δy (mm)	Δθ (°)	Δx (mm)	Δy (mm)	Δθ (°)
Physical Shifts	0.0	0.0	3.0	0.0	0.0	5.0	0.0	0.0	8.0
Portal Films	0.3	-0.3	3.4	0.6	-0.6	4.9	0.3	-0.9	7.6
EPID Images	-1.0	0.0	4.5	0.0	-1.0	5.2	-1.0	-1.0	8.6

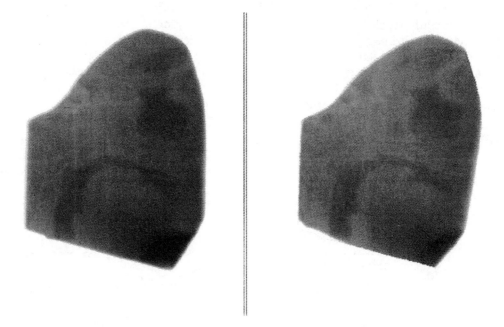

Figure 33-8. *Both the radiation field and the internal structure (anatomy) inside the radiation field was aligned by the two-step moments-correlation procedure for the test image on the right with the reference image on the left. Note, a blank space was added to the radiation field of the aligned test image because the information outside of the original radiation field was unknown.*

Conclusion

The combination of a moments method and the correlation method can be used to effectively align radiation fields and internal structure inside the radiation field. The computing time is fast enough to allow on-line EPID image registration. We estimated the accuracy of this procedure for rigid structures to be about 1mm in translational shifts and 1.5° for in-plane rotation angles. The moments-correlation procedure does not rely on the site of the fields or any landmarks inside the image. Its operation is easy and requires little user effort. Preliminary clinical application of the method indicates that the patient internal shape changes, such as lung respiration, as well as the image quality will affect the success of this method. However, those difficulties can be addressed by chosing the ROI at a region where the shape of the structure is relatively fixed (such as bone, or the apex region of the lung), and by chosing a region where the image has better contrast for the correlation algorithm to register.

Acknowledgment

This work was supported in part by grant CA43840 from the United States National Cancer Institute.

References

1. M. G. Herman, R. A. Abrams, and R. R. Mayer, "Clinical use of on-line portal imaging for daily patient treatment verification," Int. J. Rad. Oncol Biol Phys. 24 (suppl. 1) 216 (1992).

2. I. Rabinowitz, J. Broomberg, M. Goitein, K. McCarthy, J. Leong, "Accuracy of radiation field alignment in clinical practice," Int. J. Rad. Oncol. Biol. Phys. 11, 1857-1867 (1985).

3. S. A. Rosenthal, J.M. Galvin, J.W. Goldwein, A. R. Smith, P.H. Blitzer, "Improved methods for determination of variability in patient positioning for radiation therapy using simulation and serial portal film measurements," Int. J. Rad. Oncol. Biol. Phys. 23, 621-625 (1992).

4. K.S. Lam, M. Partowmah, W.C. Lam, "An on-line electronic portal imaging system for external beam radiotherapy," Br. J. Radiol. 59, 1007-1013 (1986).

5. J. E. Marks, A. G. Haus, H. G. Sutton, M. L. Griem, "Localization Error in the radiotherapy of Hodgkin's disease and malignant lymphoma with extended mantl fields,", Cancer 34, 83-90 (1974).

6. H. Meertens, J. Bijhold, and J. Strackee, "A method for the measurement of field placement errors in digital portal imaging,", Phys. Med. Bio. 35, 299-323 (1990).

7. R. Roesecke, T. Brucknew, and G. Ende, "Landmark based correlation of medical images," Phys. Med. Biol. 35, 121-126 (1990).

8. G. Ende, H. Treuer and R. Boesecke, "Optimization and evaluation of landmark-based image correlation," Phys. Med. Biol. 37, 261-271 (1992).

9. J. M. Balter, C. A. Pelizzari, G. T. Y. Chen, "Correlation of projection radiographs in radiation therapy using open curve segments and points," Med. Phys. 19, 329-334 (1992).

10. J. Bijhold, "Three-dimensional verification of patient placement during radiotherapy using portal images," Med. Phys. 20 347-351 (1992).

11. J. Bijhold, M. Van Herk, R. Vijlbrief, J. V. Lebesque, "Fast evaluation of patient set-up during radiotherapy by aligning features in portal and simulator images," Phys. Med. Biol. 36(12), 1665-1679 (1991).

12. K.G.A. Gilhuijs and M. van Herk, "Automatic on-line inspection of patient setup in radiation therapy using digital portal images," Med. Phys. 20, 667-677 (1993).

13. S.M. Jones and A. L. Boyer, "Investigation of an FFT-based correlation technique for verification of radiation treatment setup," Med. Phys. 18, 1116-1125 (1991).

14. Hu, M.K., "Visual Pattern Recognition by Moment Invariants." IRE Trans. Info. Theory, Vol. IT-8, 179-187 (1962).

15. R. C. Gonzalez and R. E. Woods, Digital Image Processing, Addison-Wesley, 3rd ed(1992).

Chapter 34

PACS, Computer Networking for 3-D Radiation Therapy Treatment Planning and Conformal Therapy

G. James Blaine, D.Sc.

Department of Radiology, Washington University School of Medicine, St. Louis, Missouri

Rapid advancements in the fields of computation and visualization, coupled with improved dose calculations promise significant changes to the practice of treatment planning and therapy. Three-dimensional planning, visualization, on-line treatment verification and potentially dynamic control of the therapy machine are being addressed using commercially available computation and display technologies. Access to three-dimensional imaging modalities, such as CT and MR, distributed viewing and information management requirements challenge developers of therapy systems to offer system solutions which support cost-effective planning, treatment and verification. These systems must be viewed as components which are readily integrated into the rapidly evolving health care systems supporting hospital information, laboratory automation and medical imaging and information management systems.

Although the computation and visualization requirements of 3-D treatment and verification are unique to oncology, the paradigm of image acquisition, management and display is common to the field of diagnostic radiology. A brief discussion of the challenges and solutions in that area follow.

PACS Developments in Diagnostic Radiology

Medical imaging and information management systems in the support of diagnostic radiology have been the subject of considerable research and development for the past decade. These systems are often referred to as Picture Archiving and Communications Systems (PACS). [1] While CT, MR and nuclear medicine provided early examples of the importance of digital imaging, computed radiography, high-resolution film digitizers and direct detection digital mammography offer the promise of a radiology department where all the diagnostic images can be available in digital form. The model, as shown in Figure 34-1, is deceptively simple: acquisition, communication, storage and display.

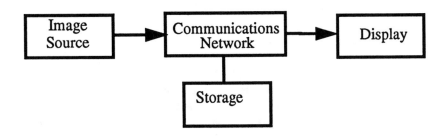

Figure 34-1. Picture Archiving and Communications System (PACS) Model

Although the PACS model is simple, implementation of a system which is acceptable from both the user's view and is deemed "cost-effective" by the hospital organization poses several challenges:

- storing and managing very large quantities of data

- maintaining image quality

- responsive delivery of medical information and images.

Data Quantity

Data quantity is a function of the sampling and quantization of data which represent the digital image, the quantity of images produced by a diagnostic exam and the volume of examinations conducted by the institution. An example set of values is provided in Table 34-1 for the most prevalent digital modalities. Table 34-2 provides a tabulation of exam volume that could be representative of a large institution which provides on the order of 1000 diagnostic exams per day. Assumptions include: MR exams of 100 images/each, CT exams of 50 images/each, and musculo-skeletal exams of 4 films/exam.

Table 34-1. Digital Image Parameters

Modality	Matrix Size-pixels	bits/pixel	bytes/image
film scan	2k x 2k to 4k x 5k	10 to 12	8Mbyte-40Mbyte
computed tomography	512 x 512 to 1k x 1k	12	0.5Mbyte-2Mbyte
magnetic resonance	256 x 256	12	0.125Mbyte

Table 34-2. Medical Imaging Data Volume Estimates Based on 1000 Exams per Day

Exam Type	Exams/Day	GBytes
chest x-ray	240	19.2
portable x-ray	220	2.2
magnetic resonance	40	0.5
computed tomography	140	3.5
mammography	90	23.0
musculo-skeletal x-ray	260	42.0
other exams	100	-
totals	1000	~90

This example 1000 study/day scenario produces a data storage requirement of approximately 90 GBytes per day and on the order of 30 Terabytes per year. System considerations of delay to access, speed of delivery and cost to store are usually addressed by an implementation based on several levels of storage hierarchy. Magnetic disk storage for minimal access delay, and responsive transfer; optical media for on-line access delays of several seconds to minutes and optical disk or tape based media for off-line access which requires operator interaction for loading the media.

Costs per Gigabyte for magnetic storage now ranges from $3000 to $900 for on-line access. Media costs for off-line storage range from $1 to $70 per Gigabyte.

Image Display

Use of soft-copy display (currently based on cathode ray tube technology) is limited by quality and cost issues, thereby impeding efforts to achieve the elusive "filmless" radiology department. While CT and MR image data are easily accommodated, displays capable of maximum luminance of 400 foot-Lamberts (fL) with a dynamic range greater than 500 to 1, are required to compete with film/light-box combinations for projection radiography. [2] Current research and development programs target goals of greater than 200 fL luminance and costs under $10,000 per display tube supporting display matrices of greater than 5Mpixels. [3]

Response Times

The required speed for image delivery has no absolute bound; the user's perception of acceptability varies with the task and experience. Coarse metrics associated with user acceptability criteria for speed of display update are show in Table 34-3.

Table 34-3. Speed of Update for Display Applications

Descriptor	Time
real-time	video ~ 30 frames/sec
near real-time	less than 1/4 sec
fast	less than 1 to 2 secs
slow	greater than 2 secs

The time to send an image from the acquisition source or the storage unit to the display is related to the bandwidth of the channel (bits/sec or b/s) and the total number of bits required to represent the image. This simple relationship, T(sec)= image size(bits)/BW(b/s), is illustrated in Figure 34-2. For example, an image size of 1024 x 1024 x 12 bits/pixel requires a transmission rate (or BW) of 12 Mb/s to achieve a delivery time of 1 sec. The line labeled "Image-1K2" provides a simple guide for varying either time or BW. Images of larger size would be represented by lines parallel to and above the "Image-1K"line. (It is assumed that the physical distance between source and display produces a propagation delay (~1.7nanosec/ft) which is much less than the transmission time and can be neglected.)

Communications Technology

Availability of communications networks, local-area (Ethernet at 10Mb/s, Fiber Distributed Data Interconnect (FDDI) at 100Mb/s and Asynchronous Transfer Mode (ATM) at 155 Mb/s), metropolitan-area (Frame Relay, Switched Multi-megabit Data Systems (SMDS) at T1=1.5Mb/s and T3=45Mb/s rates) and wide-area (Synchronous Optical Network (SONET), and ATM at multiples of 155Mb/s) offer cost-effective network alternatives to attain acceptable user response times for even the large (10 to 64 MBytes/image) data sets associated with chest and musculoskeletal radiography. [4]

A metropolitan area testbed in St. Louis supports telemedicine demonstrations and experiments in high speed information and image access and presentation. The St. Louis testbed is supported as a collaborative project between Washington University and Southwestern Bell Technology Resources Inc.[5] Image servers and ATM facilitate local-area and wide-area delivery of digital radiographic image data and full frame rate medical video.

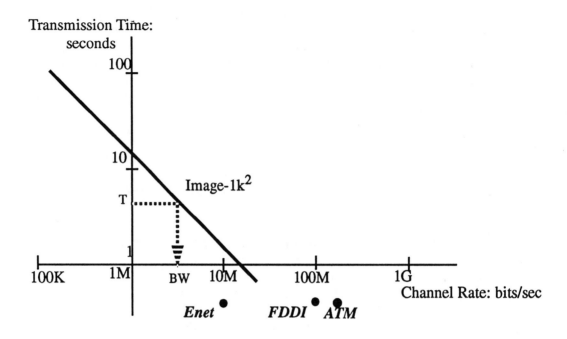

Figure 34-2. Time vs. Channel rate relationship for image transfer

Storage Technology

Image storage on magnetic and optical media can be configured with currently available storage and server products. Clinical installations of PACS targeting specific diagnostic application areas are reporting successes. [6,7]

Standards

Standards addressing the concept of "open systems" are achieving considerable support from both the user and the medical system supplier communities. The new ACR-NEMA standard for image communication, DICOM V3 [8], has been finalized this year and a rather ambitious demonstration supported by participation of multiple equipment manufacturers was presented at the RSNA scientific exhibition (infoRAD) in the fall of 1993. The current revision of HL-7, an application protocol for electronic data exchange in health care environments [9], is expected to accelerate adoption by the PACS community and both the national and international standards bodies.

Components and Requirements for 3-D RTP and CT

A simplified view of the system which supports the acquisition of data used for treatment planning, 3-D treatment planning, treatment verification, dose delivery and treatment quality assurance is shown in Figure 34-3. With the exception of the computer control component for delivery of the conformal dose of radiation, the components parallel those shown in the PACS model of Figure 34-1.

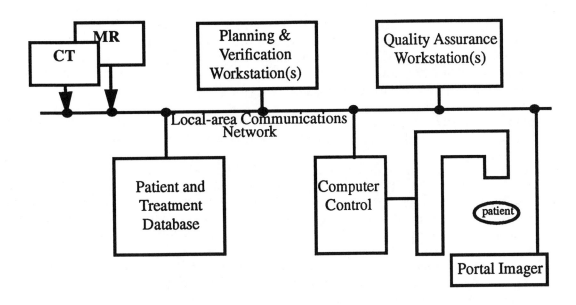

Figure 34-3. 3-D Treatment Planning and Conformal Therapy System Block Diagram

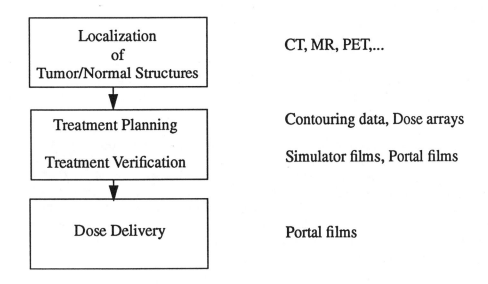

Figure 34-4. Data Model for Planning, Treatment and Verification

In order to compare the system requirements with those presented in Section 2, the processes involving data storage and communication are examined. The process of planning and treatment is represented by the data model shown in Figure 34-4.

Each of the process steps identified in the data model can be analyzed for the corresponding digital data requirements and considered in the context of both transmission and storage demands.

- localization of tumor/normal structures; assuming a computed tomography study may consist of 50 to 100 cross-sectional slices in order to visualize normal structures and the specific region of interest which defines the tumor volume. Each slice is represented by an image of 512 by 512 pixels at 2 bytes/pixel requiring 0.5 Mbytes/slice or a study data set of between 25 MBytes and 50 MBytes.

- plan and verify data sets consisting of contouring data, dose array, annotations and digitized simulator films are assumed to require 15 Mbytes to 30 Mbytes of data.

- representation of the dose delivery process may produce portal images of 512 x 512 or 1024 x 1024 pixels, at 8 bit/pixel. To establish bounds on the quantity of data, it is assumed that between 4 and 10 fields per fraction of the treatment and between 20 and 30 fractions per treatment are representative. This results in generation of a data set with a size between 20 Mbytes and 300 Mbytes during the dose delivery process.

Responsive access to treatment plans and patient images is usually facilitated by storing the digital data on magnetic disks. Assuming a department load of 1000 cases per year, or an average of 20 new cases per week, and an average treatment duration of 3 weeks, implies a requirement to maintain approximately 60 data sets on-line. This would require a capacity of between 3.6 and 23 GBytes of capacity; which is well within the capability of currently available disk storage systems.

Archival storage requirements are readily calculated for the previous assumptions of 1000 cases per year and totaling the needs specified in the single case model of Figure 34-4. The total digital data is found to be of the order of 60 to 380 GBytes per year. While this is a substantial requirement for a storage system it is a relatively small percentage of the requirements estimated for an "all digital radiology department." Assuming a total of 400,000 exams per year, the archival storage is estimated to be between 10 and 100 Terabytes per year.

Summary

The communications and storage requirements of 3-D treatment planning and conformal therapy are quite similar to those identified and addressed by PACS components and modules developed and marketed for diagnostic radiology.

Hopefully users, specifiers and developers of the treatment planning and verification systems will recognize the importance of the data import and export functionality and the advantages of adopting the existing imaging and communications standards, such as DICOM v .3.0. Early attention to the requirements for system integration can provide the seamless import of the anatomical information, integration of the patient information with the hospital/radiology information systems and support for distributed access to subsets of the treatment and verification information at other PACS image presentation stations, and thus reduce the economic penalties associated with equipment replication.

References

1. Medical Imaging VI: PACS Design and Evaluation, R. Gilbert Jost, M.D., editor, Proceedings of the Society of Photo-Optical Instrumentation Engineers, Volume 1654, February 1992.

2. H. Blume, H. Roehrig, T. Ji, M. Browne, Very-High-Resolution Monochrome CRT Displays: How Good Are They Really?, SID 91, Digest.

3. Softcopy Review, National Information Display Laboratory, publication number 711892-001, August 1992, Princeton, NJ.

4. Medical Communications, T.P. McGarty, G. J. Blaine, M. Goldberg, editors, IEEE Journal on Selected Areas in Communications, Vol 10, No 7, September 1992.

5. J. R. Cox, G.J. Blaine, et al. A Demonstration of Medical Communications on an ATM Broadband Network Technology, Medical Imaging VI: PACS Design and Evaluation, SPIE volume 1654, 1992.

6. B.K. Stewart, S.J. Dwyer III, H. Kangarloo, Design of a High-Speed, High-resolution Teleradiology Network, Journal of Digital Imaging, Vol 5 No 3, August 1992.

7. D.V. Smith, S. Smith, F. Sauls, Design Strategy and Implementation of the Medical Diagnostic Image Support System (MDIS) at Two Large Military Medical Centers, SPIE vol 1654, pp 148-157, 1992.

8. American College of Radiology-National Electrical Manufacturers Association, Digital Imaging and Communication in Medicine Standard, DICOM Version 3.0, November 1993.

9. Health Level-Seven (HL-7) an Application Protocol for Electronic Data Exchange in Healthcare Environments, Health Level Seven, Ann Arbor, MI.

Chapter 35

A Picture Archival and Communication System for Radiotherapy

George Starkschall, Ph.D.,* Stanley W. Bujnowski, M.S.,* Xuan-Jian Li, M.S.,* Ngiam W. Wong, M.S.,* Adam S. Garden, M.D.,** and Kenneth R. Hogstrom, Ph.D.*

Departments of Radiation Physics* and Clinical Radiotherapy, **
The University of Texas, M. D. Anderson Cancer Center, Houston, Texas

The purpose of this paper is to describe a picture archival and communication system for radiotherapy (RT-PACS) that is currently under development at The University of Texas M. D. Anderson Cancer Center. The RT-PACS is a system for acquiring, transmitting, storing, and operating on patient images and image-related information that are specifically used in radiotherapy. Inherent in the system's design is the premise that an RT-PACS contains functions that are unique to radiotherapy. In addition, the RT-PACS may function independently of a conventional picture archival and communication systems (PACS).

Several features make an RT-PACS different from a conventional PACS. The first difference is that fewer images are required for an RT-PACS than for a conventional PACS. Images typically required in radiotherapy include several simulation images; a set of initial portal images, with additional sets of portal images acquired during treatment; a set of computed-tomography (CT) images for treatment planning; and, possibly, a set of digitally reconstructed radiographs. Moreover, the number of patients for which images are acquired in radiotherapy is significantly fewer than the number of patients for which conventional images are acquired. As a consequence, the communications and storage requirements are far less stringent for an RT-PACS than for a conventional PACS. The second difference is that radiotherapy images require less resolution than do diagnostic images. The purpose of images used in radiotherapy is not to detect pathologic characteristics, but to identify anatomical characteristics. Thus, a resolution of 512 x 512 appears to provide more than adequate resolution for radiotherapy images. A third difference is that scalar and vector data as well as character strings must be included with images in the RT-PACS database and communicated along with the images. Scalar data include geometric parameters such as source-to-isocenter distance, source-to-image receptor distance, collimator settings, and gantry angle. Vector data include outlines of treatment portals on simulation images and target volumes and dose volumes on CT images. Character strings include annotations on images and messages. Finally, different users of the RT-PACS require different interactions with the PACS. For example, tasks of a simulator technologist include entering patient demographic information into the RT-PACS and generating digitized simulator images, whereas tasks of a staff physician include specifying a dose prescription, delineating one or more treatment portals on a simulator image, delineating one or more target volumes on CT or magnetic resonance (MR) images, and approving simulator and portal images and treatment plans.

The components of the RT-PACS at M. D. Anderson Cancer Center are shown in Figure 35-1. Simulator images can be acquired either indirectly by digitizing film or directly from the image intensifier through a frame grabber. These images can then be reviewed by the physician. One or more treatment portals can then be delineated on the image. In addition, annotations can be made on the image. Multileaf collimator (MLC) settings can be generated from the treatment portal outlines, and the settings can be transferred to an MLC workstation, where they can be set on a linear accelerator. Coordinates for treatment portal outlines are stored in a file, from which they could be extracted for use in a computer-driven hot-wire cutter, although this aspect of the RT-PACS has not yet been implemented. Portal images from the treatment machine can be entered on the RT-PACS either by digitizing film or through an electronic portal imaging device (EPID). These portal images can be displayed alongside and compared with either simulator images, other portal images, or digitally reconstructed radiographs. Image comparison is accomplished with either side-by-side viewing or image comparison tools.

MDACC RADIOTHERAPY PACS

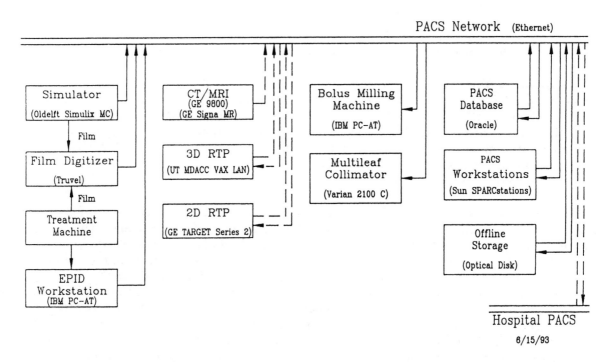

Figure 35-1. *The components of M. D. Anderson's RT-PACS. Solid lines indicate components presently included in the RT-PACS, and dashed lines represent proposed components.*

Another planned function of the RT-PACS,.which has not yet been implemented, is its integration with both two-dimensional (2-D) and three-dimensional (3-D) radiotherapy treatment planning systems. Patient images acquired from CT can be displayed on the RT-PACS, on which target volumes and critical structure outlines can be delineated. Digitally reconstructed radiographs can also be displayed on the RT-PACS for delineation of treatment portals or MLC settings. The 3-D treatment planning system can automatically design an electron bolus to deliver electron-beam conformal therapy, and the bolus design parameters can be transferred to a computer-driven milling machine. Dose distributions generated on the treatment planning system can then be displayed through the RT-PACS for physician approval.

Users of the RT-PACS

One of the differences between the RT-PACS and a conventional PACS is that different users of the RT-PACS have different interactions with the PACS. Eight classes of users have been identified for the RT-PACS (1): clerk, simulator technologist, machine technologist, dosimetrist, staff physician, resident physician, PACS manager, and demonstrator. The roles and functions of each of these users will be discussed.

When a user logs into the RT-PACS, the system identifies the user with one of the eight user classes and enables the user to access only those functions identified for the appropriate class.

The first user class is that of clerk. At the present time, a clerk can only enter patient demographic information onto the RT-PACS, although in the future the clerk may be assigned to digitize film images (simulator or portal) into the RT-PACS and to generate hard copy of PACS information for patient charts. When the clerk logs onto the RT-PACS, a window is displayed allowing the clerk to select a patient from a menu of patients, to enter a new patient, or to send messages through an internal mail system to other RT-PACS users. Figure 35-2 shows this window.

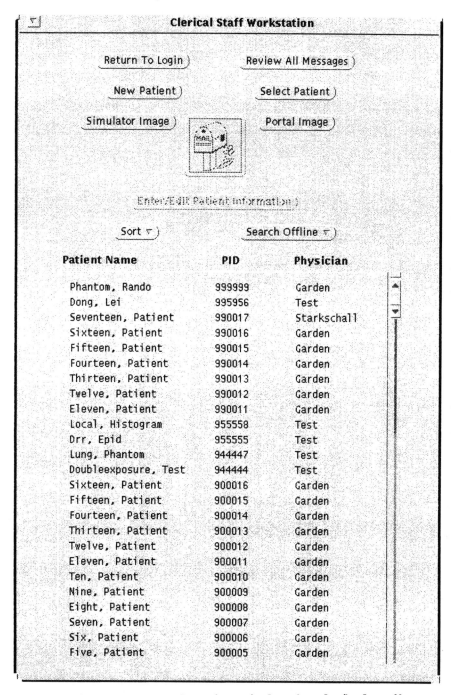

Figure 35-2. Workstation window for clerical staff

The next user class is that of simulator technologist. The simulator technologist's main task is to acquire simulation images. These may be obtained either directly from the image intensifier of the simulator, by digitizing a simulator radiograph, or by calculating a digitally reconstructed radiograph by ray-tracing through a 3-D CT array. In addition to acquiring a simulation image from the image intensifier, the simulator technologist can enter or edit patient demographic information, view existing simulation images, or send mail messages to other RT-PACS users. Figure 35-3 illustrates the window displayed to the simulator technologist upon logging onto the system.

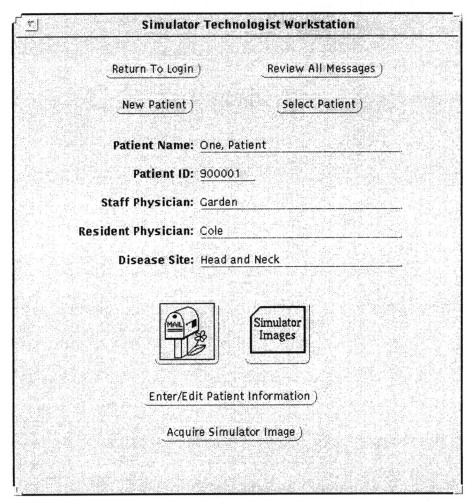

Figure 35-3. Workstation window for the simulator technologist

The treatment machine technologist's primary interaction with the RT-PACS is to acquire portal images. Portal images may be acquired either directly from an EPID or by digitizing portal radiographs. In addition to capturing EPID images. the treatment. machine technologist can enter or edit patient demographic information or send mail messages to other RT-PACS users.

The dosimetrist's interactions with the RT-PACS involve images related to treatment planning. Before planning a treatment, the dosimetrist displays CT images and outlines anatomical structures on the CT images. After beams and beam geometries have been selected and doses calculated using the treatment planning system, the dosimetrist can use the RT-PACS to display dose calculation results such as dose distributions and dose volume histograms. In addition, the dosimetrist directs output from the RT-PACS to various fabrication devices for block cutting, bolus fabrication, or compensating filter fabrication.

Two classes of physicians are identified, staff and resident physicians. For the most part, the tasks available to these two classes are identical. Physicians can review simulation images, draw one or more treatment portals on these images, and make annotations on these images. They can delineate target volumes and other patient anatomy on CT images. They can review portal images and compare them with simulation and other portal images. Staff physicians differ from resident physicians in that they also are allowed to approve images, treatment portals and treatment plans. When the physician user logs onto the system, a menu is displayed from which they can select a patient from a menu of patients that are on the RT-PACS. In addition, the status of the patient on the RT-PACS is displayed, informing the physician of the tasks that he or she needs to perform. Figure 35-4 shows this window.

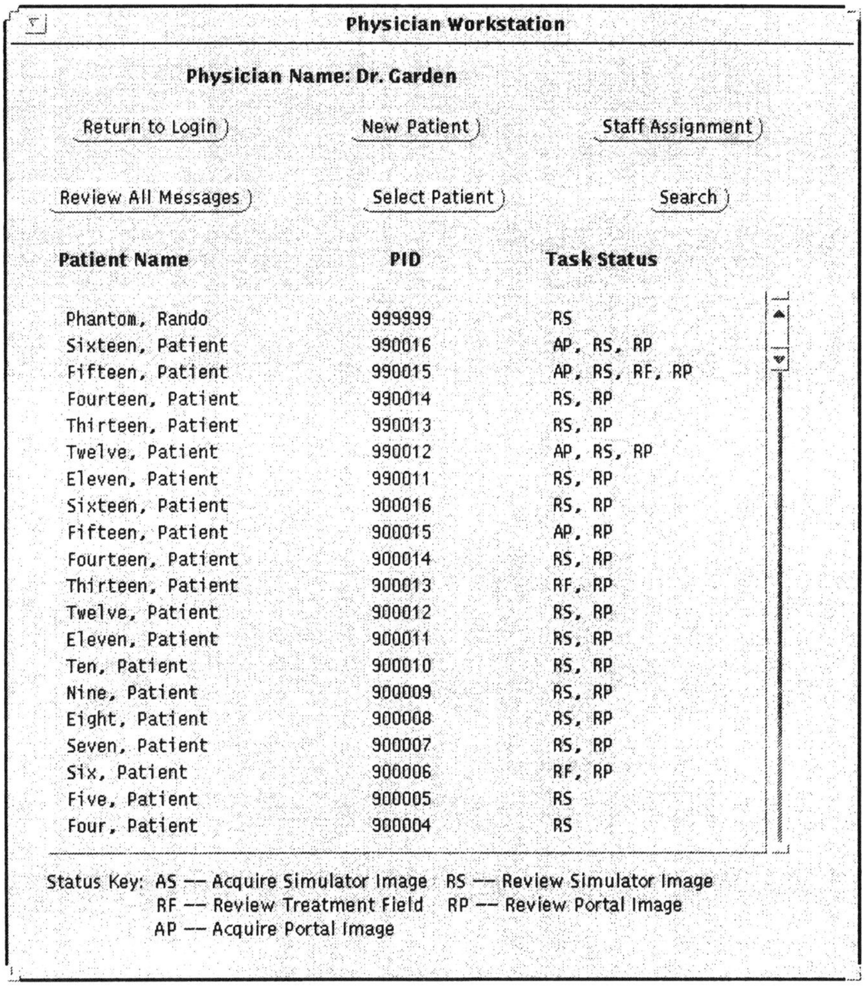

Figure 35-4. Workstation window for physicians

The PACS manager acts as the system manager for the RT-PACS. In addition to being able to simulate any other class of user on the RT-PACS, the PACS manager must perform two other classes of tasks that are unique to the PACS manager. One class of tasks is to update databases. The PACS manager may add or delete PACS users, assigning passwords to the users and assigning the users to the appropriate user class. The PACS manager can also change physician assignments of residents to staff. The second class of tasks is archiving and archival retrieval. The PACS manager archives image sets to and retrieves them from optical disks. Figure 35-5 shows the window available to the PACS manager upon logging in.

The last user class of the RT-PACS is the demonstrator. The demonstrator is used when the RT-PACS is to be demonstrated. This user class has the ability to simulate any other user, but the demonstrator may not save any information on the PACS database or approve images, treatment

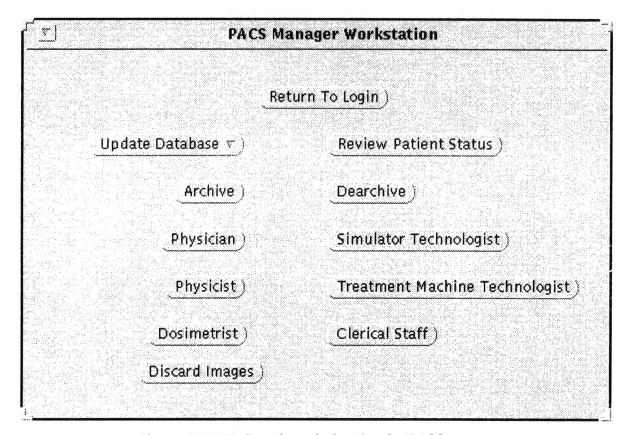

Figure 35-5. Workstation window for the PACS manager

RT-PACS Hardware and Software

Workstations

RT-PACS workstations (PACStations) currently consist of Sun SPARCstation 2 and Sun SPARCstation 10 workstations connected by an Ethernet network. These workstations are running under SunOS 4.1.1 and SunOS 4.1.3, respectively. Workstations are located in each of the areas in which the various classes of RT-PACS users work. For example, a PACStation is located in the simulator room so that the simulator technologist may acquire simulation images. In addition to the PACStations, the RT-PACS also requires space to store large amounts of patient image data. Currently these images are stored on disks connected to a MicroVAX 3800 file server. This VAX is running VAX/VMS version 5.4 and Ultrix Connection, which allows it to act as an NFS file server.

Peripherals

The RT-PACS requires that patient image data be acquired. Images currently can be acquired with two tools: a frame grabber and a film scanner (2). The Analogic DASM-FGM SCSI frame grabber acquires images from an image intensifier. This frame grabber is attached through an SCSI interface to a SPARCstation 10 and produces 8-bit 512 x 480 images. Digitization of simulation and portal films is implemented with a Truvel Truscan TZ-3X film scanner, which is connected to a Dell

486 PC. The scanner also produces 8-bit images, and the spatial resolution is variable from 75 to 900 dots per inch (dpi). It has been our experience that the low-end resolution of 75 dpi is more than adequate for the purposes of the RT-PACS. An X-Windows interface will be implemented between the PC and the Sun workstations. In the near future, some portal images will be acquired using an EPID. This system will be able to acquire and store 12-bit 256 x 256 portal images on a 486 PC as 16-bit images.

Networking

With its multitude of workstations and file servers, the RT-PACS must be a networked system. The RT-PACS network is implemented on the hospital-wide Ethernet network. All nodes in the RT-PACS run the TCP/IP protocol, and the file servers have their disks mounted through NFS.

Local Storage

Patient image data come from many sources including frame grabber, film scanner, EPID, CT images, and digitally reconstructed radiographs. A significant amount of disk space is required to store data for a typical patient. For example, a patient undergoing radiotherapy using a four-field technique and 3-D treatment planning would require approximately 1 megabyte (MB) for simulation images (4 images x 0.25 MB/image), 30 MB for CT images (60 images x 0.5 MB/image and 2 MB for digitally reconstructed radiographs (4 images x 0.5 MB/image). If portal images are taken of all four treatment fields once a week for a six-week treatment regimen, then an additional 3 MB (4 images x 6 weeks x 0.125 MB/image) are required for EPID images. In addition to this patient image data, the treatment planning system part of the RT-PACS produces dose files and stored plan files. In the case of the four-field technique given above this would add the following amount of diskspace: 8 MB for dose files (4 beams x 2 MB/beam) and 2 MB for a stored plan. Thus data for each patient requires from 10 to 50 MB of disk space, depending on whether or not the patient has received a 3-D treatment plan.

Our prototype RT-PACS currently uses four on-line magnetic hard disks for a total of 7.5 gigabytes (GB) of on-line disk space. At 20 MB per patient, this represents a capacity of 375 patients. This disk space will need to be increased when the PACS becomes available for handling clinical data. With a patient load of 3500 patients per year that requires that patient images be stored on-line on the RT-PACS for at least 6 months after the start of treatment, we estimate that on-line storage will require a minimum of 35 GB.

Archival Storage

In addition to on-line disk storage, patient files on the RT-PACS are archived to an optical disk system. Our RT-PACS uses a Tahiti optical disk drive that can accept optical disks with either a 600-MB or 1-GB capacity.

Graphical User Interface

The RT-PACS software was written in C, and the user interface was developed with the Xview toolkit from Sun that implements the Open Look GUI. Future plans include converting from OpenLook to Motif GUI.

Database

The RT-PACS uses the Oracle database to store all nonimage data. The database resides on one of the PACStations and can be accessed through the network from other PACStations. We currently use Oracle version 6.0, and the actual PACS C program accesses it through embedded sequential query language (SQL) calls.

Functions available on the RT-PACS

The RT-PACS must be capable of performing several functions in addition to acquiring and viewing images. Functions functions include drawing outlines, sending messages, and approving entities. Additional functions include enhancing and comparing images.

A local message utility is available on the RT-PACS and is accessible to all PACS users. The message utility is accessed by selecting a "mail" icon from a user window. This utility allows a user to send and receive textual or voice messages. These messages are stored in the database and can be extracted at any time for review.

At present, physicians can use the RT-PACS to outline treatment portals, but in the future, the RT-PACS will also be used to delineate target volumes and outlines of critical structures. Outlining is done by using the mouse to move a cursor across the image at deposit points at designated locations on the image. Points may be deposited continuously in stream mode or discretely by pressing a button on the mouse. Lines may be color-coded by selecting colors from a menu. An edit mode is also available, which allows outline points to be added, deleted, or moved. The outline points are stored in a file, which may be used to generate mold outlines to cast shielding blocks or to generate multileaf collimator (MLC) settings.

Treatment portals delineated on simulation images must be approved before beam limitation devices can be fabricated. The ability to approve portals is only granted to staff physicians and is accomplished by the physician entering a password in response to a prompt. If the password is not recognized, approval is denied. Approval is also required for portal images and treatment plans and is recognized in the same manner.

One advantage of displaying a digital image with a PACS instead of film is that digital images can be processed to improve image quality. Enhancement of simulation images is often necessary because of the wide dynamic range between images of heavy bony structures and thin soft-tissue regions in the same simulation image. Visualization on conventional simulator films is accomplished with "hot lights," but software can be used to enhance digital simulation images. Several image enhancement tools presently being investigated for the RT-PACS include adjustments of gray-scale window (contrast) and level (brightness), histogram equalization, and edge enhancement. The enhancement capabilities are available to any image and are accessed from an image-enhancement window (color Plate 24).

Another advantage of digital images is that two images can be compared. One of the major functions of portal imaging is to compare a portal image with a simulation image of the same treatment portal before beginning treatments. At the very least. this task can be done on the RT-PACS in a manner analogous to conventional viewing by displaying images next to each other and visually assessing their correlation. Figure 35-6 shows a simulator image placed adjacent to a portal image on the RT-PACS. The ability to digitize images also enables the development of software tools for assessing image correlation. One such tool prompts the user to enter coordinates of landmarks on a simulation image with corresponding landmarks on a portal image. A transformation from these points on the simulation image to the points on the portal image is then generated (3). The coordinates defining the treatment portal are then transformed from the simulation image to the portal image using the transformation. The transformed treatment portal on the portal image is then compared with the actual image of the treatment portal. Similar techniques can be used to compare portal images with digitally reconstructed radiographs.

Another way in which images are evaluated is to compare successive portal images to ensure consistency of patient setup. We are currently investigating several correlation based image comparison tools (4,5) developed for these tasks.

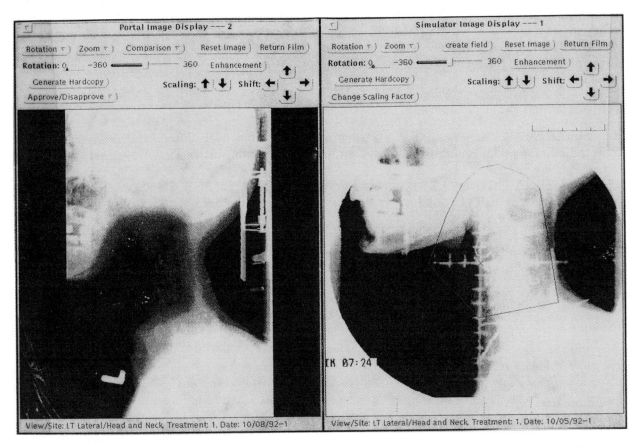

Figure 35-6. Windows that enable the physician to compare a simulator image with a portal image

Potential Benefits of an RT-PACS

While the clinical implementation of an RT-PACS in radiotherapy is still in the future, incorporation of the RT-PACS into the radiotherapy clinic may have significant potential benefits. The elimination of film in favor of digital images greatly reduces storage needs. A typical optical disk, with a capacity of 500 MB, can hold approximately 2000 8-bit images. Film storage and retrieval is a far less serious problem with digital images, and with images stored electronically along with backup files, the problems of lost or misplaced films is mitigated.

Department efficiency can also be improved with use of an RT-PACS because it generates tasking queues that indicate the status of each patient's images. Users of the RT-PACS can then determine what tasks need to be performed, making it less likely that a particular patient is overlooked. Moreover, once a task has been performed, results of that task are instantaneously posted in the RT-PACS, preparing the patient's images for the next task in the queue. Also, once a task has been performed, it is quite feasible for the RT-PACS to generate appropriate patient billing for that particular task.

Digital imaging allows for certain benefits in image processing. Various image-enhancement tools can be applied to aid the user in performing imaging tasks. Algorithms are being developed that can compare images and aid the physician in determining the accuracy of a treatment portal.

Implementation of an RT-PACS may also provide benefits to the overall care of the radiotherapy patient. With the application of the RT-PACS and the image processing tools, more accurate patient treatment is likely, as a result of tools to improve patient positioning and field verification. With the ready accessibility of RT-PACS images, as well as the tasking queue, the amount of time patients are kept waiting is likely to be reduced. The consequence of these benefits is likely to be improved care and reduced treatment cost for the radiotherapy patient.

References

1.   Starkschall, G., Bujnowski, S.W., Garden, A.S., Hogstrom, K.R., Functional relationships in a radiotherapy picture archival and communications system (Abstr.). Med. Phys. 20:922 (1993).

2.   Starkschall, G., Boyer, A.L., Bujnowski, S.W., Ewton, J.R., Li, X.-J., Steadham, R.E., Wong, N.-W., Hogstrom, K.R., Simulator image acquisition for a radiotherapy PACS (Abstr.). Med. Phys. 20:898 (1993).

3.   Balter, J.M., Pelizzari, C.A., Chen, G.T.Y., Correlation of projection radiographs in radiation therapy using open curve segments and points Med. Phys. 19:329-334 (1992).

4.   Jones, S.M., Boyer, A.L., Investigation of an FFT-based correlation technique for verification of radiation treatment setup Med. Phys. 18:1116-1125 (1991).

5.   Boyer, A.L., Dong, L., Starkschall, G., Hogstrom, K.R., A portal image correlation procedure (Abstr.). Med. Phys. 19:802 (1992).

Chapter 36

Computer-Controlled Conformal Radiation Therapy

Benedick A. Fraass, Ph.D., Daniel L. McShan, Ph.D., Marc K. Kessler, Ph.D., Gwynne M. Matrone, B.S. and Tamar Weaver, B.S.

Department of Radiation Oncology, University of Michigan Medical Center, Ann Arbor, Michigan

In recent years, there has been a large amount of interest in the use of computer-controlled treatment techniques in order to perform 3-D conformal therapy. This interest is due to several recent developments, including 1) the development and use of 3-D treatment planning, and the increasingly complex treatment plans which are developed with 3-D planning techniques, 2) the development of multileaf collimators (MLC) by many different manufacturers, 3) the increasingly interesting theoretical work on automated and semi-automated plan optimization techniques, many of which use models of sophisticated treatment delivery systems in order to implement the optimized plans, and 4) the widespread dissemination of computer control systems for accelerator treatment machines, and 5) the excellent early results of the first clinical trials which have been studying whether conformal therapy can decrease normal tissue complications and/or increase local control rates.

The use of all of this new technology may require changes to the process with which treatment planning and treatment occurs. Here, we review some of the important aspects of work with computer-controlled treatment technology, and briefly discuss a comprehensive approach to this problem which we have called the "Computer Controlled Radiotherapy System (CCRS)" project. Work on the CCRS system has included the development of a somewhat expanded model for the treatment planning and delivery process that allows routine clinical implementation of these techniques. In addition, the CCRS system makes possible the investigation of improvements in the accuracy, efficiency, or sophistication of the treatment and delivery techniques.

In order to discuss the area of computer-controlled conformal therapy, it is appropriate to first define some specific terms to describe the various kinds of activities which are relevant to the discussions. Conformal therapy is a term which is widely used, but is often used to mean different things. In this work, we define conformal therapy to be "therapy that creates a dose distribution that closely conforms to the shape of the target volume in three dimensions."

In general, most conformal therapy has been delivered with "static conformal therapy," (i.e., a series of fixed, shaped fields). In this mode of treatment, the treatment therapist goes in and out of the room to change the machine angle, field size, and insert the new blocks and other field modifiers, and each treatment is given in a standard static fashion. To create complex and conformal dose distributions, typically between four to eight static fields are treated. Each of the fields is shaped using a shaped block which has been designed to conform to the shape of the target volume as viewed from that particular beam position, typically using Beam's Eye View display techniques [1], and often computer-designed blocks [1,2].

The next level of sophistication in treatment delivery has been termed "segmental conformal therapy." This term refers to treatment of the patient using individual fixed field portals ("segments"), as with static conformal therapy, except that computer control capabilities are used to deliver a series of segments automatically without the therapist entering the treatment room to set each portal individually. This kind of multi-segment therapy is now available on commercially available equipment [3,4].

421

The final and most sophisticated level of computer-controlled conformal therapy is terms "dynamic conformal therapy." This type of treatment delivery involves dynamic motion of one or more mechanical motions of the machine (multi-leaf collimator, gantry, table, collimator angle) while the machine delivers radiation to the patient. This is clearly a logical extension from the segmental conformal situation, in which multiple fixed segments are delivered. It is also much more involved, since now the exact trajectory of each mechanical motion must be coupled to the dose delivery, whereas for segmental delivery, the dose delivery is not directly tied to mechanical motion velocity tolerances.

Each of the three methods above may be termed computer-controlled therapy, as any therapy that is delivered by a machine which is under computer control may use that term. In fact, delivery of a simple AP-PA pair of square fields can be termed computer-controlled therapy if the machine which delivers the radiation is computer controlled, even if everything is essentially still set-up directly by the treatment therapists. Therefore, we use the term Computer-controlled Conformal Radiation Therapy (CCRT) to describe the use of computer-controlled delivery techniques for plans which use conformal field shaping to shape each field individually, typically through use of a multileaf collimator.

Interestingly, it is dynamic conformal therapy, the most sophisticated of the three different techniques, which has been worked on for the longest time. 3-D treatment planning and three-dimensional dose delivery have been stated goals in radiation oncology for over forty years. As far back as 1948, Takahashi in Nagoya, Japan began preliminary work in the area of three-dimensional treatment planning and computer-controlled radiotherapy. Multileaf collimators were developed many years ago, with the leaves set using mechanical devices to allow dynamic therapy in the era before computer control was available[5]. This has led to a great deal of work on this rotational conformational therapy, particularly in Japan [6-10]. Another early participant in conformal radiotherapy was the group at the Royal Free Hospital in London. Their work, called the Tracking Cobalt Project, used table translations along with rotation of the machine about the table, also initially performed using mechanical tracking devices [11-15]. This work was a precursor to the computer-controlled therapy work at the Joint Center for Radiation Therapy in Boston, in which a computer-control system was developed for a linear accelerator, and was then used for dynamic conformal therapy treatments [16-18].

There has clearly been a large amount of work in the past, particularly on dynamic therapy techniques. This work has shown that there are several feasible approaches to full conformal radiotherapy dose delivery. However, these early efforts have not created a system for the practical treatment of large numbers of patients using these techniques in a day-to-day clinical setting. Therefore, we next discuss the capabilities needed for the routine use of CCRT techniques.

Needs for Computer-Controlled Conformal Radiation Therapy (CCRT)

In order to develop and/or implement CCRT treatment techniques for routine clinical use, the following equipment and/or capabilities are necessary.

- Multileaf Collimators. Multileaf collimators (MLCs) are a recent technological advance which is quickly becoming quite common throughout the radiotherapy community. A multileaf collimator typically consists of a number of tungsten leaves which move under computer control to make a beam shaping aperture used with megavoltage photon beams. Leaf widths for most commercially-available MLCs are between 1 and 1.25 cm (projected to the isocenter), and the number of leaves varies from 56 to 80. Some early reports on MLCs have been published [19-26]. The computer-controlled field shaping capabilities are a very significant part of the technology needed for CCRT.

- Computer Control of the Treatment Machine. One clearly needs a computer-controlled radiotherapy machine to perform CCRT, and most workers expect to use computer-controlled multileaf collimators for automated field shaping. Most new commercial linear accelerator systems have some degree of computer control as part of their control system, although there is large variability on how many computer-controlled treatment features are available to users at this point.

- New Techniques for Beam Arrangements and Plan Optimization. One clearly needs a full three-dimensional treatment planning system in order to develop plans which require CCRT treatment techniques in order to be clinically delivered. One also needs the ability to automatically optimize plans for CCRT. With beam angles coming from almost any direction and multiple fields able to be treated rapidly through a computer-controlled sequence, manual trial and error treatment planning is extremely time consuming. The computer must help design field configurations that will satisfy dose constraints to target and normal tissues that are the essential feature of conformal therapy plan optimization. See references [27-33] for further information on this area.

- Clinical Delivery of CCRT. Aside from the computer control capability described above, a clinic also requires a treatment planning and delivery process that is able to perform clinical routine treatments. The treatment plan must be transferred from the planning system to the computer control system of the therapy machine. Dozens of quality assurance issues must be addressed. For example, what if one wants to make a change in a field or fields during therapy, or change the dose distribution somewhat to shield an organ more precisely? In current practice, one can design a new block or change the dose rate with a simple note in the patient's chart. If all treatment parameters are in the computer, how does one go in and change one or more of the parameters for the next day's treatment? Should the old plan be destroyed and only the new treatment parameters be saved in the computer? If not, how does the system know which plan is valid for that particular day? How does one chart all these treatments—in a paper record such as we use today or in a computerized record? Addressing these issues are a significant part of the reason for the development of the CCRS system that is described below.

- Intensity Modulation. A very important part, at least conceptually, of the research into CCRT treatment techniques is related to the use of various types of intensity modulation techniques. In routine therapy, we use wedges and other compensators for intensity modulation routinely, but within the context of CCRT techniques, the machinery is now capable of developing quite complex intensity patterns. These patterns can then be designed individually for each segment and treated using computer-controlled features of the machinery. Some early work on MLC-based intensity modulation has already begun [34,35], as well as the introduction of the idea of the use of the scanned beam in the racetrack microtron system for intensity modulation [36,37]. Further discussion of this very interesting aspect of computer-controlled conformal therapy is beyond the scope of the current article.

- Treatment Uncertainties. Treatment verification and portal imaging for CCRT will be quite complex. There may be five, ten, or more fields or segments treated per day on many patients. The idea of using standard port film technology to verify treatment accuracy will be quite time consuming, and probably not accurate enough to be consistent with the overall goals of clinical use of CCRT technology. There is therefore a critical need for real-time portal imaging and verification systems [38] as an essential part of the CCRT system.

- QA for CCRT. As with all complex technologies, the quality assurance program and testing required by this new technology are extensive. These include: QA of the machine control system, QA of the new features of the machinery, and QA of the much more automated treatment process.

Multileaf Collimators

Virtually all major manufacturers of radiotherapy equipment are creating machines that are capable of operating under computer control. Collimator shape and rotation, gantry angle and rotation, motions of the table, and in fact monitor, dose rate and energy, are, in theory, capable of being driven by an external computer. In some machines, these accelerator functions can be driven while beam is actually being delivered (dynamic CCRT), while others only permit these motions to occur in between actual dose delivery (segmental CCRT).

A key feature in all modern CCRT approaches is the use of a computer-controlled multileaf collimator. While it is possible to create any field shape with poured blocks, one often cannot use treatment plans that routinely employ more than four to six fields with fixed blocks because of the time that it takes the therapist to enter the room, manually switch the blocks, and leave the room. If one is to perform therapy that comes from multiple directions and conforms as tightly as possible the high dose volume to the shape of the target, one will need multiple fields and the ability to change the shape of the field in complex ways without entering the accelerator room. Computer control of a multileaf collimator makes this possible. Dose calculation and treatment planning related aspects of MLC use have been discussed recently by a number of authors [20, 22-25].

Different manufacturers are taking different approaches to creating multileaf collimators (MLC). Some MLC designs are incorporated into the machine design, while others are specifically designed to be detachable from the normal head of the machine. Table 36-1 illustrates the range of specifications which are available on typical MLCs. One of the critical features of MLC systems with respect to CCRT is the extent of integration of their control system with that of the treatment machine. At the present time, many of the commercially available MLC systems are controlled by standalone workstations which have little or no link with the accelerator control system. This lack of integration makes CCRT treatments much more difficult than for an integrated system. The next section contains more information on control system integration.

Table 36-1. Multileaf Collimator Design Features

Feature	Minimum	Maximum
Leaf thickness	1.0 cm	1.25 cm
Leaf positioning	0.2 mm	2 mm
Focusing	Round leaf ends, linear motion	Double focused
Field size coverage	26 x 40	40 x 40
Control System	Standalone wkst, no link	Complete integration
Motion control	Fixed, per field	Segmental, Dynamic
Length of Clinical Experience	- 2 years	10 years

Computer Control Systems

The computer control systems of various treatment machines each have significant differences from each other. Although computers have been used in the control systems of most vendor's accelerators, only a few of those computers are used to really allow computer-controlled treatments. So current computer-control systems range from computers which replace the function of the console only, to completely integrated systems which can perform completely automatic CCRT.

In order to perform routine clinical CCRT, the computer-controlled treatment machine must have a direct connection between the control system and an external computer which can send the treatment plan to the control system. After a plan is downloaded to the control computer, the control computer then directs the machine as it proceeds through the treatment. Redundant sensor readouts, a separate verification system, and good user interface are all important parts of a good computer-control system for CCRT.

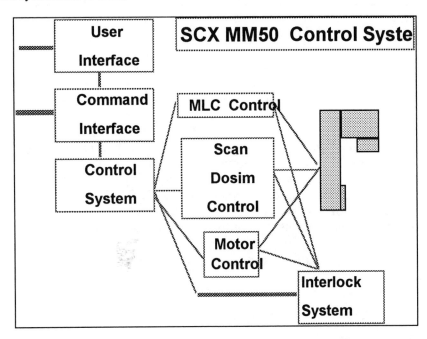

Figure 36-1. Control System for the MM50 Racetrack Microtron

In order to perform routine clinical CCRT, the computer-controlled treatment machine must have a direct connection between the control system and an external computer which can send the treatment plan to the control system. After a plan is downloaded to the control computer, the control computer then directs the machine as it proceeds through the treatment. Redundant sensor readouts, a separate verification system, and good user interface are all important parts of a good computer-control system for CCRT.

The control system for the Scanditronix MM50 Racetrack Microtron[36], shown in Figure 36-1, illustrates a number of useful control system concepts and design strategies for a CCRT machine. The MM50 has a totally integrated computer control system, and it is capable of performing automated segmental therapy. Useful design features include:

- The user interface is separate from the control system functionality.

- There is an external command interface to allow sophisticated communication and control with an external computer system.

- Major functions of the machine are controlled by separate processors, which work independently.

- The "control system" oversees and monitors the activities of all the separate processors.

- There is a separate interlock system which monitors the status of all hardware and software interlocks, and which can shut off the machine (in hardware) if fault situations develop.

Parameters which are controlled through the control system, and by use of an external command interface, are listed in Table 36-2.

Table 36-2. MM50 Computer Control

Gantry angle	Collimator angle	Table Angle
MLC	Upper Jaws	Table X, Y, Z
MU	Dose Rate	Scan Pattern
Energy	Mode	Wedge(s)
Room (2 gantries)		

A critical feature for much of the CCRT work described here has been the use of a command interface, shown in Figure 36-1. This command interface allows the use of a limited number of commands and other communication to be passed between an external computer and the machine's control system. Some of these commands are listed in Table 36-3. Through the use of this simple interface, it has been possible to determine appropriate and efficient ways to perform CCRT treatments, patient set-ups, simulations, and automated quality assurance tests.

Table 36-3. MM50 Command Interface

Download Segment	Set-up Geometry	Set-up Accelerator
Set-up MLC	Read_Actual_Values	Beam_On
Pause (Beam)	Beam_Off	STOP !
Reset_ID	etc.	

Approaches to the CCRT Treatment Process: The UM-CCRS Project

The ability to routinely deliver clinical CCRT treatments will depend on a complex system for creation, transfer, control, verification, and documentation of the CCRT therapy. This system may be mostly manual, as most normal fixed field treatments are today, where the therapists set up the patient and machine, and set the machine to deliver the appropriate fields. However, due to the much increased complexity of the CCRT plans which will be used, it is expected that a more sophisticated computer-based system will be used. A prototypical system, called the Computer-controlled Conformal Radiotherapy System ("CCRS"), to help clinical perform CCRT treatments has been developed in our institution, and will be described below.

The basic hypothesis of the CCRS approach is that the large amount of information required for accurate and safe routine clinical use of computer-controlled conformal therapy forces a major change in the entire treatment process. The overall goals of the CCRS project are two-fold:

- A standard approach to interfacing and use of all CCRT machines.

- A comprehensive approach to all chart, data transfer, and database needs of CCRT therapy.

The CCRS system is designed to be vendor-independent, in that the system will be used with conformal machines from a number of different vendors. Currently, it is being developed for use with the Varian CLinac 2100C with MLC as well as the Scanditronix MM50 Racetrack Microtron system. This system has been under design and development for five years, and an initial version is currently in use with the MM50 system. Note that there are certainly a number of other approaches to clinical use of CCRT (see the recent paper by Mageras [39] et al. on a different approach to the use of the same machine (MM50) as described here).

The conceptual organization of the CCRS system consists of several major processes:

- Sequence Processor (SP). The SP acts as the common user interface for all conformal machines. It directs the conformal treatment process, by control or interface with the machine control system.

- Integrated Simulation and Verification System (ISV). The ISV system has a large number of functions, including 1) graphical plan simulation to allow therapists to perform an exact graphical simulation of the treatment procedure, 2) collision avoidance checks, 3) record and verify functions during treatment, 4) graphical plan presentation to the therapists, and 5) real time imager interface, among others.

- CCRS Gateway and Databases. A complete electronic chart, including electronic prescriptions and plan descriptions, will be required to handle the large amount of information associated with the complex conformal plans which will be used.

The hardware architecture of the CCRS system is designed to provide a secure and flexible set of platforms to allow the development and analysis of the use of the system in a research environment (at least initially) while at the same time providing a very secure and safe environment for clinical CCRT treatments. For example, the SP and ISV systems are currently maintained on separate workstations, in order to 1) assure careful attention to security and system usage, especially in a situation where some development (especially of ISV functions) is expected to continue, and 2) to maintain a clear focus and philosophical division between the SP which controls the patient treatment, and the ISV system which monitors, checks, and records the treatments. The CCRS gateway and the various databases associated with the CCRS system are maintained in a series of linked databases which reside on various computers which are part of the main departmental VAX-cluster. Figure 36-2 illustrates the basic layout of the CCRS system.

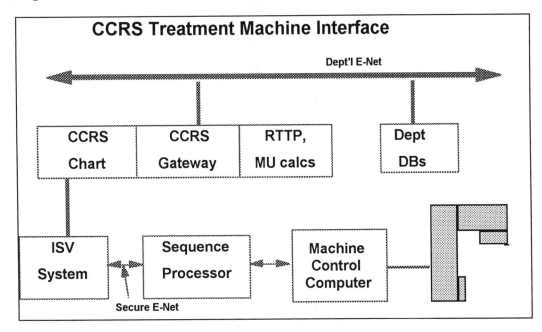

Figure 36-2. CCRS System Architecture. See text for description of components.

Components of the CCRS system, shown in Figure 36-2, include:

- CC: Machine control computer. Vendor's computer which controls the machine.

- SP: Sequence Processor. Computer which directs the sequence of activities required to treat a conformal plan.

- ISV: Integrated Simulation/Verification System. Plan data, treatment data, record and verify, graphical simulator, portal imager interface.

- CCRS Chart: Electronic Chart. Data and Procedures.

- CCRS Gateway: Overall database and installation procedures which control access to and from the CCRS electronic chart, and outside systems.

- RTTP, MU Calcs: The conformal therapy treatment planning system, integrated with monitor unit calculations.

- Other departmental databases include Master Accession, Scheduling, Billing, Archival, and other databases.

The Sequence Processor (SP) has a number of important tasks in the design of the CCRS system. The first and most important is that the therapist uses the SP to control the CCRT machine. The user interface will thus be the same for each CCRT machine, even though different machines will have different kinds of CCRT capabilities. In addition, the use of the SP clearly separates the control of the machine, a critical and real-time function, from the patient, dose, and plan-related information which must be handled correctly in order to assure that the correct treatment. Thus the SP contains a treatment plan database which contains only the plans actually being treated on the machine, and the control computer (CC) does not know at all about patients and plans, it just treats fields and segments. Although a network link exists between the SP and the other systems shown in Figure 36-2, network access to the SP is rigidly controlled from the outside. There is no unrequested access from the outside, so no one can download a plan to the SP database without the help of the operator on the SP. The SP functionally corresponds to the machine treatment console and paper chart that the therapist carries into the room to set up a manually controlled machine.

While the main task of the SP is to direct the treatments, the Integrated Simulation/Verification (ISV) system is used to prepare the plan for the SP, and then to monitor the accuracy of the treatments as they are performed. The ISV software uses sophisticated 3-D graphics to perform some of its tasks, so it requires the presence of a powerful workstation (currently VAXstation 4000/90 workstations are used). The ISV contains a copy of the plan database which is accessible to others in the department (for viewing and/or changes, if allowed), and it controls all access to and from the SP over the network. It is used for graphical simulation of the treatment before it is given (see below), collision avoidance checks, and for graphical and quantitative verification checks during treatment. Other functions designed for the system include access to the dose prescription database, automated consistency and redundancy checks of the SP plan database, interface to the real-time imager and its analysis package, etc.

The third main part of the CCRS system is the CCRS main database and gateway. All of the electronic chart information which is distributed around the department to all of the various machine-specific ISV and SP computers is maintained in the main CCRS database also. Access into this database is controlled by the CCRS Gateway process. In order to transfer a plan from the treatment planning system into the CCRS system, the plan is sent through the gateway into the main CCRS database. The gateway can be understood in analogy to how the paper chart is used. During treatment planning many plans may be investigated. When one of those plans is chosen to be used for treatment, the treatment planner performs a monitor unit calculation and then writes the plan description into the patient's treatment chart. Sending a plan through the gateway installs the plan in the CCRS database, and is equivalent to writing the plan into the chart.

Treatment with CCRT Techniques

The procedure used for CCRT treatments differs in a number of ways from the usual procedures used in the clinic. In addition, various different treatment delivery procedures are used in different departments, even when using the same treatment machine for the CCRT treatments. For CCRT, it is clear that process by which treatment plans get implemented on the treatment machine differs from the usual process. The method utilized in our clinic is summarized below:

- Treatment plan completion. In the context of this discussion, completion of the planning phase includes the plan verification procedure which is performed on the physical simulator to check patient immobilization, registration of the patient and CT data, isocenter definition and shifts, BEV patient alignment checks, and films of treatment portals.

- Dose Prescription. Physician treatment prescription must be carefully defined and input into the dose prescription database.

- MU Calculation. Monitor Unit calculations will eventually be totally integrated into the treatment planning and dose prescription aspects of the process, since MU calculations for MLC-shaped segmental fields, with or without intensity modulation, become too difficult to perform without all of the information contained within the planning system.

- Transfer of plan and MU information into CCRS system through the CCRS Gateway. This step is analogous to writing the treatment setup and MU into the paper chart (see Table 36-4). The consistency and accuracy of the transfers of treatment information must be assured and checked.

Table 36-4.   *Example CCRT Treatment Procedure. Note that this 9 segment treatment procedure contains only two treatment fields.*

Seg #	Name	Type	MU	Comments
1.1	AP Setup	Setup	-	set new isocenter reference
1.2	V_AP_1	Film	3.0	localization portal image
1.3	Move1	Move	-	move to first Tx Segment
1.4	RAO	Tx	132.2	treat Right Ant. Oblique
1.5	Move2	Move	-	shift table lat, rotate gantry
1.6	Move3	Move	-	put table lat back, rotate pedestal
1.7	LSPO	Tx	122.8	treat Left Superior Posterior Oblique
1.8	Move4	Move	-	move to intermediate position
1.9	Dsmnt	Move	-	move table to dismount position

- CCRS Tx Procedure Planning. A totally new step in the process is the definition of the procedure which will be used day by day to treat the patient. This will include definition of the segments used to perform patient set-up, verification (portal imaging) checks, motion segments (getting the machine from one place to another) and treatment segments. Different treatment procedures are defined for the first day of treatment (additional simulation and verification steps), verification checks (days on which treatment port or localization portal imaging is performed), and normal treatments. See example treatment procedure below.

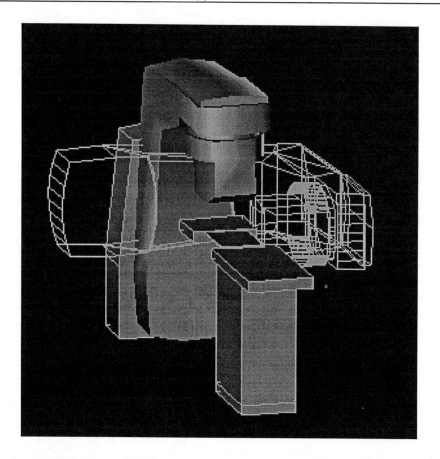

Figure 36-3. *Use of Graphical Simulator for Treatment Simulation. The wire frame shows the destination, while the solid surface shows the actual position of the gantry and table.*

- Graphical Simulation. This new step uses a complete graphical simulator as a check (and aid) for the definition of the treatment procedure. A computer graphics model of the treatment machine, treatment table, treatment room, and patient (eventually) are used to 1) plan the treatment procedure, including adding segments for portal verification and move segments (for defining the trajectory between one beam position and the next), and 2) to review the current procedure defined for the plan, and 3) to perform collision avoidance checks. An image from one of the windows used in the graphical simulator is shown in Figure 36-3. These kinds of graphics displays are also used in the record and verify functionality which is a part of the ISV system.

- Tx Machine Simulation. Another important procedure used as part of the CCRS process (currently, at least) is a formal physical simulation of the complete CCRT treatment procedure, performed on the treatment machine. Typically this is done twice in our department: once with the immobilization device in place, but without the patient, and then a second time with the patient in place. The first simulation assures that all the bugs in the plan procedure are removed before one actually involves the patient. The simulation which includes the patient in their immobilization device is used for a final check of the accuracy of the entire treatment prescription.

- Patient Start. As usual, additional checks and/or changes occasionally occur at the actual start procedure for the patient. These changes must be reflected back up through the CCRS system, so that all the different plans are consistent.

- Physics Review of Plan Implementation. The initial review of the plan which is performed by the physicist within a few days of the patient start involves a number of new checks which are not often a part of routine treatment delivery for most machines. The additional information used by the CCRS system, including dose and/or fractionation data, treatment procedure data including the segments used for portal imaging, and motion segments which move the table out of the way of the rotating gantry, should all be carefully reviewed by the physics checks.

QA for CCRT Treatments

Several areas of quality assurance are very important considerations for the use of CCRT treatment techniques. Machine control system QA involves all the checks which are associated with the relatively new technology of computer control of the accelerator. There are also many new features of the CCRT machinery which require new QA checks and procedures. Finally, one must spend significant effort checking the semi-automated QA which is performed for the new parts of the treatment planning and delivery process such as the dose prescription information and the graphical simulation and treatment procedure planning performed for each patient.

Safety is a major issue in computer-controlled therapy, whether or not sophisticated conformal treatment techniques. There have been well publicized accidents in machines that used fairly rudimentary computer control for very simple treatments not at all related to CCRT. A great deal of attention is focused on these safety issues, and it is clear that this is a significant factor in any use of the new computer-controlled capabilities which are now available, whether for simple standard treatments or sophisticated CCRT methods.

A complete analysis of one set of treatment problems which are related (to some degree) to the computer-control system of a particular machine (Therac 25) has recently been published by Levinson and Turner [40]. This report is extremely instructive in several ways: 1) it describes in detail the failures which occurred, 2) it illustrates to radiation oncology workers (physicists, physicians, etc.) the way software engineering attempts to address the question of reliability of sophisticated software-controlled systems, and 3) it addresses some of the other non-software-related aspects of quality assurance for these systems. For example, the authors state: "Most accidents involving complex technology are caused by a combination of organizational, managerial, technical, and sometime sociological or political factors. Preventing accidents requires paying attention to *all* the root causes ..." This is an extremely important point to be remembered as each institution develops the quality assurance procedures appropriate to its particular treatment process.

One such attempt to address the safety issues for computer-controlled accelerators is the recently published report by the AAPM Task Group 35: "Medical Accelerator Safety Considerations: Report of AAPM Radiation Therapy Committee Task Group 35" [41]. The report contains several important discussions and/or sets of recommendations:

- Classification of Potentially Dangerous Problems
- Procedures for Medical Physicists in Responding to Potential Safety Hazards
- Radiation Therapy Technologist Training
- Computer-Controlled Machines: Software Errors, Testing, and Documentation Issues.

Much additional work on the design of quality assurance procedures and testing is necessary as work in the field continues. See for example [42-44].

Summary

The use of computer-controlled treatment machines equipped with multileaf collimators to perform CCRT therapy, in either segmental or dynamic modes, is now possible with commercially available treatment machines. Clinical use of these techniques requires development of new methodology and techniques for the treatment planning and delivery process, as well as new quality assurance testing and procedures. Much further work is necessary in order to fully utilize the new computer-controlled conformal therapy technologies which are now becoming available.

References

1. McShan DL, Fraass BA, Lichter AS: Full integration of the beam's eye view concept in clinical treatment planning. Int J Rad Oncol Biol Phys 18: 1485-1494, 1990.

2. Brewster L, Mageras GS, Mohan R: Automatic generation of beam apertures: Med Phys 20: 1337-1342, 1993.

3. Masterson ME, Mageras GS, LoSasso TJ, Joreskog E, Larsson LG, Febo R, Mohan R, Ling CC, Fuks Z, Kutcher GJ: Pre-clinical evaluation of the reliability of a 50 MeV racetrack microtron. Int J Rad Oncol Biol Phys, in press, 1993.

4. Fraass BA, McShan DL, Kessler ML, Lewis JD, Matrone G, Weaver T: A vendor-independent system for the control of the set-up, treatment and verification processes used in computer-controlled conformal therapy. Med Phys 18: 836, 1992 [Abstract].

5. Takahashi S: Conformation radiotherapy-rotation techniques as applied to radiography and radiotherapy of cancer. Acta Radiologica (supplement 242), 1965.

6. Kitabatake T, Takahashi S: Conformational radiotherapy by means of 6-MeV linear accelerator. Tohoku J Exp Med, 94:37-43, 1968.

7. Morita K, Kawabe Y: Late effects on the eye of conformation radiotherapy for carcinoma of the paranasal sinuses and nasal cavity[1]. Radiology, 130:227-232, 1979.

8. Morita K, Takahashi S: Rotatory conformation radiotherapy of cancer of larynx. Studies on telecobalt therapy. II. Report. Studies on rotatory conformation radiotherapy. 3. Report. Nippon Acta radiol, 21;13, 1961.

9. Sasaki T: The clinical use of CT-images and computer-assisted radiation therapy planning system with a special reference to conformation radiotherapy. in Proc. 7th Int. Conf. on Computers in Radiation Therapy, ed. Umegaki Y, p 230-234, 1980.

10. Takahashi S: A new device of Co-60 rotation therapy. Clin Radiol, 5:653-658, 1960.

11. Brace JA, Davy TJ, Skeggs DBL: Computer-controlled cobalt unit for radiotherapy. Med & Biol Eng & Comput, 19:612-616, 1981.

12. Brace JA, Davy TJ, Skeggs DBL, Williams HS: Conformation therapy at the Royal Free Hospital. A progress report on the tracking cobalt project. Br J Radiol, 54:1068-1074, 1981.

13. Davy TJ, Johnson PK, Redford R, and Williams JR: Conformation therapy using the tracking cobalt unit. Br J Radiol, 48:122-130, 1975.

14. Green A, Jennings WA, Christie HM: Radiotherapy by tracking the spread of disease. Transactions of the Ninth International Congress of Radiology, Munchen 1959, Verlag, Stuttgart pp 766-772, 1960.

15. Green A: Tracking cobalt project. Nature, 207:1311, 1946.

16. Chin LM, Kijewski PK, Svensson GK, Chaffey JR, Levene MB, Bjarngard BE: A computer-controlled radiation therapy machine for pelvic and paraaortic nodal areas. Int J Rad Oncol Biol Phys 7:61-70, 1981.

17. Chin LM, Kijewski PK, Svensson GK, Bjarngard BE: Dose optimization with computer-controlled gantry rotation, collimator motion and dose-rate variation. Int J Rad Oncol Biol Phys 9:723-729, 1983.

18. Levene MB, Kijewski PK, Chin LM, Bengt SM, Bjarngard E, Hellman S: Computer-controlled radiation therapy. Radiology, 129:769-775, 1978.

19. Boesecke R, Becker G, Alandt K, Pastyr O, Doll J, Schlegel W, Lorenz WJ: Modification of a three-dimensional treatment planning system for the use of multi-leaf collimators in conformation therapy. Rad. and Oncol 21: 261-268, 1991.

20. Boyer AL, Ochran TG, Nyerick CE, Waldron TJ, Huntzinger CJ: Clinical dosimetry for implementation of a multileaf collimator, Med Phys 19: 1255-1261, 1992.

21. Brahme A, Eenmaa J, Lindback S, Montelius A, Wootton P: Neutron beam characteristics from 50 MeV photons on beryllium using a contiuously variable multileaf collimator. Radiother Oncol 1:65-76, 1983.

22. Galvin JM, Smith AR, Lally B: Characterization of a multileaf collimator system, Int J Rad Oncol Biol Phys 25: 181-192, 1993.

23. Galvin JM, Smith AR, Moeller RD, Goodman RL, Powlis WD, Rubenstein J, Solin LJ, Michael B, Needham M, Huntzinger CJ, Kligerman MM: Evaluation of multileaf collimator design for a photon beam. Int J Rad Onc Biol Phys 23:789-801, 1992.

24. LoSasso T, Chen CS, Kutcher GJ, Leibel SA, Fuks Z, Ling CC: The use of a multi-leaf collimator for conformal radiotherapy of the carcinomas of the prostate and nsaopharynx, Int J Rad Onc Biol Phys 25: 161-170, 1993.

25. Powlis WD, Smith AR, Cheng E, Galvin JM, Villari F, Bolch P, Kligerman M: Initiation of multileaf conformal radiation therapy, Int J Rad Oncol Biol Phys 25: 171-179, 1993.

26. Zhu Y, Boyer AL, Desobry GE: Dose distributions of x-ray fields as shaped with multileaf collimators. Phys Med Biol 37:163-173, 1992.

27. Brahme A: Optimization of stationary and moving beam radiation therapy techniques. Radiotherapy and Oncology 12: 129-140, 1988.

28. Holmes T, Mackie TR, Simpkin D, Reckwerdt P: A unified approach to the optimization of brachytherapy and external beam therapy. Int J Rad Oncol Biol Phys 20: 859-873, 1991.

29. Mageras GS, Mohan R: Application of fast simulated annealing to optimization for conformal radiation treatments, Med Phys 20: 639-647, 1993.

30. Mohan R, Mageras GS, Baldwin B, Brewster LJ, Kutcher GJ, Leibel S, Burman CM, Ling CC, Fuks Z: Clinically relevant optimization of 3-D conformal treatments. Med Phys 19: 933-944, 1992.

31. Webb S: Optimisation of conformal radiation therapy dose distributions by simulated annealing. Phys Med Biol 34: 1349-1370, 1989.

32. Webb S: Optimization by simulated annealing of three-dimensional treatment planning for radiation fields defined by a multileaf collimator. Phys Med Biol 36: 1201-1226, 1991.

33. Webb S: Optimization of conformal radiotherapy dose distributions by simulated annealing: 2. Inclusion of scatter in the 2-D technique. Phys Med Biol 36: 1227-1237, 1991.

34. Galvin JM, Chen X-G, Smith RM: Combining multileaf fields to modulate fluence distributions. Int J Rad Oncol Biol Phys 27: 697-705, 1993.

35. Boyer AL, Bortfeld T, Kahler D, Starkschall G, Waldron T: X-ray field compensation with multileaf collimation. Int J Rad Oncol Biol Phys 27 (s1): 208, 1993 [Abstract].

36. Brahme A: "Design Principles and clinical possibilities for a new genereation of radiation therapy equipment. Acta Oncol. 26: 403-412, 1987.

37. Nafstadius P, Brahme A, Nordell B: Computer assisted dosimetry of scanned beams for radiation therapy. Radiotherapy and Oncology 2: 261-269, 1984.

38. Boyer AL, Antonuk LE, Fenster A et al: A Review of Electronic Portal Imaging Devices (EPIDs). Med Phys 19: 1-16, 1992.

39. Mageras GS, Podmaniczky KC, Mohan R, A model for computer-controlled delivery of 3-D conformal treatments. Med Phys 19(4), 1992.

40. Levinson NG, Turner CS: An investigation of the Therac-25 Accidents. IEEE Computer, July 1993, pp. 18-41, 1993.

41. Purdy JA, Biggs PJ, Bowers C, Dally E, Downs W, Fraass BA, Karzmark CJ, Khan F, Morgan P, Morton R, Palta J, Rosen II, Thorson T, Svensson G, Ting J: Medical accelerator safety considerations: Report of AAPM Radiation Therapy Committee Task Group 35, Med Phys 20: 1261-1275, 1993.

42. Rosen II, Purdy JA: Computer-controlled medical accelerators. in Advances in Radiation Oncology Physics: Dosimetry, Treatment Planning and Brachytherapy, ed. JA Purdy, American Inst. Physics, Woodbury NY, 1992. pp. 1-18.

43. Weinhous MS, Purdy JA, Granda CO: Testing of a linear accelerator's computer-control system, Med Phys 17: 95-102, 1990.

44. Zacarias AS, Lane RG, Rosen II: Assessment of a linear accelerator for segmented conformal radiation therapy, Med Phys 20: 193-198, 1993.

Chapter 37

Beam Modulation Conformal Radiotherapy

Mark P. Carol, M.D.

NOMOS Corporation, Sewickley, Pennsylvania

The effectiveness of radiation therapy in today's clinical practice is limited by the oncologist's ability to restrict the treatment beam to diseased tissue only. Theoretically, if one could deliver radiation in such a way that only the target, regardless of its shape, received a lethal dose, then the impact radiation therapy has on many cancers might be significantly increased. This hypothesis is the basis for conformal therapy—delivering a high dose of radiation in a spatial distribution conforming to the shape of the target volume while concomitantly decreasing the volume of the surrounding normal tissue receiving that same dose.[8]

The most commonly employed technique for implementing conformal dose delivery is beam shaping. Beam shaping involves modifying the linear accelerator beam as defined by the primary and secondary jaws so that it more accurately conforms to the beam's eye view (BEV) of the target volume. Traditionally accomplished through the use of manually created cerrobend blocks, the process of beam shaping has been brought into the computer age by multileaf collimators (MLC). MLCs consist of a large number of paired vanes each of which can be independently moved under computer control.[1,6,7,9] Each pair of leaves defines a strip of radiation, usually 1.0 cm to 1.5 cm in width projected to isocenter, which is matched to the projected area of the target in a slice of the patient.

Although the MLC, designed to be a cornerstone of generalized conformal therapy, can in theory dynamically shape the field as the gantry arcs around the patient, a changing of the beam shape while the gantry is in the process of arcing is not commonly performed. In addition, although BEV field shaping, be it by an MLC or manual blocking techniques, can be a satisfactory approach when the target is geometrically well separated from surrounding organs at risk and/or when the target is convex in shape, it is less than satisfactory when the target wraps itself around organs at risk. In such situations, it is impossible to generate a BEV which "looks" at the target volume without "seeing" the organs at risk.[15]

Beam Intensity Modulation Conformal Therapy

A recent development in external beam radiotherapy treatment implementation exploits the use of fields in which intensity is varied across the beam.[1,2,4,5,14,15,16,17,18] Considered the foundation for true 3-D conformal therapy,[15] beam intensity modulation has been proposed as a means for generating concave dose distributions and to providing specific sparing of sensitive volumes (organs at risk) within complex treatment geometries.[4] The beam intensity is made to be proportional to the target thickness as assessed from a beam's eye view as the beam rotates around the patient. Where the target is "thickest," the beam intensity is at its greatest; where it is at its thinnest, the intensity is at its lowest. Unfortunately, the computer software and implementation hardware for such an approach has until recently been available only in theory,[6,12,14,15,16] in custom designed systems,[2,5,13,14] or in scanning beam accelerators and heavy particle units which cost far more than is affordable by most treatment sites.

Peacock, a linear accelerator-based three-dimensional conformal radiation therapy planning and treatment system currently under development (Figure 37-1), is an approach to intensity modulation radiation therapy with potential application in the general clinic. Peacock can be viewed as a treatment-oriented mirror image of computed tomography.[5] Both systems utilize variations on computer implementations of filtered backprojection algorithms to generate their data; both systems interact with the patient in a "slice-by-slice" fashion. However, whereas CT delivers a spatially uniform radiation exposure to the patient, measuring the spatially nonuniform attenuation of the exit beam, Peacock delivers a spatially nonuniform radiation exposure to the patient to create a uniform dose distribution at the target site (Figure 37-2).

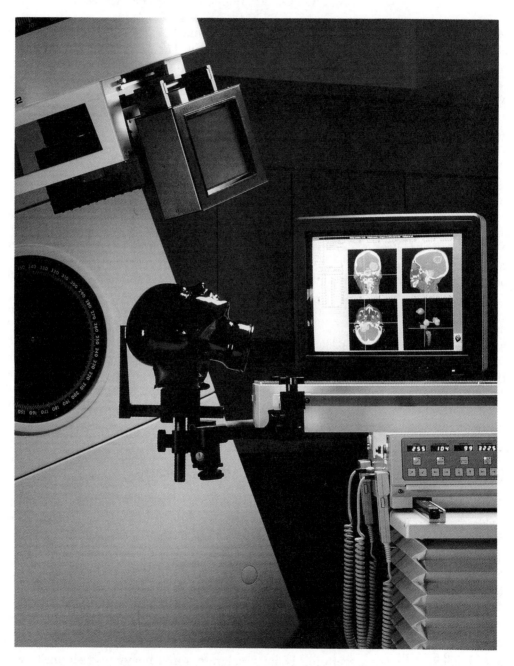

Figure 37-1. *Photograph of complete Peacock system (Planning computer, immobilization, and mini-collimation system attached to accelerator)*

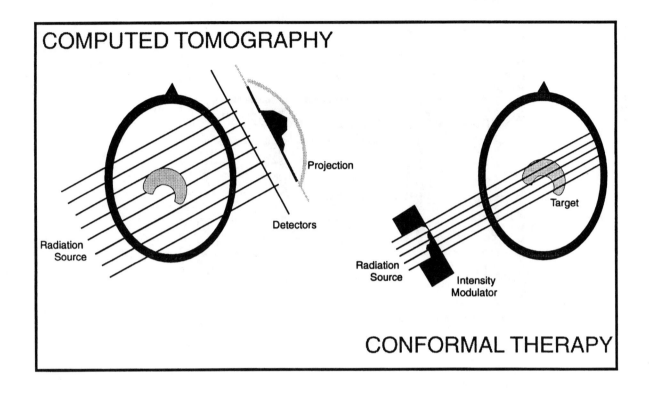

Figure 37-2. Computed Tomography Compared to Intensity Modulation Conformal Therapy

Peacock uses an electro-mechanical implementation device called MIMiC which attaches to the wedge tray slot on the treatment machine and which is used to dose the patient in a "slice-by-slice" fashion. The MIMiC functionally narrows the beam coming from the accelerator down into two thin "slices," further dividing these "slices" into 40 "smaller" beams, 20 for each slice (Figure 37-3). The MIMiC consists of 40 tungsten vanes 8 cm tall. Each vane is powered by a miniature pneumatic piston controlled by a solenoid valve. Turning the valve on causes air to flow to the front side of the piston, which drives the vane out of the field. When the valve is turned off, constant air pressure applied to the backside of the piston drives the vane back into the field (20 millisecond movement in either direction). Each vane has associated with it a set of sensors which track absolute amount of movement as well as speed of movement in/out of the field.

A treatment is delivered in a rotational fashion functionally viewed as a series of fixed ports; every five degrees of rotation is treated as a separate field. As the gantry rotates around the patient with the accelerator turned on, each of the 40 small "beams" defined by the MIMiC is turned on/off independent of the others by driving the beam's vane out of/into the beam path. Turning the individual beams "on/off" for variable periods of time during the five degree arc controls the effective attenuation of each beam segment for that five degrees of arc treated as if it were an individual port—spatial modulation through temporally variable attenuation of the treatment beam results. Since this modulation is produced in a slice-by-slice fashion and a complete treatment is accomplished by stacking a series of slices, the term "STACed Slice RT" (spatial-temporal attenuation-modulated conformal radiation therapy) has been coined to describe Peacock's implementation technique.

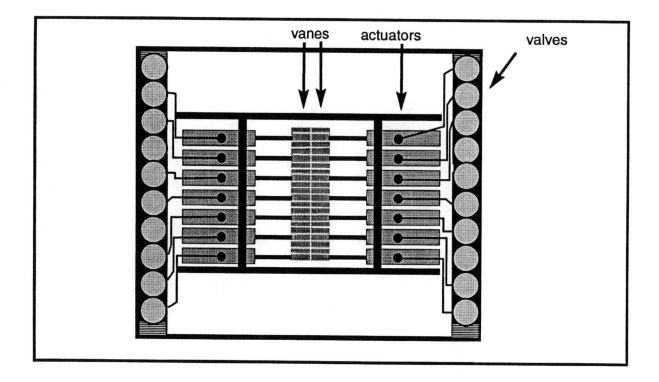

Figure 37-3. Schematic of MIMiC

After a complete rotation of the gantry, which treats the equivalent of two slices through the target, the table is indexed forward in relation to the MIMiC to treat the next two slices. A complete treatment of the patient consists of a single set of arcs or of several sets of arcs spaced around the patient's head or body (spacing produced by rotating the patient table with respect to the gantry). The use of multiple arc sets distributes the incident dose of radiation over as great an area as possible, maximizing the dose to the target while minimizing the dose to normal or sensitive tissue. Rate of dose fall-off is equivalent to that of a standard radiosurgical treatment delivered with the same number of arcs through a circular collimator.

Treatment Planning

The 3-D treatment planning and viewing program (Peacock Plan) which creates the beam weights delivered by the MIMiC is an automatic one. Rather than verifying a user-designed program, as is the norm in conventional radiation therapy and radiosurgery treatment planning, the system creates the plan itself. Peacock starts with the desired dose distribution and works in reverse to generate the beam weights needed to produce this distribution. Considered an inverse approach, it is a computer implementation of the filtered backprojection algorithms used in computer tomography.[1,10,12,13,14,15,16,17,18] In the radiation therapy application of these principles, an iterative process [15] is used to determining a set of beam weights which, when backprojected into the treatment space, will deliver not only the prescribed dose to the identified target volume but also will keep the dose to avoidance and sensitive volumes below user-defined limits.(Figure 37-4)

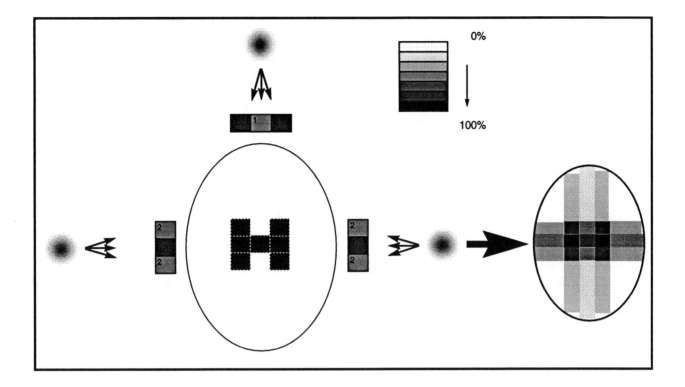

Figure 37-4. Beam weightings proportional to target thickness for three ports

Planning is done on a "slice-by-slice" basis; the beam weights for a rotation around a single slice through the target are generated independently of all other slices through the target. Dose simulation, however, is volumetric. Dosage is calculated using a modified path length algorithm based on delivered characterization data from sample beam sizes as measured by film and TLDs.11 The dose calculation matrix is set to be the same as the degree of image resolution. Scatter to planes outside the plane of each treatment arc has been incorporated into the dose model so that the dose delivered by multiple translations of the isocenter and by multiple table angles is correctly calculated. The dose to each point is calculated to be that received from all beams from all gantry angles from all slices.

Planning and dose simulation is very computer-intensive; 5,000 or more iterations encompassing greater than 1015 calculations may be required to produce an acceptable plan. A one-table angle fractionated boost for an intracranial metastatic lesion takes approximately 20 minutes to plan and dose simulate on a standard system configuration; a five-table angle radiosurgical treatment may take up to two hours or more. However, since user-interaction with the system is conducted on a physically contiguous but functionally separate compute engine from the one performing the intensive automatic plan optimization, the user may concurrently input and process data for a second or third case while the system is generating the beam weights for the first plan entered.

Once a plan has been accepted, the control parameters for beam modulation necessary to implement rotational plans are printed by the workstation on a floppy disc used as a data file by the Peacock Controller. The Controller, through an on-board microprocessor and gantry angle sensors, coordinates the disc-dictated vane movements of the MIMiC with the position of the treatment head as it rotates around the patient.

All Peacock Plans are implemented with a single effective isocenter (linear translation of the table between pairs of slices makes the isocenter effectively an "isoline"), an isocenter which is generally in the center of the treatment volume but not necessarily inside the target volume. Any number of distinct target volumes within the total treatment volume can be planned for and treated at the same time. Each of these targets can have a separate dose prescription; all targets will be treated simultaneously by the MIMiC. The system is designed to treat target volumes up to 20 centimeters in diameter. Treatment slice thickness may range from five millimeters to two centimeters; individual beam width is one centimeter.

Because Peacock has a requirement for precise movement of the treatment table between slices, a special table indexing device—the Crane—has been developed. The Crane consists of a large vertical column which supports two ball-bearing driven arms each equipped with a digital scale. The system stands at the side of the treatment table; clamps mounted to one of the arms lock the Crane to the rail supports on the side of the table. By releasing the locks on the table, movement of the table can be controlled by adjusting the position of either or both of the arms. Once the table has been properly indexed, the arms and the table top can be locked in place. The three hundred (300) pound weight of the indexing system prevents the backlash commonly found in treatment tables from affecting precise positioning of the table top. As a stand-alone device, the Crane is capable of delivering 0.01 mm indexed movements as measured by the digital scales. In practice, the accurate indexed table movement of 0.1 mm required by Peacock can be reliably achieved.

Initial validation studies showed a qualitative ability of the MIMiC to deliver the dose distributions predicted by Peacock (Figure 37-5); subsequent studies have shown dose simulation to be within 2-4% of the dose delivered to phantom targets. As with all partial transmission (beam modulation) systems, the number of monitor units required to deliver a specific dose to the patient is increased by a factor of from 2 to 3. Although this increases beam-on time for a given treatment, it does not significantly increase the time a patient spends in the room due to the efficient nature of rotational setups. Sample cases which display the application of Peacock are presented in Figure 37-6.

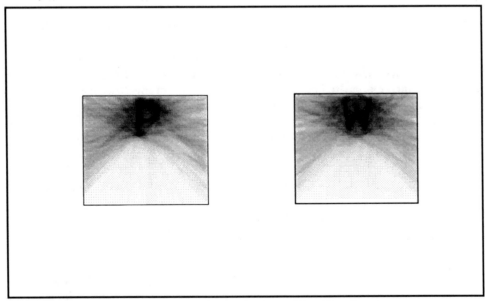

Figure 37-5. Sample dose distributions

The first patient treatments with Peacock began in March of 1994 - eleven patients had been treated as of December, 1994.[1] In general, fixation and CT scanning was performed on day 1, treatment planning and phantom Q/A on day 2-3 and treatments begun on day 4. Invasive fixation was employed in each case - a screw fixation device (Talon) consisting of two self-tapping inserts threaded into the inner table of the skull to which the actual fixation bracket was secured. The inserts were left in place throughout the course of treatment; the Talon was reapplied on a daily basis. Supplemental bead-bag support of the neck was utilized for head and neck cases where indicated. Initial set-up and Q/A time was approximately 10 to 20 minutes per patient, with treatment times varying from 10 minutes to 80 minutes depending on lesion size and dose. Film verification indicated repeat alignment to be within 1 mm in all but one case (1.5 mm).

Targets ranged in size from 2.7 cc to 69 cc (mean of 37.1 cc). Five patients had malignant lesions; six had benign lesions (one patient had two benign lesions). Eight patient had primary CNS disease, three had lesions of the head and neck, and one had an isolated lesion of the cervical spine. Patient age ranged from 10 years to 74 years (mean of 54); eight patients were male and 3 female.

The number of fractions ranged from 4 to 28 delivered over from 2 to 35 days; the dose per fraction was from 150 to 850. The number of table indexes required for complete target coverage ranged from 1 to 7 (mean of 3). The total number of fractions delivered was over 200 encompassing greater than 1,000 rotations of the gantry.

---

[1] Clinical trials are being conducted under IDEs at the Methodist Hospital, Baylor College of Medicine under the direction of Walter Grant, PH.D., Brian Butler, M.D., Shaio Woo, M.D., Robert Grossman, M.D. and at The Western Pennsylvania Hospital under the direction of Peggy Eddy, M.S., Dan Pavord, M.S., Judith Figura, M.D. and Robert Selker, M.D.

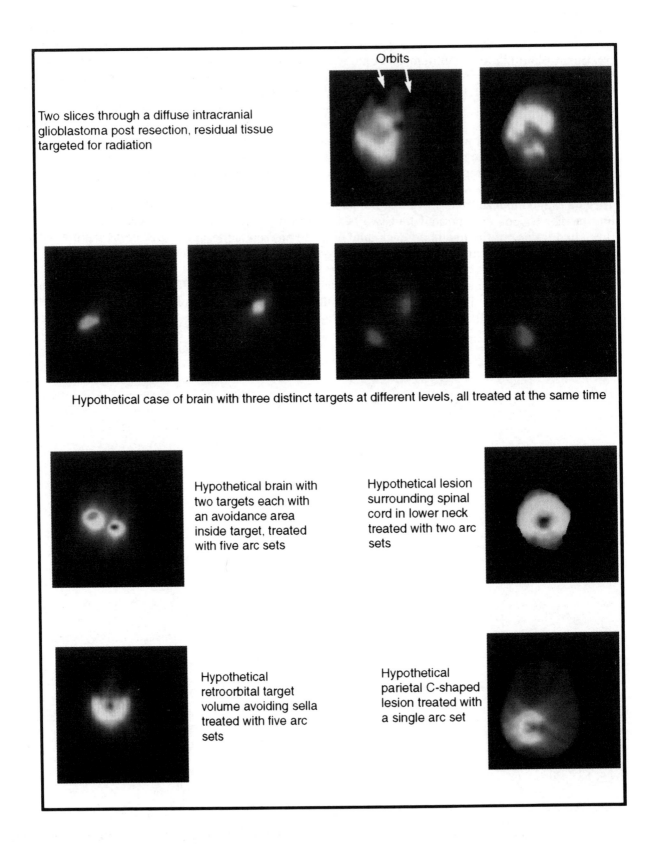

Figure 37-6. Dose distributions for sample target volumes planned for by Peacock

Discussion

The need for more conformal dose delivery systems is commonly recognized. New technologies are being bought to bear which improve the ability to conform to irregularly shaped target volumes. BEV shaping devices such as the MLC can be expected to improve dose distributions in those situations where the target is well separated from the organ at risk. However, where the target volume is integral to avoidance or sensitive volumes, simply BEV conformal protocols may produce less than satisfactory dose distributions. In such instances, beam modulation techniques may prove to be more successful for delivering 3-D conformal therapy.

Although much validation work and system fine-tuning remains to be done, the Peacock system appears to have the ability to generate and implement true 3-dimensional conformal treatment plans, plans which can adequately differentiate target volume from organs at risk even when the target wraps itself around the organs at risk. Plans can be generated and implemented which treat multiple targets in a given treatment volume at the same time with each target potentially receiving a different dose. Fractionated treatments can be delivered in a more time-effective fashion due to Peacock's optimization and normalization of each table angle independent of all others; only a single table angle need be used to deliver a full fraction dose to the target volume while keeping the dose delivered to normal structures below accepted limits.

Regardless of the approach, conformal systems, providing the ability to conform tightly to the target volume may allow the target dose to be escalated without increasing the risk to non-target tissue. They may also allow the treatment of larger target volumes than is currently possible. A limiting factor in attempts to increase field size with standard accelerator based systems is the increase in the amount of normal tissue which falls within the high dose region. Because conformal systems can shape the high dose region so it conforms to the target volume regardless of its size, the amount of normal tissue which falls within that high dose region may be reduced, allowing such volumes to be safely treated.

Multicenter, randomized, prospective studies will be required to determine whether such dose escalations and conformal dose deliveries will affect the overall course of malignant disease. However, it would seem that the aggressive use of conformal techniques should reduce the risks associated with current treatment protocols, thus decreasing the cost not only to the patient but to the institution as well.

In summary, conformal systems such as *Peacock* and those being developed by others provide the oncologist with a tool which may have the potential to improve the risk/benefit ratio associated with treating a wide range of lesions occurring not only in the central nervous system but also anywhere in the body. As such, these systems present the oncologist and the diagnostic radiologist with an interesting problem. In the past, delivery instruments for radiation therapy have not been able to restrict the delivered dose precisely to a suspected volume of abnormal tissue. Thus, diagnostic tools which approximated abnormal target margins were adequate. However, as the stereotactic principles of precise localization and immobilization gain more general acceptance, and as conformal tools become available which can precisely tailor a delivered dose to the target volume, the need to know precisely what that target volume is becomes of utmost importance. Current diagnostic techniques cannot provide that information. Perhaps conformal radiosurgical systems will be a stimulus for achieving it.

References

1. Brahme, A. Optimization of Stationary and moving beam radiation therapy techniques. Radiother. Oncol. 12: 129-140. 1988.

2. Carol, M. P. Harris Targovnik, H, Donald Smith, D., Cahill, D. 3-D planning and delivery system for optimized conformal therapy. IJROBP. 24:159. 1992.

3. Chin, L., Kijewski, P., Svensson, G., Bjarngard, B. Dose optimization with computer-controlled gantry rotation, collimator motion, and dose-rate variation. IJRO 9: 723 - 72. 1983.

4. Convery, D., Rosenbloom, M. The generation of intensity-modulated fields for conformal radiotherapy by dynamic collimation Phys. Med. Biol. 37 (6) 1359-1374. 1992.

5. Goitein, M., Abrams, M., Rowell, D., Pollari, H., Wiles, J. Multidimensional treatment planning. 2: Beam's eye view, back projection and projection through CT sections. IJROBP. 9: 789 - 797. 1983.

6. Kijewski, P., Chin, L., Bjarngard, B. Wedge-shaped dose distributions by computer-controlled collimator motion. Medical Physics. 5(5) 426-429. 1978.

7. Kobayashi, H., Sakuma, S., Kaii, O. Yogo, H. Computer-assisted conformation radiotherapy with a variable thickness multi-leaf filter. IJRO 16: 1631-1635. 1989.

8. Leibel, S., Ling, C., Kutcher, G., Mohan, R., Cordon-Cordo, C., Fuks, Z. The biological basis for conformal three-dimensional radiation therapy. IJRO 21: 805-811. 1991.

9. Levene, M., Kijewski, P., Chin, L., Bjarngard, B., Hellman, S. Computer-controlled radiation therapy. Radiology 129: 769-775. 1978.

10. Lind, B., Brahme, A. Optimization of radiation therapy dose distributions using scanned electron and photon beams and multileaf collimators. pgs.235-239 in Bruinvis, I.A.D. et al. The use of computers in radiation therapy. 1987. Elsevier Science Publishers B.V. (North Holland).

11. Luxton, G., Jozsef, G., Astrahan, M. Algorithm for dosimetry of multiarc linear-accelerator stereotactic radiosurgery. Med Phys. 18 (6) 1211 - 1221. 1991.

12. Morrill, S.M., Lane, R.G., Jacobson, G., Rosen, I.I. Treatment planning optimization using constrained simulated annealing. Phys. Med Biol. 36 (10) 1341-1361. 1991.

13. Soderstrom, S., Brahme, A. Selection of suitable beam orientations in radiation therapy using entropy and Fourier transform measures. Phys Med Biol. 37(4) 911-924. 1992.

14. Starkschall, G., Eifel, P., An interactive beam-weight optimization tool for three-dimensional radiotherapy treatment planning. Med Phys. 19 (10) 155-164. 1992.

15. Webb, S. Optimization of conformal radiotherapy dose distributions by simulated annealing. Phys. Med. Biol. 34 (10) 1359-1370. 1989.

16. Webb, S. Optimization by simulated annealing of three-dimensional conformal treatment plan-ning for radiation fields defined by a multileaf collimator. Phy. Med. Biol. 36 (9) 1201-1226. 1991.

17. Webb, S. Optimization of conformal radiotherapy dose distributions by simulated annealing: 2. Inclusion of scatter in the 2-D technique. Phys. Med. Biol., 36 (9) 1227-1237. 1991.

18. Webb, S. Beam geometry and beam shaping. Presented at the European Association Radiology meeting on Three-Dimensional Treatment Planning. Geneva. October, 1992.

Chapter 38

Clinical Decision-Support Systems in Radiation Therapy[1]

Nilesh L. Jain, D.Sc.[*] and Michael G. Kahn, M.D., Ph.D.

Section of Medical Informatics, Department of Internal Medicine,
Washington University School of Medicine, St. Louis, Missouri

Computers have been used in medicine since the late 1950s, about a decade after the appearance of the first electronic computer (44). The first systems were developed primarily for repetitious and labor-intensive tasks, such as processing medical data (7). The need for and success of these early systems along with the phenomenal advances in computer technology has led to the proliferation of computer-based systems in delivering health care. At present, computers are being used mainly to perform medical tasks which can be easily automated. These systems include medical-record systems, hospital information systems, nursing information systems, laboratory systems, pharmacy systems, radiology systems, patient-monitoring systems, and bibliographic-retrieval systems (84).

Radiation therapy, with its need for computation-intensive dose calculations and image processing, was one of the first medical fields to make extensive clinical use of computers (25). Comprehensive treatment planning systems made their appearance in the middle of the 1960s, incorporating the repetitive tasks of calculating dose distributions for various kinds of external beam radiation treatment. Due to the limitations of computer technology, most early treatment planning was two-dimensional. However, with the availability of very fast computers at a reasonable cost and with the advances in graphics, imaging and display technologies, three-dimensional (3-D) treatment planning systems are becoming possible (75). The report of National Cancer Institute's Photon Treatment Planning Collaborative Working Group (85) concluded that 3-D radiation treatment planning (RTP) is valuable because it provides a better view of the anatomical relationships and dose distributions (66, 67).

Researchers in medical informatics are interested in using computers to assist physicians and other health care personnel in difficult medical decision making tasks such as diagnosis, therapy selection, and therapy evaluation. *Clinical decision-support systems* are computer programs designed to help health care personnel in making clinical decisions (82). Since one of the first reported systems in 1964 (93), the field has matured considerably and has produced systems for various medical domains. Notable among these are MYCIN for the selection of antibiotic therapy (83), INTERNIST-1 for diagnosis in general internal medicine (51), and ONCOCIN for management of cancer patients (91). The two primary techniques used to construct clinical decision-support systems are *artificial intelligence* and *decision theory*.

Artificial intelligence (AI) is a branch of computer science concerned with the automation of intelligent behavior (45), attempting to make computers do things which people currently do better (73). One of the most visible and commercially-successful products of AI research are *expert systems* (63). An expert system is a computer program that relies on knowledge and reasoning to perform a task that is usually performed by human experts. Knowledge is stored in a knowledge base using various representation techniques. The most common representation technique is IF-THEN rules,

[1] Supported in part by the National Library of Medicine Grant 5-R29-LM05387, National Cancer Institute Contract N01-CM97564, and Office of Human Genome Research Grant 1-R01-HG00223.
[*] Present Address: Department of Medical Informatics, Columbia Presbyterian Medical Center, N.Y., N.Y.

hence the term rule-based expert systems. Figure 38-1 contains a typical rule that might be used in radiation therapy treatment selection. Other representation techniques include frames, semantic networks, conceptual graphs, and scripts. *Knowledge acquisition* is the process of eliciting a knowledge base from a domain expert (19). Different reasoning strategies are used to arrive at conclusions based on the problem data and the knowledge base. In rule-based expert systems, the reasoning strategies used are forward chaining where the data are used to arrive at a conclusion, and backward chaining where a conclusion is tentatively assumed and the data are used to justify it. Other applications of AI include planning, vision, learning, and natural language understanding.

IF   the primary tumor site is lung

THEN   use parallel opposed AP/PA beams to deliver 4500 cGy to the target volume and oblique (off-spinal cord) beams to deliver an additional 200 cGy to the target volume

---

Figure 38-1. A simple IF-THEN rule that can be used in radiation therapy

Artificial intelligence has been applied to medical problems for the past two decades (10, 50, 89, 90). Most of the applications concentrate on diagnosis, therapy recommendation, and critiquing management plans. Researchers in medical AI have contributed significantly to advancing the state-of-the-art of AI research. They have developed probabilistic reasoning techniques to handle uncertainty (9, 21), and temporal reasoning techniques to handle time (32), all of which are inherent in routine medical decision making.

Decision theory is a branch of operations research which provides an explicit methodology to handle preferences and uncertainty in making optimal decisions depending on the objectives of the decision maker (22, 72). The decision problem is structured as a decision tree starting with the available options (Figure 38-2). At each stage, either the decision maker has a choice of other options, or a previous option can lead to few different events. In the latter case, the probability of each event is elicited. The tree is expanded until the final outcomes are reached. If the decision problem has a single objective, the *utility* (desirability) of each final outcome is elicited, the expected utility (based on multiplying utilities and probabilities) of each initial option is computed, and by the principles of normative decision theory, the option with the highest expected utility is chosen. Most non-trivial decision problems require the decision maker to fulfill multiple and often conflicting objectives. In these cases, it is difficult to elicit a single utility value for each outcome. In this setting, each outcome is divided into a number of attributes, each attribute usually corresponding to one of the objectives. Techniques of *multiattribute utility theory* are used for these problems (38, 92). In addition to the utility of each attribute, multiattribute *weights* are elicited to make trade-offs among the conflicting objectives. The overall utility of each outcome is computed by using a suitable combining function for the utilities and weights of the attributes.

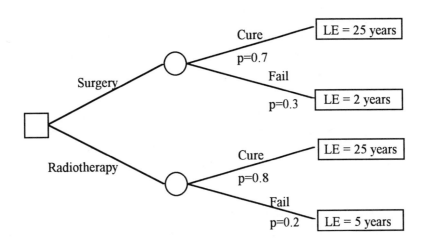

Figure 38-2. *A simple decision tree for choosing between surgery and radiotherapy. Squares represent choices or decisions, circles represent uncertain events, and rectangles represent final outcomes. (LE = life expectancy)*

Clinical decision analysis has been applied to medical decision making problems for the past three decades (37, 65, 86, 94). Representative applications include choosing among treatments, choosing between treatment and no treatment, choosing between treatment and testing, and sequencing of therapy. Researchers developed Markov models to handle large decision trees with time-dependent events (4), uniform outcome measurement scales such as quality-adjusted life years (69), and cost-effectiveness and cost-benefit analyses to trade-off expected health benefits versus costs (95).

With the advent of 3-D conformal radiation therapy (CRT), treatment planning has become more difficult as the class solutions which were used in 2-D RTP are no longer optimal (75). Instead of two or three potential plans based on 2-D RTP standard solutions, hundreds or thousands of potential plans can be generated in 3-D CRT. With the availability of real-time dose calculation, generating each plan is not as time-consuming as it used to be (74). However, current manual treatment planning methods are inadequate to generate all clinically-plausible plans. Hence, researchers have pointed out the need for AI applications to assist in automatically generating treatment plans (33, 36, 43, 97). In addition, the problem of automatic treatment plan optimization has gained renewed interest (52, 56). With the use of unconventional beam arrangements such as non-coplanar beams, the treatment planner can no longer use intuition to infer dose distributions in other planes by looking at the dose distribution in only one plane. Also, 3-D CRT produces large data sets which must be used in the evaluation phase of treatment planning. The task of evaluating potential 3-D treatment plans has become very difficult (15). Hence, researchers have been pointing out the need for objective plan-evaluation methods which can use this data (76). Since the evaluation of potential plans involves making trade-offs between the doses delivered to the target volumes and to the normal tissues, decision theory can be used for developing such models. The potential use of decision theory in radiation therapy evaluation was first pointed out two decades ago (57, 77). However, nearly ten years passed before the first such model was developed (79).

The past decade has seen an increasing number of decision-support systems in radiation therapy which can be classified into four categories — AI-based systems for target volume generation, AI-based systems for automatically generating treatment plans, decision-theoretic systems for evaluating competing treatment plans, and AI-based systems for diagnosing treatment machine failures. Although decision-support systems have been developed for other aspects of oncology such as diagnosis (3, 11, 13, 46, 64) and selection of treatment modality (47, 48, 49, 53, 54, 68, 87), we review the key features of a selection of systems designed specifically for radiation therapy decision-making.

Target Volume Definition

The consistent addition of margins to the gross tumor to account for possible microextensions of the tumor and patient motion is a difficult problem. We have identified one research group currently developing an AI-based system for the automatic generation of the planning target volume.

PTVT

PTVT (Planning Target Volume Tool) is a rule-based expert system to generate the planning target volume developed by Kromhout-Schiro et al. at the University of Washington, Seattle (40). This system is one of a set of 3-D CRT tools developed as part of National Cancer Institute's Radiotherapy Treatment Planning Tools Contract (71). PTVT calculates the planning target volume by adding a region of tissue to the gross tumor volume.

Four factors are considered in computing this additional region:
1. areas of tissue adjacent to the visible tumor that may contain microscopic amounts of tumor;
2. errors in positioning the patient for treatment;
3. patient movement during treatment;
4. movement of tumor due to physiologic processes such as breathing.

Data concerning these four factors were gathered from the literature as well as from local radiation oncologists, and were indexed according to the clinical condition of the patient and the clinical characteristics of the tumor. Preliminary evaluation found the generated planning target volumes to be consistent with those manually outlined by the radiation oncologists.

Automatic Treatment Planning

The step in RTP investigated by most decision-support investigators is the automatic generation of plausible or optimal radiation treatment plans. We describe the efforts of six research groups which either have developed or are currently developing AI-based systems for automatic treatment planning. Each of these systems focuses on a particular tumor site to make knowledge acquisition manageable. However, the techniques used in these systems can be applied to other tumor sites by suitable augmentation to the knowledge base.

ROENTGEN

ROENTGEN is a case-based reasoning system for lung cancer currently being developed by Berger et al. at the University of Chicago (5, 6). Case-based reasoning is an AI technique where the solution to the current problem is found by adapting the solution of a previously-solved similar problem (18). All problems and solutions are stored in an indexed case library, the indices are used to retrieve a similar problem, its solution is repaired to account for the differences between the current and the retrieved problem, and the new solution is stored in the case library enabling the system to learn from its problem-solving experience.

ROENTGEN has five modules for the five steps it follows in designing a treatment plan. Given the description of the current patient and the desired prescribed target dose, the *Retriever* module finds a similar prior case from the case library. To facilitate the retrieval, therapy plans have preconditions for their selection based on tumor location and patient geometry. If more than one prior plan satisfies the preconditions, other plan-specific features are used and the prior plan with the best match is retrieved. If this still yields more than one plan, the simplest prior plan based on the number of beams, and the number of beam energies, is chosen. The *Adapter* module then modifies this retrieved plan to account for the differences between the current patient and the previous patient whose plan was retrieved. The adaptation process also uses the plan-specific features used by the *Retriever* by changing them until they are correct for the current patient. Having obtained a potential current plan, the *Detector* module tries to determine the result of applying the plan by using the resulting dose distribution. It then produces a list of faults indicating areas in the treatment field containing hot spots or cold spots. This list is compared with expected failures which is the fault list of the retrieved prior plan. If an unexpected fault occurs, the *Corrector* module asks a human expert for the relevant knowledge to repair the plan so that this unexpected fault will be eliminated. This plan is passed through the *Detector* again to make sure no new unexpected fault develops. At this point, a new treatment plan has been designed for the current patient, and it is added to the case base by the *Storer* module along with the plan-specific features and other information. Figure 38-3 contains a simplified system diagram explaining the relationships among the various modules and the working of the system.

It is important to note that ROENTGEN only designs a plausible treatment plan, and leaves it up to the human designer to decide whether this plan is optimal or not. Individual modules can be used for different tasks. The *Retriever* and *Adapter* can suggest plans to a novice designer. The *Detector* can be used as a critic for manually generated plans.

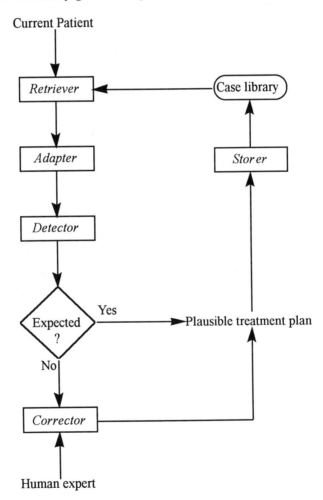

Figure 38-3. *Simplified system diagram for ROENTGEN. (Modified from: Berger, J. ROENTGEN: Case-based reasoning and radiation therapy planning. In: Frisse, M. E., ed. Proceedings of the Sixteenth Annual Symposium on Computer Applications in Medical Care. New York, NY: McGraw-Hill; 1992:210–214.)*

RADEK

RADEK is a rule-based expert system for head and neck tumors developed by et al. at the University of Washington, Seattle (58). Initially, a simple rule-based system determines the treatment modality and the prescription dose for the primary tumor and nodal metastases (35). In RADEK, treatment planning begins by selecting one or more prototypic plans from a library of standard starting plans traditionally used by the local treatment planners, and placing them on a list of *promising* plans (34, 60). This selection is based on the tumor site, shape and size of the patient, and prescription dose.

RADEK must evaluate *promising* plans to determine if they are clinically acceptable, if they can lead to acceptable plans, or if they should be discarded. The system performs this evaluation by plan simulation which involves calculating the dose distribution, determining the volume of hot and/or cold spots, and comparing the peak doses and integral doses in the various tissues (59). Based on the results of this evaluation, some *promising* plans are modified to create new treatment plans which are marked as *unexplored*. Because this step can generate a large number of *unexplored* plans and the evaluation can become time-consuming, *unexplored* plans are compared to previously evaluated *promising* plans to prune plans that are very similar (59). Only dissimilar plans are placed on the *promising* list to be evaluated. The planning process stops when no new plans are placed on the *promising* list after the similarity-based pruning. This resulting plan is presented to the treatment planner. Figure 38-4 contains a simplified system diagram.

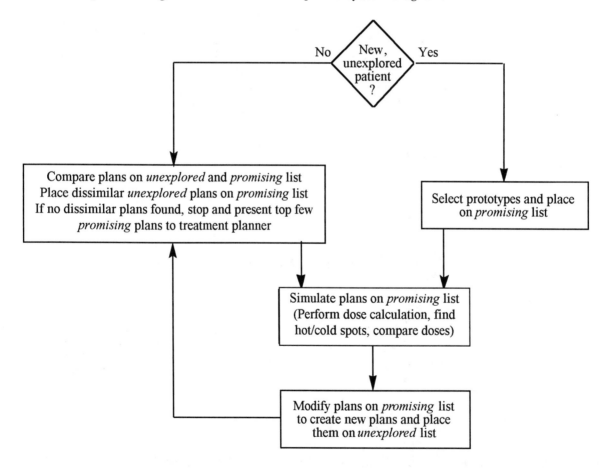

Figure 38-4. *Simplified system diagram for RADEK. (Modified from: Paluszynski, W. Designing Radiation Therapy for Cancer: An Approach to Knowledge-Based Optimization. Ph.D. Dissertation, Department of Computer Science. Seattle, WA: University of Washington; 1990.)*

CARTES

CARTES (Computer Aided RadioTherapy Expert System) is a decision-support system for inoperable non-small cell lung cancer developed by Hyödynmaa, Kolari et al. at the Technical Research Center, Finland (39). It is a part of the Nordic program CART (Computer Aided RadioTherapy) to develop an integrated information system for radiotherapy (42). Three stages in cancer therapy were identified where AI techniques could be applied — treatment decision making, design of new treatment protocols, and analysis of treatment results. CARTES is a prototype of the first and third stages, and no prototype was built for the second stage.

The prototype for the first stage (treatment decision making) uses relevant data and information about the social and medical history of the patient, clinical signs and symptoms, results of various tests and examinations, and the intention of the therapy (23, 39). The information is obtained automatically from an integrated clinical database, or directly from the user. CARTES acts as a critiquing system by checking if the diagnosis made by the physician agrees with the patient's clinical data, and whether the chosen therapy intent is appropriate in this case. It also determines if the patient has any symptoms which would indicate immediate treatment. The intended users of this first stage prototype are young physicians without much experience in cancer therapy.

The prototype for the third stage (analysis of treatment results) uses the treatment results and follow-up data gathered from a set of treated patients (24). This data comes from the clinical register which acts as a data bank for all therapeutic information. The goal is to provide the oncologist with an intelligent user interface to a statistical analysis software package to assist in preparation and specification of data, problem formulation, and interpretation of the outcome. This statistical analysis helps in quality assurance of the therapy and can provide feedback to the prototype for the first stage performing treatment decision making.

RADONCOL

RADONCOL is a rule-based system for head and neck tumors developed by Ionescu-Farca et al. at Rätisches Kantons- und Regionalspital, Switzerland (27, 28). It uses clinical information such as the case description, tumor site, extent of disease, staging, Karnofsky performance of the patient and other factors to recommend the appropriate treatment. The system is built using a commercial expert system shell and has about 300 rules. It uses backward chaining — it reasons from the goal of finding the appropriate therapy to the available clinical data. Certainty factors are used to handle multiple solutions. RADONCOL provides explanation about its reasoning, and the knowledge base can be modified and augmented.

Given the clinical data, RADONCOL determines the primary treatment modality, and the chronological order when more than one modality is indicated. If radiation therapy is one of the selected modalities, the system prescribes the dose and fractionation, and recommends a basic or standard beam arrangement based on a library of prototypical plans.

CAVCAV

CAVCAV is a rule-based expert system for cavum cancers developed by Aletti et al. at the Alexis Vautrin Center, France and Haton et al. at the University of Nancy, France (1, 2, 20). The system performs treatment planning in three phases. The first phase consists of the basic treatment up to 40 Grays. Using information about the tumor and abnormal ganglions, the system specifies a beam arrangement, nature and energy of the beams, and protective devices needed for sensitive organs such as the eye. In the second or boost phase ranging from 40 to 50 Grays, the precise location and shape of the target volume is used to arrive at an optimal treatment plan. The criteria used to determine optimality include maximization of tumor coverage, and minimization of surface inside the 90% isodose. The third phase consists of scheduling the extra irradiation based on the tumor irradiation in the first two phases and the patient's availability for treatment.

National Institute for Cancer Research, Italy

Paoli et al. at the National Institute of Cancer Research, Italy have developed an expert system for head and neck cancers (62, 78). The expert system consists of two parts: (1) a neural network to arrive at a general treatment plan; (2) a rule-based system to define the complete treatment plan.

The neural network uses anatomical, morphological and functional data obtained from CT images to determine the standard treatment plan which has the highest probability of success. The rule-based expert system then starts with this plan, uses clinical and dosimetric data from a relational database, and a heuristic knowledge base encoding the treatment planning expertise of local experts to arrive at a complete treatment plan.

This group is currently working on a rule-based expert system for total body irradiation in leukemia (61).

Treatment Plan Evaluation

In addition to generating treatment plans, another significant and interesting problem is the evaluation of competing radiation treatment plans. Currently, most treatment plan evaluation is performed manually by radiation oncologists using subjective techniques. We describe two research projects which have used multiattribute utility theory for the objective evaluation of competing radiation treatment plans.

Schultheiss' Model

Schultheiss at Eastern Virginia Medical School, Norfolk, used multiattribute utility theory for the evaluation and optimization of radiation treatment plans (79, 80, 81). The component attributes of his multiattribute model were the possible clinical complications of treatment such as non-eradication of the tumor and radiation-induced damage to the healthy normal tissues appearing in the treatment field. For each attribute, he computed its *utility* by combining the *probability* that the associated complication occurs with a *weight* representing the morbidity of the complication. The utilities of all the attributes were multiplied together to arrive at the overall utility for the plan known as its *Figure of merit (FOM)* using:

$$FOM = \prod_i^{\text{complications}} (1 - probability_i \times weight_i)$$

The *FOM* was used as an objective function for an automatic optimization algorithm that attempted to obtain a statistically optimal treatment plan. Complication probabilities were obtained from dose-response models developed by Schultheiss. Weights were the subjective judgment of the physician about the morbidity of the complication. However, while evaluating his decision-theoretic model, Schultheiss set $weight_i = 1$ so that the *FOM* effectively computed the probability that no complication occurs.

Jain's Model

Jain et al. at Washington University, St. Louis extended Schultheiss' model to include the treatment preferences of the radiation oncologist as well as the clinical condition of the patient (30, 31). The model extension was done by making the weight a function of two quantities: *prototypical weight* and *modifier*. The prototypical weight represents the morbidity of the complication for an average patient for the treating radiation oncologist. The modifier encodes the clinical condition of the patient which would change the prototypical weight. The probability of complication was computed from radiobiological probability computation models such as the Tumor Control Probability (TCP) (16) and the Normal Tissue Complication Probability (NTCP) (41).

Unlike Schultheiss, Jain elicited weights from radiation oncologists for three tumor sites — prostate, lung, and head and neck. Two different methodologies were used — Level of Concern (30) and Level of Enthusiasm (31) — both of which were variants of the direct rating method of multiattribute weight elicitation. In response to physicians' concerns, additional attributes were added to the model to handle different fractions of the volume of a tissue exceeding threshold dose. A clinical study is underway to validate this model in the context of three-dimensional radiation treatment of non-small cell lung cancer (17).

Preliminary evaluation of the model indicated some shortcomings due to the unreliability of the TCP and NTCP models as well as the low values for the complication probabilities. Research is underway to investigate a new model which eliminates the shortcomings in the current model (29).

Treatment Machine Diagnosis

In addition to the clinical systems described in the previous three sections, researchers have also focused on the non-clinical aspects of radiation therapy such as delivery of the radiation. This step can be hindered by the failure of the treatment machine. Two research groups have developed expert systems for the diagnosis and troubleshooting of different treatment machines.

TROUBLESHOOTER

TROUBLESHOOTER is a rule-based expert system developed by Curran et al. at the Tufts–New England Medical Center to handle hardware failures and operator errors that may occur with Varian Clinac 4/100 and 6/100 linear accelerators during clinical operation (12, 88). The system is built using a commercial expert system shell and has about 400 rules. The system first elicits the symptoms from the user through a series of menus. Backward chaining is used to evaluate the possible malfunctions using a pre-specified list of potential subsystem failures. Forward chaining is then used to arrive at the precise diagnosis and to make repair suggestions.

Philips SL-25 Linac Diagnostics

Myers (currently at University of Pennsylvania, Philadelphia) et al. at University of California, Los Angeles developed a rule-based expert system for general machine diagnosis and troubleshooting of the Philips SL-25 Linac (55). Knowledge is organized in a hybrid of object-oriented and rule-based framework. The objects include components arranged in a semantic network, as well as symptoms and tests. The system assists the user in navigating through the semantic net to find the minimum replaceable component. The knowledge base is updated after each session so that the system becomes more efficient as it is used.

Future Directions

A patient diagnosed with cancer is treated using one or more of surgery, radiotherapy and chemotherapy. If radiation therapy is one of the selected treatment modalities, the following steps are undertaken to deliver appropriate therapy:

1. The patient undergoes imaging using computerized tomography (CT) or magnetic resonance imaging (MRI) to determine his/her internal anatomy. Typically 20-30 slices/scans are taken to cover the region of interest.

2. The radiation oncologist delineates the target volumes on all images and prescribes a radiation dose.

3. Normal tissues occurring near the target volume are also contoured as the dose delivered to them needs to be minimized to prevent radiation-induced damage.

4. Various treatment plans are designed for the patient.

5. The competing plans are evaluated to select an optimal plan.

6. The patient is filmed in the proposed treatment position to simulate the treatment and verify that the treatment achieves its goal.

7. The treatment is delivered.

The systems described in this paper represent promising prototypes for steps 2, 4, 5, and 7. However, most of these steps will have to be revisited in the 3-D CRT era because of new unforeseen challenges requiring computer-based decision-support. In this section, we outline some of the opportunities or "grand challenges" for future decision-support systems in radiation therapy.

Target Volume Delineation

The International Commission on Radiation Units and Measurements (ICRU) published its report defining the three target volumes which should be specified by the radiation oncologists for treatment planning (26). The Gross Tumor Volume (GTV) refers to the gross palpable or visible/demonstrable extent and location of the tumor. The Clinical Target Volume (CTV) extends the GTV to include the microscopic extensions that need to be treated. The Planning Target Volume (PTV) adds margins to the CTV to account for organ and patient movement, and inaccuracies in beam and patient set up. Additionally, ICRU requires investigators to report three dose values for the target dose – maximum dose, minimum dose, and dose at the ICRU reference point which is a point in the PTV where the dose can be accurately measured and is not in a region having a steep dose gradient. Such standardization is necessary for meaningful comparison of tumor control data from clinical trials performed at different institutions. Radiation oncologists will need assistance to consistently follow these guidelines in defining GTV, CTV and PTV, and reporting target volume doses (70).

Initial difficulty for the radiation oncologists in following these recommendations will occur as most institutions currently follow their own standard. Knowledge-based decision-support systems like PTVT will be invaluable for consistent use of the ICRU recommendations. Although PTVT is a prescriptive tool, it could be modified into a critiquing-based tool which ensures that the volumes being used by the radiation oncologist are consistent with the ICRU terminology.

Normal Tissue Contouring

Outlining normal tissues on all CT or MR images is a labor-intensive and time-consuming task (14). Research is underway in structural biology to build a knowledge base about the anatomical structure of the human body (8). The knowledge base will have two kinds of information — spatial and symbolic. The spatial information will be in the form of CT slices of a male and female cadaver to encode the physical structure of the human body. This will be annotated by symbolic information containing the names of the tissues, their hierarchy and other anatomical facts. Such a knowledge base can be used to enhance automatic contouring algorithms which attempt to perform the time-consuming task of contouring normal tissues on each image. Since the anatomical knowledge base will be composed of CT slices, the location of the image within the body will give information on the tissues expected on that slice along with their approximate shape. This will enable edge-detection algorithms to make intelligent choices when the image contrast is not that high on a particular portion of the slice. The knowledge base will also facilitate consistent inclusion or exclusion of tissue in the low contrast regions to develop a consistent 3-D reconstruction of the tissue.

Treatment Plan Generation

Perhaps the most challenging task in the radiation therapy process is treatment plan generation, bringing to bear all the skills and experience of the treatment planners. The advent of 3-D CRT makes heavy demands on treatment planners as the class solutions used in traditional 2-D RTP are not optimal. Also, treatment planners no longer are restricted to a single plane, but can plan and deliver treatments having non-coplanar beams. The relaxing of these restrictions makes the solution space of plausible 3-D treatment plans much larger than that for 2-D RTP. Conservative estimates of simple four beam plans suggest that the number of possible treatment plans may run into the millions of millions, though not all of them will be clinically plausible. Even with real-time 3-D dose calculation, the time required to examine each of them automatically to find the optimal solution will be impractical. Clearly, there is need for knowledge-based techniques to generate plausible treatment plans automatically.

The systems described in the section **Automatic Treatment Planning** use ad hoc rules to move or add beams to generate treatment plans, giving rise to the possibility of generating clinically implausible plans. The anatomical knowledge base described in the previous subsection could be used to perform the kind of anatomical reasoning performed by treatment planners while manually designing treatment plans. Such a system would reason about the shape and position of the various tissues in the treatment field, and attempt to design beams which spare the critical normal tissues as much as possible, and at the same time deliver the prescribed dose to the planning target volume. The system can also be given information about the relative importance of the various tissues in the treatment field to make tradeoffs among the tissues while positioning a beam. Anatomical reasoning is similar to the spatial reasoning problem being investigated by researchers in robotic planning.

Systems performing anatomical reasoning will endeavor to generate a treatment plan from scratch, and thus will need to contain a vast amount of treatment planning knowledge. An alternative to this approach uses case-based reasoning, as exemplified by ROENTGEN. By sharing treatment plans across institutions, it would be possible to build large case libraries containing many of the possible variation in the types and locations of tumors. The decision-support challenge will then be to devise a suitable metric to categorize patients, tumors and treatment plans to facilitate the accurate retrieval of one or more similar treatment plans.

Treatment Plan Evaluation

The treatment plan evaluation systems described here, as well as the mathematical optimization algorithms investigated by other researchers, are increasingly relying on TCP and NTCP values to characterize outcomes. While these concepts represent the ultimate bottom line for outcomes, state-of-the-art TCP and NTCP models are still not reliable and have not gained clinical acceptance. This lack of reliability is evident from the caveats mentioned by most authors while defending the use of current TCP and NTCP models (15, 31, 56). One way of getting more realistic outcomes data may be to construct a national (or international) outcome database of patients which contains image data along with dose distributions of the administered treatment plan. Patient follow-up and outcomes will allow researchers to use actual outcomes data for treatment plan evaluation and optimization. This data also can assist in validating current and future TCP and NTCP models.

With 3-D CRT, it is possible to deliver higher doses to the target volume while keeping normal tissues below acceptable thresholds. This new capability is allowing radiation oncologists to increase the target dose to test the hypothesis that increased target dose improves local control (96). Such dose escalation studies are a major focus of current clinical radiation oncology research. NCI is sponsoring multi-institutional clinical trial to study the impact of dose escalation in carcinoma of the prostate. One project goal is to create a national outcomes resource database for 3-D CRT prostate treatment planning data.

Evaluating treatment plans at escalated dose levels is difficult for two reasons — TCP models which are unreliable at normal prescription dose levels are equally or perhaps more unreliable at higher levels, and not enough clinical data is available to make subjective estimates of the tumor control rate. Hence the evaluation of plans has to rely on other criteria to characterize the outcomes. Treatment objectives can be stated in terms of prescribed target dose and the desire to minimize dose to the normal tissues. Decision theory provides the framework to elicit utility functions to indicate how closely these objectives are met. This information could be used to compute the overall utility of the plan or its figure of merit and could be used for treatment plan evaluation.

Treatment Optimization

We have highlighted the difficulty of manually generating all the clinically plausible 3-D treatment plans and the need for decision-support systems to perform this task. A similar argument could be made for the manual optimization of 3-D plans as the treatment planner would have to consider all plausible plans to select the most optimal plan. Objective plan-evaluation models could be used for the automatic optimization of treatment plans by detecting the clinically plausible 3-D plan with the highest figure of merit. Since 3-D dose calculations can be performed in real-time, the computational cost of performing such optimization will not be very high (74).

Decision-support systems can also be developed to assist in the manual or semi-automated optimization of treatment plans. Using an anatomical knowledge base, a critiquing system could examine a proposed treatment plan and suggest possible improvements to it. By combining this critiquing system with objective plan-evaluation models, it could suggest the change which would result in the greatest improvement in the figure of merit of the plan. This design would be the best kind of decision-support system for treatment planners who remain in the optimization loop as it would work using the starting points suggested by the treatment planner.

Treatment Delivery

One of the neglected issues in treatment plan evaluation and optimization has been the complexity of delivering the treatment plan. The use of multiple energies, or other complex maneuvers, leads to an increased chance of error in delivering the treatment. While there has been a steady increase in the number of computer-controlled treatment machines, the need to incorporate the treatment plan complexity into the evaluation and optimization of radiation treatment plans is still required. Artificial intelligence techniques such as case-based reasoning possibly could be used for computing the complexity of a treatment plan. Research also needs to be done on decision-support systems for diagnosis and repair of treatment machines.

Conclusion

This paper examines eleven prototype decision-support systems developed to assist in various steps in the radiation therapy of a cancer patient. With the imminent 3-D CRT era, a complete transformation will occur in the way in which radiation therapy personnel perform their tasks. The increased number of possibilities and amount of information will require radiation therapy to use decision-support technology to best exploit the advantages of 3-D conformal therapy. We have described some of the specific advances that we foresee or that are necessary for better decision-support. Completely untapped is the potential pedagogical use for the tools that could be developed to instruct residents in the art of designing, evaluating and optimizing 3-D radiation treatment plans.

Acknowledgments

We thank Pierre Aletti, Jeffrey Berger, Bruce Curran, Florica Ionescu, Ira Kalet, Pentti Kolari, Lee Myers, Gabriella Paoli, Niilo Saranummi, and others who helped us gather the material for this review. We also thank Dr. Bahman Emami and Dr. James A. Purdy of the Mallinckrodt Institute of Radiology, St. Louis MO for allowing us to contribute to the First International Symposium on 3-D Radiation Treatment Planning and Conformal Therapy.

References

1. Aletti, P.; Chauvet, M. P.; Haton, M.-C.; Malissard, L. An application of expert systems in the radiation therapy planning (Abstr.). Med. Biol. Eng. Comput. 29 (Suppl.):440; 1991.

2. Aletti, P.; Malissard, L.; Jacquot, P.; Meresse, L.; Haton, M.-C.; Haton, J. P. An aid in treatment simulation: Radiotherapy expert system (Abstr.). Med. Phys. 15:789; 1988.

3. Alvey, P. L.; Preston, N. J.; Greaves, M. F. High performance expert systems: II. A system for leukaemia diagnosis. Med. Inform. 12:97–114; 1987.

4. Beck, J. R.; Pauker, S. G. The Markov process in medical prognosis. Med. Decis. Making 3:419–458; 1983.

5. Berger, J. ROENTGEN: Case-based reasoning and radiation therapy planning. In: Frisse, M. E., ed. Proceedings of the Sixteenth Symposium on Computer Applications in Medical Care. New York, NY: McGraw-Hill; 1992:210–214.

6. Berger, J.; Hammond, K. J. ROENTGEN: A memory-based approach to radiation therapy treatment design. In: Bareiss, R., ed. Proceedings: Case-based Reasoning Workshop-1991. San Mateo, CA: Morgan Kaufmann; 1991:203–214.

7. Blum, B. I. Clinical Information Systems. New York, NY: Springer-Verlag; 1986.

8. Brinkley, J. F.; Prothero, J. S.; Prothero, J. W.; Rosse, C. A framework for the design of knowledge-based systems in structural biology. In: Kingsland, L. C., ed. Proceedings of the Thirteenth Annual Symposium on Computer Applications in Medical Care. Washington, DC: IEEE Computer Society Press. 1989:61–65.

9. Chavez, R. M.; Cooper, G. F. A randomized approximation algorithm for probabilistic inference on Bayesian belief networks. Networks 20:661–685; 1990.

10. Clancey, W. J.; Shortliffe, E. H., eds. Readings in Medical Artificial Intelligence: The First Decade. Reading, MA: Addison-Wesley; 1984.

11. Cook, H. M.; Fox, M. D. Application of expert systems to mammographic image analysis. Am. J. Physiol. Imag. 4:16–22; 1989.

12. Curran, B.; Sternick, E. S. The development of an expert system in radiation oncology. In: Bruinvis, I. A. D.; van der Giessen, P. H.; van Kleffens, H. J.; Wittkämper, F. W., eds. The Use of Computers in Radiation Therapy. Amsterdam: Elsevier Science; 1987:557–559.

13. Dhawan, A. P. An expert system for the early detection of melanoma using knowledge-based image analysis. Anal. Quant. Cytol. Hist. 10:405–416; 1988.

14. Dowsett, R. J.; Galvin, J. M.; Cheng, E.; Smith, R.; Epperson, R.; Harris, R.; Henze, G.; Needham, M.; Payne, R.; Peterson, M. A.; Skinner, A. L.; Reynolds, A. Contouring structures for 3-dimensional treatment planning. Int. J. Radiat. Oncol. Biol. Phys. 22:1083–1088; 1992.

15. Goitein, M. The comparison of treatment plans. Semin. Radiat. Oncol. 2:246–256; 1992.

16. Goitein, M.; Schultheiss, T. E. Strategies for treating possible tumor extension: Some theoretical considerations. Int. J. Radiat. Oncol. Biol. Phys. 11:1519–1528; 1985.

17. Graham, M. V.; Jain, N. L.; Kahn, M. G.; Drzymala, R. E.; Mackey, M. A.; Purdy, J. A. Validation and clinical usefulness of an objective plan evaluation model in the three-dimensional treatment of non-small cell lung cancer (Abstr.). IJROBP 27(1):240; 1993.

18. Hammond, K. J. Case-Based Planning: Viewing Planning as a Memory Task. Boston, MA: Academic Press; 1989.

19. Hart, A. Knowledge Acquisition for Expert Systems, Second Edition. New York, NY: McGraw-Hill; 1992.

20. Haton, M.-C. Knowledge-based decision making for radiotherapy planning. In: Morucci, J. P.; Plonsey, R.; Coatrieux, J. L.; Laxminarayan, S., eds. Proceedings of the Fourteenth Annual International Conference of the IEEE Engineering in Medicine and Biology Society. New York, NY: IEEE Press; 1992:916–917.

21. Heckerman, D. E. Probabilistic Similarity Networks. Cambridge, MA: MIT Press; 1991.

22. Howard, R. A.; Matheson, J. E., eds. Readings on the Principles and Applications of Decision Analysis. Menlo Park, CA: Strategic Decisions Group; 1983.

23. Hyödynmaa, S.; Kolari, P.; Näriäinen, K.; Ojala, A.; Rantanen, J.; Saranummi, N. Decision support system in oncology. In: Rienhoff, O.; Piccolo, U.; Schneider, B., eds. Expert Systems and Decision Support in Medicine. Berlin: Springer-Verlag; 1988:65–68.

24. Hyödynmaa, S.; Ojala, A.; Kolari, P.; Yliaho, J.; Rantanen, J.; Oksanen, H.; Saranummi, N. Decision support for treatment decision making and treatment result evaluation in radiation oncology. In: Minet, P., ed. Impact of Personal Computers (PCs) on Radio-Oncology Departments. Liege, Belgium: European Association of Radiology; 1990:89–95.

25. International Atomic Energy Agency. Computer Calculation of Dose Distributions in Radiotherapy. Vienna, Austria: IAEA; 1966.

26. International Commission on Radiation Units and Measurements. Prescribing, Recording, and Reporting Photon Beam Therapy (Report No. 50). Washington, DC; 1993.

27. Ionescu-Farca, F.; Willi, A. RADONCOL: An expert system for treatment advice in radiation oncology. In: Proceedings of the Annual Meeting of the Swiss Society of Radiation Biology and Medical Physics. Kerzers, Switzerland: Max Huber Verlag; 1991:29–36.

28. Ionescu-Farca, F.; Willi, A. Towards the simulation of clinical cognition: Development of an expert system for radiation oncology (Abstr.). Med. Biol. Eng. Comput. 29 (Suppl.):515; 1991.

29. Jain, N. L.; Kahn, M. G. Objective evaluation of radiation therapy plans. In: Safran, NY: McGraw Hill; 1993:134-138. c., Ed. Proceedings of the Seventeenth Symposium on Computer Applications in Medical Care.

30. Jain, N. L.; Kahn, M. G. Ranking radiotherapy treatment plans using decision-analytic and heuristic techniques. Comput. Biomed. Res. 25:374–383; 1992.

31. Jain, N. L.; Kahn, M. G.; Drzymala, R. E.; Emami, B.; Purdy, J. A. Objective evaluation of 3-D radiation treatment plans: A decision-analytic tool incorporating treatment preferences of radiation oncologists. Int. J. Radiat. Oncol. Biol. Phys. 26:321–333; 1993.

32. Kahn, M. G. Modeling time in medical decision-support programs. Med. Decis. Making 11:249–264; 1991.

33. Kalet, I. J. AI applications in radiation therapy. In: Purdy, J. A., ed. Advances in Radiation Oncology Physics: Dosimetry, Treatment Planning, and Brachytherapy. Woodbury, NY: American Institute of Physics; 1992:1058–1085.

34. Kalet, I. J.; Jacky, J. P. Knowledge-based computer simulation for radiation therapy planning. In: Bruinvis, I. A. D.; van der Giessen, P. H.; van Kleffens, H. J.; Wittkämper, F. W., eds. The Use of Computers in Radiation Therapy. Amsterdam: Elsevier Science; 1987:553–556.

35. Kalet, I. J.; Paluszynski, W. A production expert system for radiation therapy planning. In: Levy, A. J.; Williams, B. T., eds. Proceedings of the Congress of Medical Informatics. Washington, DC: American Association for Medical Systems and Informatics; 1985:315–319.

36. Kalet, I. J.; Paluszynski, W. Knowledge-based computer systems for radiotherapy planning. Am. J. Clin. Oncol. 13:344–351; 1990.

37. Kassirer, J. P.; Moskowitz, A. J.; Lau, J.; Pauker, S. G. Decision analysis: A progress report. Ann. Intern. Med. 106:275–291; 1987.

38. Keeney, R. L.; Raiffa, H. Decisions with Multiple Objectives: Preferences and Value Tradeoffs. New York, NY: John Wiley; 1976.

39. Kolari, P.; Yliaho, J.; Näriäinen, K.; Hyödynmaa, S.; Ojala, A.; Rantanen, J.; Saranummi, N. CARTES—a prototype decision support system in oncology. In: Talmon, J. L.; Fox, J., eds. Knowledge Based Systems in Medicine: Methods, Applications and Evaluations. Berlin: Springer-Verlag; 1991:148–158.

40. Kromhout-Schiro, S. E. Development and Evaluation of a Model of Radiotherapy Planning Target Volume Generation. Ph.D. Dissertation, Center for Bioengineering. Seattle, WA: University of Washington; 1993.

41. Kutcher, G. J.; Burman, C. Calculation of complication probability factors for non-uniform normal tissue irradiation: The effective volume method. Int. J. Radiat. Oncol. Biol. Phys. 16:1623–1630; 1989.

42. Lamm, I. J. CART — Report on the Nordic co-operation program. In: Bruinvis, I. A. D.; van der Giessen, P. H.; van Kleffens, H. J.; Wittkämper, F. W., eds. The Use of Computers in Radiation Therapy. Amsterdam: Elsevier Science; 1987:257–260.

43. Laramore, G. E.; Altschuler, M. D.; Banks, G.; Kalet, I. J.; Pajak, T. F.; Schultheiss, T. E.; Zink, S. Applications of data bases and AI/expert systems in radiation therapy. Am. J. Clin. Oncol. 11:387–393; 1988.

44. Ledley, R. S. Use of Computers in Biology and Medicine. New York, NY: McGraw-Hill; 1965.

45. Luger, G. F.; Stubblefield, W. A. Artificial Intelligence and the Design of Expert Systems. Redwood City, CA: Benjamin/Cummins; 1989.

46. Maceratini, R.; Rafanelli, M.; Pisanelli, D. M.; Crollari, S. Expert systems and the pancreatic cancer problem: Decision support in the pre-operative diagnosis. J. Biomed. Eng. 11:487–510; 1989.

47. McNeil, B. J.; Pauker, S. G.; Sox, Jr., H. C.; Tversky, A. On the elicitation of preferences for alternative therapies. N. Engl. J. Med. 306:1259–1262; 1982.

48. McNeil, B. J.; Weichselbaum, R.; Pauker, S. G. Fallacy of the five-year survival in lung cancer. N. Engl. J. Med. 299:1397–1401; 1978.

49. McNeil, B. J.; Weichselbaum, R.; Pauker, S. G. Speech and survival. Tradeoffs between quality and quantity of life in laryngeal cancer. N. Engl. J. Med. 305:982–987; 1981.

50. Miller, P. L., ed. Selected Topics in Medical Artificial Intelligence. New York, NY: Springer-Verlag; 1988.

51. Miller, R. A.; Pople, Jr., H. E.; Myers, J. D. INTERNIST-1: An experimental computer-based diagnostic consultant for general internal medicine. N. Engl. J. Med. 307:468–476; 1982.

52. Mohan, R.; Mageras, G. S.; Baldwin, B.; Brewster, L. J.; Kutcher, G. J.; Leibel, S.; Burman, C. M.; Ling, C. C.; Fuks, Z. Clinically relevant optimization of 3-D conformal treatments. Med. Phys. 19:933–944; 1992.

53. Munro, A. J. A graphical method for the analysis of decisions in clinical oncology. Clin. Radiol. 37:263–266; 1986.

54. Munro, A. J. Decision analysis in oncology: Panacea or chimera? Clin. Oncol. 4:306–312; 1992.

55. Myers, L. T.; Debebe, B. A prototype knowledge-based system for machine diagnostics based on the Philips SL-25 Linac (Abstr.). Med. Phys. 19:811; 1992.

56. Niemierko, A.; Urie, M.; Goitein, M. Optimization of 3-D radiation therapy with both physical and biological end points and constraints. Int. J. Radiat. Oncol. Biol. Phys. 23:99–108; 1992.

57. Orr, J. S. Optimization of radiation therapy treatment planning. Comput. Prog. Biomed. 2:216–220; 1972.

58. Paluszynski, W. Designing Radiation Therapy for Cancer: An Approach to Knowledge-Based Optimization. Ph.D. Dissertation, Department of Computer Science. Seattle, WA: University of Washington; 1990.

59. Paluszynski, W.; Kalet, I. Design optimization using dynamic evaluation. In: Sridharan, N. S., ed. Proceedings of the Eleventh International Joint Conference of Artificial Intelligence. San Mateo, CA: Morgan Kaufmann; 1989:1408–1412.

60. Paluszynski, W.; Kalet, I. Radiation therapy planning: A design-oriented expert system. In: Proceedings of the Second Western Expert Systems Conference. 1987:169–176.

61. Paoli, G.; Schenone, A.; Bacigalupo, A.; Andreucci, L.; Foppiano, F.; Barra, S. An AI application in total body irradiation therapy (Abstr.). Submitted to ESTRO; 1993.

62. Paoli, G.; Schenone, A.; Lemmi, G. L.; Andreucci, L. A knowledge base support system for decision making for radiotherapy planning based on artificial techniques (Abstr.). Radiother. Oncol. 24 (Suppl.):S71; 1992.

63. Parsaye, K.; Chignell, M. Expert Systems for Experts. New York, NY: John Wiley; 1988.

64. Patrick, E. A.; Moskowitz, M.; Mansukhani, V. T.; Gruenstein, E. I. Expert learning system network for diagnosis of breast calcifications. Invest. Radiol. 26:534–539; 1991.

65. Pauker, S. G.; Kassirer, J. P. Decision analysis. N. Engl. J. Med. 316:250–258; 1987.

66. Photon Treatment Planning Collaborative Working Group. Evaluation of high energy photon external beam treatment planning: Project summary. Int. J. Radiat. Oncol. Biol. Phys. 21:3–8; 1991.

67. Photon Treatment Planning Collaborative Working Group. Three-dimensional dose calculations for radiation treatment planning. Int. J. Radiat. Oncol. Biol. Phys. 21:25–36; 1991.

68. Plante, D. A.; Piccirillo, J. F.; Sofferman, R. A. Decision analysis of treatment options in pyriform sinus carcinoma. Med. Decis. Making 7:74–83; 1987.

69. Pliskin, J. S.; Shepard, D. S.; Weinstein, M. C. Utility functions for life years and health status. Oper. Res. 28:206–224; 1980.

70. Purdy, J. A. Volume and dose specification for 3-D conformal radiation therapy. Presented at the First International Symposium on 3-D Radiation Treatment Planning and Conformal Therapy, 1993. This volume.

71. Purdy, J. A.; Kalet, I. J.; Chaney, E. L.; Zink, S. Radiotherapy treatment planning tools: A collaborative project of the National Cancer Institute (Abstr.). Med. Phys. 18:666–667; 1991.

72. Raiffa, H. Decision Analysis: Introductory Lectures on Choice under Uncertainty. New York, NY: Random House; 1968.

73. Rich, E.; Knight, K. Artificial Intelligence, Second Edition. New York, NY: McGraw-Hill; 1991.

74. Rosenberger, F. U.; Matthews, J. W.; Johns, G. C.; Drzymala, R. E.; Purdy, J. A. Use of transputers for real time dose calculation and presentation for three-dimensional radiation treatment planning. Int. J. Radiat. Oncol. Biol. Phys. 25:709–719; 1993.

75. Rosenman, J.; Chaney, E. L.; Sailer, S.; Sherouse, G. W.; Tepper, J. E. Recent advances in radiotherapy treatment planning. Cancer Invest. 9:465–481; 1991.

76. Rosenman, J.; Cullip, T. High-performance computing in radiation cancer treatment. In: Pilkington, T. C.; Loftis, B.; Thompson, J. F.; Woo, S. L-Y.; Palmer, T. C.; Budinger, T. F., eds., High-Performance Computing in Biomedical Research. Boca Raton, FL: CRC Press; 1993:466–476.

77. Rubin, P. Multidiscipline clinical trials in cancer centers. Front. Radiat. Ther. Oncol. 8:145–174; 1973.

78. Schenone, A.; Paoli, G.; Puzone, R.; Ghiso, G.; Pellecchia, G. L.; Foppiano, F.; Bagnera, M. C.; Andreucci, L. A support system for decision-making in radiotherapy based on artificial intelligence techniques. In: Andreucci, L.; Schenone, A., eds. Topics in Biomedical Physics. Singapore: World Scientific; 1991:452–454.

79. Schultheiss, T. E. Treatment planning by computer decision. In: Cunningham, J. R.; Ragan, D.; Van Dyk, J., eds., Proceedings of the Eighth International Conference on the Use of Computers in Radiation Therapy. Silver Spring, MD: IEEE Computer Society Press; 1984:225–229.

80. Schultheiss, T. E.; El-Mahdi, A. M. Statistical decision theory applied to radiation therapy treatment decisions. In: Blum, B. I., ed., Proceedings of the Sixth Symposium on Computer Applications in Medical Care. Los Angeles, CA: IEEE Computer Society Press; 1982:978–982.

81. Schultheiss, T. E.; Orton, C. G. Models in radiotherapy: Definition of decision criteria. Med. Phys. 12:183–187; 1985.

82. Shortliffe, E. H. Clinical decision-support systems. In: Shortliffe, E. H.; Perreault, L. E.; Wiederhold, G.; Fagan, L. M., eds. Medical Informatics: Computer Applications in Health Care. Reading, MA: Addison-Wesley; 1990:466–502.

83. Shortliffe, E. H. Computer-Based Medical Consultations: MYCIN. New York, NY: Elsevier; 1976.

84. Shortliffe, E. H.; Perreault, L. E.; Wiederhold, G.; Fagan, L. M., eds., Medical Informatics: Computer Applications in Health Care. Reading, MA: Addison-Wesley; 1990.

85. Smith, A. R.; Purdy, J. A., eds. Three-Dimensional Photon Treatment Planning: Report of the Collaborative Working Group on the Evaluation of Treatment Planning for External Photon Beam Radiotherapy. Special Issue: Int. J. Radiat. Oncol. Biol. Phys. 21(1); 1991.

86. Sox, Jr., H. C.; Blatt, M. A.; Higgins, M. C.; Marton, K. I. Medical Decision Making. Boston, MA: Butterworths; 1988.

87. Stalpers, L. J.; Verbeek, A. L.; van Daal, W. A. Radiotherapy or surgery for $T_2N_0M_0$ glottic carcinoma? A decision-analytic approach. Radiother. Oncol. 14:209–217; 1989.

88. Sternick, E. S.; Curran, B. H. An expert system for diagnosing linear accelerator technical problems (Abstr.). Med. Phys. 13:610; 1986.

89. Szolovits, P., ed. Artificial Intelligence in Medicine. Boulder, CO: Westview Press; 1982.

90. Szolovits, P.; Patil, R. S.; Schwartz, W. B. Artificial intelligence in medical diagnosis. Ann. Intern. Med. 108:80–87; 1988.

91. Tu, S. W.; Kahn, M. G.; Musen, M. A.; Ferguson, J. C.; Shortliffe, E. H.; Fagan, L. M. Episodic skeletal-plan refinement based on temporal data. Commun. ACM 32:1439–1455; 1989.

92. von Winterfeldt, D.; Edwards, E. Decision Analysis and Behavioral Research. Cambridge, UK: Cambridge University Press; 1986.

93. Warner, H. R.; Toronto, A.; Veasy, L. Experience with Bayes' theorem for computer diagnosis of congenital heart disease. Ann. New York Acad. Sci. 115:2–16; 1964.

94. Weinstein, M. C.; Fineberg, H. V. Clinical Decision Analysis. Philadelphia, PA: W. B. Saunders; 1980.

95. Weinstein, M. C.; Stason, W. B. Foundations of cost-effectiveness analysis for health and medical practices. N. Engl. J. Med. 296:716–721; 1977.

96. Zelefsky, M. J.; Leibel, S. A.; Fuks, Z. Conventional external beam radiation therapy for prostatic cancer: Where do we go from here? Int. J. Radiat. Oncol. Biol. Phys. 26:365–367; 1993.

97. Zink, S. The promise of a new technology: Knowledge-based systems in radiation oncology and diagnostic radiology. Comput. Med. Imaging Graph. 13:281–293; 1989.